EMERGENCY
MEDICINE

MCQs

EMERGENCY MEDICINE

MCQs

WARUNA DE ALWIS
YOLANDE WEINER

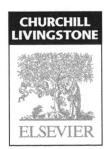

CHURCHILL
LIVINGSTONE

ELSEVIER

Sydney   Edinburgh   London   New York   Philadelphia   St Louis   Toronto

Churchill Livingstone
is an imprint of Elsevier

Elsevier Australia. ACN 001 002 357
(a division of Reed International Books Australia Pty Ltd)
Tower 1, 475 Victoria Avenue, Chatswood, NSW 2067

This edition © 2012 Elsevier Australia

ISBN 9780729541046

National Library of Australia Cataloguing-in-Publication entry

Author:	De Alwis, Waruna.
Title:	Emergency medicine MCQs / Waruna de Alwis, Yolande Weiner.
ISBN:	9780729541046 (pbk.)
Subjects:	Emergency medicine–Australasia–Problems, exercises, etc.
	Medical emergencies–Australasia–Problems, exercises, etc.
	Hospitals–Emergency services–Australasia.
Other Authors/Contributors:	
	Weiner, Yolande.
Dewey Number: 616.025	

Publishing Director: *Luisa Cecotti*
Publisher: *Sophie Kaliniecki*
Developmental Editor: *Neli Bryant*
Project Coordinator: *Liz Malcolm*
Project Manager: *Nayagi Athmanathan*
Edited by: *Matt Davies*
Proofread by: *Sarah Newton-John*
Cover and internal design by: *Stella Vassiliou*
Typeset by Toppan Best-set Premedia Ltd.
Printed in China by China Translation & Printing Services Limited.

CONTENTS

List of Authors and Contributors   vii

List of Reviewers   ix

Dedication   xi

Preface   xiii

Acknowledgements   xv

Section 1   Questions   **1**

Chapter 1   Resuscitation   3

Chapter 2   Cardiovascular emergencies   11

Chapter 3   Respiratory emergencies   18

Chapter 4   Neurological and neurosurgical emergencies   24

Chapter 5   Endocrine emergencies   28

Chapter 6   Gastroenterological emergencies   32

Chapter 7   Renal emergencies   37

Chapter 8   Haematological and oncological emergencies   41

Chapter 9   Infectious diseases   44

Chapter 10   Dermatological emergencies   49

Chapter 11   Electrolyte and acid–base disorders   51

Chapter 12   Emergency anaesthesia and pain management   54

Chapter 13   Trauma and burns   57

Chapter 14   Orthopaedic emergencies   64

Chapter 15   Surgical emergencies   70

Chapter 16   Eye, ENT and dental emergencies   76

Chapter 17   Urological emergencies   80

Chapter 18   Obstetric and gynaecological emergencies   82

Chapter 19   Toxicology and toxinology   86

Chapter 20   Environmental emergencies   92

Chapter 21   Psychiatric emergencies   94

Chapter 22   Paediatric emergencies   97

Chapter 23   Disaster management   105

Chapter 24   ED management and medicolegal issues   107

Section 2   Answers   **113**

Chapter 1   Resuscitation   115

Chapter 2   Cardiovascular emergencies   133

Chapter 3   Respiratory emergencies   146

Chapter 4   Neurological and neurosurgical emergencies   162

Chapter 5   Endocrine emergencies   172

Chapter 6   Gastroenterological emergencies   182

Chapter 7   Renal emergencies   198

Chapter 8   Haematological and oncological emergencies   207

Chapter 9   Infectious diseases   218

Chapter 10 Dermatological emergencies   229

Chapter 11 Electrolyte and acid–base disorders   233

Chapter 12 Emergency anaesthesia and pain management   241

Chapter 13 Trauma and burns   250

Chapter 14 Orthopaedic emergencies   267

Chapter 15 Surgical emergencies   281

Chapter 16 Eye, ENT and dental emergencies   301

Chapter 17 Urological emergencies   310

Chapter 18 Obstetric and gynaecological emergencies   317

Chapter 19 Toxicology and toxinology   330

Chapter 20 Environmental emergencies   348

Chapter 21 Psychiatric emergencies   353

Chapter 22 Paediatric emergencies   361

Chapter 23 Disaster management   391

Chapter 24 ED management and medicolegal issues   395

Index   407

LIST OF AUTHORS AND CONTRIBUTORS

Authors

Waruna de Alwis MBBS, FACEM
Emergency Medicine Consultant, Director of Emergency Medicine Training, Logan Hospital, Meadowbrook, QLD, Australia

Yolande Weiner MBChB, MMed EM (UCT), FCEM (SA), FACEM
Emergency Medicine Consultant, Logan Hospital, Meadowbrook, QLD, Australia

Contributors

Alison Boyle MBBCh, BAO, FACEM
Emergency Medicine Consultant, Logan Hospital, Meadowbrook, Queensland

Kanchana de Alwis MBBS FRANZCP
Consultant Psychiatrist, New Farm Clinic, Brisbane, Queensland

Deepak Doshi FACEM, FCEM, DCH, MRCS A&E (Edin), MRCS (Glasgow), MS, MBBS
Emergency Medicine Consultant, Logan Hospital, Meadowbrook, Queensland

Katie Gallop BSc, MBBS, FACEM
Emergency Medicine Consultant, Logan Hospital, Meadowbrook, Queensland
Senior Lecturer, Griffith University, Gold Coast, Queensland

Melissa Gan BSc (UQ), MBBS (Hons 1), BSc (Med) (UNSW), FACEM
Emergency Medicine Consultant, Gold Coast Hospital, Gold Coast, Queensland

Jonathon Isoardi MBBS FACEM
Emergency Medicine Consultant, The Princess Alexandra Hospital, Senior Lecturer, The University of Queensland, Brisbane, Queensland

Sean Lawrence MBBS FACEM
Senior Emergency Medicine Consultant, The Princess Alexandra Hospital, Brisbane, Queensland, Emergency Medicine Lead Faculty, Qld Health Clinical Skills Development Service, Brisbane, Queensland

Larry McGuire MBChB, MRCP (UK), FFAEM, FACEM
Senior Emergency Medicine Consultant, Logan Hospital, Meadowbrook, Queensland

Yogesh Nataly MBBS FACEM
Emergency Medicine Consultant, Redlands Hospital, Cleveland, Queensland
Royal Children's Hospital, Brisbane, Queensland

Zaahid Pandie MBChB (UCT), FRACP (PEM), FACEM
Emergency Medicine Consultant and Paediatric Emergency Medicine Specialist, Logan Hospital, Meadowbrook, Queensland
Mater Children's Hospital, Brisbane, Queensland

Glenn Ryan BSc, Grad Dip Psych, MBBS (Hons), FACEM
Emergency Medicine Consultant, Princess Alexandra Hospital, Senior Lecturer, The University of Queensland, Brisbane, Queensland

LIST OF REVIEWERS

S Javad Mojtahed Najafi MD, FACEM
Emergency Medicine Consultant, St George Hospital, Sydney, New South Wales

Mary Stevens MBBS
Emergency Registrar, St George Hospital, Sydney, New South Wales

Sarah Bombell MBBS
Resident Medical Officer, The Canberra Hospital, Australian Capital Territory

Selina Watchorn MBBS, BNursing, BArts
The Canberra Hospital/Australian National University

DEDICATION

To my amazing husband, Michael, for his unlimited support, patience and encouragement.
YW

To my wife, Kanchana, for your love, resilience and strength, and to my children, Mahima
and Ruveen, for reminding me what's really important.
WD

PREFACE

The practice of emergency medicine has expanded over the past two decades in Australasia. The expanding emergency medicine workforce includes both specialists and non-specialists, some of whom are in training positions. The locations of practice range from rural and regional emergency departments (EDs) to tertiary university-affiliated departments. For everybody, a knowledge that covers both the breadth and depth and a wide range of skills are essential to deliver a high standard of clinical emergency medical care.

Multiple choice questions (MCQs) form an essential part of many formal assessment processes; however, they are notoriously difficult to study for. While helping many residents and registrars over the past years prepare for various examinations we recognised a gap in the availability of resources relevant to Australasian emergency medicine practice. With time we also realised the value of MCQs to clinical practice, even for someone who is not in a formal training program, as MCQs can target clinically relevant and practical questions. It would therefore be useful to have an evidence-based answer readily available when on the emergency floor without having to read through many textbooks.

The book will also be accompanied by an app as a separate product, which will contain another 180 MCQs covering all topics. We have used the ACEM fellowship MCQ matrix to organise these questions as 3 MCQ papers. Once again detailed explanations are provided for each question.

With generous contributions from other contributors we subsequently prepared this book using our combined experience gained through working in busy non-tertiary and tertiary EDs. We used well-known textbooks in emergency medicine, both Australasian and international, peer-reviewed journal articles, and web resources. The chapters are structured in keeping with the topics covered in the core curriculum of the Australasian College for Emergency Medicine fellowship program.

HOW TO USE THIS BOOK

This book contains single-answer MCQs covering both adult and paediatric emergency medicine. Try each question and select the answer that is most relevant according to the question. For each question we have formulated an evidence-based explanation that is structured in such a way that core knowledge is given in an easily available and understandable format. We have referenced the answers to textbooks as well as other resources, and also have provided a relevant additional reading list.

This book is aimed at enhancing your knowledge and improving your critical thinking skills while helping you to identify gaps in your knowledge. We hope this book will be useful in your everyday clinical practice as well as during your preparation for examinations.

We wish you the very best in your career in emergency medicine.

Waruna de Alwis and Yolande Weiner

ACKNOWLEDGEMENTS

We would like to thank all contributors for their invaluable efforts and for the numerous hours they spent preparing the manuscript while attending to increasingly busy clinical practices. We thank Dr Stuart Young, director of emergency medicine at Logan Hospital, and Dr James Collier, co-director of emergency medicine and emergency medicine training at Princess Alexandra Hospital for their support.

We also thank Sophie Kaliniecki, publisher, and Neli Bryant, developmental editor, at Elsevier Australia for their help in developing this publication, as well as our panel of reviewers for their critical review and valuable suggestions.

Lastly, a special thanks to our families and friends for their patience and support in the face of the numerous hours we took preparing this book.

QUESTIONS

Adult resuscitation

Yolande Weiner

1. For confirming endotracheal tube placement following intubation of a patient in cardiac arrest, which ONE of the following methods is the most reliable?

    A. Waveform capnography

    B. Calorimetric end-tidal carbon dioxide (ETCO$_2$)

    C. Oesophageal detector device

    D. Pulse oximetry

2. Regarding the use of bilevel positive airway pressure (BiPAP) in acute hypercapnic respiratory failure in chronic obstructive pulmonary disease (COPD), adjustment of which ONE of the following parameters will most effectively reduce PCO$_2$ levels?

    A. Increase positive end-expiratory pressure (PEEP)

    B. Increase inspiratory positive airway pressure (IPAP)

    C. Increase PEEP and IPAP proportionally

    D. Decrease the timed ventilations when in spontaneous/timed (S/T) mode

3. Regarding non-invasive ventilation (NIV) in acute cardiogenic pulmonary oedema, which ONE of the following is TRUE?

    A. BiPAP has been shown to be superior to continuous positive airway pressure (CPAP)

    B. PEEP should never be increased above 5 cm H$_2$O

    C. It has a proven short-term mortality benefit

    D. It improves cardiac output

4. Regarding NIV in COPD, which ONE of the following is FALSE?

    A. It has no mortality benefit in hospital, but there may be a survival advantage after discharge

    B. It reduces preload and therefore may reduce cardiac output

    C. Oxygen saturation of 85–90% is acceptable

    D. Application of external PEEP worsens intrinsic PEEP and lung hyperinflation and should not be used

5. Regarding severe life-threatening asthma, which ONE of the following is the most appropriate indication for intubation?

    A. PCO$_2$ > 70 mmHg

    B. pH < 7.35

    C. SaO$_2$ 85%

    D. Respiratory exhaustion

6. Regarding mechanical ventilation in the acute asthmatic, which ONE of the following is TRUE?

    A. Pressure-controlled ventilation is preferred over volume-controlled to prevent lung damage due to hyperinflation

    B. Peak inspiratory pressures (P$_{peak}$) should be limited to ≤25 cm H$_2$O

    C. Plateau pressures (P$_{plat}$) and not P$_{peak}$ is associated with ventilator induced lung injury (VILI)

    D. The aim of ventilation is to maintain oxygenation and correct the CO$_2$ to normal levels

7. Regarding providing ventilatory support in patients with an acute lung injury (ALI) or the adult respiratory distress syndrome (ARDS), which ONE of the following is TRUE?

    A. NIV has a high success rate and is therefore recommended over invasive ventilation

    B. The FiO$_2$ should be weaned to maintain a SaO$_2$ of at least 95%

    C. The respiratory rate should be increased to compensate for lower tidal volumes to maintain a normal PaCO$_2$ and pH

    D. Plateau pressures should be kept <30 cm H$_2$O and may require reducing tidal volumes as low as 4 mL/kg

8. The International Liaison Committee on Resuscitation (ILCOR) has published new recommendations in 2010 on CPR in adult cardiac arrest. Regarding this, which ONE of the following statements is TRUE?

    A. In an unwitnessed cardiac arrest the patient should receive 2 minutes of CPR before defibrillation is attempted

    B. Continuous ETCO$_2$ monitoring can be used to indicate the quality of CPR

C. Effective external cardiac compressions provide an output of about 40–50% of the pre-arrest value

D. The inspired concentration of oxygen should be reduced to 21–60% as hyperoxaemia is associated with worse neurological outcome

9. Regarding CPR in adult cardiac arrest for advanced life support providers, which ONE of the following is TRUE?

A. The chest compression ratio is 30 : 2 if one rescuer present and 15 : 2 if more than one rescuer

B. The internipple line is a reliable landmark for hand placement during chest compressions

C. Chest compression depths should be at least one half of the depth of the adult chest

D. When using an advanced airway, ventilation should be delivered during the relaxation phase of a chest compression

10. Regarding defibrillation with a manual biphasic defibrillator using pads in patients with cardiac arrest, which ONE of the following statements is TRUE?

A. For rescuer safety, chest compressions should briefly be stopped while charging the defibrillator in preparation for delivery of a shock

B. After delivery of a shock, one should check for the presence or absence of a pulse before restarting chest compressions

C. Three stacked shocks should initially be delivered in all patients suffering from a ventricular fibrillation (VF) arrest

D. The default energy level for adults should be set at 200 J for all shocks

11. When comparing monophasic and biphasic defibrillators, all of the following statements are correct regarding biphasic defibrillators EXCEPT:

A. They are more effective at terminating ventricular arrhythmias at lower energy levels

B. They are more effective for cardioversion of atrial fibrillation

C. They have a greater first-shock efficacy for long duration VF/VT

D. They are associated with a better survival to hospital discharge outcome

12. A 63-year-old male suffered a VF cardiac arrest and the first shock was delivered on arrival in the emergency department (ED). After a further 2 minutes of CPR, he was noted to be still in VF on the monitor. What is the next MOST appropriate step to take?

A. Feel for the presence or absence of a pulse

B. Give adrenaline 1 mL of 1 : 1000 intravenously

C. Deliver a second shock at 200 J

D. Give amiodarone 300 mg intravenously

13. A 70-year-old male suffered an out-of-hospital cardiac arrest (OHCA). On arrival in the ED CPR is in progress and a laryngeal mask airway (LMA) is in situ. IV access was not obtained prehospital. The initial rhythm on arrival in the ED showed a pulseless electrical activity (PEA) at 30 bpm. What is the MOST appropriate next step to be performed?

A. Confirm correct placement of LMA and adequacy of chest compressions

B. High-dose adrenaline should be administered via the LMA

C. Establish IV access and give 1 mg of atropine

D. Establish IV access and give 1 mL of adrenaline 1 : 1000

14. Regarding the use of vasopressors during cardiac arrest in adults with a shockable rhythm, which ONE of the following is TRUE?

A. It improves return of spontaneous circulation (ROSC) and survival to hospital discharge

B. Vasopressin is associated with a better neurological outcome compared with adrenaline

C. Current evidence suggests that the optimal dose of adrenaline is 1 mg given after the second shock and then every second cycle if there is no response to defibrillation

D. High-dose adrenaline has shown improvement in ROSC but no change in survival outcome compared with standard-dose adrenaline

15. A 30-week pregnant female suffers a cardiac arrest. Which ONE of the following statements is TRUE?

A. Aortacaval decompression is best achieved with a left lateral tilt manoeuvre compared with manual displacement of the uterus to the left

B. Strong evidence exists that aortacaval decompression improves maternal haemodynamics and fetal wellbeing

C. Perimortem caesarean section performed after 5 minutes of maternal arrest may improve infant survival

D. Therapeutic hypothermia is proven to be safe and effective in pregnancy after ROSC and is strongly recommended

16. Regarding cardiac arrest secondary to hypothermia, which ONE of the following statements is TRUE?

A. Defibrillation should only be attempted when temperature is >30°C

B. Temperature of gas delivered to facemask or endotracheal tube (ETT) as well as IV fluids should be warmed to 40°C

C. Endotracheal intubation should be delayed due to myocardial irritability and subsequent predisposition to VF

D. Adrenaline dose should be reduced due to decreased drug metabolism and potential toxicity

17. Which ONE of the following statements is TRUE regarding post cardiac arrest care in adults?

A. Provide 100% oxygen in all cases after ROSC

B. Maintain a systolic BP > 90 mmHg

C. Maintain a tight glucose control with blood sugar levels between 4 and 6 mmol/L

D. Immediate emergent angiography and PCI should be considered even in the absence of ST elevation or left bundle branch block (LBBB) on electrocardiogram (ECG)

18. Which ONE of the following statements is TRUE regarding therapeutic hypothermia in patients with return of spontaneous circulation after a cardiac arrest?

A. It has no benefit in neurological outcome in comatose patients after cardiac arrest from a non-shockable rhythm

B. It can be safely initiated with a rapid infusion of 4°C normal saline at 30 mL/kg over 2 hours

C. Hypothermia should be sustained for a period of 24–48 hours

D. The recommended temperature to be achieved in therapeutic hypothermia is 30–32°C

19. Regarding prognostication after resuscitation in adults, which ONE of the following reliably predicts poor outcome?

A. Absent vestibulo-ocular reflexes within 24 hours in a patient who had NOT been treated with therapeutic hypothermia

B. Absent pupillary light and corneal reflexes at >72 hours in a patient who had NOT been treated with therapeutic hypothermia

C. A GCS motor score of ≤2 at >72 hours in a patient who had been treated with therapeutic hypothermia

D. EEG used within 24 hours after sustained ROSC in a patient who had been treated with therapeutic hypothermia

20. Regarding emergency transcutaneous pacing (TCP), which ONE of the following statements is TRUE?

A. Once mechanical capture is achieved, pacing should continue at an output 10% higher than the threshold of initial electrical capture

B. Successful electrical capture is achieved if each pacing spike is followed by a wide QRS complex

C. Current recommendations support routine use of TCP in asystolic arrest within 10 minutes

D. The presence of an arterial pulse confirms successful mechanical capture

21. Regarding lactic acidosis, which ONE of the following is TRUE?

A. Lactic acidosis is defined as the combination of increased blood lactate concentration >2 mmol/L and acidaemia (arterial blood pH < 7.35)

B. There is no correlation between the degree of elevation of serum lactate and the severity of shock

C. Normalisation of acidaemia with bicarbonate is recommended to improve cardiac dysfunction

D. Adrenaline can cause hyperlactaemia

22. Regarding the management of septic shock in the ED, which ONE of the following statements is TRUE?

A. Crystalloids are superior to colloids and should be used for initial volume resuscitation

B. Current recommendations suggest the maintenance of mean arterial blood pressure (MAP) ≥55 mmHg

C. Both noradrenaline and dopamine are good initial vasopressor choices

D. The use of high-dose steroids is associated with decreased requirements for vasopressor agents and improves survival

23. Regarding haemodynamic monitoring in critically ill patients, which ONE of the following statements is TRUE?

A. The Trendelenberg position improves cardiopulmonary performance compared with the supine position

B. Passive leg raising above the level of the heart is an inaccurate test in assessing fluid responsiveness

C. Pulse pressure variation can be used to estimate fluid responsiveness in patients during positive pressure ventilation

D. The respiratory variability of the arterial waveform can accurately predict fluid responsiveness in spontaneously breathing patients

24. Early goal-directed therapy in sepsis has been associated with decreased mortality rates. Regarding early goal-directed therapy in sepsis, which ONE of the following is NOT included in the end points of resuscitation?

A. Urine output >0.5 mL/kg/hr

B. Mixed venous oxygen saturation ($SmvO_2$) ≥65%

C. Heart rate <100 bpm

D. Central venous pressure (CVP) 8–12 mmHg

25. Regarding the use of vasoactive agents in shock, which ONE of the following is FALSE?

A. Noradrenaline is a potent α-agonist with significant activity at β1 receptors and minimal or no activity at β2 receptors

B. Metaraminol can cause reflex bradycardia and increased left ventricular (LV) afterload, which may be harmful in patients with cardiogenic shock

C. Isoprenaline is a non-selective β-agonist that causes peripheral vasodilation with subsequent fall in diastolic and mean arterial blood pressure

D. Dopamine at doses of 5–10 µg/kg/min predominantly acts on α-receptors with a profile similar to noradrenaline

26. Regarding the use of vasoactive agents in the ED, which ONE of the following statements is TRUE?

A. Safe infusion of dobutamine requires central venous access

B. The lack of inotropic effects make metaraminol a useful drug for managing hypotension in patients with severe aortic stenosis

C. Noradrenaline causes an increase in systolic but not diastolic blood pressure

D. Noradrenaline is preferred over adrenaline in patients with septic shock due to its proven mortality benefit

27. Regarding the use of hypertonic saline in traumatic brain injury (TBI), which ONE of the following statements is TRUE?

A. It reliably decreases intracranial pressure and significantly improves cerebral blood flow

B. It is as effective as mannitol when osmotherapy is indicated

C. There is good evidence showing an outcome benefit in traumatic brain injury

D. It is the preferred crystalloid if severe traumatic brain injury occurs with hypotension

28. Which ONE of the following subset of trauma patients will MOST likely benefit from 'hypotensive resuscitation'?

A. A 40-year-old male with a penetrating chest injury

B. A 32-year-old female with multisite blunt trauma following a road traffic collision with GCS 15

C. A 50-year-old male with blunt abdominal trauma and severe closed head injury

D. A 22-year-old with a compound femur fracture

29. Regarding resuscitative thoracotomy in penetrating trauma due to a precordial stab wound, which ONE of the following statements is TRUE?

A. The survival rate may be >40%

B. It should only be performed by trained cardiothoracic surgeons

C. It should only be performed if the arrest is witnessed in the ED

D. It is contraindicated in the absence of cardiac arrest

30. Regarding transfusion-related acute lung injury (TRALI), which ONE of the following is TRUE?

A. Usually occurs ≥24 hours after transfusion

B. It is the leading cause of transfusion-related mortality

C. TRALI is associated with transfusion of packed red cells only

D. It has a higher mortality than other causes of ALI

31. A 42-year-old female presents to the ED in shock after suffering a massive pulmonary embolus (PE). Bedside echocardiography shows unequivocal signs of right ventricular (RV) overload. Regarding this case, which ONE of the following statements is TRUE?

A. Untreated, she has a mortality of approximately 30%

B. Fluid resuscitation should be performed carefully as excessive fluids might worsen RV failure

C. A CT pulmonary angiogram must be performed to confirm the diagnosis prior to urgent thrombolysis

D. When thrombolysis are considered, tPA should be given intravenously at a dose of 0.9 mg/kg – 10% as a bolus dose over 2 minutes and the rest as a continuous infusion over 1 hour

32. Regarding the use of focused echocardiography in the ED to examine pericardial effusions in a critically ill patient, which ONE of the following is TRUE?

A. A probe with a frequency of 5–10 mHz is the most appropriate

B. An effusion of <15 mm excludes tamponade

C. LV diastolic collapse is an early sign of tamponade

D. An apical approach is usually preferred over the subxiphoid approach as the optimum needle insertion site for pericardiocentesis

Paediatric resuscitation

Zaahid Pandie

1. Regarding current paediatric resuscitation guidelines in the prehospital and hospital environment, which ONE of the following statements is TRUE?

A. Infants more than a few hours beyond birth should receive CPR with a compression-ventilation ratio of 3:1

B. A 10-year-old child should be treated according to paediatric resuscitation guidelines

C. A 2-week-old infant in cardiac arrest secondary to hypoxaemia may be treated initially with positive pressure ventilation and oxygen

D. LMAs have been shown to be superior to bag–valve–mask (BVM) ventilation during resuscitation of children

2. Prevention of cardiopulmonary arrest in children is an important aspect of paediatric critical care. In this regard, which ONE of the following is FALSE?

A. Early warning systems, such as a medical emergency team (MET), allow prompt medical assessment and treatment, preventing cardiopulmonary arrest

B. The introduction of a MET is associated with a decrease in the number of respiratory arrests and the total number of arrests

C. Cardiorespiratory arrest in children is usually preceded by a recognisable phase of deterioration and is usually of cardiac origin

D. Children with fluid refractory septic shock should be managed with a sepsis protocol

3. Regarding paediatric arrhythmia in the setting of critical illness and cardiorespiratory arrest, which ONE of the following is INCORRECT?

A. The initial cardiac rhythm discovered is often asystole

B. The incidence of VF as the initial rhythm is approximately 20%

C. Up to 10% of sudden infant death syndrome (SIDS) deaths in infants may be attributable to inherited channelopathies

D. In the setting of VF or pulseless VT, doses higher than 4 J/kg, if delivered with a biphasic defibrillator are safe and effective

4. In recognising cardiopulmonary arrest in infants and commencing appropriate CPR, which ONE of the following is TRUE?

A. Radial pulse palpation is an important part of assessment and CPR should be commenced immediately if a pulse is not identified within 10 seconds

B. The depth of compression should be less than a third of the anteroposterior dimension of the chest to avoid harm from compressions

C. The two-finger technique is more effective in providing cardiac output in Infants than the two-thumb technique

D. 50% of a compression cycle should be devoted to compression and 50% to relaxation to enable recoil of the chest wall

5. Intravenous access during resuscitation is a vital part of management. Which ONE of the following is TRUE?

A. All resuscitative drugs may be given via the intravenous, intraosseous (IO) or endotracheal route

B. Current evidence suggests that newer IO devices, such as drills and bone injection guns, improve the outcome in paediatric resuscitation

C. IO blood can be used reliably for biochemical, haematological and venous blood gas analyses

D. IO access is often achieved more rapidly and successfully than IV access in cardiopulmonary arrest in children

6. Regarding the assessment and management of the airway and breathing in children during resuscitation, which ONE of the following is TRUE?

A. Protection of an airway may be achieved by an endotracheal tube or laryngeal mask airway

B. Current evidence shows a clear benefit of endotracheal intubation over BVM ventilation in out-of-hospital paediatric arrests

C. A nasopharyngeal airway of appropriate length is the equivalent distance from the tip of the nose to the tragus of the ear

D. Differences in the anatomy of the airway of a child compared with an adult include a more posterior and cephalad larynx, a long floppy epiglottis and a shorter trachea

7. Regarding providing effective ventilation during paediatric resuscitation, which ONE of the following is INCORRECT?

A. Routine use of cricoid pressure during endotracheal intubation may not protect against aspiration and may make intubation more difficult

B. BVM ventilation was associated with fewer complications than endotracheal intubation in out-of-hospital prospective controlled studies

C. If a cuffed tracheal tube is used in an infant with a weight >3.5 kg and <1 year of age, a tube with an ID of 3.0 mm should be used

D. After the age of 2, to estimate the cuffed tracheal tube size the correct formulae is with the formula ID (mm) = (age in years/4) +3   (Khine formula)

8. In the initial management of cardiac arrest in children, which ONE of the following is TRUE?

A. A single rescuer encountering an unwitnessed collapse of an infant or child should obtain assistance first, then start CPR

B. A rescuer witnessing a sudden collapse should start CPR immediately

C. An automated external defibrillator (AED) with dose attenuation is preferred over a manual defibrillator in children who suffered an OHCA

D. The safety of AEDs in infants 1 year of age is unknown but successful defibrillations have been achieved using AEDs in infants

9. A 5-year-old boy has an unwitnessed collapse in a shopping centre. Bystanders attempt CPR with a compression ventilation ratio of 30:2. Which ONE of the following is TRUE?

A. When paramedic staff arrive they should continue the above compression ventilation ratio

B. If paramedic staff insert an LMA for ventilation, pauses to administer breaths are not required

C. If the resuscitation guidelines are followed, basic life support (BLS) will deliver a ventilation ratio that is about half the normal respiratory rate for age

D. If resuscitation guidelines are adhered to, advanced life support (ALS) BVM ventilation will provide approximately five breaths per minute

10. When estimating drug dosages in children in the resuscitation room, which ONE of the following is INCORRECT?

A. In non-obese children, doses can be estimated according to the body weight in kilograms derived from the formulae: [2 (age +4)] in young children *or* age x 3.3 in older children

B. In obese patients, the ideal weight should be used, estimated from height

C. Recent evidence confirms that traditional weight formulae are accurate in estimating weight in children

D. Doses of drugs, energy of DC shock and volume of fluid therapy may be prescribed on the basis of height

11. Which ONE of the following is TRUE in relation to the use of a defibrillator in children?

A. An adult AED with the dose attenuated to 50 J is preferred to manual defibrillators in infants and children ≤ 8 years of age

B. The initial dose for children in VF or VT arrest who are unresponsive is 4 J/kg given as a synchronised shock

C. If neither a manual defibrillator nor an adult AED with an attenuated energy level is available, an AED with an adult preset dose may be used

D. Adult AED devices are all unable to accurately distinguish between a shockable and nonshockable rhythm in infants and children

12. A 3-year-old boy presents to the ED with septic shock. His respiratory rate (RR) is 55 with SaO_2 of 89% in room air. His pulse rate is 33/min, capillary refill time is 4 seconds, and BP is unrecordable. He is lethargic but easily rousable and has a GCS of 13. Respiratory examination suggests a right-sided pneumonia. Resuscitation is initiated with BVM ventilation with 100% oxygen, which improves his SaO_2 to 100%. An intravenous fluid bolus of normal saline is given and antibiotics administered. His HR remains at 33/min with unrecordable BP. Which one of the following is the MOST appropriate next step?

   A. Perform rapid sequence intubation

   B. Commence an adrenaline infusion

   C. Administer atropine 20 mcg/kg IV

   D. B followed by A

13. Regarding the use of IO cannulae to establish circulatory access during resuscitation, which ONE of the following is TRUE?

   A. Complications have been reported in 20% of patients after IO infusion

   B. IO catheterisation has been used successfully in term neonates but has not been studied in preterm babies

   C. Development of osteomyelitis is associated with prolonged IO use and the administration of hypertonic fluids

   D. Injury to the epiphyseal growth plate with poor bone growth is a common complication

14. Regarding neonatal resuscitation, which ONE of the following is TRUE?

   A. Newborn term babies who are breathing or crying but who have had meconium-stained amniotic fluid should have their nares and oropharynx suctioned

   B. Term babies who are depressed in terms of crying, breathing or tone immediately after birth should be given oxygen as the initial resuscitation step

   C. The most important indicator of the need for resuscitation in the newborn is a heart rate below 100

   D. Auscultation of the heart is a sensitive method in assessing the heart rate after 90 seconds

15. In assessing the initial need for resuscitation of a newborn, which ONE of the following is the BEST option?

   A. The Apgar score should remain the primary assessment tool to judge the need for resuscitation

   B. Palpation of the umbilicus is a good means of assessing heart rate

   C. In assessing the heart rate, both palpation of the umbilicus and the auscultation of the heart are equally insensitive methods

   D. The pulse oximeter should be used with the probe attached to the left hand to account for the preductal difference in blood flow

16. A precipitous delivery has occurred in the ED and a term neonate has been delivered by vaginal delivery. Meconium-stained liquor was present. Currently the baby appears floppy and is not crying. Which ONE of the following is TRUE?

   A. Initial provision of warmth, stimulation and drying should be followed by tracheal suctioning to prevent meconium aspiration syndrome

   B. Warm and dry the baby, open the airway, and stimulate breathing. If the heart rate is below 60 following this step, positive pressure ventilation using a BVM is the next step

   C. If this baby remains depressed, it should initially be resuscitated using 100% oxygen

   D. If initial effective ventilation with air does not improve the heart rate or oxygenation, use of a higher concentration of oxygen should be considered

17. Regarding ventilation strategies in newborn resuscitation, which ONE of the following is TRUE?

   A. Initial peak inflating pressures necessary to achieve an increase in heart rate or movement of the chest are variable

   B. An initial inflation pressure of 40 cm H_2O is recommended in preterm babies

   C. Continuous positive airway pressure (CPAP) is more effective than standard mechanical ventilation in reducing mortality and oxygen requirement in preterm babies

   D. Positive end-expiratory pressure (PEEP) is contraindicated in the preterm neonate due to the high incidence of barotraumas induced in this age group

18. Regarding ongoing monitoring during resuscitation of children, which ONE of the following is TRUE?

A. If the end-tidal CO_2 ($ETCO_2$) is consistently >15 mmHg, it may indicate that chest compressions may be inadequate or of poor quality

B. Current evidence suggests that it is appropriate to terminate advanced life support measures if $ETCO_2$ is <15 mmHg

C. The $ETCO_2$ has been shown to decrease for 1–2 minutes after administration of adrenaline and should be interpreted cautiously during these periods

D. The routine use of focused echocardiography to detect reversible causes of cardiac arrest is strongly recommended

CHAPTER 2
CARDIOVASCULAR EMERGENCIES

QUESTIONS

Jonathon Isoardi, Glenn Ryan and Waruna de Alwis

1. Regarding chest pain, which ONE of the following statements is TRUE?

A. Pain radiating to the right arm or shoulder is more predictive of myocardial infarction than pain radiating to the left arm or shoulder

B. Burning or indigestion pain is rarely associated with acute coronary syndrome (ACS)

C. Pain that is reproducible by chest wall palpation excludes ACS

D. Unremitting pain of constant nature lasting more than 12 hours is less likely to be due to ACS

2. Regarding investigations for chest pain, which ONE of the following statements is TRUE?

A. A new ST segment elevation ≥1 mm in two contiguous leads on electrocardiogram (ECG) has a 50% positive predictive value for diagnosis of acute myocardial infarction (AMI)

B. Troponin is specific to myocardial damage and is infrequently elevated in other pathology

C. Any troponin elevation above threshold has prognostic significance in patients presenting with ACS

D. Exercise stress testing has a high sensitivity and specificity for coronary heart disease and is a useful investigation to diagnose coronary artery disease

3. Regarding risk stratification for patients with suspected non-ST segment elevated ACS (NSTEAC), which ONE of the following statements is TRUE?

A. The thrombolysis in myocardial infarction (TIMI) score is a useful tool to identify which NSTEAC patients will benefit from early invasive therapy

B. Patients with a TIMI score of <2 have a very low (<2%) 14-day risk of adverse events including subsequent myocardial infarction

C. Prior aspirin use has no bearing on risk stratification

D. Diabetes and age have no bearing on risk stratification

4. Regarding ST elevation myocardial infarction, all of the following are true EXCEPT:

A. ST elevation in leads II, III and aVF may be associated with occlusion of the right coronary artery or circumflex artery

B. Posterior infarction, characterised by ST elevation in V1 and V2, is associated with occlusion of the right coronary artery or occasionally the circumflex artery

C. Inferior and posterior infarction may be associated with right ventricular (RV) infarction

D. An early marker of inferior infarction may be ST depression in lead aVL

5. Regarding the ECG in ST segment elevation myocardial infarction, which ONE of the following statements is TRUE?

A. ST segment elevation in lead aVR in a patient with ischaemic pain is a marker of left main coronary artery stenosis

B. Posterior ST segment elevation myocardial infarction (STEMI) is suggested by ST elevation in V1–3, R wave in V1 and V2, R/S ratio <1 in V1 and V2, and upright T waves in V1 and V2

C. Wellen's syndrome is characterised by ST segment elevation in V1–V4

D. ST segment elevation of ≥1 mm in two or more contiguous chest leads is an indication for reperfusion therapy

6. Regarding ACS which of ONE the following statements is TRUE?

A. Negative serial troponin excludes ACS

B. Troponin has a high early sensitivity for myocardial infarction

C. The ECG is the only investigation required to determine whether a patient requires emergency reperfusion

D. A chest X-ray (CXR) should be performed before thrombolysis in every patient

7. Regarding ECG changes associated with ACS, which ONE of the following statements is TRUE?

A. 70% of patients with AMI have a diagnostic ECG

B. Pseudoinfarction patterns mimicking STEMI on an ECG may be secondary to pulmonary embolus (PE) and subarachnoid haemorrhage

C. Discordance of the QRS complex and ST segment or T wave in the left bundle branch block (LBBB) is suggestive of myocardial ischaemia

D. ST segment elevation of 1 mm in 2 or more contiguous chest leads meets reperfusion criteria

8. Regarding myocardial infarction, which ONE of the following statements is TRUE?

A. Anterior or anteroseptal myocardial infarction is the least common, has the worst prognosis and occurs secondary to occlusion of the left anterior descending artery.

B. Inferior myocardial infarction is the most common infarction and may be associated with RV involvement and heart block

C. Lateral infarction occurs as a consequence of occlusion of posterior descending artery

D. Posterior infarction occurs as a consequence of occlusion of the posterior descending artery or occasionally from the circumflex artery in patients with dominant left-sided coronary circulation

9. Regarding contraindications to thrombolysis in STEMI, which ONE of the following statements is TRUE?

A. Known malignant intracranial neoplasm is a relative contraindication

B. Current use of anticoagulants is an absolute contraindication

C. Recent (within 4 weeks) internal bleeding (gastrointestinal tract or urinary tract) is an absolute contraindication

D. Chest pain with new left upper-limb weakness is an absolute contraindication

10. Regarding reperfusion therapy in AMI, which ONE of the following is TRUE?

A. Recent research has suggested that prehospital thrombolysis within 2 hours of symptom onset has superior outcomes compared with percutaneous coronary intervention, and similar outcomes if given within 4 hours of symptom onset

B. Early thrombolysis is as effective as percutaneous coronary intervention in patients with cardiogenic shock

C. Thrombolysis has the same risk of bleeding-related complications for all patients

D. The number needed to treat with thrombolytics for inferior STEMI to save one life is approximately 20

11. Regarding pharmacological management of ACS, which ONE of the following statements is TRUE?

A. Aspirin alone has no mortality benefit

B. There is strong evidence to support the early use of oral or IV metoprolol in the management of STEMI

C. A loading dose of clopidogrel has been shown to be safe in patients older than 75 years of age

D. Enoxaparin has been shown to be superior to unfractionated heparin when used for STEMI patients treated with fibrinolysis

12. A 75-year-old man presents to the emergency department (ED) with a gradual new onset dyspnoea on exertion. Regarding assessment for heart failure in this patient, all of the following statements are true EXCEPT:

A. The patient may have significant heart failure even if the ejection fraction on echocardiography is normal

B. Clinical features such as orthopnoea, paroxysmal nocturnal dyspnoea, raised jugular venous pressure and third heart sound have a low specificity for diagnosis of heart failure

C. Looking for evidence for diastolic dysfunction is essential

D. Uncontrolled hypertension may promote fluid retention

13. Regarding acute pulmonary oedema, which ONE of the following statements is TRUE?

A. Diastolic heart failure is responsible for two-thirds of cases

B. Normotensive or hypertensive acute pulmonary oedema is most commonly associated with fluid maldistribution rather than fluid overload

C. Diuretics remain the mainstay of treatment of normotensive or hypertensive acute pulmonary oedema

D. A brain natriuretic peptide (BNP) value between 100 and 500 pg/mL is diagnostic of pulmonary oedema

14. Regarding cardiogenic shock, which ONE of the following is TRUE?

A. Cardiogenic shock complicates 25% of patients with AMI

B. Vasopressors or inotropes have been shown to have a mortality benefit in cardiogenic shock

C. Early reperfusion with thrombolytics is as effective as percutaneous coronary intervention or coronary artery bypass grafting in the management of cardiogenic shock complicating ST segment elevation myocardial infarction

D. Early revascularisation with percutaneous coronary intervention or coronary artery bypass grafting is indicated in ST segment elevation myocardial infarction or new LBBB

15. Regarding cardiogenic shock in AMI, which ONE of the following is FALSE?

A. Cardiogenic shock complicating myocardial infarction carries a mortality of approximately 80%

B. The early use of inotropes is associated with reduced mortality

C. Arranging urgent reperfusion is critical when left anterior descending artery occlusion causing myocardial infarction is responsible

D. Intra-aortic balloon counterpulsation is only useful when combined with revascularisation

16. Regarding management of cardiogenic shock, which ONE of the following is TRUE?

A. IV fluids should never be first-line therapy

B. Vasodilators should be part of the treatment in acute mitral regurgitation

C. Endotracheal intubation will usually alleviate hypotension and improve perfusion

D. Intra-aortic ballon counterpulsation provides haemodynamic support by decreasing diastolic blood pressure (BP) and thereby decreasing afterload

17. Regarding hypertensive crises, which ONE of the following is TRUE?

A. There is good evidence to suggest that severe hypertension should be treated in ischaemic stroke

B. Hypertensive encephalopathy is largely irreversible

C. Treatment of hypertensive encephalopathy should aim to reduce the mean arterial pressure by approximately 25% over 1–2 hours

D. A patient with a BP of 220/130 would be classified as having malignant hypertension

18. In the pharmacological treatment of hypertensive crises in the ED, which ONE of the following is TRUE?

A. Aortic dissection initially requires rapid minimisation of BP with a vasodilator

B. Hydralazine is a direct arteriolar vasodilating agent

C. Due to its rapid onset of action and long duration of action, sodium nitroprusside is usually given as sequential boluses

D. Glyceryl trinitrate (GTN) predominantly reduces afterload and as such is ideal for pulmonary oedema caused by severe hypertension

19. Regarding ECG changes in pericarditis, which ONE of the following statements is TRUE?

A. ST segment elevation is invariably associated with reciprocal changes

B. The ECG in pericarditis is characterised by concave ST segment elevation across multiple anatomical areas of arterial perfusion and PR depression

C. Pericarditis can be differentiated from benign early repolarisation by the presence of concave upward ST segment elevation

D. Tall-tented T waves are diagnostic

20. With respect to pericarditis, which ONE of the following is TRUE regarding ECG findings?

A. ECG is not useful in the diagnosis of cardiac tamponade

B. The ECG will return to normal within 2–3 days

C. Q waves may be caused by acute pericarditis

D. PR segment depression is useful to discriminate between pericarditis and AMI

21. In non-traumatic pericardial tamponade, which ONE of the following is TRUE?

A. Metastatic malignancy accounts for 80–90% of cases

B. CXR is a reliable diagnostic test

C. Tachycardia is usually present

D. Pulsus paradoxus is pathognomonic of pericardial tamponade

22. Regarding infective endocarditis, which ONE of the following statements is TRUE?

A. Duke major criteria include fever and positive blood culture

B. The major pathogens involved are streptococcal species, Staphylococcus aureus and enterococcus species

C. Involvement of the aortic valve is rare in intravenous drug users

D. A single blood culture is helpful in identifying the causative pathogen when a patient has been treated with antibiotics for fewer than 3 days

23. Regarding endocarditis, which ONE of the following statements is TRUE?

A. In intravenous drug users with right-sided endocarditis, coagulase negative staphylococci account for most of the cases

B. The pulmonary valve is most commonly involved in right-sided endocarditis in intravenous drug users

C. In the absence of prior antibiotics, blood cultures will be positive in at least 95% of cases, where 3–5 sets are taken

D. Overall mortality for native and prosthetic valve endocarditis is <10%

24. In patients presenting to the ED with syncope, which ONE of the following is TRUE?

A. Clinical examination alone will identify the diagnosis in up to 45% of patients

B. A clear diagnosis will be established in approximately 75% of patients

C. The San Francisco syncope rule suggests that a systolic BP of <110 mmHg places the patient in a high-risk group

D. ECG is usually a high-yield test in this group of patients

25. Regarding patients presenting to the ED with syncope, which ONE of the following is TRUE?

A. A decrease in systolic BP of at least 30 mmHg on standing is required to diagnose orthostatic hypotension

B. Patients with orthostatic hypotension have a raised 30-day mortality

C. Routine CT scan of the brain is recommended in most guidelines for investigation of syncope

D. The disposition of patients with unexplained syncope largely revolves around identifying those at high risk for cardiac events

26. With respect to heart block, which ONE of the following is TRUE?

A. First-degree heart block refers to a PR interval >180 ms

B. The PR interval in Mobitz type I second-degree heart block should be constant

C. Third-degree heart block with nodal escape will display a broad QRS interval

D. Third-degree heart block complicating AMI confers an increased mortality, even when rate is controlled

27. Regarding atrioventricular block, which ONE of the following statements is TRUE?

A. Mobitz type I (Wenckebach) is characterised by increased refractoriness of the His-Purkinje system, resulting in progressive lengthening of the PR interval until a QRS complex is dropped

B. The most common conduction defect found in AMI patients is Mobitz type II

C. The most frequent unstable rhythm found in AMI patients is complete heart block

D. Complete heart block is always associated with a wide QRS complex

28. Regarding VT, which ONE of the following statements is TRUE?

A. AV dissociation is the hallmark of VT, and is seen in >50% of cases of VT

B. A QRS axis of −90 to +180 (negative QRS complex in I and aVF) is the only axis that has specificity for VT

C. Right bundle branch block (RBBB) morphology in QRS complex in V1 excludes VT

D. VT never has a rate <140 beats per minute

29. Regarding broad-complex tachycardia, which ONE of the following is TRUE?

A. Cannon A waves in the jugular venous pressure (JVP) are more likely to indicate ventricular tachycardia than supraventricular tachycardia (SVT) with aberrancy

B. In the ED, SVT with aberrancy is about equally as common as ventricular tachycardia

C. The presence of retrograde P waves on the ECG is a reliable indicator of ventricular tachycardia

D. Myocardial ischaemia is not known to cause torsades de pointes

30. Regarding broad-complex tachycardia, which ONE of the following characteristics would favour a diagnosis of VT rather than SVT with aberrancy?

A. A preceding ectopic P wave

B. Response to carotid sinus massage

C. The patient is aged 55 years

D. An rSR pattern in lead V1 of the ECG

31. The following are associated with causing torsades de pointes EXCEPT:

  A. Midazolam

  B. Sotalol

  C. Hypomagnesemia

  D. Organophosphates

32. Regarding the pharmacological treatment of cardiac dysrhythmias, which ONE of the following statements is TRUE?

  A. Lignocaine is a class 1a antiarrhythmic drug in the Vaughan Williams Classification system

  B. Isoprenaline may be effective in the treatment of torsades de pointes

  C. The dose of adenosine may need to be decreased in those patients taking theophylline

  D. Sotalol is a third-line agent in the treatment of torsades de pointes

33. Regarding Brugada syndrome, which ONE of the following statements is FALSE?

  A. Brugada syndrome is associated with syncope and sudden cardiac death in young patients with a structurally normal heart

  B. It is characterised by incomplete or complete RBBB and ST segment elevation in V1–V3 that may be downsloping or concave

  C. When untreated, it has a mortality of 20% at 2 years

  D. It is best treated with a sodium channel blocking agent

34. Which ONE of the following drugs can safely be used in patients with Brugada syndrome?

  A. Flecainide

  B. Bupivacaine

  C. Isoprenaline

  D. Amitriptyline

35. Regarding use of adenosine in the treatment of SVT, which ONE of the following statements is TRUE?

  A. Efficacy of adenosine in converting stable SVT to sinus rhythm is <30%

  B. Adenosine is equally effective in converting SVT both in slower and faster heart rates

  C. In one-third of patients with SVT, failure of treatment with return of SVT can be expected following initial conversion

  D. Adenosine is a less reliable drug with a lower conversion rate compared with intravenous magnesium infusion in SVT

36. Regarding preexcitation syndromes, which ONE of the following statements is TRUE?

  A. Tachycardia associated with Wolff-Parkinson-White syndrome (WPW) is always wide complex

  B. Antidromic reentry tachycardia is the most common of the paroxysmal tachycardias seen in WPW

  C. Verapamil is indicated for managing rapid atrial fibrillation (AF) with preexcitation in patients without haemodynamic instability

  D. Adenosine and beta-blockers may convert a rapid atrial rate to a rapid ventricular rate and precipitate ventricular fibrillation (VF) in atrial fibrillation with preexcitation

37. Regarding reentrant SVT, which ONE of the following is TRUE?

  A. Most patients have reentry involving a bypass tract

  B. Adenosine has been shown to convert 70% of reentrant SVT

  C. In WPW, anti-dromic reentrant SVT is more common than orthodromic reentrant SVT

  D. Of all reentrant SVT, about 60% have reentry within the atrioventricular node (AV node)

38. Regarding WPW, all of the following statements are correct EXCEPT:

  A. 15–30% of arrhythmias are atrial fibrillation

  B. A prominent R wave in V1 is one of the recognised ECG features

  C. AV reentrant tachycardia is a common presentation

  D. More than 50% of the patients with WPW present with an arrhythmia

39. According to the Australian Resuscitation Council recommendations for management of AF, which ONE of the following is TRUE?

  A. Amiodarone is recommended for rate control of patients with AF and heart failure who do not have an accessory pathway

  B. Intravenous beta-blockers or dihydropyridine calcium channel blockers are recommended for rate control of AF in the acute setting, exercising control in patients with hypotension or heart failure

C. Cardioversion may be attempted safely in patients with new AF of up to 72 hours' duration

D. Intravenous administration of digoxin is recommended as first line for rate control of AF in those patients with a preexcitation syndrome

40. With respect to AF in the ED, which ONE of the following is TRUE?

A. Electrical cardioversion usually requires more than 100 J of energy

B. Electrical cardioversion needs to be delayed until echocardiography has demonstrated no evidence of atrial thrombus

C. Rhythm control should be the goal of treatment when chronic AF is suspected

D. In the absence of structural heart disease or underlying illness, patients with paroxysmal AF have a 90% chance of reverting to sinus rhythm in the next 48 hours without any treatment

41. When AF is associated with WPW, which ONE of the following statements is TRUE?

A. QRS complexes are narrow

B. Ventricular rate remains relatively slow

C. It is associated with long AV node refractory periods

D. Heart rate can be over 250/min

42. Regarding recognition of atrial flutter on a 12-lead ECG, which ONE of the following statements is TRUE?

A. Atrial rate does not usually exceed 300/min

B. Regularity of atrial complexes can vary

C. A very short isoelectric period can be seen between atrial complexes

D. The intersection between a flutter wave and the QRS complex can be identified at the base (isoelectric) line

43. Regarding artificial pacemaker code, which ONE of the following is INCORRECT?

A. The first letter refers to the chamber paced

B. The third letter refers to the response to sensing

C. 'T' in the third letter position indicates pacemaker termination in response to sensing

D. 'R' refers to the ability of the pacemaker to modulate its response to sensing depending on rate

44. Which ONE of the following statements is FALSE regarding failure of electrical and mechanical capture in a patient with a pacemaker?

A. Inadequate energy generation in the pacemaker, such as due to battery failure, may contribute

B. Increased electrical resistance at the electrode–myocardial interface secondary to fibrosis is a cause

C. Flecainide is known to cause failure to capture

D. A shortened refractory period of the myocardium is a recognised cause

45. Regarding artificial pacemakers, when the pacemaker fails to provide output, which ONE of the following statements is FALSE?

A. Lack of pacing activity can be detected on the ECG when the patient is pacemaker dependent, i.e. when patient's heart rate is lower than the target rate

B. Oversensing of P and T waves and skeletal muscle activity as QRS complexes is a cause for failure of pacemaker output

C. Modern bipolar pacemakers can cause more oversensing of inappropriate signals

D. Suxamethonium can cause failure of output by a pacemaker

46. For a child known to have uncorrected tetralogy of Fallot presenting with a cyanotic episode, which ONE of the following would NOT be appropriate treatment?

A. Allowing the child to sit calmly in the mother's lap

B. Encouraging the child to stand, in an effort to decrease right-to-left shunting

C. A small fluid bolus of 5–10 mL/kg

D. A bolus dose of metaraminol

47. Regarding paroxysmal SVT in an infant, which ONE of the following statements is TRUE?

A. Infants usually present late (after 48 hours from the onset) as they tolerate SVT well

B. Vagal manoeuvres are ineffective in infants

C. Use of verapamil may cause cardiovascular collapse and death

D. AV nodal reentry is a more common mechanism in this age group

48. Regarding a neonate with an undiagnosed congenital heart disease presenting for the first time to the ED, which ONE of the following statements is TRUE?

A. Soft early systolic murmur indicates a strong suspicion for an undiagnosed congenital heart disease

B. A shocked neonate of 1–2 weeks of age may be due to a duct dependent lesion

C. Coarctation of the aorta frequently presents during the first month with hypertension

D. The most common presentation in a neonate is with features of congestive cardiac failure

49. Regarding the hyperoxia test in a neonate with suspected congenital heart disease, which ONE of the following statements is FALSE?

A. Pulse oxymetry can reliably substitute for arterial blood gas sampling

B. A passed hyperoxia test means $PaO_2 >$ 250 mmHg and it excludes hypoxia secondary to congenital heart disease

C. First the neonate should be tested on room air and then tested on 100% oxygen given for 15 minutes

D. A neonate with a failed hyperoxia test should be considered for immediate prostaglandin E1 therapy

50. Regarding the assessment of children with hypertension, all of the following statements are true EXCEPT:

A. Acute glomerulonephritis is a common cause in early infancy

B. The diagnosis of essential hypertension in an adolescent requires thorough assessment to exclude secondary causes

C. Hypertension is defined as systolic or diastolic BP ≥95th percentile of the age and height matched normal value

D. Hyperthyroidism and hypercortisol states are life-threatening causes

Waruna de Alwis and Sean Lawrence

1. Regarding assessment of a patient presenting to the emergency department (ED) with undifferentiated dyspnoea, which ONE of the following statements is TRUE?

A. The presence of dyspnoea on exertion, orthopnoea and paroxysmal nocturnal dyspnoea strongly suggests a cardiac origin

B. In the presence of a $PaCO_2 > 45$ mm Hg on arterial blood gas, a rise in HCO_3 of 1 mmol/L for each 10 mm Hg $PaCO_2$ indicates chronic CO_2 retention

C. Finger-clubbing found on examination is specific to lung pathology

D. Presence of a third heart sound (S3 or gallop rhythm) on auscultation has a high positive likelihood ratio for congestive heart failure

2. Venous blood gas (VBG) analysis is increasingly being used in the place of arterial blood gas (ABG) analysis in the ED. Which ONE of the following statements is TRUE regarding its use?

A. VBG can substitute ABG to obtain pH, HCO_3 and base excess in a patient in a shock state

B. There is a good agreement between venous and arterial PCO_2

C. Use of venous PCO_2 to screen for the presence of arterial hypercarbia may reduce the need to do ABG analysis

D. The difference between arterial and venous pH is approximately 0.1 pH units

3. The chest X-ray (CXR) of a 65-year-old female smoker presenting to the ED with a history of recent onset worsening dyspnoea reveals a moderately large left-sided pleural effusion. In determining the cause of this pleural effusion, which ONE of the following statements is TRUE?

A. Measurement of pleural fluid protein and lactate dehydrogenase (LDH) levels have no value in establishing the cause of the effusion

B. Pulmonary oedema is unlikely to be the cause if the effusion is unilateral

C. Pulmonary embolism (PE) alone does not cause pleural effusions

D. Empyema is often loculated and seen as a pleural-based collection

4. Regarding life-threatening massive haemoptysis in an elderly patient, which ONE of the following statements is TRUE?

A. Selective intubation of the bleeding lung may be attempted

B. If the bleeding side can be identified, the patient should be positioned with that side down

C. Exsanguination is the usual cause of death

D. 90% of bleeding originates from systemic circulation

5. Regarding a patient presenting to the ED with haemoptysis, which ONE of the following statements is TRUE?

A. CXR is usually normal in most patients with lung malignancy

B. PE is a common cause of severe haemoptysis

C. Early bronchoscopy, within the first 48 hours, is more valuable in identifying the bleeding site than late bronchoscopy

D. When it is associated with right upper lobe collapse on CXR, it is usually due to pneumonia

6. Regarding the diagnosis and management of pertussis which ONE of the following is TRUE?

A. Positive serology (IgM) is the gold standard for diagnosis

B. Maternal antibodies produce robust protection for infants in the first 6 months of life

C. Treatment with macrolide antibiotic shortens the clinical course but does not alter the transmission rate

D. The illness is highly communicable early in the illness with attack rates of 75–100% from symptomatic individuals to susceptible contacts

7. Regarding assessment of severity of a patient with community-acquired pneumonia (CAP) in the ED, which ONE of the following statements is TRUE?

A. Assessment based on a single validated severity scoring system is often adequate

B. The SMART-COP score identifies patients who require ventilatory and haemodynamic support

C. Pneumonia severity index (PSI) mainly predicts clinical deterioration in patients with CAP

D. Determining the severity of CAP is useful in distinguishing typical from atypical aetiology

8. Regarding use of blood culture and sensitivity in a patient with CAP, which ONE of the following statements is TRUE?

A. Results are positive in up to half of the patients

B. Empiric antibiotic therapy initiated in the ED will need to be changed in the medical ward for the majority of patients once results are available

C. When positive it does not confirm the causative organism of pneumonia

D. Blood cultures are of low value if the patient is likely to be discharged from the ED for outpatient antibiotic therapy

9. Regarding the aetiological diagnosis of CAP, which ONE of the following statements is FALSE?

A. The causative organism of pneumonia can be predicted via a CXR

B. Correctly collected sputum for gram stain and culture may have a diagnostic yield of up to 40%

C. Pneumococcal urinary antigen assay is a useful assay where *Streptococcus pneumoniae* is suspected

D. Throat swab polymerase chain reaction (PCR) is useful to identify a virus aetiology

10. Regarding pneumonia caused by *Staphylococcus aureus*, all of the following statements are correct EXCEPT:

A. It is more common during influenza epidemics

B. It does not usually occur in patients other than recently hospitalised patients and nursing home residents

C. Empyema and cavity formation are not common radiological features

D. It is associated with a comparatively higher incidence of septic shock than that caused by other bacterial pathogens

11. Regarding pneumonia caused by methicillin-resistant *S. aureus* (MRSA), all of the following statements are correct EXCEPT:

A. It is more likely to be present as severe CAP in children and young adults

B. It should be suspected when it is associated with a history of furunculosis or folliculitis

C. It is caused by community-associated *S. aureus* strains in many parts of Australia

D. Severe sepsis is unlikely in these patients

12. Regarding aspiration pneumonitis, which ONE of the following statements is TRUE?

A. CXR at presentation is nearly always normal

B. It is secondary to aspiration of sterile gastric contents

C. It usually presents after 24–48 hours

D. *S. aureus* is the most common causative pathogen

13. Regarding the management of an elderly patient with suspected pulmonary aspiration, which ONE of the following statements is TRUE?

A. Antibiotic treatment is recommended in all elderly patients

B. Rigid bronchoscopy may be indicated

C. Intravenous hydrocortisone 200 mg is beneficial

D. The patient can often be discharged from the ED with oral antibiotics

14. Regarding a patient with diagnosed bronchiectasis presenting to the ED with recent onset cough and increasing dyspnoea, which ONE of the following statements is TRUE?

A. Empiric antibiotic treatment should be directed at a previous *Pseudomonas aeruginosa* infection if present

B. Bronchodilator therapy with salbutamol is not likely to be beneficial

C. There is minimal risk for severe haemoptysis in these patients

D. Mucolytic agents should be prescribed early for better clearance of airway secretions

15. Regarding recurrence of a spontaneous pneumothorax, which ONE the following statements is TRUE?

A. The expected rate of recurrence is lower if the first pneumothorax reexpanded within 24 hours

B. Definitive treatment such as pleurodesis with or without video-assisted thoracoscopy (VAT) procedure is not indicated after the first pneumothorax

C. Approximately 20% of all secondary spontaneous pneumothoraces recur

D. Cessation of cigarette smoking after the first pneumothorax reduces the chance of recurrence

16. It is often difficult to identify a pneumothorax on a supine CXR in a ventilated patient. All of the following signs on the CXR suggest the presence of pneumothorax EXCEPT:

A. Deep sulcus sign at costophrenic angle

B. A sharp outline of the pericardial fat (pericardial fat pad sign)

C. Oligaemic lung field

D. Lucency over liver and upper abdomen not explained by an abdominal structure

17. Regarding the diagnosis of a spontaneous pneumothorax in a patient with severe **chronic obstructive pulmonary disease** (COPD), which ONE of the following statements is TRUE?

A. Expiratory films are more sensitive than inspiratory films

B. A bulla can be differentiated from a pneumothorax on CXR because the bulla has a concave inner margin but pneumothorax does not

C. CXR is equally sensitive as CT for detecting a pneumothorax

D. Differentiation between a large bulla and a pneumothorax is not important because both can be drained using the same principles

18. All of the following statements are correct regarding detection of a pneumothorax in a supine patient using bedside ultrasound in the ED EXCEPT:

A. The 'lung point' sign when present is highly specific for a pneumothorax

B. The lung sliding cannot be seen with a linear or curvilinear probe when there is a pneumothorax

C. The comet tail artefacts are due to pneumothorax

D. A horizontal linear pattern both superficial and deep to the pleural line on M-mode indicates a pneumothorax

19. Regarding management of a patient presenting with a first episode of primary spontaneous pneumothorax, which ONE of the following statements is TRUE?

A. 100% oxygen treatment prevents reexpansion pulmonary oedema

B. Supplemental oxygen increases the pressure gradient for nitrogen from pleural space (pneumothorax) to alveoli

C. Chest tube drainage is more effective than aspiration

D. Aspiration has been shown to be equally successful across all age groups

20. Regarding the selection of an appropriately sized intercostal catheter or tube when treating a spontaneous pneumothorax, which ONE of the statements is TRUE?

A. Size should be based on the anticipated amount of air leak from the lung because a smaller sized tube could cause a tension pneumothorax

B. Smaller tubes should be selected to prevent scarring at the insertion site

C. Inserting a larger tube is not indicated in the management of a spontaneous pneumothorax

D. The catheter or tube diameter is indicated in French sizes where 1 French equals 1 mm

21. Regarding reexpansion pulmonary oedema following treatment of a spontaneous pneumothorax, all of the following statements are true EXCEPT:

A. It usually occurs with needle aspiration

B. There is a high risk in a patient who presents late with a larger pneumothorax

C. Treatment includes aggressive fluid resuscitation

D. Intubation and ventilation may be needed for severe hypoxaemia

22. Which ONE of the following factors is LEAST likely to predict the risk for a fatal or near-fatal episode of asthma?

A. A life-threatening admission within the previous 12 months

B. Arterial desaturation

C. Normal $PaCO_2$ on ABG analysis

D. Current use of corticosteroids

23. Regarding bronchodilator therapy in severe asthma, which ONE of the following statements is TRUE?

A. Intravenous adrenaline infusion is preferable to nebulised salbutamol in life-threatening asthma

B. Intravenous salbutamol causes significant reduction of airway oedema

C. The only indication for intravenous salbutamol therapy in adults is a critically unwell asthma patient who cannot effectively have inhaled therapy

D. Up to 50% of the salbutamol dose placed in the chamber is delivered to the bronchioles during nebulisation therapy

24. Regarding the use of magnesium sulphate in severe asthma, which ONE of the following statements is TRUE?

A. The greatest response to intravenous magnesium sulphate is seen in patients with the most severe bronchospasm compared with less severe bronchospasm

B. It reduces the rate of hospital admission in severe asthma

C. Nebulised therapy is as effective as intravenous magnesium sulphate

D. It is not recommended for use in children

25. Regarding intubation of a patient with severe asthma, which ONE of the following is the MOST appropriate option?

A. Intubation of a patient with a normal level of consciousness and severe hypercapnoea and fatigue

B. Intravenous fluid bolus prior to intubation and careful adjustment of the induction dosage

C. Use of ketamine 1–2 mg/kg alone without use of a paralytic agent

D. Brisk bagging using bag–valve–mask ventilation prior to induction and soon after intubation to maintain oxygen saturation

26. Regarding invasive ventilation of a patient with severe life-threatening asthma, all of the following statements are correct EXCEPT:

A. A tidal volume of 5–6 mL/kg is recommended

B. The ventilator graph should show expiration to be complete before the next breath is delivered

C. Hypercarbia is generally not detrimental except in patients with myocardial dysfunction

D. Pressure control ventilation is considered ideal

27. Regarding the management of acute asthma in adults, which ONE of the following is TRUE?

A. High-inspiratory flow rates are recommended in patients requiring mechanical ventilation

B. Measurement of plateau pressures is not helpful in ventilated asthmatics because dynamic hyperinflation makes the reading unreliable

C. Non-invasive ventilation (NIV) should currently be avoided because available evidence suggests it is associated with poorer outcomes

D. Parenteral (IV) salbutamol has no benefit over continuous nebulised salbutamol

28. A young adult male was intubated in the ED for a near-fatal asthma episode. A few minutes after connecting to the ventilator, significant oxygen desaturation was observed on the monitor. If the ventilator, ventilator circuit, oxygen delivery and tube placement are found to be functioning well and correct, which ONE of the following statements is TRUE regarding the patient's hypoxaemia?

A. CXR alone cannot exclude a pneumothorax when it's due to barotrauma

B. Dynamic hyperinflation is not usually contributory

C. Suction may cause further bronchospasm and worsen hypoxaemia

D. Mucus plugging is often the cause

29. Regarding the treatment of acute asthma in children, which ONE of the following is TRUE?

A. Evidence suggests that intravenous salbutamol is the parenteral bronchodilator of choice for life-threatening asthma due to its minimal side effect profile

B. Salbutamol administered via nebuliser has a higher incidence of side effects than when administered via a metered dose inhaler (MDI) and spacer

C. Aminophylline has no role in the management of acute severe asthma

D. NIV is not indicated in children with severe asthma because it does not alter outcomes

30. Regarding the management of acute severe exacerbation of COPD, all of the following statements are correct EXCEPT:

A. Spirometry should be obtained in all patients on presentation

B. ABGs are not routinely required

C. A hypoxic patient should be treated with nasal prong oxygen at 0.5–2.0 L/min or a Venturi mask at 24% or 28%

D. 5 mg of nebulised S-salbutamol is equivalent to 10 puffs of 100 mcg salbutamol delivered with an MDI and a spacer

31. All of the following clinical features may suggest hypercapnic rather than normocapnic COPD EXCEPT:

A. Obesity

B. Use of central nervous system depressants such as sedatives

C. Obstructive sleep apnoea

D. Diagnosis of emphysema rather than chronic bronchitis

32. Regarding the investigation of patients presenting with an apparent exacerbation of COPD, which ONE of the following is TRUE?

A. All patients with acute exacerbations have major reductions in peak expiratory flow rate (PEFR) or FEV1 measurements

B. A very low B-type natriuretic peptide (BNP) < 100 pg/mL is useful in excluding coexistent congestive heart failure

C. Uncertainty regarding the presence or absence of pneumothorax in a patient with bullous emphysema is best resolved using a combination of inspiratory and expiratory films and bedside ultrasonography

D. D-dimer is an unreliable test for excluding PE in patients with moderate to severe COPD

33. Regarding the use of supportive ventilation in the management of patients presenting with an acute exacerbation of COPD, which ONE of the following is FALSE?

A. NIV should not be initiated unless pH is <7.30

B. NIV is associated with a reduction in mortality

C. Patients with a pH between 7.25 and 7.30 appear to receive the greatest benefit

D. The main benefit of NIV is in providing reduced work of breathing

34. Regarding the management of patients presenting with an exacerbation of COPD, which ONE of the following is TRUE?

A. There is evidence that a combination of anticholinergic and beta-sympathomimetic bronchodilators is more effective than either agent alone

B. Antibiotics have little role

C. Systemic corticosteroid use reduces the length of hospital stay

D. The inpatient mortality of patients requiring invasive mechanical ventilation is approximately 75%.

35. All of the following factors contribute to increased mortality rate among haemodynamically stable patients with PE EXCEPT:

A. Elevated serum troponin levels

B. Immobilisation due to neurological disease

C. Current use of the oral contraceptive pill

D. Right ventricle dilatation as assessed by echocardiography

36. Regarding venous thromboembolism in a pregnant woman all of the following statements are correct EXCEPT:

A. There a is an increased predisposition for deep venous thrombosis (DVT) to occur in the left leg

B. Thrombophilia screening should be done in pregnant patients diagnosed to have a current DVT or PE as it determines further management

C. Isolated iliac vein thrombosis may present with abdominal pain and back pain

D. Magnetic resonance direct thrombus imaging (MRDTI) has a high-sensitivity and specificity for diagnosis of iliac vein thrombosis in pregnancy

37. Regarding diagnosis of PE in a pregnant patient, which ONE of the following statements is TRUE?

A. Ventilation/perfusion (V/Q) lung scanning delivers a lower fetal dose of radiation than the dose delivered in CT pulmonary angiogram (CTPA)

B. A normal compression ultrasound of the lower limbs can rule out PE

C. The risk of childhood cancer is higher with V/Q scan than with CTPA

D. When clinical features are suggestive of PE and compressive ultrasound of the lower limbs is positive, confirmation of PE should be done with further testing

38. Regarding the use of the pulmonary embolism rule-out criteria (PERC), which ONE of the following statements is FALSE?

A. PERC is a validated rule that can be applied to all patients with suspected PE

B. Patients falling above the acceptable testing threshold should be tested further

C. Testing threshold is the pretest probability below which a clinician may safely not perform diagnostic testing

D. When pretest probability is lower than the testing threshold, the potential harm to the patient may be more than the benefit of a diagnostic test

39. Regarding management of a haemodynamically stable patient with acute PE, which ONE of the following statements is TRUE?

A. Unfractionated heparin should be given for a patient with creatinine clearance of 40 mL/min

B. Unfractionated heparin should be used in pregnancy in place of low molecular weight heparin

C. Warfarin should be commenced preferably on the first day of treatment and should be continued for at least 3 months

D. Low molecular weight heparin is the appropriate treatment in morbid obesity

40. Regarding DVT affecting the upper extremity, which ONE of the following statements is TRUE?

A. Patients are more likely to have cancer than patients with a DVT of the legs

B. It is not associated with PE

C. In suspected patients with low pretest probability, a D-dimer test is as reliable as in DVT of the legs for screening

D. Up to 20% of the cases are due to secondary causes such as central venous lines, pacemaker or defibrillator leads and malignancy

Waruna de Alwis

1. Which ONE of the following features is LEAST likely to be helpful in making a clinical diagnosis of migraine?

A. A gradual onset hemiparaesthesia preceding or accompanied by headache that lasts <60 minutes

B. Onset of lethargy and yawning a few hours before the onset of headache

C. Bilateral headache

D. External ocular muscle palsy associated with headache

2. Which ONE of the following statements is TRUE regarding a patient aged over 50 years who presents to the emergency department (ED) with a severe headache?

A. The occipitonuchal location of the headache has a high positive predictive value (PPV) for a critical secondary cause

B. Ischaemic optic neuritis can be a complication in this patient

C. Headache onset associated with exertion is not a predictor of subarachnoid haemorrhage

D. Secondary causes of headaches are more common in this age group than primary causes

3. Regarding secondary causes of headache, all of the following statements are true EXCEPT:

A. Pregnancy and the postpartum period increases the risk for cerebral venous thrombosis

B. Abnormal findings on neurological examination are present in the majority of patients with brain tumours

C. Diastolic hypertension is a recognised cause of severe headache

D. 10–25% of ischaemic stroke in the young and middle-aged population is secondary to spontaneous cervical arterial dissection

4. Regarding temporal arteritis, all of the following statements are correct EXCEPT:

A. It is almost exclusive to the over-50 age group

B. The classic headache is an essential diagnostic criterion

C. Jaw claudication may be a prominent feature

D. Scalp necrosis may be found on examination

5. Regarding subarachnoid haemorrhage (SAH), which ONE of the following is TRUE?

A. Non-contrast CT is useful in predicting the site of aneurysmal rupture

B. More than 50% of patients with SAH have an additional aneurysm that has not ruptured

C. Subhyaloid retinal haemorrhage is pathognomonic and can be identified in most patients on careful fundoscopy

D. Syncope as a sole symptom, without any other neurological features, can be a presenting feature

6. Regarding the diagnosis of SAH, which ONE of the following is TRUE?

A. When performed within 12 hours of the onset of symptoms, the sensitivity of non-contrast CT in detecting subarachnoid blood is up to 98%

B. Magnetic resonance imaging (MRI) is an equally sensitive substitute to non-contrast CT

C. In the presence of red blood cells (RBCs) in the cerebrospinal fluid (CSF), the absence of xanthrochromia reliably excludes SAH

D. Currently available evidence suggests that CT angiography is suitable as a first-line investigation

7. Regarding complications associated with SAH, which ONE of the following is TRUE?

A. Vasospasm is maximal in the first 24 hours

B. Seizure prophylaxis is indicated in the ED for all patients

C. Delayed cerebral ischaemia is usually associated with hyperglycaemia and suboptimal maintenance of body temperature

D. Rebleeding is generally independent of the patient's blood pressure control

8. A 56-year-old woman presents to the ED with a 2-day history of sudden onset severe headache. Which ONE of the following findings is MOST likely to suggest SAH?

A. Homogenously bloody CSF in all tubes

B. Normal opening pressure at lumbar puncture

C. Maximal headache at 6 hours after the onset

D. Absence of white cells in the CSF

9. A 34-year-old man presents with an ongoing moderately severe headache that had a sudden severe onset 8 days ago. Which ONE of the following statements is TRUE regarding investigations to exclude SAH?

A. Appearance of xanthochromia in CSF obtained through LP is not reliable because of the delayed presentation from the onset of headache

B. CSF oxyhaemoglobin produced in vitro due to a traumatic tap does not contribute to xanthochromia

C. Progressively reducing RBC count in successive tubes confirms the LP as a traumatic tap

D. Negative xanthochromia with >5 RBC count should require further evaluation to exclude SAH

10. Which ONE of the following clinical features is LEAST likely to be associated with an embolic stroke?

A. Previous transient neurological deficits involving more than one vascular distribution area

B. Current intravenous drug use

C. Fluctuating severity of neurological deficit

D. A recent ST segment elevation myocardial infarction (STEMI) treated with primary angioplasty

11. Regarding the use of the National Institute of Health Stroke Scale (NIHSS) to assess a patient presenting with a stroke to the ED, which ONE of the following statements is FALSE?

A. The neurological assessment of both anterior and posterior circulations are given similar weights in the NIHSS

B. A score over 22 is considered a severe stroke

C. The score correlates with infarct volume

D. NIHSS has a high interrater reliability

12. Regarding an ischaemic stroke involving the middle cerebral artery territory, which ONE of the following is TRUE?

A. If more than one-third of the territory is involved on an emergent head CT, the patient should be considered for thrombolysis, unless contraindications for thrombolysis exist

B. Less than 50% of strokes involve this territory

C. Spatial neglect and constructional apraxia are due to left hemispheric involvement in a right-handed person

D. Hyperdense sign of the middle cerebral artery on non-contrast head CT indicates the presence of a thrombus at that location

13. Regarding symptoms of a posterior circulation stroke, which ONE of the following is TRUE?

A. A patient may infrequently present with a headache

B. A major alteration of consciousness is due to involvement of the medulla

C. Symptoms are nearly always unilateral

D. Homonymous hemianopia is not a recognised symptom

14. Regarding the prediction of stroke in a patient with symptoms of a transient ischemic attack (TIA), which ONE of the following is TRUE?

A. The overall risk of stroke at 2 days after a TIA is approximately 4%

B. The ABCD^2 score predicts long-term risk of ischaemic stroke

C. The incidence of cerebral ischaemia is equal in both people with diabetes and those without

D. Diagnostic studies such as a head CT and MRI do not help to predict increased short-term risk

15. The following conditions are likely to result in poor outcome in ischaemic stroke, EXCEPT:

A. Hypertension at the time of presentation with a systolic pressure over 220 mmHg and diastolic pressure over 120 mmHg

B. Delayed oxygen administration in the ED

C. Inadequate hydration in the ED

D. Too aggressive control of blood pressure at the time of presentation

16. Regarding ischaemic stroke in a young adult, which ONE of the following statements is INCORRECT?

A. There is a strong association between ischaemic stroke risk and migraine episodes with aura

B. Pregnancy-related stroke is rare but risk rises in the late third trimester and until 6 weeks postpartum

C. CT angiography has a very high sensitivity in detecting both carotid and vertebral artery dissection

D. Unlike in older people, cardioembolism is the least important cause of ischaemic stroke in young adults

17. Regarding cervical artery dissection in a young patient, which ONE of the following statements is TRUE?

A. Transient unilateral posterior neck pain and occipital headache exclude vertebral artery dissection

B. Patients with atherosclerotic disease are more prone to this condition

C. Unilateral headache that may mimic migraine is a typical early symptom in internal carotid artery dissection

D. The neurological deficits must occur in the first 24 hours

18. Regarding intracerebral haemorrhage in an elderly patient, all of the following statements are true EXCEPT:

A. Cerebral amyloid angiopathy is the second most important risk factor in the elderly population

B. Mortality is determined by the presence or absence of blood in the ventricles

C. If it is secondary to chronic hypertension, it is usually localised to the putamen, thalamus, pons or cerebellum

D. If the patient is on warfarin, reversal is not required if the INR is below 3

19. Regarding spontaneous intracerebral haemorrhage, which ONE of the following statements is TRUE?

A. Cerebral angiography has a limited role to play in the investigations

B. For haemorrhage in the cerebral hemispheres, haematoma evacuation with open craniotomy reduces mortality

C. Urgent neurosurgical consultation for possible surgical evacuation is indicated for cerebellar haemorrhage

D. Routine use of intravenous mannitol to reduce mass effect is well supported by clinical trials

20. Which ONE of the following is the MOST LIKELY cause in a 72-year-old woman who presents with severe vertigo and positive examination findings for otitis media?

A. Ménière's disease

B. Bacterial labyrinthitis

C. Ramsay Hunt syndrome

D. Cerebellopontine angle tumour

21. Regarding vertigo in an elderly man, which ONE of the following statements is TRUE?

A. Vertibrobasilar insufficiency can be ruled out if the patient presents with a positional vertigo

B. Dix-Hallpike position test is positive in the majority of patients with benign paroxysmal positional vertigo (BPPV)

C. Peripheral vertigo is nearly always associated with tinnitus and hearing loss

D. Negative examination findings on the middle ear are a hallmark of vertigo due to labyrinthitis

22. Regarding generalised convulsive status epilepticus, which ONE of the following statements is TRUE?

A. Permanent neuronal injury is rare due to generalised status epilepticus

B. Prolonged episodes are more refractory to treatment

C. Incidence is equally distributed throughout adult life

D. Mortality remains approximately 5% when seizures last more than 1 hour

23. Regarding the use of phenytoin for a young adult presenting with generalised convulsive status epilepticus, which ONE of the statements is TRUE?

A. Faster intravenous rate of delivery is preferred to terminate the seizure activity early

B. Full intravenous loading dose should be considered when the patient is known to be on regular phenytoin

C. It may cause QT shortening

D. Most adults will have adequate seizure control with 1 g of phenytoin given intravenously

24. Regarding a patient with a known history of alcohol abuse presenting with generalised seizures, which ONE of the following is TRUE?

A. Generalised seizures do not occur in the first 24 hours due to minor alcohol withdrawal from abstinence

B. A patient with continuing seizures should be ventilated with adequate use of sedation and paralysis

C. A fluctuating level of consciousness with eye deviation and blinking during postictal period is more likely to be due to non-convulsive status epilepticus

D. Delirium tremens is common in the first 72 hours since abstinence

25. Regarding absence seizures, all of the following statements are true EXCEPT:

  A. Sudden loss of consciousness

  B. No loss of postural tone

  C. Intact consciousness and mentation

  D. Frequent recurrent attacks as many as 100 times daily

26. Which ONE of the following features of pseudoseizures is LEAST helpful in differentiating it from a true seizure?

  A. No high anion gap (AG) metabolic acidosis checked at 15 minutes from cessation of seizure activity

  B. Clonic seizure movements of the limbs that are alternating and non-symmetrical

  C. Abrupt onset or termination of seizure activity

  D. Lack of postictal confusion

27. Regarding a first seizure in a 36-year-old man with human immunodeficiency virus (HIV) infection, all of the following statements are correct EXCEPT:

  A. Cerebral lymphoma is a recognised cause

  B. MRI is the first-line investigation and may avoid the need for lumbar puncture

  C. Non-contrast head CT may miss a small lesion due to cerebral toxoplasmosis

  D. The majority of patients don't have an identifiable cause

28. Regarding the diagnosis of Guillain-Barré syndrome in a 10-year-old child, which ONE of the following statements is TRUE?

  A. Distal muscular weakness in the limbs is more prevalent than proximal muscular weakness

  B. Antibody testing for *Campylobacter jejuni* can confirm the diagnosis in a suspected case

  C. Dyspnoea is a feature when the respiratory muscles are affected

  D. CSF examination will typically show high protein content and more than 50×10^6 cells/l that are mainly mononuclear cells

29. A 10-year-old child with a **ventriculoperitoneal** shunt presents to the ED with increasing headache, nausea, vomiting and unsteady gait that has developed over the past 48 hours. Which ONE of the following statements is correct regarding his initial management?

  A. If the shunt chamber refills when compressed, shunt series X-rays are not indicated

  B. The combination of shunt series X-rays and a head CT has a high sensitivity for detecting shunt malfunction

  C. If there is no evidence of increased intracranial pressure on a head CT, lumbar puncture is indicated to rule out shunt infection

  D. Absence of fever and meningism does not reliably exclude shunt infection

30. Regarding the diagnosis of botulism in infancy, which ONE of the following statements is TRUE?

  A. An ascending paralysis may be seen in the infant

  B. It is not associated with an altered level of consciousness

  C. Fever is a significant clinical feature

  D. Sucking and feeding is not usually affected in the infant

Larry McGuire and Waruna de Alwis

1. Regarding lower limb examination findings of a patient with diabetes, which ONE of the following statements is TRUE?

A. Pretibial myxoedema is a purplish-pink plaque on the front of the shins associated with type 2 diabetes

B. Diabetic peripheral neuropathy causes loss of fine touch, pain and temperature sensation with preserved vibratory and position sense

C. Neuropathic arthropathy presents as an acutely painful swollen joint

D. Diabetic foot ulcers are most commonly seen under the metatarsal heads

2. Regarding ophthalmic complications in a patient with diabetes, which ONE of the following statements is INCORRECT?

A. There is a higher risk of vitreous haemorrhage than in the general population

B. Ocular haemorrhage is common in patients with diabetic retinopathy, following thrombolysis for acute myocardial infarction

C. Diabetic retinopathy may cause retinal detachment

D. Measurement of intraocular pressure is important because glaucoma is more common in diabetics

3. In considering a patient with diabetes with unstable blood glucose, which ONE of the following statements is TRUE?

A. Octreotide reverses hypoglycaemia secondary to insulin toxicity

B. Excess nocturnal insulin may result in reactive hyperglycaemia

C. Acarbose stabilises blood glucose levels by promoting intracellular intake

D. Strict glycaemic control (BSL < 7 mmol/L) has been shown to reverse early vascular disease

4. Regarding hypoglycaemia in a patient with diabetes, which ONE of the following is TRUE?

A. Symptoms of hypoglycaemia may be concealed by concomitant use of calcium channel blockers

B. Symptoms of hypoglycaemia begin to appear at blood glucose of <4 mmol/L

C. Oral glucose preparations will return blood glucose to normal more rapidly than intramuscular glucagon

D. Intramuscular glucagon is useful in therapy of patients with low liver glycogen stores

5. Regarding management of an episode of hypoglycaemia in a 65-year-old who is on sulfonylurea therapy, which ONE of the following is TRUE?

A. Initial oral or intravenous glucose therapy can be omitted because it is likely to fail

B. Octreotide should be considered for recurrent or persistent hypoglycaemia

C. Hypoglycaemia in a stable diabetic on a regular sulfonylurea dose is not usually due to a precipitating event

D. There is a more sustained response to intravenous glucose therapy in sulfonylurea-induced hypoglycaemia than in insulin-induced hypoglycaemia

6. With respect to diabetic ketoacidosis (DKA), which ONE of the following statements is TRUE?

A. Kussmaul breathing (deep rapid respiration) is the result of elevated serum osmolality due to hyperglycaemia

B. Standard urine ward tests detect acetoacetate but not beta-hydroxybutyrate

C. The presence of metabolic alkalosis with normal or elevated HCO_3 excludes the diagnosis

D. Hyperkalaemia is likely to develop because the acidosis is corrected with treatment

7. Regarding the management of DKA, which ONE of the following statements is TRUE?

A. A loading dose of insulin is recommended in both adults and children

B. The water deficit of an average adult is approximately 100 mL/kg or 5–10 L

C. Initial hypokalaemia <3.5 mmol/L indicates less severe disease

D. When venous pH is <7.2, sodium bicarbonate is recommended to correct metabolic acidosis

8. Regarding complications that may occur due to treatment of DKA, all of the following are true EXCEPT:

A. Severe hypokalaemia may cause cardiac arrest

B. Hyperchloraemic normal anion gap (AG) metabolic acidosis may develop

C. If the neurological state is altered during therapy, intravenous mannitol should be given only when a head CT confirms cerebral oedema

D. Hypophosphataemia is a feature

9. Regarding hyperglycaemic hyperosmolar state (HHS), which ONE of the following statements is TRUE?

A. HHS is associated with significantly higher mortality than DKA

B. Onset is often rapid following intercurrent illness

C. Blood glucose is generally elevated to the same level as in patients with DKA

D. Serum osmolality remains in the normal range

10. In the management of HHS, which ONE of the following statements is TRUE?

A. Since patients have a degree of insulin resistance, initial insulin therapy is indicated at a higher rate than for management of DKA

B. Potassium deficit is lower than in DKA, so replacement therapy is not usually required

C. Initial corrected hypernatraemia indicates a good prognosis

D. Heparin is indicated preventing thromboembolic events

11. In the assessment of a foot ulcer in a patient with diabetes presenting to the emergency department (ED), which ONE of the following features is MOST LIKELY to be associated with underlying osteomyelitis?

A. Ulcer <2 cm^2 in area

B. Presence of Charcot's arthropathy

C. Bacterial growth on a wound swab

D. An ulcer extending to the underlying bone on sterile surgical probing

12. Regarding ED management of a lower extremity ulcer in a patient with type 1 diabetes, which ONE of the following is TRUE?

A. Antibiotic treatment is indicated even without significant discharge or surrounding cellulitis

B. Deep ulceration with 5 cm of surrounding cellulitis without systemic toxicity may be appropriately managed on an outpatient basis

C. When peripheral pulses are not palpable, further vascular assessment is not required because this is a frequent finding in people with diabetes

D. Immediate surgical debridement is a priority for an ulcer with >2 cm of surrounding cellulitis, lymphangitis or purulent or malodorous discharge

13. In the diagnosis of alcoholic ketoacidosis, which ONE of the following statements is TRUE?

A. Marked confusion often accompanies severe acidosis

B. Elevated ketone bodies levels are confirmed by positive Ketostix testing

C. Presentation is commonly several days after ceasing alcohol consumption

D. Blood glucose is mildly elevated

14. In the management of alcoholic ketoacidosis, which ONE of the following is TRUE?

A. Intravenous insulin infusion is required to support resolution of metabolic changes

B. Intravenous glucose resolves metabolic disturbances more rapidly than saline alone

C. Rapid intravenous saline may induce metabolic alkalosis

D. Vitamin B6 administration prevents subsequent Wernicke's encephalopathy

15. Regarding examination findings in a patient with adrenal insufficiency, which ONE of the following statements is CORRECT?

A. Generalised hyperpigmentation of the skin and mucosal surfaces suggests secondary adrenal insufficiency due to pituitary failure

B. The presence of vitiligo suggests a primary adrenal insufficiency

C. Cushingoid features may be found in primary adrenal insufficiency

D. Marked hypotension is a usual finding in secondary adrenal insufficiency

16. Regarding the diagnosis of adrenal crisis, which ONE of the following statements is TRUE?

A. Adrenal crisis does not occur in patients with primary adrenocortical insufficiency

B. Hypotension nearly always responds to fluid resuscitation

C. Adrenal crisis may be precipitated by intercurrent sepsis during long-term steroid therapy in a compliant patient

D. Glucocorticoid deficiency results in profound hypoglycaemia

17. Regarding the management of adrenal crisis, which ONE of the following is TRUE?

A. Intravenous hydrocortisone is given because of its glucocorticoid and mineralocorticoid actions

B. Intravenous dexamethasone should be avoided in unconfirmed cases because it interferes with laboratory investigations

C. Slow fluid replacement with both normal saline and 5% dextrose is adequate

D. Fludrocortisone supplementation is required to retain replaced salt and fluid treatment

18. An adult patient presents to the ED with sepsis and hypotension, secondary to right lower lobe pneumonia. He is on immunosuppressant therapy, including long-term prednisolone, as treatment for a previous liver transplant. Which ONE of the following is MOST appropriate in the initial management of this patient?

A. Increase of daily oral prednisolone dose to 50 mg

B. 8 mg of dexamethasone as a single dose intravenously

C. 200 mg of hydrocortisone as a single dose intravenously

D. 100 mg of hydrocortisone every 6 hours and 50 mcg of fludrocortisone daily until the shock resolves

19. Regarding ocular examination findings in thyroid disease, which ONE of the following statements is TRUE?

A. Lid lag is best viewed with the patient gazing upwards

B. Lid lag and proptosis are symptomatic of Hashimoto thyroiditis

C. Lid retraction is determined by visibility of the sclera above the iris

D. Lid lag may require surgical correction

20. In considering Graves' disease, which ONE of the following statements is TRUE?

A. IgA antibodies stimulate thyroid-stimulating hormone (TSH) receptors on thyroid follicular cells

B. Hyperthyroidism may present with acute generalised weakness

C. The mainstay of management of thyroid ophthalmopathy is treatment of the hyperactive thyroid

D. Pretibial myxoedema appears as a long-term sequela of therapy for Graves' disease, caused by induced hypothyroidism

21. Regarding the treatment of thyrotoxic crisis, which ONE of the following statementsis TRUE?

A. Potassium iodide should be given first to inhibit thyroid hormone release

B. Intravenous propranolol is rapidly effective in blocking cardiovascular and peripheral effects

C. Propylthiouracil (PTU) blocks the release of stored thyroxine (T_4) from follicular cells

D. Salicylates are effective in managing hyperthermia

22. In a patient who presents to the ED with a high suspicion for having a thyroid storm, which ONE of the following conditions is LEAST likely to be considered in the differential diagnosis?

A. Intravenous amphetamine use

B. Alcohol withdrawal

C. Salicylate overdose

D. Neuroleptic malignant syndrome

23. Regarding elderly patients with clinical suspicion of myxoedema crisis (myxoedema coma), which ONE of the following statements is TRUE?

A. Normal body temperature suggests an underlying infection

B. Arterial PCO_2 is usually low

C. Hypothermia occurs in <20% of patients

D. Hypernatraemia is a common finding

24. Regarding ED management of a patient with myxoedema crisis (myxoedema coma), which ONE of the following is the LEAST appropriate management step?

A. 200 mg of hydrocortisone intravenously

B. Noradrenaline infusion

C. Commencement of intravenous T_4 (levothyroxine) before thyroid function test results are available from the laboratory

D. Active rewarming for hypothermia

25. In the management of an elderly patient with hypothyroidism, which ONE of the following statements is TRUE?

A. Initiating thyroxine replacement at standard doses may precipitate myocardial ischaemia

B. Oral thyroxin is most effective in a twice-daily dose to mirror circadian variation

C. Thyroxin should always be given as an intravenous dose before initiating oral replacement

D. T_3 (liothyronine) is the recommended choice for replacement

26. A patient presents to the ED with a known diagnosis of hypopituitarism. He appears ill but remains slightly tachycardic and normotensive. Which ONE of the following interventions should take the HIGHEST priority?

A. Treatment with intravenous hydrocortisone

B. Urgent thyroid hormone replacement

C. Correction of hyponatraemia

D. Correction of hyperkalaemia

27. Regarding primary hyperaldosteronism, which ONE of the following statements is TRUE?

A. Hyponatraemia is a feature

B. Increased renal excretion of potassium results in a metabolic alkalosis

C. Muscle weakness and polyuria are due to hypercalcaemia

D. Patients may present with profound hypotension

28. In a patient with severe hypercalcaemia due to primary hyperparathyroidism, which ONE of the following statements is TRUE?

A. Rapid rehydration using 4–6 L of normal saline is indicated as a first-line treatment

B. IV bisphosphonates reduce serum calcium by enhancing renal excretion

C. Parathyroid adenomas are typically palpable in the anterior triangle of the neck

D. Electrocardiogram (ECG) changes typically include a widened QRS complex and prolonged QT interval

29. All of the following features in patients presenting to the ED raise suspicion of an undiagnosed phaeochromocytoma EXCEPT:

A. Paroxysmal episodes of severe hypertension on a background of normal blood pressure or sustained hypertension

B. Recurrent unexplained urinary retention

C. Unexplained refractory shock

D. Unexplained orthostatic hypotension in a patient with sustained hypertension

30. A patient with type 2 diabetes who is on intensive insulin treatment presents to the ED with uncomplicated hyperglycaemia > 20 mmol/L. Regarding the initial stat (supplemental) doses of insulin she would receive in the ED, which ONE of the following statements is TRUE?

A. Subcutaneous rapid-acting insulin (e.g. insulin aspart, lispro or glulisine) should not be used

B. When determining the initial stat dose, the patient's current total daily insulin dose has no bearing

C. Insulin infusion should be started in a patient who is eating normally

D. Hyperglycaemia should be managed with supplemental rapid or short-acting insulin doses based on both blood glucose level and previous total daily insulin dose

1. Regarding the assessment and classification of dehydration in children with acute gastroenteritis, which ONE of the following is TRUE?

A. The degree of dehydration can accurately be determined on the basis of symptoms and signs

B. Modern classification systems describe the degree of dehydration as mild, moderate or severe

C. Prolonged capillary refill time, abnormal skin turgor and abnormal respiratory pattern are the three best clinical signs for identifying dehydration

D. Renal function and electrolytes are useful in determining the degree of dehydration

2. An 18-month-old boy is diagnosed with acute gastroenteritis. On examination he appears miserable but alert, has sunken eyes, dry mucous membranes and reduced skin turgor. His vital signs are normal with good peripheral pulses and capillary refill < 2 seconds. He refuses to drink oral rehydration solution (ORS) offered to him. Which ONE of the following is the MOST appropriate next step?

A. He should be offered fruit juice or lemonade to encourage oral intake

B. An intravenous line should be inserted and his deficit replaced over the next 8–12 hours

C. He should receive an intravenous fluid bolus with 10–20 mL/kg of 0.9% saline

D. A nasogastric tube should be inserted and the deficit replaced with a hypotonic rehydration solution over 4 hours

3. Regarding the management of children with acute gastroenteritis after successful rehydration, which ONE of the following statements is MOST appropriate?

A. A period of fasting is recommended

B. Clear fluid should be given until the diarrhoea settles followed by full-strength milk

C. Formula-fed infants should initially receive diluted milk, after which the concentration should gradually be increased to full-strength milk (graded feeding)

D. Children receiving cow's milk as part of their diet should be given full-strength cow's milk

4. A 4-year-old boy presents with two episodes of bloody diarrhoea in the preceding 24 hours. He is apyrexial and clinically well with no travel history. His mother has just recovered from gastroenteritis. Which ONE of the following is the MOST appropriate answer?

A. He should be treated with antibiotics if *Escherichia coli* O157:H7 is isolated on his stool sample to prevent development of haemolytic uremic syndrome (HUS)

B. He should be admitted and empiric antibiotics started

C. Stool should be collected for microscopy and culture and he can be discharged with follow-up within 24–48 hours

D. Stool should be collected for microscopy and culture and he can be discharged with empiric antibiotic therapy until follow-up in 24–48 hours

5. A 23-year-old female presents with 2 days' history of watery, non-bloody diarrhoea. She is otherwise well. She has recently returned from a visit to South-East Asia and will return there in 1 month on an important business trip. Which ONE of the following is TRUE?

A. *Campylobacter* is a common pathogen in this scenario

B. Short-course antibiotic treatment with a fluoroquinolone should be commenced early to prevent protracted illness

C. Combination therapy with antibiotics and loperamide is limited to patients with a fever and bloody diarrhoea

D. There is no role for antibiotic prophylaxis to prevent traveller's diarrhoea

6. A 66-year-old female presents with severe watery diarrhoea and a fever of 38.5°C. She is currently on a day 5 of a 10-day course of clindamycin for leg cellulitis. Which ONE of the following statements is TRUE regarding *Clostridium difficile* (*C. difficile*)-associated diarrhoea?

A. Clindamycin is infrequently implicated

B. This infection accounts for 50–60% of cases of antibiotic-associated diarrhoea

C. It is more commonly associated with oral than parenteral antibiotic administration

D. Intravenous vancomycin is not effective against *C. difficile*

7. A 19-year-old man presents with violent vomiting, abdominal cramps and mild diarrhoea 2 hours after the consumption of leftover fried rice and meat. Which ONE of the following is the MOST likely responsible organism?

A. Staphylococcus

B. Vibrio

C. Bacillus cereus

D. Clostridium perfringens

8. Regarding the clinical features of inflammatory bowel disease (IBD), which ONE of the following statements is FALSE?

A. Both Crohn's disease (CD) and ulcerative colitis (UC) are associated with an equivalent increased risk of colonic carcinoma

B. UC more commonly presents with bloody diarrhoea than CD

C. Systemic symptoms of malaise, anorexia or fever are more common in UC

D. The incidence of extraintestinal manifestations are higher in CD than UC

9. A 26-year-old male has known IBD. He presents with a fever of 38°C, increased stool frequency and abdominal pain. Regarding exacerbations and complications in patients with IBD, which ONE of the following statements is TRUE?

A. An erythrocyte sedimentation rate (ESR) >30 mm/hr indicates severe colitis

B. Toxic megacolon is unlikely if the transverse colon is <12 cm on abdominal X-ray

C. Both selective and non-selective nonsteroidal anti-inflammatory drugs (NSAIDs) have been shown to be safe and effective in patients with IBD

D. There is a limited role for stool cultures in patients with an exacerbation of IBD

10. A 42-year-old female presents late at night to the ED with right upper quadrant (RUQ) pain. You perform a focused ultrasound of the RUQ to look for biliary disease. Regarding ultrasonographic assessment of the biliary system, which ONE of the following is FALSE?

A. A sonographic Murphy's sign refers to pain on compression of the fundus of the gallbladder with the probe tip

B. When measuring gallbladder thickness, the posterior gallbladder wall should be measured

C. Gall bladder wall thickness >3 mm is abnormal

D. The common bile duct is typically <6 mm in diameter

11. Which ONE of the following statements is TRUE regarding the aetiology of peptic ulcer disease (PUD)?

A. NSAIDs are more commonly associated with gastric rather than duodenal ulceration

B. 90–95% of patients with gastric and duodenal ulcers are infected with *Helicobacter pylori* (*H. pylori*)

C. Prevalence of *H. pylori* is higher in patients with complicated duodenal ulcers (bleeding or perforation) than in those with uncomplicated disease

D. Up to 80% of people infected with *H. pylori* will develop PUD

12. A 35-year-old female presents to the ED with mild epigastric pain and dyspepsia. She has no other symptoms and denies weight loss. Her physical examination is unremarkable and she doesn't have anaemia. You make the presumptive diagnosis of uncomplicated PUD. Which ONE of the following statements is the MOST appropriate?

A. She should be empirically treated with *H. pylori* eradication therapy

B. She should be prescribed a proton pump inhibitor (PPI) and advised to take it with meals

C. She should be referred as an outpatient for an upper gastrointestinal endoscopy

D. A negative urea breath test excludes PUD

13. Regarding the aetiology of upper gastrointestinal tract (GIT) bleeding in adults, which ONE of the following is TRUE?

A. Mallory-Weiss tears are associated with repeated vomiting in only one-third of cases

B. Erosive gastritis, oesophagitis and duodenitis are responsible for the majority of bleeds

C. Bleeding originates proximal to the ileocecal junction

D. Initial bleeding due to aortoenteric fistula is usually massive

14. Which ONE of the following is TRUE regarding the clinical manifestations of upper GIT bleeding?

 A. The presence of melena is associated with poorer outcomes

 B. It is always accompanied by haematemesis, melena or haematochezia

 C. A negative nasogastric aspirate for blood as well as the absence of haematemesis excludes upper GIT bleed

 D. The presence of melena requires at least 150–200 mL of blood

15. Investigations are commonly performed in patients with upper gastrointestinal bleeding. Regarding this, which ONE of the following is TRUE?

 A. A chest X-ray (CXR) should routinely be requested in all patients

 B. A normal haemoglobin essentially excludes a large bleed

 C. A CXR is 70–80% sensitive for picking up a perforated peptic ulcer

 D. An elevated serum urea compared with creatinine is more suggestive of lower than upper GIT bleed

16. A 76-year-old male presents with a small amount of coffee-ground vomitus earlier in the day. He has no ongoing vomiting, his vital signs are normal and he has a negative guaiac test for faecal occult blood. Which ONE of the following is the MOST appropriate answer?

 A. He can safely be discharged after initiation of a PPI

 B. He should be observed for at least 6 hours and an outpatient endoscopy booked within the next 2 weeks

 C. He should be admitted and an endoscopy performed within 24 hours

 D. It is unlikely to be due to PUD in the absence of abdominal pain and preceding symptoms

17. Regarding the management of a 40-year-old male presenting with massive haematemesis, which ONE of the following is TRUE?

 A. Gastric lavage should be performed, preferably with ice-cold water to decrease bleeding and the risk of rebleeding

 B. PPIs reduce bleeding but not the risk of rebleeding from peptic ulcers

 C. Octreotide may decrease the risk of persistent bleeding and rebleeding in non-variceal bleeds

 D. A nasogastric tube should not be inserted if varices are suspected as it may provoke bleeding

18. Regarding a 45-year-old male with liver cirrhosis and known oesophageal varices presenting with haematemesis, which ONE of the following is TRUE?

 A. Injection sclerotherapy is superior to intravenous octreotide in terms of bleeding control and survival

 B. After insertion of a Sengstaken-Blakemore tube, one should inflate the gastric balloon first followed by the oesophageal balloon if control is not achieved

 C. There is no role for antibiotics

 D. There is limited role for PPIs

19. Regarding the clinical examination of patients with suspected liver disease, which ONE of the following is TRUE?

 A. A palpable liver edge is most likely due to hepatomegaly

 B. Bulging flanks are more sensitive and specific for the detection of ascites than the presence of a fluid thrill

 C. The presence of >2 spider naevi is abnormal

 D. Percussion is the only clinical method to measure liver span

20. Regarding the detection of ascites and interpretation of ascitic fluid results, which ONE of the following is TRUE?

 A. A serum-ascites albumin gradient (SAAG) ≥11 g/L suggests portal hypertension

 B. Up to 1000 WBC/mm³ is acceptable in uncomplicated cirrhosis

 C. Approximately 500 mL of fluid has to be present for flank dullness to be detected

 D. Ascitic fluid protein concentration of <30 g/L is more accurate in predicting the presence of portal hypertension than the SAAG

21. A 45-year-old male with known alcoholic liver cirrhosis presents with worsening ascites. Which ONE of the following is the next MOST appropriate management step?

 A. Commence oral frusemide at 80 mg daily

 B. Serial therapeutic paracentesis should be performed as needed

C. He should be advised to restrict his fluid intake to 1000 mL/day

D. He should be advised to restrict his salt intake

22. Regarding serial therapeutic paracentesis performed in patients with liver cirrhosis and recurrent ascites, which ONE of the following is TRUE?

A. An acceptable needle insertion site is approximately 2 cm below the umbilicus in the midline through the avascular linea alba

B. Not more than 2 L of fluid should be tapped at a single occasion unless a concurrent albumin infusion is given

C. A coagulation screen should be routinely performed prior to paracentesis

D. Current recommendations support an albumin infusion of 20 g/L of ascitic fluid removed regardless of the volume tapped

23. A 51-year-old male presents with decompensated chronic liver disease. He has tense ascites and slight confusion and you want to perform a diagnostic as well as therapeutic paracentesis to exclude peritonitis. Which ONE of the following statements is TRUE?

A. Continuous manual aspiration during the procedure is recommended to detect vascular or bowel injury early

B. An 18-guage metal needle can safely be used and left in the abdomen during the therapeutic tap

C. Spontaneous bacterial peritonitis (SBP) can be excluded in the absence of fever or abdominal pain

D. Evidence supports the use of fresh frozen plasma (FFP) if the international normalised ratio (INR) ≥ 1.5

24. A 42-year-old female with known liver cirrhosis and ascites presents with an unexplained fever. You perform an ascitic tap. Which ONE of the following is TRUE?

A. Ascitic fluid should be inoculated in blood culture bottles to increase sensitivity

B. She should receive empiric antibiotics only if the ascitic fluid polymorphoneuclear (PMN) count is ≥250 cells/mm^3

C. Ascitic fluid analysis is not useful to distinguish between SBP and secondary bacterial peritonitis

D. SBP is usually caused by polymicrobial and anaerobic infections

25. A 44-year-old female with known liver cirrhosis and portal hypertension presents with acute hepatic encephalopathy. She is apyrexial with no clinical evidence of infection. Regarding her management, which ONE of the following is TRUE?

A. Protein restriction is recommended

B. 10 mL of lactulose should be given 3–4 times daily

C. Empiric antibiotic therapy should be commenced

D. 6 g of neomycin per day should be commenced

26. A 27-year-old male presents with a 1-day history of jaundice, fever, nausea and RUQ pain 4 weeks after returning from India. Viral studies show anti-hepatitis A virus (anti-HAV) IgM positive. He has a wife and a 6-year-old child at home. They are not vaccinated. Which ONE of the following is TRUE?

A. He is currently not infectious because he had already developed jaundice

B. His family should receive normal human immunoglobulin (NHIG) only, to prevent secondary cases

C. His family should receive a hepatitis A vaccine only, to prevent secondary cases

D. There is no need for NHIG or vaccine in this scenario

27. Regarding liver function tests, which ONE of the following is TRUE?

A. An elevated conjugated bilirubin level is pathognomonic of extrahepatic cholestasis

B. An ALT:AST ratio > 2 is common in alcoholic hepatitis

C. In cholestatic disorders, AST increases before ALT

D. The absence of urobilinogen on urine dipstix excludes biliary obstruction

28. You are requested to insert a nasogastric tube (NGT) into a 48-year-old male with a small bowel obstruction. Which ONE of the following statements is TRUE?

A. Estimation of tube insertion length is estimated by measuring the distance from the tip of the xiphoid to the tip of the nose

B. A size 24 Fr sump tube is a good initial choice

C. To ameliorate the pain associated with NGT passage, the tube should be lubricated with anaesthetic jelly

D. Aspiration of stomach contents and measuring pH is more reliable than insufflation with air

29. Regarding a patient presenting to the ED with a fever who has a history of a liver transplant and who is on immunosuppressant therapy, which ONE of the following is TRUE?

A. Simultaneous treatment with antibiotics and large-dose corticosteroid is appropriate

B. Infection occurring in the first month after transplant is usually due to opportunistic infections

C. The presence or absence of fever is useful in distinguishing between infection and rejection

D. NSAIDs, but not paracetamol, can safely be prescribed for pain and fever

30. A 29-year-old female with a liver transplant requires transfusion of blood products in the ED. Which ONE of the following is TRUE?

A. Solid-organ transplant recipients are at minimally increased risk of developing transfusion-associated graft-versus-host disease

B. Packed red blood cells should routinely be irradiated

C. Transfusion-associated graft-versus-host disease manifests within 6 hours of transfusion

D. Fresh frozen plasma requires irradiation before administration

QUESTIONS   Yolande Weiner

1. Which ONE of the following statements is TRUE regarding clinical features that are MOST consistent with the associated underlying cause of acute renal failure (ARF)?

   A. Acute renal artery occlusion is usually asymptomatic

   B. Arthralgia and rash are uncommon with acute interstitial nephritis

   C. Papillary necrosis may present with fever, flank pain and haematuria

   D. An autoimmune aetiology rarely presents with fever

2. Regarding the causes of ARF, which ONE of the following statements is TRUE?

   A. Prerenal causes are responsible for 20% of community-acquired ARF

   B. Infection is the most common cause of acute interstitial nephritis

   C. Up to 90% of community-acquired cases have a potentially reversible cause

   D. Glomerular disease is the most common cause of intrinsic renal failure

3. Which ONE of the following statements is TRUE regarding mortality associated with ARF?

   A. Mortality has improved over the past few decades due to the introduction of dialysis

   B. The most common cause of death associated with ARF is sepsis

   C. Mortality rates are higher in older patients compared with those of young adults

   D. Mortality rates in children with ARF average 5%

4. Medications may precipitate renal failure. Which ONE of the following statements is TRUE?

   A. Development of hyperkalemia shortly after initiation of angiotensin-converting enzyme (ACE) inhibitor therapy is an indicator of imminent renal failure

   B. Volume depletion is a common precipitant of nonsteroidal anti-inflammatory drug (NSAID)-induced ARF but not ACE inhibitor therapy

   C. Angiotensin-receptor blockers, unlike ACE inhibitors, do not precipitate renal failure

   D. Renal effects of selective cyclooxygenase –2 inhibitors (most new generation NSAIDs) are similar to those of non-selective cyclooxygenase inhibitors

5. Regarding investigations performed in renal failure, which ONE of the following is TRUE?

   A. Serum markers of myocardial damage (CK and troponin) are reliable in the diagnosis of myocardial damage in dialysis patients

   B. Serum urea can be used as an accurate marker of the clinical syndrome of uraemia

   C. Fractional excretion of sodium (FeNa) >1% is suggestive of prerenal causes of ARF

   D. The presence of hyaline casts in the urine suggests acute tubular necrosis

6. Regarding contrast-induced nephropathy (CIN), which ONE of the following statements is FALSE?

   A. An eGFR <60 mL/min/1.73m² is associated with a significant risk for developing CIN

   B. Diabetes, age >75 years and the presence of congestive cardiac failure are all risk factors for the development of CIN

   C. Administration of periprocedural parenteral fluids has been shown to not reduce the risk of CIN in high-risk patients

   D. Patients at high risk of developing CIN should have a repeat creatinine at 24–48 hours after discharge from the emergency department (ED)

7. Regarding pericarditis in patients with end-stage renal disease (ESRD) requiring chronic dialysis, which ONE of the following statements is TRUE?

   A. Dialysis-related pericarditis is responsible for about 75% of cases

   B. The absence of a pericardial friction rub is a feature of uraemic pericarditis

   C. Typical electrocardiogram (ECG) changes of acute pericarditis are usually absent in uraemic pericarditis

   D. Anterior pericardectomy is the treatment of choice in haemodynamically stable patients with a large pericardial effusion

8. Which ONE of the following statements is TRUE regarding complications of vascular access associated with haemodialysis?

A. Grafts are associated with a higher complication rate compared with natural arteriovenous (AV) fistulas

B. Bleeding is the most common complication

C. Thrombosis of AV fistula with failure to provide adequate flow for dialysis is an emergency and requires immediate vascular intervention

D. Infection usually presents with the classic signs of pain, erythema and swelling of an infected vascular abcess

9. Regarding renal transplant patients presenting to the ED, which ONE of the following is FALSE?

A. The transplanted kidney is placed in the right or left lower quadrant of the abdomen and is easily palpable on abdominal examination

B. The serum creatinine level is a poor prognostic marker of graft function after transplantation

C. Immunosuppressant drugs are a common cause of ARF after kidney transplantation

D. Opportunistic infections are uncommon in the first post-transplant month

10. Regarding calcium administration in severe hyperkalemia in patients with renal failure, which ONE of the following statements is TRUE?

A. CaCl 10% is more potent than Ca-gluconate 10% and is the calcium preparation of choice

B. Improvement in the ECG is visible within 1–3 minutes

C. Ca-gluconate 10% is more likely than CaCl 10% to cause tissue necrosis if it extravasates

D. Ca^{2+} administration does not potentiate cardiac toxicity to digoxin if initial serum Ca^{2+} levels are normal

11. Regarding the treatment of hyperkalemia in patients with renal failure, which ONE of the following statements is TRUE?

A. $NaHCO_3$ is regarded as the first-line therapy

B. The effective dose of β-receptor agonists is the same as typically used for bronchodilation

C. Cation exchange resins promotes elimination of total body potassium by renal excretion

D. Intravenous insulin reliably lowers serum potassium in patients with ESRD

12. Regarding the aetiology of rhabdomyolysis, which ONE of the following is TRUE?

A. Crush injuries are the most common cause in adults

B. Rhabdomyolysis as a complication of statins occurs in about 10% of patients

C. Influenza virus is the most common infectious cause

D. Endurance-based exercise is more prone to cause rhabdomyolysis than strength training or heavy lifting

13. Regarding the diagnosis of rhabdomyolysis, which ONE of the following is TRUE?

A. Musculoskeletal symptoms are present in 80% of cases

B. Serum myoglobin is a sensitive marker for rhabdomyolysis

C. Serum CK levels more than 5 times normal, in the absence of myocardial or cerebral injury, generally indicates rhabdomyolysis

D. Serum CK levels >2000 U/L correlates well with the development of renal failure

14. Regarding haemolytic uremic syndrome (HUS) in children, which ONE of the following statements is TRUE?

A. The majority of cases are associated with *Shigella* infectious diarrhoea

B. HUS classically occurs in children over 4 years of age

C. HUS is an uncommon cause of ARF in children

D. Antibiotic use in diarrhoeal illness may increase the risk of HUS

15. Which ONE of the following features is MOST consistent with HUS in children?

A. HUS is associated with fever in the majority of cases

B. Stools are usually watery; bloody stools are reported in the minority of cases

C. Central nervous system irritability and seizures occur in about one-third of patients

D. Anaemia is typically mild and haemoglobin never drops <90 g/L

16. Regarding the diagnosis of acute post-streptococcal glomerulonephritis (APSGN), which ONE of the following statements is TRUE?

A. Presence of peripheral oedema indicates development of nephrotic syndrome

B. A positive throat culture confirms the diagnosis

C. The antistreptolysin O (ASO) titer is commonly elevated after *Streptococcal* pharyngeal and skin infections

D. The serum C3 level is significantly reduced in the majority of patients, with C4 most often normal

17. Which ONE of the following features is NOT consistent with nephrotic syndrome?

A. ARF is rare in primary nephrotic syndrome

B. The characteristics of nephrotic syndrome include oedema, hypoalbuminaemia, proteinuria and hyperlipidaemia

C. Microscopic haematuria is typically absent and distinguishes the disease from glomerulonephritis

D. Nephrotic children are at high risk of thromboembolic complications

18. Which ONE of the following statements is TRUE regarding haematuria?

A. Haematuria associated with pain during urination is often due to a neoplastic cause

B. Gross macroscopic haematuria is more often associated with a renal than postrenal cause

C. The incidence of underlying disease in patients who develop haematuria while on anticoagulants is approximately 10%

D. Most patients aged over 40 years with a first episode of asymptomatic microscopic haematuria should be further investigated

19. Which ONE of the following is INCORRECT regarding prostatitis?

A. Gram-negative bacilli such as *Escherichia coli* are commonly implicated in acute bacterial prostatitis

B. Prostatic massage with sampling of prostatic fluid should be performed to confirm the diagnosis of acute bacterial prostatitis

C. Acute prostatitis can be due to sexually transmitted infections

D. Chronic bacterial prostatitis occurs in adults who usually have a history of recurrent urinary tract infections (UTIs)

20. Regarding the aetiology of urinary tract infections (UTIs), which ONE of the following is TRUE?

A. Reinfection within 1–6 months after treatment is usually by the same organism

B. *E. coli* is the causative organism in at least 70% of complicated UTIs

C. *Klebsiella* is common in dysuria-pyuria syndrome (culture negative pyuria) in which sterile or low-colony count culture results are obtained

D. *Pseudomonas* species have a low virulence for the urinary tract and its presence suggests that normal host defenses have been altered

21. Regarding urinalysis in patients with dysuria-frequency syndrome, which ONE of the following statements is TRUE?

A. Cloudy or malodorous urine is a good predictor of infection

B. Nitrate reaction by dipstix is unlikely to be positive in *Pseudomonas* infection

C. The absence of pyuria and bacteriuria excludes pyelonephritis

D. A midstream urine specimen should be obtained routinely at triage, especially in young males

22. Which ONE of the following statements is TRUE regarding asymptomatic bacteriuria?

A. Asymptomatic bacteriuria is the presence of $>10^3$ CFU/mL of a single bacterial species on two successive urine cultures in patients without symptoms

B. Screening is recommended in pregnancy, nursing home residents and patients with indwelling urinary catheters due to the high incidence

C. Treatment is recommended in patients with indwelling urinary catheters

D. Treatment in pregnancy reduces the incidence of pyelonephritis

23. Regarding a UTI diagnosis, which ONE of the following statements is TRUE?

A. Flank pain, costovertebral angle tenderness and renal tenderness to deep palpation are pathognomonic of pyelonephritis

B. Gross haematuria (haemorrhagic cystitis) is present in 30–40% of female cases

C. External dysuria is most likely due to UTI

D. Clinical findings can reliably differentiate between upper and lower tract infections

24. Regarding the epidemiology of UTI in children, which ONE of the following is TRUE?

A. Most cases of UTI in girls occur before the age of 2 years

B. Children with UTI are more likely to have a family history of UTI in first-degree relatives than children without UTI

C. Vesicoureteric reflux (VUR) is present in at least 5% of children having their first UTI

D. Having a first UTI at a young age is not associated with recurrence

25. Regarding the diagnostic evaluation of a first UTI in children, which ONE of the following statements is TRUE?

A. A renal ultrasound is recommended within 6 weeks in young children after an initial febrile UTI

B. Micturating cystourethrogram (MCUG) is indicated in most children under the age of 4 years

C. A technetium 99m-dimercaptosuccinicacid (DMSA) scan should ideally be performed in the first month after diagnosis to detect renal scarring

D. Suprapubic aspiration (SPA) should not be performed in children >6 months of age

Yolande Weiner

1. A 31-year-old male requires an emergency blood transfusion. Which ONE of the following statements is TRUE?

A. O negative blood must be given if cross-matching can't be performed

B. O positive blood can safely be given in this scenario

C. Uncross-matched O positive blood should not be given in this case due to the higher risk of acute haemolytic reaction compared with O negative blood

D. Type-specific blood takes approximately 20 minutes

2. Regarding a multi-trauma patient with critical bleeding requiring a massive blood transfusion, which ONE of the following statements is TRUE?

A. Administration of recombinant activated factor VII (rFVIIa) for critical bleeding in trauma patients significantly improves morbidity, mortality and lowers transfusion rates

B. Administration of packed red blood cells (PRBC) and fresh frozen plasma (FFP) in a ratio of 1:4 is recommended during massive transfusion

C. Platelets should only be transfused if count falls <50 × 10⁹/L

D. Administration of tranexamic acid (TXA) early after injury reduces the risk of death from bleeding

3. A 35-year-old female receives a blood transfusion in the emergency department (ED) for symptomatic chronic anaemia. A full cross-match was performed prior to administration. One hour into the transfusion the nurse informs you that the patient has developed a fever of 38.3°C. She is otherwise well with normal vital signs. Which ONE of the following is TRUE?

A. The transfusion should be stopped immediately and blood samples sent to the lab for investigation of transfusion reaction

B. Transfusion should be continued at a slower rate if the patient is otherwise well with normal vital signs

C. The temperature is unlikely due to a transfusion reaction because the blood was fully cross-matched

D. The transfusion should be stopped and if the fever settles and the patient remains well, it can be restarted

4. Regarding anticoagulation therapy with warfarin, which ONE of the following statements is TRUE?

A. Age is not a risk factor for over-coagulation

B. The two available brands of warfarin, Coumadin and Marevan, are bioequivalent and interchangeable

C. About 50% of bleeding episodes occur while the international normalised ratio (INR) is <4.0

D. Unfractionated or low molecular weight heparin should always be given concurrently until the INR is therapeutic

5. A 60-year-old male is referred by his general practitioner (GP) with an INR of >10. He has no active bleeding. He is on warfarin for atrial fibrillation. Which ONE of the following is the MOST appropriate action?

A. He should receive FFP, prothrombinex and 5–10 mg vitamin K intravenously

B. He should be given 5 mg of the intravenous preparation of vitamin K orally

C. He should be admitted and observed with daily INR testing

D. Vitamin K 5–10 mg should be given intravenously

6. Which ONE of the following is TRUE regarding complications associated with the use of heparin?

A. Bleeding is a major complication of heparin-induced thrombocytopaenia (HIT)

B. Protamine is not indicated in bleeding associated with low molecular weight heparin (LMWH)

C. A drop of 50% or more from baseline is considered evidence of HIT, even if the platelet count is within normal range

D. Unfractionated heparin (UFH) should be substituted with LMWH if HIT occurs and ongoing anticoagulation is required

7. Regarding thrombolytic therapy for acute ischaemic stroke, which ONE of the following is TRUE?

A. Tenecteplase, a third generation fibrinolytic, is approved for treatment of acute ischaemic stroke

B. Intravenous alteplase (rtPA) is given as a weight-based dose via an infusion over 60 minutes

C. Aspirin should be given immediately once an intracranial bleed is excluded on CT

D. After thrombolysis, patients should receive heparin anticoagulation at a reduced dose

8. Regarding laboratory tests in the evaluation of anaemia, which ONE of the following is FALSE?

A. Direct Coombs' test is used to detect antibodies in the serum and is positive in autoimmune haemolytic anaemia

B. An increased red cell distribution width (RDW) can indicate an early deficiency anaemia (iron, vitamin B12 or folate)

C. The hallmark of thalassaemia is microcytic, hypochromic haemolytic anaemia

D. RDW is useful in differentiating iron deficiency from thalassaemia

9. Which ONE of the following statements is TRUE regarding sickle cell disease (SCD)?

A. Nonsteroidal anti-inflammatory drugs (NSAIDs) should be avoided in the management of vaso-occlusive crisis

B. Aplastic crisis is recognised by a sudden drop in all cell lines

C. Transfusion should be avoided in acute splenic sequestration due to underlying haemolysis

D. Baseline haemoglobin (Hb) level is often 60–90 g/L

10. Regarding idiopathic thrombocytopaenic purpura (ITP), which ONE of the following is TRUE?

A. It is caused by an autoimmune destruction of platelets

B. The presence of a large spleen supports the diagnoses of ITP

C. Usually associated with palpable petechiae or purpura

D. The laboratory hallmark of ITP is isolated thrombocytopaenia with platelet fragments on the peripheral smear

11. A 5-year-old previously healthy boy presents to the ED with diffuse petechiae. His mother states he had a viral respiratory illness 2 weeks ago but is now well. He has a normal physical examination. His blood film shows an isolated thrombocytopaenia with a platelet count of 8 x 10⁹/L. Which ONE of the following is TRUE?

A. The risk of intracranial haemorrhage is high if the platelet count is <10 x 10⁹/L

B. He should receive a platelet transfusion because his risk of serious bleeding is high

C. He should receive a platelet transfusion only if mucosal bleeding is present

D. His condition is likely to resolve spontaneously within the next 2 months

12. Regarding bleeding disorders, which ONE of the following statements is TRUE?

A. Haemarthrosis and epistaxis are typical of von Willebrand's disease

B. In patients with haemophilia, the prothrombin time will usually be abnormal

C. Recurrent bleeding into muscles are associated with both haemophilia A and B

D. Spontaneous bleeding from the oropharyngeal tract is common in patients with haemophilia A

13. A 45-year-old female presents with fever. She is known to have breast carcinoma and has recently received chemotherapy. Which ONE of the following is MOST correct?

A. Fever in cancer patients are defined as a temperature ≥37.5°C

B. Rectal measurement of temperature most accurately reflects core body temperature and is the recommended route

C. Most fevers occurring in cancer patients are due to antineoplastics and/or tumour necrosis

D. The lowest neutrophil count is typically seen 5–10 days after the last dose of chemotherapy

14. Regarding febrile neutropenia in cancer patients, which ONE of the following is TRUE?

A. Gram-negative enteric bacteria currently account for 60–70% of microbiologically confirmed infections

B. *Staphylococcus epidermidis* cultured in the blood is usually not a contaminant

C. Indwelling vascular catheters should immediately be removed if no other source of infection is found on initial examination

D. *Pseudomonas* is the most common pathogen

15. Regarding tumour lysis syndrome, which ONE of the following is TRUE?

A. It is characterised by increased serum uric acid, potassium and calcium

B. It is more commonly associated with haematologic tumours than solid tumours

C. It is a complication only associated with chemotherapy

D. The mainstay of therapy is frusemide and mannitol

16. Regarding the clinical manifestation of malignant spinal cord compression (MSCC), which ONE of the following is TRUE?

A. Back pain occurs in 90% of cases

B. Paralysis is the presenting complaint in a majority of cases

C. Bladder or bowel dysfunction are early findings

D. Sensory deficits usually occur before motor deficit

17. Regarding hypercalcaemia associated with malignancy, which ONE of the following is TRUE?

A. The most common cause of hypercalcaemia in malignancy is bone metastases

B. Symptoms usually correlate with acuity of the rise as opposed to actual calcium level

C. Biphosphonates should be simultaneously administered with fluid hydration for maximal effect

D. Pamidronate, when indicated, should ideally be given as a bolus injection

18. Regarding the assessment of haematological malignancies in children, which ONE of the following is TRUE?

A. Bone pain caused by marrow displacement in acute leukaemia is typically tender to palpation

B. Gingival hyperplasia occurs more commonly in acute lymphoblastic leukemia (ALL) than acute myeloid leukaemia (AML)

C. The absence of a raised white cell count (WCC) excludes leukaemia

D. Disseminated intravascular coagulopathy may occur in newly diagnosed AML

19. Regarding hyperleucocytosis in children with acute leukaemia, which ONE of the following is TRUE?

A. Hyperleukocytosis is diagnosed with a WCC > 50×10^9/L

B. Leukostasis commonly presents with dyspnoea or respiratory distress

C. Platelet transfusions should be avoided because they may increase the blood viscosity

D. It is more common in older children

20. Regarding solid tumours in children, which ONE of the following is TRUE?

A. Wilms' tumour usually presents with abdominal pain

B. Brain tumours are rare in children

C. Neuroblastoma often presents as an abdominal mass

D. Headache in children is rare and requires further imaging to exclude a brain tumour

1. A 15-year-old girl was brought to the emergency department (ED) by friends; she was at a party and began to feel unwell with a headache and fever. By the time she arrived she had deteriorated significantly and was obtunded, requiring intubation and aggressive fluid resuscitation. She has been transferred to the intensive care unit (ICU) with a working diagnosis of meningococcaemia. You contact public health authorities to initiate contact tracing. Who of the following should receive clearance antibiotics?

A. The staff member who intubated the patient if a mask was not worn

B. The patient's classmates

C. All staff who came within 1 m of the patient

D. The friends who brought the patient to the ED when she was symptomatic

2. An 18-year-old male has presented to the ED with a rapid-onset febrile illness associated with myalgia. You consider meningococcaemia as a potential diagnosis. Which ONE of the following is INCORRECT regarding meningococcaemia?

A. The rash of meningococcaemia may be urticarial, macular or maculopapular

B. Carriers have some immunity against invasive disease

C. Serogroup C causes the most disease in Australia

D. The mortality of a patient with meningococcal meningitis is higher than that of patients with invasive meningococcal disease

3. A 42-year-old female presents to the ED with a cough and a fever of 38.9°C; she is found to have mild community-acquired pneumonia. Which ONE of the following is correct regarding blood cultures in this patient?

A. Aerobic and anaerobic cultures are indicated

B. If multiple bacteria are isolated on culture, these are likely to be pathogenic

C. The most likely organism to be cultured is *Chlamydia pneumoniae*

D. The primary determinant in detecting bacteraemia is the volume of blood collected

4. A 57-year-old woman presents to the ED in Cairns with symptoms of pneumonia. She has no medical history, medications or allergies. She is a non-smoker and drinks 35 standard drinks per week. Her observations are: respiratory rate 32, heart rate 122, blood pressure (BP) 100/56 mmHg, SaO2 90% on 15l O$_2$/min, temperature 38.2°C, Glasgow Coma Scale (GCS) 14. Chest X-ray (CXR) confirms a right middle lobe (RML) and right lower lobe (RLL) pneumonia. What is the most appropriate initial regime of antibiotics for this patient?

A. Benzylpenicillin 1.2 g IV 4-hourly plus azithromycin 500 mg IV daily plus gentamicin 4–6 mg/kg IV daily

B. Ceftriaxone 1 g IV daily plus azithromycin 500 mg IV daily

C. Moxifloxacin 400 mg IV daily plus azithromycin 500mg IV daily

D. Meropenem 1 g IV 8-hourly plus azithromycin 500 mg IV daily

5. A 26-year-old female who is 39 weeks pregnant presents to a rural ED with an itchy vesicular rash of 24 hours' duration. She has no past history and this is her first pregnancy, which has, so far, been uncomplicated. You diagnose chickenpox and find that this patient has not been immunised or exposed to varicella in the past. What should you do prior to discharging her?

A. Give her a dose of varicella zoster immunoglobulin

B. Counsel her regarding the risk of congenital varicella syndrome

C. Commence a course of oral acyclovir

D. Arrange in utero transfer to a larger centre for caesarean section to reduce transmission at delivery

6. A 28-year-old man is brought to the ED with a 10-day history of fevers, myalgia, headache and malaise. Today he is feeling much worse, is confused and lethargic. He has recently returned from a holiday in South-East Asia; prior to the trip he had all necessary vaccinations and took Malarone (atavaquone-proguanil) as chemoprophylaxis against malaria. Which ONE of the following is correct regarding malaria?

A. The full blood count (FBC) in patients with malaria typically shows a microcytic anaemia with an elevated white cell count and thrombocytopenia

B. The cerebrospinal fluid (CSF) usually shows markedly raised white cells and a reduced protein and glucose level

C. A negative blood smear (thick and thin film) indicates that the diagnosis is unlikely to be malaria

D. Artesunate or quinine would be a suitable treatment for this patient if he had *Plasmodium falciparum* malaria

7. A 32-year-old female presents to the ED with a history of fever and malaise. She has recently returned from travelling in Africa for 3 months. She took doxycycline as malaria prophylaxis throughout her trip and had all mandatory vaccinations prior to the trip. Further questioning reveals she has additional symptoms including constipation, abdominal pain and a pale red macular rash. Which ONE of the following infections is most likely to be causing her symptoms?

A. Yellow fever

B. Dengue

C. Typhoid

D. Malaria

8. A 42-year-old man who has human immunodeficiency virus (HIV) is brought to the ED with a 2-day history of increasing headaches and fever; prior to this he had no symptoms. He takes HAART regularly; his last CD4+ count was 150 cells/μl. A contrast-enhanced CT shows multiple ring-enhancing lesions. What is the most likely pathology causing these findings?

A. Cryptococcal meningitis

B. Lymphoma

C. AIDS dementia complex

D. Toxoplasmosis

9. A staff member presents to the ED shortly after a needlestick exposure. The exposure involved a solid needle, which had just been used to suture the source patient; it entered the staff member's gloved thumb. The source patient is a 35-year-old injecting drug user who has refused to give consent for serological testing. The staff member has been vaccinated for hepatitis B and is a responder. Which ONE of the following is CORRECT?

A. The overall risk of HIV transmission in this scenario is relatively low because the risk of HIV among injecting drug users in Australasia is 1–2%

B. The staff member should be treated with hepatitis B immune globulin (HBIG)

C. The risk of hepatitis C virus (HCV) transmission would be substantially reduced by giving the staff member a combination of immunoglobulin and α-interferon

D. HIV post-exposure prophylaxis (PEP) with a single agent should be prescribed in this scenario

10. A patient presents to the ED requesting rabies PEP after he woke up to find a bat in the bedroom. The incident occurred 2 days ago; at the time there was a small scratch on the arm which is barely visible today. He has never been immunised for rabies and is fit and well with no allergies. Which ONE of the following is CORRECT?

A. The patient does not require PEP because the only injury appears to be a small scratch

B. The patient has presented too late to begin PEP

C. The patient requires rabies immunoglobulin and rabies vaccine

D. Rabies is not a concern in Australasia

11. You are informed by the infectious diseases director at your hospital that a patient admitted 2 days ago via the ED has a confirmed case of measles. Which ONE of the following is INCORRECT?

A. Susceptible contacts of the patient, including staff, who are at high risk of complications, should receive passive immunisation with immunoglobulin

B. Treatment of the patient is largely supportive

C. Droplet precautions plus nursing the patient in a negative pressure room are required when suspected measles patients present to the ED

D. The rash of measles typically begins on the limbs and spreads to involve the trunk and face

12. A 30-year-old man presents to the ED with fever, malaise and painful hands. He has no history of trauma or prior joint disease, takes no medications and has no allergies. On examination he is systemically well and his observations are normal (temp 37.5°C). He has tenosynovitis and arthritis of the right wrist and hand with no other arthritis, and he also has several small pustules over the hands and wrists. What is the MOST likely diagnosis in this patient?

A. Lyme disease

B. Disseminated gonococcal infection (DGI)

C. Reactive arthritis

D. Acute HIV infection

13. A patient presents with a painful thigh; there is no history of trauma, heavy exercise or prior skin lesion. On examination he is tachycardic and has a low-grade fever, but there are no clinical signs in the affected leg. He is admitted for observation and is subsequently diagnosed with necrotising fasciitis. Which ONE of the following regarding necrotizing fasciitis is INCORRECT?

A. Infections due to group A streptococcus should be managed with high-dose benzylpenicillin and clindamycin

B. Gas formation may be seen in infections caused by organisms other than *Clostridia*

C. Pain is typically severe in early infection

D. Clostridial infections are the most common cause

14. Parents bring a 6-month-old infant to the ED with a history of poor feeding and a fever. On examination there are ulcerated lesions throughout the mouth and on the lips; the remainder of the examination is unremarkable. Which ONE of the following is CORRECT?

A. This is likely to be herpangina

B. Topical acyclovir is ineffective

C. The likely causative organism is HSV-2, transmitted from the mother's genital tract during delivery

D. The patient is not at risk of encephalitis because only the skin and mucosa are involved

15. You are working in an ED which is in an area affected by severe floods. A 32-year-old man who has been helping his neighbours clear debris from flood-affected properties presents unwell with fever, rash, aching joints and lethargy. Which ONE of the following is LEAST likely to be the causative illness in this patient?

A. Barmah Forest virus

B. Melioidosis

C. Cholera

D. Dengue fever

16. A patient presents with cellulitis of the lower limb. Which ONE of the following is TRUE regarding cellulitis?

A. Aeromonas species are implicated in infections associated with fresh water

B. Mild to moderate chronic diabetic foot infections should be treated with amoxicillin-clavulanate 875/125 mg po bd or ciprofloxacin 500 mg bd in penicillin-allergic patients

C. Laboratory tests can accurately differentiate between cellulitis and deep venous thrombosis (DVT) of the lower limb

D. Previous venous harvest is not a risk factor for cellulitis

17. A 40-year-old childcare worker presents to the ED with 2 weeks of malaise and intermittent fevers. She has recently had a positive Mantoux test as part of a screening test for tuberculosis (TB) performed because her mother, who lives with her, has been diagnosed with TB and commenced on treatment. Which ONE of the following is correct?

A. A positive Mantoux test indicates active disease only

B. This patient should be off work to prevent transmission to staff and children at work

C. Primary tuberculosis infection may be asymptomatic or may resemble a viral pneumonitis

D. Absence of an apical or cavitating lesion on chest X-ray may be used to rule out TB in patients with positive skin tests

18. You are involved in ensuring the hospital's infection control policy is implemented in the ED and are planning an education session for medical and nursing staff in the ED. Which ONE of the following is correct regarding infection control principles?

A. Airborne, droplet and contact precautions should be used in place of standard precautions

B. Handwashing with soap and water is effective in preventing spread of infection of multidrug-resistant organisms

C. Patients suspected of having pertussis require isolation in a negative pressure room while in the ED

D. Policies regarding protection of staff from infectious agents should advocate the use of equipment that lowers the risk of percutaneous exposure to infection

19. An ED resident comes to ask your advice on what antimicrobial treatment to start in the ED for a patient with a febrile illness of unknown source. The patient, a 62-year-old woman on sulfasalazine for rheumatoid arthritis, has a systemic inflammatory response. Which ONE of the following is CORRECT?

A. If this patient had chronic kidney disease, the first dose of gentamicin should be reduced

B. If prescribing a fluoroquinolone antibiotic for this patient, there is no need to review her regular medications, which include a calcium-containing antacid

C. If the patient had had a recent significant pseudomonal infection, ceftazidime would be a better choice of empiric antibiotic than ceftriaxone

D. If the source of infection was thought to be a deep tissue infection from a 2-week-old wound sustained in shallow marine water, benzylpenicillin would be sufficient cover

20. A 17-year-old male presents to the ED with a 6-hour history of vomiting and profuse diarrhoea and blurred vision. He has no past medical history, medications or allergies and lives with two other college students, neither of whom have symptoms. On examination he is mildly dehydrated; he is unable to tolerate oral fluids due to difficulty in swallowing, and his power is 3/5 in the upper limbs and 4/5 in the lower limbs. What is the most likely causative organism?

A. *Botulinum toxin*

B. *Salmonella*

C. *Shigella*

D. Enterohaemorrhagic *E. coli*

21. A 14-year-old boy is brought by his mother with a fever, sore throat and malaise. On examination he has an exudative pharyngitis with cervical lymphadenopathy. You order laboratory testing including a monospot test, which is positive. Which ONE of the following is correct regarding Epstein-Barr virus (EBV)?

A. Screening tests used in the ED test for EBV-specific antibodies

B. Splenomegaly develops in a small proportion of patients but in these patients there is a high chance of complications

C. Patients may develop haematological complications including haemolytic anaemia and thrombocytopenia

D. Patients should remain off school or work until their symptoms have completely resolved

22. A 12-year-old boy is referred to the ED by his GP with symptoms of a lower respiratory tract infection. Which ONE of the following would be LEAST likely to support a diagnosis of Mycoplasma pneumonia?

A. A non-productive cough that has been present for 3 weeks

B. A CXR that shows patchy lung infiltrates

C. Elevated cold agglutinins

D. The presence of pet birds in the home

23. Which ONE of the following is CORRECT regarding patients with HIV presenting with gastrointestinal symptoms?

A. Oesophageal *Candidiasis* is seen early in the disease

B. Oral hairy leukoplakia is caused by EBV

C. *Cryptosporidium* typically causes bloody diarrhoea

D. Proctitis is not associated with *Neisseria gonorrhoeae*

24. A 24-year-old woman presents with a 5-day history of mild lower abdominal pain. As part of her ED examination she is found to have cervicitis but no discharge or signs of pelvic inflammatory disease. Which ONE of the following is INCORRECT regarding this patient?

A. She should be treated with azithromycin and ceftriaxone

B. Ectopic pregnancy is a recognised complication of this condition

C. The likely cause is *Candida albicans*

D. Diagnosis involves PCR of an endocervical swab

25. A 3-year-old unimmunised girl is brought to the ED by her parents with a 1-day history of a mild fever, with refusal to eat or drink today. On examination she appears unwell, is sitting up and has a very swollen neck. Her pharynx is red with a thick grey-white coating over the posterior pharyngeal wall and tonsils. Which ONE of the following is CORRECT regarding this patient?

A. Specific treatment requires antitoxin and antibiotics

B. Cutaneous lesions are a common precursor to pharyngeal involvement

C. Limb weakness would be expected at the time of presentation

D. The most likely diagnosis is measles

1. Target or target-like lesions are seen in all of the following conditions EXCEPT:

A. Erythema multiforme

B. Toxic epidermal necrolysis (TEN)

C. Stevens-Johnson syndrome (SJS)

D. Pyoderma gangrenosum

2. Which ONE of the following statements is TRUE regarding SJS and toxic epidermal necrolysis?

A. In these conditions more than one mucous membrane surface is affected

B. The epidermal detachment involves more than 50% of the body surface area

C. Bacterial infections are the usual cause of both conditions

D. Eyes are spared in both conditions

3. Regarding Staphylococcal scalded skin syndrome (SSSS), which ONE of the following statements is INCORRECT?

A. This condition should be considered in the differential diagnosis of SJS and TEN

B. There is no mucosal involvement

C. In adults it is more likely to affect the elderly with renal failure

D. There is extensive primary skin infection

4. Which ONE of the following conditions is LEAST likely to cause erythroderma in a patient presenting to the emergency department (ED)?

A. Systemic lupus erythematosus (SLE)

B. Human immunodeficiency virus (HIV) infection

C. Drug eruption

D. Dermatitis

5. Causes of pustules in the skin of a noonate include all of the following EXCEPT:

A. Group B streptococcal infection

B. Neutropenia

C. Milia

D. Toxic erythema of the newborn

6. Regarding disseminated gonococcal infection, which ONE of the following statements is TRUE?

A. The typical rash consists of generalised petechiae

B. It should be suspected in a sexually active person with typical skin rash, tenosynovitis and arthralgia

C. The diagnosis can be confirmed with culture of organisms from mucosal surfaces such as cervical, vaginal or urethral surfaces

D. It is often associated with systemic toxicity

7. Regarding drug eruptions seen in the ED, which ONE of the following statements is INCORRECT?

A. Exanthematous drug reactions are more likely in patients infected with Epstein-Barr virus (EBV), HIV and patients with leukaemia

B. Urticaria in a patient, if drug induced, should arise within 1 week from the time of first exposure to the medication

C. Fixed drug eruptions have solitary or multiple oval plaques with central blisters

D. Type II and type IV hypersensitivity reactions may cause TEN

8. Regarding blistering skin disorders that may be encountered in the ED, which ONE of the following statements is TRUE?

A. The morphological appearance of a blister depends on the site of intercellular split in the epidermis

B. Blistering diseases are not due to immunological reactions

C. Bullous pemphigoid mainly affects children

D. The diagnosis is complex in blistering disorders in children as a wide differential diagnoses have to be considered

9. Regarding hand, foot and mouth disease in children, which ONE of the following statements is INCORRECT?

A. It is caused by both coxackievirus A16 and enterovirus 71

B. When a rash appears the condition is non-infectious

C. Erythema multiforme and pustular psoriasis are important differential diagnoses to consider

D. Infection is usually spread by faeco-oral contamination

10. Regarding herpes simplex infections in children, which ONE of the following statements is INCORRECT?

　A. Herpes simplex virus (HSV) type 1 is commonly involved in skin infections of the face

　B. Herpetic whitlow is often misdiagnosed as bacterial infection

C. Eczema herpeticum is the disseminated herpes simplex infection associated with atopic eczema

D. Typical herpes vesicles can often be seen in eczema herpeticum

Melissa Gan

1. Which ONE of the following is a cause for pseudohyponatraemia?

   A. Hyperglycaemia

   B. Syndrome of inappropriate antidiuretic hormone (SIADH)

   C. Hyperlipidaemia

   D. Liver cirrhosis

2. Which ONE of the following is NOT one of the criteria required in making a diagnosis of SIADH?

   A. Hypotonicity

   B. Urinary osmolality > plasma osmolality

   C. Normovolaemia

   D. Urinary [Na⁺] <20 mmol/L

3. A 68-year-old man is brought in seizing from a nursing home. His initial [Na⁺] on a venous blood gas is found to be 176 mmol/L. Which ONE of the following drugs may be responsible for this finding?

   A. Morphine

   B. Lithium

   C. Nonsteroidal anti-inflammatory drugs (NSAIDs)

   D. Carbamazepine

4. Which ONE of the following treatments is NOT recommended in the treatment of hypercalcaemia?

   A. Thiazide diuretics

   B. Corticosteroids

   C. Bisphosphonates

   D. Normal saline

5. A 53-year-old woman is brought to the emergency department (ED) with confusion. Her only past medical history is that of breast cancer. Her serum calcium level has returned as 3.63 mmol/L. Which ONE of the following would you NOT expect to see during her ED work-up?

   A. Polyuria

   B. Hyporeflexia

   C. Constipation

   D. Prolonged QTc on electrocardiogram (ECG)

6. Which ONE of the following statements is TRUE regarding the anion gap (AG)?

   A. It represents the amount of excess amount of positive charge in plasma

   B. Causes of a low AG (<6) include conditions of increased unmeasured cations such as hypercalcaemia, hypermagnesaemia and lithium intoxication

   C. To correct for hypoalbuminaemia you must subtract 2.5 from the AG for every 10 g/L below normal

   D. It is only ever present in metabolic acidosis

7. Which ONE of the following statements is FALSE regarding the delta gap?

   A. The delta gap is equal to the ratio of change in AG and the change in bicarbonate

   B. A delta gap of 1 indicates a pure high AG metabolic acidosis

   C. If the rise in the AG is greater than the fall in the bicarbonate level, then a mixed high AG metabolic acidosis must coexist with a metabolic alkalosis

   D. If the rise in the AG is greater than the fall in the bicarbonate level, then a mixed high AG metabolic acidosis and normal AG metabolic acidosis coexist

8. Which ONE of the following is a cause for metabolic alkalosis?

   A. Adrenal insufficiency

   B. Cushing's syndrome

   C. Acetazolamide

   D. Profuse diarrhoea

9. A 28-year-old man is brought into the ED with a Glasgow Coma Scale (GCS) of 12/15 and having ingested an unknown substance. His blood results are as follows:

- pH 7.15 mmol/L (7.35–7.45)
- HCO_3^- 8 mmol/L (20–24)
- PCO_2 28 mmol/L (35–45)
- Na⁺ 141 mmol/L (135–145)
- K⁺ 4.5 mmol/L (3.5–5.0)
- Cl⁻ 92 mmol/L (95–105)
- Ur 10 mmol/L (2–7)
- Cr 100 mmol/L (60–110)
- BSL 7.5 mmol/L (3.6–5.8)
- lactate 16 mmol/L (< 2.2)
- Osm measured = 375 mOsm/L (275–295)
- ethanol 30 mmol/L.

Which ONE of the following drugs/poisons would NOT typically explain the above results?

A. Paracetamol

B. Ethanol

C. Cyanide

D. Acetone

10. Which ONE of the following is a cause of saline unresponsive metabolic alkalosis?

A. Thiazide diuretic use

B. Protracted vomiting

C. Primary hyperaldosteronism

D. Cystic fibrosis

11. Which ONE of the following conditions is associated with hypokalaemia?

A. Beta-blockers

B. Metabolic alkalosis

C. Addisonian crisis

D. Digoxin intoxication

12. A 48-year-old alcoholic man presents to the ED after an episode of syncope. An ECG is performed that shows a QTc of 523 ms. Which ONE of the following electrolyte imbalances would LEAST likely be a cause for his prolonged QTc?

A. Hypomagnesaemia secondary to nutritional deficiency

B. Hypokalaemia secondary to vomiting

C. Hyponatraemia secondary to liver cirrhosis

D. Hypocalcaemia secondary to increased calcium excretion

13. Which ONE of the following ECG findings would you LEAST expect to see in a patient with hyperkalaemia?

A. Tall, symmetrical peaked T waves

B. Shortened PR interval

C. Shortened QT interval

D. Widening of QRS complex

14. Which ONE of the following is NOT a potential complication in the treatment of metabolic acidosis with sodium bicarbonate?

A. Dehydration

B. Overshoot alkalosis

C. Cerebrospinal fluid (CSF) acidosis

D. Hypercapnoea and respiratory failure

15. Which ONE of the following conditions is NOT an indication for the use of bicarbonate therapy in metabolic acidosis?

A. Tricyclic antidepressant overdose

B. Severe hyperchloraemic acidaemia

C. Diabetic ketoacidosis

D. Hyperkalaemia with cardiac toxicity

16. An 8-week-old boy is brought to the ED with a 3-day history of vomiting. His venous blood gas shows:

- pH 7.55 (7.35–7.45)
- HCO_3^- 40 mmol/L (22–24)
- PCO_2 48 mmol/L (35–45)
- K^+ 2.8 mmol/L (3.5–5.0)
- Na^+ 135 mmol/L (135–145)
- Cl^- 85 mmol/L (95–105).

His gas improves with normal saline therapy. Which ONE of the following conditions is the MOST likely cause of his blood gas result?

A. Sepsis

B. Adrenogenital syndrome

C. Adrenal insufficiency

D. Pyloric stenosis

17. A 78-year-old man is brought in from home after a 3-day history of diarrhoea. His venous blood gas shows:

- pH 7.27 (7.35–7.45)
- HCO_3^- 14 mmol/L (22–24)
- PCO_2 28 mmol/L (35–45)
- K^+ 2.6 mmol/L (3.5–5.0)
- Na^+ 134 mmol/L (135–145)
- Cl^- 113 mmol/L (95–105)
- Ur 14 mmol/L (2–7)
- Cr 320 mmol/L (50–100)
- lactate 1.5 mmol/L (<2.2).

Which ONE of the following options would BEST explain the clinical scenario?

A. High AG metabolic acidosis secondary to renal failure

B. High AG metabolic acidosis secondary to dehydration and lactic acidosis

C. Normal AG metabolic acidosis secondary to diarrhoea

D. Concurrent normal AG metabolic acidosis and respiratory alkalosis

18. Which ONE of the following blood gas pictures would you expect to see in a 6-year-old boy being treated for acute life-threatening asthma?

A. pH 7.21, CO_2 = 76, HCO_3 = 27, K^+ 3.3
B. pH 7.21, CO_2 = 76, HCO_3 = 27, K^+ 5.3
C. pH 7.55, CO_2 = 26, HCO_3 = 21, K^+ 5.3
D. pH 7.55, CO_2 = 26, HCO_3 = 35, K^+ 3.3

19. A 48-year-old man presents to the ED with a right middle lobe pneumonia. His arterial blood gas on room air taken on arrival is as follows:

- pH 7.55 (7.35–7.45)
- PCO_2 18 mmol/L (35–45)
- PO_2 70 mmol/L (80–100)
- HCO_3^- 18 mmol/L (22–24)

Which ONE of the following is his A-a gradient?

A. 127 mmHg
B. 47 mmHg
C. 57 mmHg
D. 77 mmHg

20. The concentration of sodium ions in a 1 L bag of normal saline is:

A. 115 mmol/L
B. 130 mmol/L
C. 154 mmol/L
D. 290 mmol/L

21. Which ONE of the following would NOT cause a high AG metabolic acidosis?

A. Paracetamol ingestion
B. Diabetic ketoacidosis (DKA)
C. Fanconi's syndrome
D. Carbon monoxide poisoning

22. Rapid overcorrection of hyponatraemia can lead to all of the following EXCEPT:

A. Quadriparesis
B. Seizures
C. Ataxia
D. Cardiac arrhythmias

23. Which ONE of the following conditions is a cause of hypocalcaemia?

A. Hyperparathyroidism
B. Thiazide diuretics
C. Rhabdomyolysis
D. Sarcoidosis

24. Which ONE of the following statements is FALSE regarding rhabdomyolysis?

A. Hypercalcaemia is the most common metabolic abnormality
B. Renal function is the most important determinant of the degree of potassium elevation
C. Hyperphosphataemia occurs initially then hypophosphataemia later in the disease course
D. Uric acid levels usually correlate well with CK levels

25. A 35-year-old female presents with a prolonged seizure. Her initial ABG is shown.

- pH 7.25 (7.35–7.45)
- PCO_2 55 mmol/L (35–45)
- PO_2 100 mmol/L (80–100)
- HCO_3 15 mmol/L (22–24)
- Na^+ 135 mmol/L (135–145)
- K^+ 4.5 mmol/L (3.5–5)
- Cl^- 98 mmol/L (95–105).

Which ONE of the following explains the above blood gas?

A. Mixed normal AG metabolic acidosis and respiratory acidosis
B. High AG metabolic acidosis
C. Mixed high AG metabolic acidosis and metabolic alkalosis
D. Mixed high AG metabolic acidosis and respiratory acidosis

Yolande Weiner and Zaahid Pandie

1. Which ONE of the following techniques provides the best visualisation of the vocal cords during rapid sequence intubation (RSI)?

   A. Backwards-upwards-rightwards pressure on thyroid cartilage (BURP manoeuvre)

   B. Bimanual laryngoscopy

   C. Retraction of the right side of the mouth laterally by an assistant

   D. Sellick's manoeuvre

2. Cricoid pressure using Sellick's manoeuvre is commonly used during RSI. Which ONE of the following is TRUE?

   A. It reliably prevents regurgitation and aspiration

   B. It is helpful in improving the quality of the laryngoscopic view

   C. It should always be used in patients during RSI

   D. It can adversely affect ventilation during bag–valve–mask (BVM) ventilation

3. Regarding laryngospasm as a cause of upper airway obstruction, which ONE of the following is TRUE?

   A. It is most common in children aged 1–3 years

   B. Bradycardia is an unlikely complication in children

   C. It can cause pulmonary oedema

   D. It resolves as soon as the causative stimulus has ceased

4. The laryngeal mask airway (LMA) is a successful rescue device in emergency airway management. Which ONE of the following statements is TRUE regarding the LMA?

   A. Positioning of the patient into the 'sniffing' position is essential

   B. It is a useful alternative to an endotracheal tube (ETT) for establishing a definitive airway

   C. Cricoid pressure almost always impedes insertion of an LMA

   D. The device should be held firmly in place during inflation to allow the LMA to seat properly

5. Regarding the management of the airway and ventilation in a morbidly obese patient, which ONE of the following statements is TRUE?

   A. Ventilation should be performed with initial tidal volumes of 10 mL/kg based on ideal body weight

   B. The 'sniffing' position provides the best laryngoscopic view

   C. Suxamethonium should be dosed according to ideal body weight

   D. Vecuronium should be dosed according to lean body weight

6. Regarding pretreatment agents given prior to RSI, which ONE of the following statements is TRUE?

   A. Adverse reactions such as chest wall rigidity and respiratory depression are minimised when fentanyl is given over 30–60 seconds

   B. Atropine 0.02 mg/kg is routinely recommended in children < 5 years of age to prevent significant bradycardia

   C. Lignocaine attenuates the adverse physiologic response to intubation and has been shown to improve outcome in patients with asthma but not head injury

   D. Pretreatment with a small dose (defasciculating dose) of a non-depolarising muscle relaxant significantly reduces muscle pain associated with suxamethonium

7. Regarding the use of propofol as an induction agent during RSI, which ONE of the following is TRUE?

   A. It causes hypotension due to histamine release

   B. Vomiting is a common side effect

   C. It can safely be given to patients with an egg allergy

   D. It should be discarded within 6 hours of opening

8. Regarding the use of suxamethonium as a paralytic agent in RSI, which ONE of the following is TRUE?

   A. The use of a higher dose (1.5 mg/kg) results in more fasciculation and myalgia than a low dose (1.0 mg/kg) but better intubation conditions

   B. Prophylactic atropine should be administered to all infants < 1 year of age

   C. It can safely be used in patients with suspected raised intracranial pressure

   D. The dose in neonates and infants is 1.5 mg/kg

9. Regarding the use of lignocaine as a local anaesthetic agent, which ONE of the following is TRUE?

A. Alkalinisation of the anaesthetic solution reduces the pain of injection but does not hasten the onset of action

B. Lignocaine remains effective for up to 4 hours when administered as a regional nerve block

C. The safe dose of lignocaine without adrenaline is 5–7 mg/kg

D. The dose should not exceed 300 mg at a single injection

10. Which ONE of the following is TRUE regarding the use of bupivacaine as a local anaesthetic agent?

A. The duration of anaesthesia is twice as long with bupivacaine than lignocaine

B. Total dose of bupivacaine should not exceed more than 400 mg in a 24-hour period

C. Bupivacaine is as likely as lignocaine to cause cardiotoxicity

D. The safe dose of bupivacaine with adrenaline is 3–5 mg/kg

11. Regarding intravenous regional anaesthesia (Bier's block), which ONE of the following statements is TRUE?

A. Prilocaine can safely be infused at a dose of 5 mg/kg

B. Lignocaine injected as a 0.5% solution is an acceptable alternative to prilocaine

C. The anaesthetic agent should always be injected distal to the site of injury to be effective

D. Minimum tourniquet inflation time should be at least 10 minutes

12. Femoral nerve blocks are performed for the management of pain in femoral shaft fractures. Which ONE of the following statements is TRUE?

A. Ultrasound guided femoral nerve block provides a more complete block and requires less local anaesthetic volume

B. It is inappropriate to use a nerve stimulator in the trauma setting because it will aggravate pain

C. When the blind technique is performed, a local anaesthetic should be injected as soon as paraesthesia is elicited with the needle

D. With femoral nerve block, the time to achieve the lowest pain score is similar compared with intravenous narcotics but additional parenteral analgesic requirements are reduced

13. Regarding the use of opioids for the management of acute pain in the emergency department (ED), which ONE of the following is TRUE?

A. Fentanyl provides anxiolysis at doses of 1–2 mcg/kg given intravenous

B. Respiratory depression is rare and occurs in <1% of patients

C. Pethidine is the preferred opioid in biliary colic

D. Intranasal administration of fentanyl at a dose of 0.15 mcg/kg provides pain relief comparable to intravenous opioids in children

14. Regarding agents used in procedural sedation and analgesia (PSA) in the ED, which ONE of the following statements is TRUE?

A. Propofol has good analgesic and amnestic properties

B. Vomiting associated with the use of ketamine usually occurs soon after administration

C. Hypersalivation associated with ketamine use is dose dependant

D. Flumazenil successfully reverses paradoxal agitation that can occur with midazolam

15. Regarding fasting and ED PSA, which ONE of the following is the MOST appropriate answer?

A. Evidence suggests that gastric emptying is delayed by acute stress or anxiety

B. Fasting time, gastric volume and gastric acidity is strongly associated with the probability of aspiration

C. Current fasting guidelines are evidence based

D. Aspiration risk with procedural sedation and analgesia is less likely than with operative anaesthesia

16. Regarding PSA in children, which ONE of the following principles is TRUE?

A. In preparing children for a painful procedure, children should not be exposed to aspects of the procedure that may cause stress, for example, handling procedural equipment

B. The American Society of Anesthesiology (ASA) physical status classification is applicable to children undergoing procedural sedation

C. Evidence suggests that pre-procedure fasting results in a decreased incidence of adverse events

D. Gastric emptying agents should be used routinely as it decreases the risk of aspiration

17. Pain scales and tools are used in the assessment of pain in children. Which ONE of the following is TRUE?

A. The FLACC (face, legs, activity, cry, consolation) scale is validated for pain assessment in children with cognitive impairment

B. The Pieces of Hurt tool is a self-report tool that allows children to rate their pain using coloured chips

C. Faces Pain Scale – Revised is useful from 2 to 10 years of age

D. Visual analogue scales require that children must understand number concepts and have sufficient abstract thinking ability

18. Which ONE of the following non-pharmacological techniques will most likely interfere with the child's coping ability during a painful procedure in the ED?

A. Non-procedural talk

B. Distraction methods

C. Giving the child control over when to start the procedure

D. Involving play therapists during the periprocedural phase

19. Regarding the use of anaesthetic agents in reducing pain during skin puncture in children, which ONE of the following is INCORRECT?

A. EMLA® (euteric mixture of local anaesthetics – lignocaine and prilocaine) cream is effective in relieving the pain from capillary sampling in neonates

B. Sucrose 24% in doses of 0.25 mL aliquots up to 1 mL in total decreases pain during neonatal procedures

C. AnGel® (amethocaine) cream is more potent than EMLA® in relieving pain from venepuncture in children

D. The use of EMLA® with sucrose provides further analgesic efficacy than sucrose alone in neonates undergoing skin puncture

20. Regarding management of procedure-related pain in children, which ONE of the following is INCORRECT?

A. Continuous flow nitrous oxide is more effective than oral midazolam for laceration repair

B. Laceraine® (lignocaine, amethocaine, adrenaline) is an excellent topical anaesthetic for instillation into minor lacerations

C. The combination of ketamine and midazolam provides more effective analgesia than the fentanyl and midazolam combination for fracture manipulation

D. Vapocoolant is less effective than EMLA® in reducing immunisation pain in school-aged children

CHAPTER 13
TRAUMA AND BURNS

QUESTIONS

Yogesh Nataly and Waruna de Alwis

1. Regarding anatomical and physiological features in children that should be considered in the management of trauma, which ONE of the following is TRUE?

A. Ribs contribute most to the chest expansion during breathing

B. The larynx sits more anteriorly and inferiorly than in adults

C. The tidal volume per kilogram of body weight increases through to adulthood

D. Children have a higher circulating blood volume per kilogram of body weight than adults

2. Regarding major trauma in children, which ONE of the following statements is TRUE?

A. Abdominal injury is the most common single-organ injury associated with death in children

B. Injuries to internal abdominal organs are more likely to occur in children than in adults

C. The absence of rib fractures on X-ray essentially excludes underlying lung injury

D. Bladder injuries are less common in children than in adults

3. Which ONE of the following injuries is NOT typically considered as a non-accidental injury (NAI) in a child 2 years of age?

A. Bruising over shins

B. Spiral fracture of the tibia

C. Metaphyseal fractures of long bones

D. Posterior rib fractures

4. Which ONE of the following is the MOST common manifestation of abusive head trauma in children?

A. Retinal haemorrhage

B. Brainstem infarction

C. Subdural haematoma

D. Extradural haematoma

5. Which ONE of the following statements is TRUE in the assessment of motor function in a patient with a severe head injury?

A. Decerebrate posture consists of abnormal flexor response in the arms with extension of the legs

B. Decerebrate posture consists of abnormal flexor response of the arms and legs

C. Decorticate posture consists of abnormal flexor response of the arms with extension of the legs

D. Decorticate posture consists of abnormal flexor response of the arms and legs

6. In a patient with a major head injury, which ONE of the following secondary insults should be given the HIGHEST priority for correction in the emergency department (ED)?

A. Hypoglycaemia

B. Hypercarbia

C. Hypotension

D. Temperature of 40°C

7. Prediction of an intracranial injury visible on CT is one of the main objectives in the assessment of an adult patient with head injury. Which ONE of the following statements is TRUE regarding this assessment?

A. A history of loss of consciousness is the only proven predictor

B. Isolated vomiting without a history of loss of consciousness is not a valuable predictor

C. 2% of patients without a history of loss of consciousness have CT positive intracranial injury

D. Isolated amnesia without a history of loss of consciousness in not a valuable predictor

8. Regarding a patient with diffuse axonal injury (axonal shear injury) of the brain, all of the following are correct EXCEPT:

A. This is due to severe blunt trauma and cerebral oedema may develop rapidly

B. Majority of patients show punctate haemorrhage in cerebral cortex on a head CT

C. Any rise in intracranial pressure should be prevented in the ED

D. In infants it may be due to NAI

9. Regarding intracranial haemorrhage associated with traumatic brain injury, all of the following are correct EXCEPT:

A. Traumatic subarachnoid haemorrhage (SAH) may be missed on CT scans obtained within 6–8 hours from the time of injury

QUESTIONS   57

B. Mortality from an acute subdural haematoma is higher than from an extradural haematoma

C. Subdural haematomas but not extradural haematomas cross suture lines on a CT scan

D. A history of loss of consciousness is nearly always present in patients with an extradural haematoma

10. Which ONE of the following statements is TRUE regarding cervical spine injuries in children?

A. If suspected in an infant, the cervical spine should be immobilised while placing adequate padding under the shoulders

B. The injuries usually involve the lower three cervical vertebrae

C. Transient paraesthesia or weakness in the limbs that were present immediately after injury are not considered significant if the X-ray and CT are normal

D. NEXUS and the 'Canadian cervical spine decision rules' can safely be applied to most children

11. Regarding the assessment of the cervical spine in a trauma patient, which ONE of the following statements is TRUE?

A. Both NEXUS criteria and the Canadian cervical spine decision rules have very high sensitivities and specificities in detecting cervical spine fractures in awake and alert adults

B. A focused neurological examination with checking for active range of motion of the cervical spine is essential when clearing the spine

C. If a cervical spine X-ray is technically adequate and all three views are obtained, the chance of missing a fracture is minimal

D. In the elderly, odontoid fracture is easily identifiable on plain films

12. Regarding injuries to the spine, which ONE of the following statements is CORRECT?

A. Bilateral facet joint dislocation is generally the result of hyperextension injury

B. Less than 2% of sacral injuries are associated with neurological deficits

C. Teardrop fractures to the antero-inferior aspect of the vertebra are unstable injuries

D. A Jefferson fracture is a fracture through the C2 pedicles

13. Regarding the assessment of a patient with a cervical spinal cord injury (SCI), all of the following statements are true EXCEPT:

A. Central cord syndrome, where arm weakness is more than leg weakness, is seen in older patients

B. The breathing pattern is mainly abdominal if cord injury is at C4 level

C. Hypoxaemia is uncommon during the early ED stay

D. Asystolic cardiac arrest is relatively common following tracheal suctioning in high spinal cord injuries

14. Spinal shock is characterised by which ONE of the following?

A. Hypotension

B. Hypovolaemia

C. Flaccid paralysis

D. Bradycardia

15. Regarding ED management of a young adult with an acute spinal cord injury, which ONE of the following statements is TRUE?

A. Hypotension should be managed with vasopressors as it is usually secondary to neurogenic shock

B. Suxamethonium should not be used as a paralytic agent during rapid sequence intubation

C. There is high-quality evidence to support the early use of corticosteroids

D. A nasogastric tube should be inserted early during ED management

16. Regarding zygomatic fractures due to blunt facial trauma, which ONE of the following statements is TRUE?

A. The 'tripod' fracture involves the infraorbital rim

B. Diplopia is not a feature, as the orbit is not involved

C. Associated lateral conjunctival haemorrhages is rare

D. It causes proptosis

17. Regarding the diagnosis and ED management of midfacial fractures in a patient involved in severe blunt trauma, which ONE of the following interventions is LEAST appropriate?

A. When suspected, a Le Fort fracture and midfacial instability should be clinically identified by manually rocking the hard palate

B. Early control of posterior nasal epistaxis by balloon devices is a priority

C. When there is severe intraoral bleeding from the palate, oral packing should be done to stop bleeding prior to intubation

D. If the patient is awake and maintaining the airway, the sitting-up position is most suitable once the cervical spine is cleared

18. Regarding the management of injuries in the face, which ONE of the following statements is CORRECT?

A. An avulsed primary tooth should be replaced as soon as possible to improve its chances of survival

B. Traumatic rupture of the tympanic membrane usually takes 12 weeks to heal when conservatively treated

C. Parents should be advised that a tongue laceration in a child when conservatively treated in the ED may require subsequent revision

D. Nasal septal haematoma with superimposed infection causes late cartilage necrosis

19. A 25-year-old male presents to the ED with a stab wound to the neck. During the primary survey, the emergency medicine registrar searches for the presence of any hard signs. Which ONE of the following is LEAST likely to be a hard sign in this patient?

A. Evolving stroke

B. Air bubbling through the wound

C. Subcutaneous emphysema

D. Large haematoma

20. The neck is divided into three zones to aide clinical assessment and management of penetrating neck injuries. Compared with zone II stab wounds, all of the following statements are true regarding zone I and III stab wounds EXCEPT:

A. The ED diagnosis of injuries and their extent is more difficult and less reliable in zone I and III

B. Occult vascular injuries are more likely to be present in zone I and III

C. CT angiogram has a very high sensitivity in detecting significant vascular injuries in zone I and III

D. Cervical spine injuries are more common in zone I and III

21. Regarding hanging injuries, which ONE of the following statements is INCORRECT?

A. Cervical spine injury is unlikely if the drop (fall) is less than the body height

B. Bradycardia and asystolic arrest may occur

C. Venous cerebral infarction is common and venous compression in the neck should be avoided during resuscitation

D. Tracheal compression is the likely cause of death in non-judicial hanging

22. Regarding the diagnosis and management of haemothorax in patients with thoracic trauma, which ONE of the following statements is TRUE?

A. A massive haemothorax in the adult is defined as at least 1000 mL blood in the hemithorax or blood occupying approximately one-third of the available space in the hemithorax

B. More than 1000 mL of blood in the hemithorax may be missed on a supine chest X-ray (CXR)

C. There is no indication to evacuate blood from the pleural cavity with tube thoracostomy, when the estimated amount in a stable patient is 200–500 mL

D. More than half of patients with chest trauma require intercostal tube drainage

23. Regarding a patient with a flail chest secondary to blunt trauma, which ONE of the following statements is TRUE?

A. Hypoxaemia is usually the result of increased work of breathing due to paradoxical chest wall movements of the flail segment during inspiration and expiration

B. The movement of the flail segment is most visible just after injury and less visible 24 hours later

C. In an awake patient conservative treatment with meticulous analgesia provides good recovery even with significant flail segment and underlying lung contusion

D. A patient with flail segment involving more than eight ribs has a high mortality

24. Regarding traumatic pneumothorax in a spontaneously ventilated patient, all of the following are correct EXCEPT:

A. A pneumothorax incidentally detected on chest CT or abdomen but not seen on CXR does not usually require drainage with an intercostal tube

B. If a pneumothorax is not visualised on a properly done CXR, a stable patient with an isolated stab wound to the chest can be discharged early

C. Bedside ultrasound scan (USS) is more sensitive than a supine CXR in detecting a pneumothorax in a supine trauma patient

D. A traumatic pneumothorax in a patient with moderate to severe chronic obstructive pulmonary disease (COPD) has an increasing likelihood to convert to a tension pneumothorax

25. Regarding pneumomediastinum caused by blunt chest trauma in an adult, which ONE of the following statements is TRUE?

A. A thorough search for injuries to the larynx, trachobroncheal tree, pharynx and oesophagus should be carried out

B. Electrical alternans is a classical electrocardiogram (ECG) feature

C. Auscultation over the heart during systole can be quieter than in a healthy individual

D. Hoarseness of voice and stridor are not recognised symptoms

26. A 50-year-old woman with underlying ischaemic heart disease presents to the ED following a motor vehicle crash. Her car rear-ended a stationary car at 60 km per hour and she was unrestrained. She was found to have an isolated undisplaced fracture of the sternum on a contrast-enhanced chest CT. Her vital signs and the 12-lead ECG are normal. The MOST appropriate management of this patient would be:

A. Admit the patient to a monitored area for observation for 24 hours

B. Admit the patient to a monitored area for serial cardiac enzymes

C. Observe for 6 hours and consider discharge if repeat ECG and vital signs are normal at 6 hours and pain control is adequate

D. Perform an urgent echocardiography to ensure that there is no myocardial contusion

27. Regarding ECG and troponin testing in a patient suspected of having myocardial contusion due to blunt chest trauma, which ONE of the following statements is TRUE?

A. When both 12-lead ECG and serum troponin are normal, the negative predictive value for a myocardial contusion reaches 100%

B. Right ventricular wall contusions usually cause prominent ECG abnormalities

C. Myocardial contusion does not cause troponin rise because there is no associated myocardial cell necrosis

D. Anteroseptal ST segment elevations are considered gold standard ECG abnormalities in the diagnosis of myocardial contusion in a relevant patient

28. Regarding stab wounds to the heart, which ONE of the following statements is TRUE?

A. The left side of the heart is at greatest risk of injury from a stab wound

B. Exsanguinating haemorrhage is more likely to occur if cardiac wound communicates with pleural cavity

C. Cardiac tamponade is less likely to occur from a myocardial stab wound than from a gunshot wound

D. Atrial stab wounds spontaneously seal better than ventricular wounds and therefore blood loss is limited from atrial wounds

29. Which one of the following scenarios is the MOST appropriate indication for an ED thoracotomy?

A. 30-year-old woman arrests just after arriving in the ED having had chest injuries following a motor vehicle crash

B. A 25-year-old male with a knife wound to his right precordium that arrests en route to hospital and arrives at the ED in PEA

C. 36-year-old male who presents following a motor vehicle crash and drains more than 1500 mL of blood immediately after the placement of a left intercostal tube and arrests

D. A 45-year-old male with a knife wound to his left precordium that presents with a systolic blood pressure of 85, distended neck veins and muffled heart sounds

30. Which ONE of the following is NOT an aim of ED resuscitative thoracotomy?

A. Control of bleeding from pulmonary vessels with clamping

B. Cross-clamping of the ascending aorta to stop massive intraabdominal bleeding

C. Internal cardiac massage

D. Removal of a blood clot from the pericardial sac

31. Regarding traumatic rupture of the aorta (TRA), which ONE of the following statements is TRUE?

A. Atherosclerosis or medial necrosis predisposes to traumatic rupture

B. Most blunt aortic injuries in patients who reach the hospital alive are found at the origin of the left subclavian artery

C. Widened mediastinum on a CXR has a high sensitivity and specificity for diagnosis

D. A small number of patients with blunt trauma to the aorta have fractures of bones other then ribs

32. Regarding diaphragmatic injuries, which ONE of the following statements is CORRECT?

A. As the diaphragm is a strong muscular structure and the injury is sealed early, delayed sequelae are uncommon

B. When present, early diagnosis is typical for these injuries

C. Most patients with diaphragmatic rupture have an abnormal CXR, but these findings are non-specific

D. If this is due to blunt trauma such as a motor vehicle crash it is more common on the right than on the left side

33. In the assessment of intraabdominal injuries due to blunt trauma, which ONE of the following statements is CORRECT?

A. Localised tenderness has a high sensitivity to identify intraabdominal injury but its specificity is low

B. Abdominal girth measurement has a value in predicting intraabdominal bleeding

C. Physical examination when combined with a FAST scan is reliable in identifying retroperitoneal injuries

D. There is no indication to do an abdominal CT in a haemodynamically stable patient who has a large area of abdominal wall abrasion when the FAST scan is negative

34. Regarding splenic injuries due to blunt trauma in children, which ONE of the following statements is TRUE?

A. Slow bleeding without initial haemodynamic instability is a feature

B. For the same degree of splenic injury, children are more likely to be haemodynamically unstable than adults

C. A fatal haemorrhage is more likely to be associated with a splenic injury than with a liver injury

D. About half of the children require splenectomy

35. Regarding small bowel injury due to blunt abdominal trauma, which ONE of the following statements is TRUE?

A. Mortality is usually not due to the resultant peritonitis

B. Abdominal tenderness is an early sign

C. It is not associated with intraabdominal bleeding

D. Extravasation of oral contrast on CT scan is present in the majority of the patients

36. Which one of the following is the MOST COMMON mechanism of pelvic fracture as per the Young-Burgess classification?

A. Anteroposterior compression

B. Lateral compression

C. Vertical shear

D. Mixed mechanism

37. In the management of a haemodynamically unstable patient with a pelvic fracture, which ONE of the following measures is MOST appropriate?

A. If the FAST is negative, all measures should be taken to control pelvic bleeding, which may include prompt angiography and selective embolisation

B. If the FAST is negative, patient should proceed for laparotomy because a false negative FAST is common in patients with pelvic fractures

C. If the FAST is positive, the patient should proceed to operating theatre for surgical control of bleeding from common and external iliac and common femoral arteries

D. All patients, irrespective of the FAST results, should proceed first to laparotomy and then to surgical or radiological control of pelvic bleeding

38. In the assessment of genitourinary injuries following blunt trauma, which ONE of the following statements is TRUE?

A. A contrast-enhanced CT with passive bladder filling is adequate to exclude bladder rupture

B. Anterior urethral injuries are common following straddle injuries while posterior urethral injuries are seen with pelvic fractures

C. The degree of haematuria corresponds to the degree of genitourinary injury

D. The current consensus is that all adult patients with isolated microscopic hematuria do not require further imaging studies

39. Which ONE of the following physiological changes in a pregnant woman is RELAVENT in trauma management in pregnancy?

A. An increase in blood volume of 15% in the third trimester

B. An increase in blood flow and blood volume to the gravid uterus with a decreased volume of blood in the lower limbs

C. Physiological anaemia resulting in a decrease in oxygen-carrying capacity

D. The reduced oxygen reserve, which is more due to the elevation of diaphragm than an increase in oxygen consumption related to the growing fetus

40. In the assessment of a pregnant woman of 28 weeks' gestation involved in a motor vehicle crash, which ONE of the following is TRUE?

A. In women with minor trauma, fetal outcome is predicted by USS, abdominal tenderness and blood tests

B. The most likely cause of fetal death is fetal intracranial injury

C. In the absence of restraint the fetal mortality rate is three times as high

D. A CXR causes a significant radiation exposure to the uterus

41. In the assessment and management of a pregnant woman involved in a motor vehicle crash, which ONE of the following is TRUE?

A. Signs of fetal distress include acceleration of heart rate following a uterine contraction

B. Venous blood gas HCO_3^- helps in predicting placental bleeding

C. The Kleihauer-Betke test is positive with fetomaternal haemorrhage (FMH) of <1 mL

D. Tetanus toxoid to the mother is detrimental to the fetus

42. Regarding trauma in the third trimester of pregnancy, which ONE of the following is TRUE?

A. Intercostal drains should be inserted at the usual location (5th intercostal space)

B. Clinical abdominal examination may underestimate the extent of significant intraabdominal injuries

C. Bladder injuries are less likely due to protection of the bladder by the uterus

D. Diastasis of the pubic symphysis is always due to pelvic disruption

43. In a patient who has been injured in a bomb explosion once the immediate life threats have been excluded or attended to, assessment should be done to identify the injuries due to primary blast injury. Regarding primary blast injury, which ONE of the following statements is TRUE?

A. The lung is the most commonly injured structure due to primary blast injury

B. The detection of tympanic membrane rupture with otoscopy is a sensitive marker for the presence of other significant injuries due to primary blast injury

C. Abdominal solid organ injuries are usually due to primary blast injury

D. An explosion in a confined space (e.g. a bus) is less likely to cause primary blast injury than an explosion in an open space

44. Regarding categories of injuries occurring in a bomb explosion, all of the following are correct EXCEPT:

A. Rupture of the colon or small intestine are due to primary blast injury and it is difficult to detect initially

B. Secondary blast injuries due to penetrating fragments are the leading cause of death in bomb explosions

C. Tertiary blast injuries are mainly blunt trauma caused by structural collapses and the patient being thrown away due to blast wind

D. Burns are considered as tertiary injuries and rare in a bomb explosion

45. Which ONE of the following is applicable for estimating the total body surface area (TBSA) of a burn?

A. The 'rule of 9' should not be used for children under the age of 10

B. The head of a 2-year-old child is equivalent to about 9% of TBSA

C. The palm of a patient's hand, including the fingers, is approximately 5% of the TBSA

D. The back of the trunk accounts for 9% TBSA in an adult

46. A 7-year-old child presents to the ED with 30% TBSA burns. His body weight is 22 kg. Using the Parkland formula, which ONE of the following is the initial intravenous fluid rate that needs to be added to the maintenance fluids?

   A. 220 mL/hr

   B. 440 mL/hr

   C. 165 mL/hr

   D. 62 mL/hr

47. Regarding fluid resuscitation in haemorrhagic hypovolaemia due to trauma, which ONE of the following statements is TRUE?

   A. There is evidence to suggest that albumin compared with normal saline improves mortality during resuscitation for haemorrhagic hypovolaemia

   B. Blood loss of 600 mL in adults is associated with orthostatic blood pressure (BP) changes

   C. Initial lactate level is not predictive of a patient's need for ongoing fluid resuscitation

   D. Hypotensive resuscitation is contraindicated in the presence of end-organ hypoperfusion

48. Which ONE of the following is NOT a component of damage control resuscitation (DCR)?

   A. A temporary colostomy in large bowel perforation following blunt abdominal trauma

   B. Early haemostatic resuscitation with packed red blood cells (PRBC), platelets and cryoprecipitate in a ratio of 1:1:1

   C. Keeping systolic blood pressure between 80 and 100 mm Hg

   D. Target ionised Ca^{2+} to >1.0 mEq/L

49. Considering massive transfusion, which ONE of the following statements is CORRECT?

   A. The definition of massive transfusion in an adult is replacement of >50% of a patient's blood volume in a 12 hour period

   B. Markers of successful treatment include a pH > 7.1 and INR < 2 × normal

   C. In a child, the transfusion of >40% of the blood volume is considered as massive transfusion

   D. Frequent monitoring of coagulation is not useful

50. Regarding trauma systems for timely management of patients with traumatic injuries, which ONE of the following is TRUE?

   A. A level 1 trauma centre needs a 24-hour neuroradiology and haemodialysis facilities

   B. The second peak in the bimodal distribution of trauma deaths occurs in the intensive care unit (ICU) secondary to the systemic inflammatory response syndrome (SIRS) response

   C. Mandatory trauma call should only be initiated in the presence of agreed anatomical injury and/or physiological criteria

   D. All of the above

CHAPTER 14
ORTHOPAEDIC EMERGENCIES

QUESTIONS

Waruna de Alwis

1. Regarding Salter-Harris type I growth plate injuries, which ONE of the following statements is FALSE?

A. The epiphysis separates completely from the metaphysis

B. There is tenderness over the growth plate on examination but no radiological abnormality

C. A displaced epiphysis in type I injury is usually difficult to reduce

D. Type I injuries are caused by shearing and avulsion forces compared with type V injuries, which are caused by axial compression

2. Regarding physeal (growth plate) injuries in children, which ONE of the following statements is INCORRECT?

A. The most common site for the Salter-Harris type III fracture is the distal end of the tibia

B. Fractures of the lateral condyle of the humerus can be treated conservatively

C. Injuries to the growth plate occur in one-third of all bony injuries in children

D. Avascular necrosis of the epiphysis is a complication

3. Regarding a diagnosis of nerve injuries when assessing a child with a supracondylar fracture of the humerus, all of the following statements are correct EXCEPT:

A. Inability to flex the distal interphalangeal joint of the index finger and the interphalangeal joint of the thumb indicates injury to the anterior interosseous branch of the median nerve

B. If the child is able to fully extend the thumb it excludes a radial nerve injury

C. If the child is able to fully abduct all fingers it excludes an ulnar nerve injury

D. Inability to make a fist is usually secondary to pain and should not be considered as a median nerve injury

4. Regarding emergency department (ED) management of a supracondylar humeral fracture in a child, which ONE of the following is the MOST appropriate step?

A. Immobilisation of the elbow with flexion >90 degrees in all patients

B. Immediate manipulation in the operating theatre (OT) if the radial pulse is lost during hyperflexion of the elbow for immobilisation

C. Referral for admission for relevant Gartland type 2 and all type 3 fractures

D. Immobilisation in flexion when the elbow is significantly swollen

5. Regarding vascular compromise associated with supracondylar fracture, which ONE of the following statements is INCORRECT?

A. If the hand is pulseless, cool and pale, the fracture should be reduced immediately in the ED

B. Multiple attempts at reduction in the ED is associated with increased risk of vascular damage

C. If the hand is pulseless but remains warm and pink, the fracture should be splinted to prevent further vascular compromise until urgent reduction is done in the OT

D. Vascular surgeons should be alerted if the hand is pulseless, cool and pale

6. Regarding distal humeral fractures in children, which ONE of the following statements is CORRECT?

A. A lateral condylar fracture with <2 mm of displacement requires operative management

B. Medial condylar fractures are rare in children

C. Medial epicondylar avulsion occurs in children <5 years old

D. Vascular compromise is common with lateral condylar fractures

7. During assessment of a child with a fracture in the distal one-third of the radius, which ONE of the following injuries is MOST likely to be missed in the ED?

A. Plastic deformity of the ulna without fracture

B. A proximal ulna fracture

C. Dislocation of the distal radioulnar joint

D. Dislocation of the radial head

8. Regarding femur fractures in children, which ONE of the following statements is FALSE?

A. It may be caused by minimal trauma or a twisting injury during ordinary play

B. The majority of femur fractures in children <1 year of age are secondary to accidental injury

C. Shock is common in isolated femur fractures in children

D. In toddlers (1–2 year olds) spiral fractures are common

9. Regarding Toddler's fracture, which ONE of the following statements is FALSE?

A. The fracture is usually visible on a lateral X-ray in the first week

B. Children < 2 years of age usually present with refusal to walk or a painful limp

C. When there is no history of a witnessed mechanism and the leg X-rays are normal, a full blood count (FBC) and inflammatory markers are indicated

D. It should be treated with a long leg walking cast, even if the fracture is not visible on X-ray

10. Regarding acute septic arthritis and osteomyelitis in children, which ONE of the following statements is TRUE?

A. Both conditions most commonly occur secondary to direct inoculation from an overlying local wound

B. Widening of the joint space is an early sign seen on X-ray in acute septic arthritis

C. Osteomyelitis most commonly affects metaphysis of long bones

D. *Streptococcal* species are the most commonly isolated organisms in clidren

11. When differentiating transient synovitis of the hip from septic arthritis in a child who presents with a history of inability to weight-bear, which ONE of the following features is MOST likely to be helpful towards diagnosing transient synovitis?

A. Pain-free passive movement of the hip on examination

B. Lateral displacement of the femoral epiphysis on X-ray (Waldenstrom's sign) due to a hip effusion

C. Pain in the hip, groin, medial thigh or knee

D. White cell count (WCC) < 12 × 10⁶/L in serum

12. Regarding interpretation of children's cervical spine radiographs, all of the following are correct EXCEPT:

A. Fractures of the upper cervical spine above C3–4 level is more common than that of the lower spine in children < 8 years of age

B. Anterior atlantodental space (preodontoid space) is < 5 mm in those < 8 years of age

C. C2–3 pseudosubluxation is common and can be identified by assessing posterior vertebral and spinolaminar lines

D. A fracture-like appearance at the base of the odontoid should be interpreted as incomplete ossification (synchondrosis)

13. Regarding injuries to the sternoclavicular joint and medial part of the clavicle, which ONE of the following statements is TRUE?

A. Routine clavicular radiographs have a high sensitivity for diagnosis

B. Signs of superior mediastinal impingement should be sought

C. Pneumothorax is not a recognised complication of this fracture

D. A minimal functional impairment can be expected from these injuries

14. Which ONE of the following is INCORRECT regarding an acute rotator cuff tear?

A. Forced hyperabduction or hyperextension of the shoulder is a frequent mechanism

B. The presence of chronic impingement increases the chance of having an acute tear

C. The most commonly affected component is the supraspinatus tendon and muscle

D. Most rotator cuff tears cannot be identified and assessed with ultrasound therefore MRI is required

15. Regarding the radiographic appearance of posterior dislocation of the shoulder joint, which ONE of the following statements is INCORRECT?

A. The anteroposterior (AP) view of the normal overlap between the humeral head and glenoid fossa may be lost

B. The Hill-Sachs deformity is usually present

C. Transcapular view confirms the diagnosis

D. On the AP view the humeral head is in internal rotation, producing a 'lightbulb' sign

16. Which ONE of the following abnormalities in a distal radial fracture is LEAST likely to require reduction in the ED?

A. Dorsal tilt of 20 degrees

B. Dorsal displacement

C. Volar tilt of 10 degrees

D. Radial shift

17. Regarding scapholunate dislocation, which ONE of the following statements is TRUE?

A. Scapholunate dislocation is likely if the space between the scaphoid and lunate is >1 mm in an adult on the PA view of a wrist X-ray

B. Lunate does not maintain the normal position in relation to the distal radius

C. Ischaemic necrosis of lunate (Kienbock's disease) is a complication of a missed injury

D. MRI has a high sensitivity and specificity in the diagnosis

18. Regarding perilunate dislocation, which ONE of the following statements is TRUE?

A. On lateral X-ray of the wrist, the lunate is shown to be pushed off the distal radius

B. On lateral X-ray of the wrist, the capitate is dorsally dislocated

C. This injury is seldom associated with fractures

D. This injury usually causes gross deformity at the wrist

19. Regarding emergent referral for replantation of an amputated digit which ONE of the following condition is NOT an indication?

A. Amputation proximal to flexor digitorum superficialis insertion

B. Amputation of a finger in the paediatric age group

C. Amputation of multiple digits

D. Amputation of a thumb

20. In a conscious multitrauma patient, compartment syndrome of the forearm was diagnosed a few hours after the injury, which included a fracture of the midshaft of radius and ulna. Regarding the initial management of compartment syndrome, which ONE of the following steps is LEAST likely to be beneficial?

A. Removal of the cast and dressings

B. Elevation of the forearm above the level of the heart to reduce oedema

C. Supporting BP with inotropes if the patient is hypotensive

D. Urgent surgical fasciotomy

21. Regarding the diagnosis of compartment syndrome, which ONE of the following statements is TRUE?

A. A warm limb with an easily palpable pulse may be a feature

B. Excessive pain usually develops after 48 hours

C. Motor deficit in the affected nerve distribution is usually an early feature

D. Permanent damage to the muscles and nerves in the compartment begins after 15–20 hours

22. Regarding an elderly patient with a fractured neck of femur, which of the following is the MOST appropriate ED management?

A. Skin traction should be applied early in the ED because it is proven to reduce preoperative pain

B. Oxygen therapy is not important because it has no proven benefit in reducing complications

C. A three-in-one femoral nerve block should be done in the ED because most effective analgesia can be provided with this method

D. Detailed medical assessment in the ED has no proven value

23. An 82-year-old woman presents 3 days after a mechanical fall at home. She has mild dementia. Since the fall she is able to walk but with considerable right hip pain. Her leg is not shortened or externally rotated. On examination, she has some tenderness in the right inguinal region and has restricted active range of movement due to pain. She has almost full passive range of movement with pain in that hip. Her pelvis X-ray and AP and lateral right hip X-rays appear normal. Regarding an occult neck of femur fracture, which ONE of the following is TRUE?

A. 30% of patients with normal X-ray have an occult fracture diagnosed on MRI

B. Early bone scan is indicated because it can detect fracture as well as tumours and septic hip

C. When an occult fracture is suspected, the acceptable approach is to advise bed rest and non-weight bearing, with a repeat X-ray in 7 days

D. CT should be done and, if the CT is negative, the patient can be safely discharged without further investigations

24. Regarding hip dislocation, which ONE of the following statements is INCORRECT?

A. Avascular necrosis of the femoral head is a complication

B. When a patient presents overnight to the ED, the reduction can be delayed up to 12 hours

C. An incarcerated tendon or capsule is often the cause of difficulty in reductions

D. A post-reduction CT is indicated to assess for acetabular and femoral head fractures

25. Regarding collateral ligamentous injuries of the knee, which ONE of the following statements is INCORRECT?

A. Injuries to the medial side is more common than injuries to the lateral side

B. Laxity of 1 cm with a firm end point on stress indicates a complete tear

C. Peroneal nerve injury is associated with lateral collateral ligament injury

D. Haemarthrosis is an associated feature

26. Regarding clinical diagnosis of a cruciate ligament injury, which ONE of the following statements is TRUE?

A. The majority of patients with a traumatic haemarthrosis have anterior cruciate ligament (ACL) injuries

B. Anterior drawer test, Lachman test and lateral pivot shift test have similar sensitivities in the diagnosis of an ACL injury

C. Isolated posterior cruciate ligament (PCL) tears are more common than isolated ACL tears

D. A meniscal injury is more likely to cause haemarthrosis than a cruciate ligament injury

27. Regarding the diagnostic accuracy of a physical examination in detecting a meniscal injury, which ONE of the following examinations is likely to be MOST accurate?

A. Composite examination of the knee

B. A finding of joint line tenderness

C. A positive McMurray test

D. Presence of a knee effusion

28. Regarding ankle sprains, which ONE of the following statements is TRUE?

A. Ligament sprains on the medial side of the ankle most commonly occur as isolated injuries

B. Deltoid ligament sprains are more common than anterior talofibular ligament sprains

C. A crossed-leg test to rule out injuries to the tibiofibular syndesmotic complex has no bearing in the assessment

D. Peroneal tendon subluxation or dislocation may mimic a lateral collateral ligament sprain

29. Regarding radiographic assessment of an ankle in a patient who has a clinical diagnosis of an acute ankle sprain, which ONE of the following statements is INCORRECT?

A. The lateral view is helpful in identifying a joint effusion

B. Ankle joint margins should be parallel and the medial part of the joint space should not exceed 4 mm in the mortise view

C. Avulsion fractures are often present but they do not correlate to the location of ligamentous injuries

D. Syndesmotic disruption can be identified by examining the distal tibial and fibular overlap on an AP view

30. Regarding an Achilles tendon rupture, which ONE of the following statements is INCORRECT?

A. A Thompson test and hyperdorsiflexion may be helpful in diagnosis

B. Weak plantar flexion is not possible when there is a complete tendon rupture

C. A large defect on palpation indicates a worse prognosis with non-operative management than a small defect

D. For selected patients a short leg cast can be applied, with the foot at gravity equinus position

31. Regarding fracture of the talar dome, which ONE of the following statements is TRUE?

A. Examination findings are non-specific and may mimic an ankle sprain

B. Eversion mechanisms at the ankle mainly cause this injury

C. It does not usually cause gross oedema in the ankle

D. This injury should be managed as an ankle sprain

32. Regarding ankle fractures, which ONE of the following statements is TRUE?

A. Pilon fractures of the distal tibia are frequently associated with fractures involving multiple lower limb sites

B. Medial malleolar fractures occur as isolated injuries in the majority of patients

C. A lateral malleolar fracture at or below the ankle joint line are more likely to cause distal tibiofibular syndesmosis disruption than fractures above the joint line

D. Bimalleolar fractures are considered stable injuries

33. Which ONE of the following features is LEAST likely to be associated with a significant Lisfranc's injury?

A. Associated compartment syndrome

B. Tarsal and metatarsal fractures

C. Increased foot arch height

D. Disruption of the Lisfranc's ligament

34. Regarding unilateral facet joint dislocation in the cervical spine, which ONE of the following statements is TRUE?

A. As appears on the lateral X-ray, the vertebral body is displaced anteriorly for more than 50% of its width

B. Associated spinal cord injury is common

C. The usual mechanism is hyperextension of the cervical spine

D. This is a stable injury when there is no associated fracture present

35. An adult male who had a cervical spine injury with a significant mechanism presents to the ED complaining of severe pain and limited range of motion. Fracture and dislocation have been excluded with a CT scan. Regarding *isolated ligamentous injury* to the cervical spine, which ONE of the following statements is INCORRECT?

A. Isolated ligamentous injuries are common in cervical spine injuries due to high-risk mechanisms

B. Isolated ligamentous injuries may cause delayed instability

C. Hyperextension sprain causes widening of the anterior part of the intervertebral space

D. Increased pre-dental space (the space between the odontoid process and anterior arch of the atlas vertebra) on lateral cervical spine view and CT is found in rupture of transverse ligament

36. Regarding a patient presenting with acute lumbosacral pain without sciatica, which ONE of the following statements is TRUE?

A. 60–70% take over 6 months to recover

B. Radiological imaging is nearly always likely to find the cause

C. Staying active as opposed to bed rest results in improved functional status and early pain reduction

D. This is often due to herniated nucleus pulposus

37. Regarding sciatica, which ONE of the following statements is TRUE?

A. When due to herniated nucleus pulposus (HNP) most patients require surgical intervention to resolve pain

B. In the elderly sciatica is nearly always due to disc herniation

C. In all patients presenting with sciatica CT imaging is indicated if not done prior

D. Neuropathic pain medication such as tricyclic antidepressants and selective noradrenagic reuptake inhibitors should be tried in sciatica

38. A 70-year-old female presents to the ED with acute low back pain. The report of a CT lumbar spine ordered by the general practitioner (GP) states that there is moderate to severe lumbar spinal canal stenosis with degenerative changes of the lumbar vertebrae. On examination, there is no neurological deficit. Regarding lumbar spinal canal stenosis, all of the following statements are true EXCEPT:

A. Most common symptoms are neurogenic claudication, which include mechanical low back pain radiating to the buttocks and the entire legs

B. Pain worsens with walking or standing and resolves with sitting

C. Cauda equina syndrome is common

D. The symptoms should be differentiated from vascular claudication

39. A 40-year-old man presents to the ED with a history of a penetrating injury to the palmar surface of the middle phalanx of the left middle finger. The injury happened 2 weeks ago when he was using a cordless drill during a DIY job at home. For the past 3 days his finger has become swollen and painful. There is a limited range of movement at the proximal (PIP) and distal interphalangeal (DIP) joints due to severe pain. Regarding assessment and management of this patient, which ONE of the following statements is TRUE?

A. Identifying specific areas of tenderness in the finger may not help as it is non-specific

B. Middle finger infection is unlikely to spread to the midpalmar space

C. Initial conservative management with intravenous antibiotics for 24 hours should be attempted

D. Pain during passive extension of the PIP and DIP joints indicates flexor sheath tenosynovitis

40. Regarding likely infecting organisms involved in causing acute osteomyelitis in adults, all of the following statements are true EXCEPT:

A. Polymicrobial infections, which include *Staphylococcus aureus, Staphylococcus pyogenes*, coliforms and anaerobes cause oeteomyelitis in poorly controlled diabetics

B. *Staphylococcus aureus* and *Pseudomonas* are common in injecting drug users

C. Coagulase negative *Staphylococci* are likely to be involved in causing infection associated with orthopaedic hardware

D. Gram-negative enteric bacteria is the most common cause in the elderly

CHAPTER 15
SURGICAL EMERGENCIES

QUESTIONS

Alison Boyle

1. Regarding appendicitis, which ONE of the following statements is most CORRECT?

  A. Pain may be localised to the flank or right upper quadrant

  B. Obturator sign is positive when pain is elicited on external rotation of the hip

  C. A patient with a MANTRELS score of <7 should be referred for surgery

  D. The perforation rate is high between the ages of 5 and 60 years

2. Which ONE of the following is the MOST LIKELY diagnosis for a 68-year-old male who presents to the emergency department (ED) with a history of left lower quadrant abdominal pain and tenderness, low-grade fever and altered bowel habit?

  A. Pyelonephritis

  B. Irritable bowel syndrome

  C. Sigmoid volvulus

  D. Diverticulitis

3. An elderly patient with atrial fibrillation presents with acute severe abdominal pain, nausea and vomiting. Which ONE of the following would MOST support the diagnosis of acute mesenteric ischaemia?

  A. Generalised abdominal pain, abdominal distension and last bowel movement 5 days ago

  B. Fever, generalised abdominal pain that *was* localised to the right lower quadrant

  C. Fever, generalised abdominal pain out of keeping with physical examination and pneumatosis intestinalis on abdominal X-ray

  D. Fever, abdominal pain radiating to the back, bruising around the umbilical region and an elevated serum lipase

4. A 56-year-old male patient presents to the ED with acute abdominal pain. He is a smoker and takes aspirin for a heart condition. He has severe, constant epigastric pain that radiates to the left shoulder. He has associated vomiting but no haematemesis. On examination his vital signs are HR 104, BP 135/89, RR 22, temp 37.2°. He has rebound tenderness on palpation of the abdomen. Erect chest X-ray (CXR) demonstrates a small amount of free air under the diaphragm. Which ONE of the following describes the MOST appropriate management?

  A. Nil by mouth, IV access, 2 L IV crystalloid stat, analgesia and urgent upper abdominal ultrasound scan (USS)

  B. Nil by mouth, IV access, fluid resuscitate to maintain adequate blood pressure, IV analgesia, antiemetic, nasogastric tube (NGT), urgent CT scan and surgical referral

  C. Nil by mouth, large bore IV access, IV analgesia, triple antibiotics and transfer to theatre for urgent laparotomy

  D. Nil by mouth, IV fluids to maintain adequate BP, NGT insertion, IV analgesia, antiemetic, IV esomeprazole, triple antibiotics and urgent surgical referral

5. What ONE of the following is the MOST common cause of small bowel obstruction (SBO) in the adult population?

  A. Inflammatory bowel disease

  B. Adhesions

  C. Intussusception

  D. Hernia

6. Which ONE of the following is the MOST common reason for large bowel/colonic obstruction?

  A. Adhesions

  B. Neoplasms

  C. Hernias

  D. Diverticulitis

7. A 69-year-old man presents to the ED with abdominal bloating over the past 4 hours. He has severe generalised abdominal pain and nausea but no vomiting. He has been unable to pass flatus for several hours. An abdominal X-ray demonstrates a large dilated loop of bowel that extends from the pelvis towards the right upper quadrant and looks like a bent inner tube. Multiple air fluid levels are seen within the small bowel loops.

Which ONE of the statements below describes the MOST appropriate management?

  A. IV fluids, nil by mouth, nasogastric tube insertion and triple antibiotics

B. IV fluids, nil by mouth, nasogastric tube insertion referral for laparotomy

C. IV fluids, nil by mouth, nasogastric tube insertion, sigmoidoscopy and insertion of a rectal tube

D. IV fluids, nil by mouth, nasogastric tube insertion, contrast enema

8. Use of bedside ultrasound for detecting abdominal aortic aneurysm in the ED is becoming increasingly common. Which ONE of the following statements pertaining to this is TRUE?

A. Emergency clinicians with relatively limited training can reliably detect an abdominal aortic aneurysm

B. The lumen of the aorta should be measured from inner wall to inner wall

C. The probe selected should have a frequency of 7–12 mHz

D. Bedside ultrasound can reliably exclude a ruptured abdominal aortic aneurysm

9. Abdominal aortic aneurysms (AAA) are at risk of rupture. Which ONE of the following statements is most CORRECT?

A. Risk of rupture is increased in women, non-smokers and increasing age

B. Most patients with rupture present with all of: hypotension, pain and a pulsatile mass

C. Rupture can present with gastrointestinal bleeding

D. Tenderness on palpation is a sign of rupture

10. A 63-year-old man with atrial fibrillation had pelvic radiotherapy 2 months ago. He now presents with lower abdominal pain, diarrhoea, rectal bleeding and tenesmus. What is the MOST likely diagnosis?

A. Radiation proctocolitis

B. Ulcerative colitis

C. Infective colitis

D. Ischaemic colitis

11. A 28-year-old woman who is 31 weeks pregnant presents with right lower abdominal pain and vomiting. She has a temperature of 37.8°C, HR 110 and systolic blood pressure of 120. There is tenderness and guarding in the right lower quadrant. Which ONE of the following statements Is TRUE?

A. Pain in the right lower quadrant in advanced pregnancy is uncommon in appendicitis

B. Appendicitis is more common in pregnant than non-pregnant women

C. Ultrasound has a higher sensitivity and specificity in a pregnant patient compared with that of the non-pregnant population

D. Pregnant patients in the first trimester are less likely to have perforation of the appendix than those in the second or third trimesters

12. Which ONE of the following is NOT associated with cholelithiasis?

A. Sickle cell disease

B. Rapid weight loss

C. Crohn's disease

D. Hypercalcaemia

13. A patient who is known to have cholelithiasis presents to the ED. Which ONE of the following patients does NOT have a complication of gallstones?

A. A patient with right upper quadrant pain, fever 39.1°C, jaundice, HR 124, hypotension and dilated intrahepatic ducts on ultrasound

B. A patient with vomiting, right upper quadrant pain and tenderness with a temperature of 36.6°C

C. A patient with crampy abdominal pain, bile-stained vomiting, mild abdominal distention and HR 118

D. A patient with epigastric pain, vomiting, diaphoresis and a HR 52

14. In the investigation and diagnosis of cholecystitis, which ONE of the statements below is the most CORRECT?

A. CT is a more useful test than ultrasound scan (USS) for acute cholecystitis

B. Absence of gallstones does not exclude the diagnosis

C. Laboratory investigations are frequently abnormal

D. 30% of gallstones can be see on abdominal X-ray

15. Recognised complications of pancreatitis include all of the following EXCEPT:

A. Acute respiratory distress syndrome (ARDS)

B. Pleural effusion

C. Hyperglycaemia

D. Hypercalcaemia

16. Which ONE of the following is NOT a clinical predictor in acute pancreatitis?

A. Calcium < 2 mmol/L

B. Glucose < 10 mmol/L

C. PaO$_2$ < 60 mmHg

D. AST > 250 IU/L

17. A 58-year-old male presents with pruritis and dark urine. On examination there is a mild yellow discolouration of his sclera. Which ONE of the following statements is most CORRECT?

A. Presence of urobilinogen in the urine is suggestive of biliary obstruction

B. Testicular atrophy and caput medusa are suggestive of a pancreatic tumour

C. An ultrasound examination showing the presence of a common bile duct stone with dilated intra and extra-hepatic biliary system is consistent with Mirizzi syndrome

D. Jaundice is evident clinically in tissues with high albumin concentrations

18. Which ONE of the statements regarding hernias is most CORRECT?

A. Incisional hernias have a narrow origin and complications are uncommon

B. Umbilical hernias resolve spontaneously in children

C. Direct inguinal hernias occur more frequently in the older age group, extend into the scrotum and can become strangulated requiring surgery

D. Indirect inguinal hernias occur due to a defect in the transversalis fascia and anterior abdominal wall; they may become strangulated and require surgery

19. Regarding hernias, which ONE of the following statements is the most CORRECT?

A. Reduction of an incarcerated inguinal hernia should always be attempted in the ED

B. For reduction of an incarcerated inguinal hernia the patient should be given adequate analgesia, sedation if necessary and placed in an upright position for reduction

C. An incarcerated inguinal hernia can be managed conservatively with an elastic hernia belt

D. Femoral hernias occur more commonly in women and have a high rate of strangulation

20. Which ONE of the following patients is the MOST suitable for discharge from the ED?

A. 77-year-old female, low-grade fever 37.7°C, cognitively normal, with one episode of vomiting, mild lower abdominal pain, no rebound or guarding with a urine dipstick that is positive for nitrites and large leucocytes

B. 82-year-old female who has constipation, is confused, afebrile, has central abdominal pain and a distended abdomen

C. 73-year-old male, history of hypertension with sudden onset of flank pain and a BP of 95/62

D. 86-year-old male with diarrhoea and vomiting with mild generalised abdominal pain

21. A 68-year-old gentleman with a history of ischaemic heart disease who had percutaneous coronary angiography (PCA) several weeks ago presents to the ED with a lump in the right groin. He is a keen gardener and has a history of inguinal hernia. It has been gradually increasing in size, is not reducible and is tender to palpate. He also complains of weakness in his right leg. His vital signs are HR 88, BP 132/78, temp 36.9°C. Which is the MOST likely diagnosis?

A. Incarcerated inguinal hernia

B. Incarcerated femoral hernia

C. Femoral artery pseudoaneurysm

D. Haematoma

22. Which ONE of the following is TRUE regarding Boerhaave's syndrome?

A. It is associated with rupture of the left posterior wall of the lower oesophagus

B. CXR is normal in 60% of patients

C. The classic presentation is vomiting, chest pain and shortness of breath

D. Haematemesis is common

23. A 69-year-old man who has been immobile for 3 days presents with sudden onset of painful right lower leg. The leg is pale and cool to touch. He has a past medical history that includes, hypertension, non-insulin-dependent diabetes and heavy smoking. He has recently been treated for atrial fibrillation and is now rate controlled. Which ONE of the options below is the most CORRECT? This patient should:

A. Have IV unfractionated heparin and urgent referral for embolectomy

B. Have urgent investigation with Doppler ultrasound followed by treatment with thrombolysis providing there are no contraindications

C. Have urgent investigation with Doppler ultrasound followed by treatment with therapeutic subcutaneous low molecular weight heparin

D. Have the ankle-brachial index checked, ECG, CXR, angiography and be referred to the outpatient clinic for follow up

24. A patient with a history of intravenous drug use presents with an acutely painful hand. It is cool, pale and mottled. Radial and ulnar pulses are present. The second–third fingertips are dusky in colour and there is pain on both passive and active wrist movement. Other than an elevated creatine kinase level of 3000 IU/L (35–145 IU/L normal range), laboratory investigations are all within the normal range. What is the MOST likely diagnosis?

A. Raynaud's disease

B. Inadvertent intraarterial injection of a drug

C. Acute ischaemic limb

D. Deep venous thrombosis (DVT) of the upper limb

25. A patient with a history of intravenous drug use presents with an acutely painful hand. It is cool, pale and mottled. Radial and ulnar pulses are present. The second–third fingertips are dusky in colour and there is pain on both passive and active wrist movement. Other than an elevated creatine kinase level of 3000 IU/L (35–145 IU/L normal range), laboratory investigations are all within the normal range. What is the MOST appropriate next step?

A. Request a Doppler ultrasound scan (USS) of the upper limb and commence heparin infusion

B. Rest, elevation, compression bandage and analgesia. Commence subcutaneous low molecular weight heparin and warfarin

C. Measure compartmental pressures and consider fasciotomy

D. Analgesia, heparin infusion, Doppler USS, measure compartmental pressures, consider fasciotomy

26. Which ONE of the following statements about aortic dissection is TRUE?

A. Distal dissections require surgical intervention

B. CXR is a specific investigation

C. Neurological complications occur frequently

D. The site of dissection rarely occurs at a site where atherosclerosis is present

27. Which ONE of the following statements about haemorrhoids is most CORRECT?

A. Portal hypertension is a cause of haemorrhoids

B. They can present with pruritis ani, mucoid discharge and prolapse

C. Internal haemorrhoids originate above the dentate line and have somatic innervation

D. Thrombosed external haemorrhoids can be incised and drained in the ED

28. Regarding pilonidal sinus, which ONE of the following statements is TRUE?

A. They are seen more commonly in females than males

B. Recurrence is common and can be seen in up to 40% of patients

C. They are treated primarily with antibiotics

D. They are frequently seen in the over-50 age group

29. Regarding infection of the breast, which ONE of the following statements is the most CORRECT?

A. Breast infections occur in one of every 10 lactating women

B. In non-lactating women *Staphylococcus epidermidis* is the most common causative organism

C. Risk factors include smoking, diabetes and gestational age <41weeks

D. The majority of cases in lactating women can be treated with oral co-amoxiclav and regular expression of milk from the breast

30. Which ONE of the wounds described below is MOST suitable for delayed primary closure?

A. An 8 cm wound to the medial thigh through the subcutaneous tissue from a surfboard that occurred 6 hours ago

B. A dog bite, with laceration to the finger that occurred 4 hours ago

C. Laceration to the hand from broken glass that occurred 12 hours ago

D. A pretibial skin flap in an elderly patient who fell on a curb

31. Which ONE of the flowing statements describes the CORRECT management of abdominal wound dehiscence?

A. Clean the wound, take a swab for culture and sensitivity and surgical referral for urgent wound exploration

B. Clean the wound, take a swab for culture and sensitivity, debride the edges and close the wound in the ED

C. Clean the wound, pack with sterile saline-soaked gauze, dress with an absorbent dressing, commence on oral antibiotics and general practitioner (GP) follow-up

D. Clean the wound, pack with sterile saline-soaked gauze, dress with an absorbent dressing, commence on oral antibiotics and urgent referral to surgical outpatients

32. With respect to subarachnoid haemorrhage (SAH), which ONE of the following is FALSE?

A. Risk factors include polycystic kidney disease, smoking and hypertension

B. ECG may mimic an acute myocardial infarction

C. Arteriovenous malformation is seen more often in the older population

D. Presenting signs and symptoms include seizures, focal neurological deficit and intraocular haemorrhages

33. In the investigation and management of SAH, which ONE of the following is TRUE?

A. Non-contrast CT scan is a reliable test at 48 hours

B. Xanthochromia may be present in a traumatic lumbar puncture sample

C. Nimodipine is used to prevent hypertension

D. Rebleeding, seizures, fever, electrolyte disturbances and cerebral salt wasting are all recognised complications of SAH

34. A 4-week-old baby girl presents to the ED with sudden and persistent bilious vomiting. She is lethargic and mottled. What is the next MOST appropriate step in her management?

A. Trial of oral fluids in the ED

B. Rapid rehydration either via NGT or IV fluids

C. IV access, correction of fluid and electrolyte imbalance, urgent ultrasound and elective surgical repair

D. IV fluid resuscitation with 20 mL/kg normal saline, IV antibiotics (ampicillin, gentamicin, metronidazole) and urgent surgical intervention

35. Pyloric stenosis is associated with which ONE of the following?

A. A higher incidence in the first-born child

B. Non-bilious vomiting and diarrhoea

C. Reduced appetite and weight loss

D. Hyperkalaemic, hypochloraemic metabolic alkalosis

36. Which of the following is LEAST likely to cause abdominal pain in children?

A. Migraine

B. Congenital adrenal hyperplasia

C. Lead poisoning

D. Henoch-Schönlein purpura

37. Which of the following is most CORRECT with respect to intussusception?

A. It occurs more commonly in females than males

B. The peak incidence is between ages 2 and 6 years

C. It may be associated with Henoch-Schönlein purpura

D. On examination the abdomen may be distended with a sausage-shaped mass palpable in the left upper quadrant

38. A 2-year-old boy presents with rectal bleeding, mild crampy abdominal pain and mild anaemia. Abdominal X-rays are unremarkable and a barium enema looks normal. What is the MOST likely diagnosis?

A. Meckel's diverticulum

B. Intussusception

C. Haemophilia

D. Anal fissure

39. Which ONE of the following statements relating to upper gastrointestinal tract foreign bodies is CORRECT?

A. A button battery located in the stomach 8 hours post ingestion needs urgent endoscopic removal

B. On anterior–posterior (AP) X-ray coins lying in the sagittal plane are more likely to be in the oesophagus

C. Mediastinitis is a recognised complication of an oesophageal foreign body

D. In adults an oesophageal foreign body is most likely to get stuck at the cricopharyngeal region

40. A 6-year-old girl presents with a 4-day history of a large 6.5 cm left submandibular swelling. She has a fever of 39.2°C and is lethargic, airway is not compromised, pharynx is red and inflamed, tonsils are not enlarged, no conjunctivitis or rash. The swelling is red, hot, tender and fluctuant. What is the MOST appropriate action?

A. Administer PR paracetamol 125 mg, discharge home on dicloxacillin 250 mg 6-hourly for 7 days and advise to represent if not improving

B. Administer PO ibuprofen 200 mg, take bloods for FBC and culture, IV cephazolin 400 mg 12-hourly, ultrasound neck, surgical review for incision and drainage

C. Administer ibuprofen PO 400 mg, take bloods for FBC and culture, IV flucloxacillin 1 g 6-hourly, ultrasound and needle aspiration in the ED

D. Administer PO paracetamol 300 mg, take bloods for FBC and culture, IV flucloxacillin 500 mg 6-hourly, ultrasound neck, surgical review for incision and drainage

Waruna de Alwis

1. Regarding a positive relative afferent pupillary defect (RAPD), all of the following statements are true EXCEPT:

A. The pupil on the affected side dilates when the light is swung to it from the opposite eye

B. It means there is a disturbance anywhere along the anterior afferent visual pathway

C. A patient with a positive afferent pupillary defect on testing will have a dilated pupil on the affected eye prior to testing

D. Intraocular haemorrhage, central retinal artery or vein occlusion, retinal detachment and optic tract lesions produce a positive RAPD

2. Regarding childhood conjunctivitis, which ONE of the following statements is FALSE?

A. Appropriate swabs and cultures should be done in every child with conjunctivitis who presents to the emergency department (ED)

B. Adenovirus is the most common virus causing conjunctivitis and it can be part of a viral syndrome

C. Preauricular lympadenopthy is more commonly seen in viral conjunctivitis than in bacterial conjunctivitis

D. The slit lamp examination is a difficult but necessary examination in children

3. Regarding orbital cellulitis and periorbital cellulitis in children, which ONE of the following statements is TRUE?

A. Organisms originating from paranasal sinuses usually cause both conditions

B. Pain on eye movement is present in both conditions but is worse in orbital cellulitis

C. Visual acuity is preserved in both conditions

D. In orbital cellulitis, eyelid swelling does not extend into the eyebrow beyond the superior orbital rim

4. In differentiating acute anterior uveitis from other causes of acute red eye, which ONE of the following clinical features of anterior uveitis is MOST useful?

A. Photophobia in the affected eye when a light is shone into the unaffected eye

B. Worsening of eye pain on movement and during accommodation

C. Perilimbal or circumcorneal injection

D. Unilateral red eye with a deep aching pain radiating to the periorbital and temporal region

5. Regarding the diagnosis of acute angle closure glaucoma (AACG) in the ED, which ONE of the following statements is TRUE?

A. Normal intraocular pressure is 20–30 mmHg

B. If the pupil reacts, an alternative diagnosis should be considered

C. Patients commonly present with a red eye without associated eye pain

D. The anterior chamber appears deep on slit lamp examination and flare and cells can be seen

6. Which ONE of the following conditions is NOT a cause of acute painless uniocular visual loss?

A. Central retinal artery occlusion

B. Optic neuritis

C. Posterior vitreous detachment

D. Vitreous haemorrhage

7. Regarding assessment and management of central retinal artery occlusion (CRAO) and central retinal vein occlusion (CRVO), which ONE of the following statements is INCORRECT?

A. In both conditions the visual loss can be abrupt

B. A 'blood and thunder' appearance of the retina can be seen in CRVO

C. Emergent referral to ophthalmology is indicated in both CRAO and CRVO

D. There is no evidence to suggest that emergent therapies such as pulse massage of the eyeball and intravenous acetazolamide are effective

8. Regarding central retinal artery occlusion, which ONE of the following statements is TRUE?

A. Atherosclerosis in the carotid arteries and emboli originating in the heart are the two most common causes

B. Relative afferent pupillary defect is absent

C. Local intraarterial thrombolysis has proven benefit

D. The majority of patients will recover to gain a good visual acuity

9. A 65-year-old woman presents to the ED with an isolated dilated pupil on the left side. There is no history of significant head injury. All of the following are likely causes of her isolated dilated pupil EXCEPT:

A. Adie's tonic pupil

B. Blunt trauma to the eye

C. Horner's syndrome

D. Isolated third nerve palsy

10. Regarding ED management of acid and alkali injuries to the eye, which ONE of the following is the LEAST appropriate option?

A. If visual acuity and slit lamp examination are normal, irrigation of the eye with 1 L of normal saline

B. Continuous irrigation with normal saline until normal pH is restored

C. Checking pH 30 minutes after the normal pH is restored

D. Urgent referral to ophthalmology if corneal clouding or epithelia defect is present

11. Regarding an orbital blowout fracture, which ONE of the following statements is TRUE?

A. Usually there is an extension of the fracture to the orbital rim

B. Enophthalmos and a difference in the pupillary level may be present

C. The most common complication is restriction of downward gaze

D. Periorbital ecchymosis may be present but not periorbital emphysema

12. Regarding an orbital blowout fracture, which ONE of the following statements is CORRECT?

A. An isolated blowout fracture with features of entrapment require urgent surgery within 24–48 hours

B. Significant injury to the eye is not usually associated with this fracture

C. It should be treated with oral antibiotics

D. Retrobulbar haematoma is not a recognised complication

13. Regarding a patient presenting to the ED with a suspected retrobulbar haematoma following blunt trauma to the orbit, all of the following statements are true EXCEPT:

A. If there is no visual loss, reducing elevated intraocular pressure with intravenous mannitol or acetazolamide can be attempted first

B. If there is visual loss lateral canthotomy is indicated

C. Lateral canthotomy done in the ED usually results in significant complications

D. Lateral canthotomy can be done under local anaesthetic

14. Regarding the control of bleeding in posterior epistaxis, all of the following methods may be helpful EXCEPT:

A. Inflatable balloons such as Foley catheter and Rapid Rhino®

B. Endoscopic surgical ligation or embolisation of the bleeding vessel

C. Thrombogenic foams and gels

D. Transpalatal injection of vasoconstrictor near the sphenopalatine artery

15. Regarding a patient presenting to the ED with epistaxis, which ONE of the following statements is TRUE?

A. Posterior epistaxis is more common in young patients

B. There is a clear association between hypertension and epistaxis

C. When posterior packing is done with a Foley catheter, the balloon should be fully inflated to 30 cc to achieve an effective tamponade

D. Chemical cautery should be done on one side only

16. Regarding peritonsillar abscess, which ONE of the following statements is TRUE?

A. A better outcome can be achieved with incision and drainage of a peritonsillar abscess than by needle aspiration

B. Anaerobes are the most commonly isolated organisms causing peritonsillar abscess

C. The clinical features of peritonsillar cellulitis are similar to peritonsillar abscess except there is no surrounding pus

D. Transcutaneous ultrasound scan has a low utility in the diagnosis

17. A 55-year-old adult male presents to the ED with a severe sore throat and fever of 36 hours' duration. Which ONE of the following features LEAST supports a presumptive diagnosis of adult epiglottitis (supraglottitis)?

A. Bilateral submandibular swelling

B. Soft, low-pitched inspiratory stridor

C. Tenderness caused by gentle palpation of the larynx

D. 'Thumb print' sign on the lateral soft tissue X-ray of the neck

18. Regarding removal of nasal foreign bodies in children, all of the following statements are true EXCEPT:

A. Positive pressure techniques are recommended as first-line methods of removal for most foreign bodies that are not firmly impacted

B. The 'big kiss' and 'modified big kiss' techniques often cause barotrauma to the lungs

C. The success rates with the use of a balloon catheters is high

D. During procedural sedation, the preservation of gag and cough reflexes is important to prevent aspiration

19. Regarding nasal fractures in children, which ONE of the following statements is TRUE?

A. These should be reduced within 4 days

B. Children have a lower risk for poor cosmetic outcome than adults with similar nasal fractures

C. Closed reduction under general anaesthetic is usually not required

D. Nasal obstruction that occurs due to a fracture is likely to get better as the child grows

20. Regarding malignant otitis externa, which ONE of the following statements is INCORRECT?

A. Otalgia is out of proportion to what is expected from acute otitis externa

B. It is caused by *Pseudomonas* infection in more than 90% of patients

C. It should be suspected when acute otitis externa is not improving with appropriate treatment

D. If cranial nerve involvement is present, an alternative diagnosis is more likely than malignant otitis externa

21. Regarding repair of a through-and-through laceration involving the pinna of the ear, which ONE of the following statements is TRUE?

A. If a haematoma develops a few days after suturing a laceration, it should be treated conservatively

B. As cartilage heals slowly, the skin sutures should be removed in 10–14 days

C. If the cartilage is exposed due to avulsed skin, the wound should be managed with non-adherent dressings until skin cover develops

D. A repaired large laceration should always be covered with a properly placed pressure dressing

22. Regarding Ludwig's angina, which ONE of the following statements is FALSE?

A. Awake fibre optic tracheal intubation should be considered early in the presentation

B. Dental infection is the most commonly attributed cause

C. Infection and swelling is primarily outside the submandibular space

D. CT scan may be helpful to determine if the patient needs to go to the operating theatre

23. Regarding an avulsed tooth, which ONE of the following statements is TRUE?

A. Both primary and permanent teeth should be replaced after avulsion

B. An avulsed tooth that is also fractured should be replaced into the socket

C. Milk preserves periodontal ligament cells for 4–8 hours when the tooth is placed in milk immediately after avulsion

D. An avulsed tooth should not be replaced in the prehospital setting

24. Regarding a patient presenting to the ED with continued bleeding from the tooth socket after extraction, which ONE of the following is the LEAST appropriate management?

A. Infiltrate the gingiva surrounding the bleeding socket with lignocaine and adrenaline (1 : 100,000)

B. Leave any clot inside the socket

C. Place a coagulation sponge such as Gelfoam or Surgicel in the socket

D. Close the gingiva over the socket tightly with 3-0 absorbable sutures

25. Regarding tongue lacerations, which ONE of the following statements is FALSE?

A. A lingual block or local anaesthetic infiltration are the preferred anaesthetic choices

B. A large gaping laceration if not repaired results in a grooved or a bifid tongue

C. Lignocaine with adrenaline should not be used for local anaesthesia and to achieve haemostasis

D. A deep laceration involving the muscle can be sutured with deep stitches that penetrate both the mucosa and the muscle

QUESTIONS

Alison Boyle

1. Which ONE of the following regarding percutaneous suprapubic catheterisation (SPC) is FALSE?

A. History of previous lower abdominal surgery or irradiation is a contraindication to SPC insertion

B. Recognised complications include extraperitoneal extravasation, haematuria and injury to the bowel

C. Indications include trauma to the urethra, phimosis with urinary retention and pelvic trauma

D. It is less likely to cause bacteriuria than urethral catheterisation

2. Regarding investigation of a patient with renal colic, which ONE of the following is TRUE?

A. Most stones cannot be visualised with magnetic resonance urography

B. Nearly all stones are radiolucent

C. Haematuria is not present in 40% of patients

D. A urinary pH of <5 suggests struvite stones

3. Which ONE of the following patients with a urological presentation to the emergency department (ED) requires referral for admission?

A. A patient with a single kidney who has a distal ureteric 3 mm stone with a low degree of obstruction and who is now pain free

B. An 82-year-old man who presents with macrosopic haematuria with passage of blood clots per urethra

C. An adolescent with fever, rigors, white cell casts in the urine with normal vital signs and no vomiting

D. A 13-year-old boy with gradual onset of pain over 1–2 days in the upper pole of the right testis and a blue dot sign is visible on examination

4. A young female patient presents to the ED with right flank pain, fever, rigors and vomiting. Her heart rate is 110 and systolic blood pressure (BP) is 95 mmHg. She has a penicillin allergy. Her body weight is 72 kg. Which ONE of the following is the most appropriate empiric antibiotic regime?

A. Amoxicillin 500 mg orally 8-hourly for 7 days

B. Cephalexin 500 mg orally 6-hourly for 10 days

C. Gentamicin 220 mg IV first dose

D. Cefotaxime 1 g IV 8-hourly

5. Causes of priapism include all of the following EXCEPT:

A. Papaverine injection

B. Spinal cord injury

C. Systemic sclerosis

D. Sickle cell disease

6. Regarding the management of priapism in the ED, which ONE of the following statements is most CORRECT?

A. For low-flow priapism, administer analgesia and apply ice to the shaft for 4 hours

B. If thrombosis is the cause, administer IV fluids, oxygen and analgesia, commence exchange blood tranfusion and request a urological review

C. Prescribe analgesia, insert a urethral catheter if the patient is in retention and provide reassurance

D. If the patient has high-flow priapism perform a penile block, insert an 18-gauge needle into one of the corpus cavernosum and inject phentolamine

7. Regarding urogenital trauma, which ONE of the following statements is TRUE?

A. In blunt trauma the ureter is most likely to be injured from a rapid deceleration injury

B. Renal trauma usually occurs in isolation

C. The degree of haematuria is proportional to severity of the injury sustained from blunt trauma

D. A grade III renal injury is defined as a laceration to the parenchyma >1 cm depth with urinary extravasation or rupture of the collecting system

8. Regarding testicular torsion, which ONE of the following statements is TRUE?

A. It is mostly due to lateral rotation of the spermatic cord

B. The cremasteric reflex is always absent

C. It can be reliably excluded with scrotal ultrasound scan (USS)

D. It can be associated with a fever

9. All of the following conditions cause scrotal pain EXCEPT:

A. Mumps

B. Abdominal aortic aneurysm

C. Renal colic

D. Genital warts

10. Which ONE of the following statements regarding urinary retention is TRUE?

A. If the patient is able to pass small amounts of urine, urinary retention can be excluded

B. Medications that cause urinary retention include tricyclic antidepressants, nonsteroidal anti-inflammatory drugs (NSAIDs), selective serotonin reuptake inhibitors (SSRIs) and α-blockers

C. It is infrequently associated with obstructive uropathy causing renal impairment

D. 55% of men who present with urinary retention have or will develop prostate cancer

11. Urine dipstick testing is frequently used in the ED. Which ONE of the following statements is INCORRECT?

A. The presence of nitrites on a urine dipstick is highly sensitive for diagnosis of a urinary tract infection (UTI)

B. A negative urinalysis test on a bag urine sample in a paediatric patient is sufficient to exclude a UTI

C. Urine dipstick tests in the ED frequently give false positive or false negative readings

D. Urine dipstick is an adequate test to exclude UTI

12. Regarding haematuria, which ONE of the following statements is TRUE?

A. The most common cause of macroscopic haematuria in a male patient is urothelial carcinoma of the bladder

B. Causes include benign prostatic hypertrophy, toxaemia of pregnancy, serum sickness, sickle cell disease and exercise

C. It is present in up to 70% of those patients with urolithiasis

D. Large clots suggest an upper renal tract cause

13. Regarding Fourniers's gangrene, which ONE of the following statements is TRUE?

A. It is a polymicrobial necrotising infection confined to the scrotal skin that originates from the skin

B. It may slowly progress to involve the buttocks and thighs

C. Hyperbaric oxygen is an adjunctive treatment

D. The antibiotic of choice is IV metronidazole

14. Regarding diagnosis and treatment of genital infections, which ONE of the following statements is CORRECT?

A. A 22-year-old male with dysuria, purulent urethral discharge and frequency should be treated with 500 mg IM ceftriaxone

B. The presence of clue cells on a wet mount preperation of vaginal/urethral discharge is suggestive of a trichomonas infection

C. Painful vesiculopustular lesions on the perineum should be treated with metronidazole

D. Symptoms of a UTI with perineal pain and tender prostate in a 37-year-old man should be treated with nitrofurantoin

15. Complications of a ureteric stent include all of the following EXCEPT:

A. Haematuria

B. Urinary obstruction

C. Hydronephrosis

D. Low-grade pyrexia

Yolande Weiner

1. A 24-year-old female presents to the emergency department (ED) with a history of intractable vomiting for 4 weeks. She is 13 weeks pregnant. On examination she appears dehydrated with evidence of recent weight loss. The rest of her examination is normal. Her urine shows ketones 1+ and her blood sugar level is 5.8 mmol/L. Regarding hyperemesis gravidarum in this case, which ONE of the following statements is FALSE?

A. Thiamine should be administered to prevent Wernicke's encephalopathy

B. Glucose containing (5–10%) intravenous (IV) fluids is the preferable initial choice of fluid in prolonged cases of hyperemesis

C. Piridoxine has been shown to reduce nausea in pregnancy

D. Metoclopramide is a Therapeutic Goods Administration (TGA) category A drug in pregnancy

2. Regarding ultrasound findings in early pregnancy, which ONE of the following is TRUE?

A. Evidence of an intrauterine gestational sac excludes an ectopic pregnancy

B. The absence of a yolk sac in the presence of a gestational sac >10 mm visible on a transabdominal ultrasound performed in the ED indicates a blighted ovum

C. The first evidence of an intrauterine pregnancy (IUP) includes the intradecidual sign, gestational sac and double decidual sign

D. An indeterminate ultrasound refers to an ultrasound where no signs of IUP can be demonstrated

3. Regarding the clinical features of ectopic pregnancies, which ONE of the following is TRUE?

A. Risk factors for ectopic pregnancy are present in almost all cases

B. The passage of tissue can differentiate between an ectopic and an IUP

C. Uterine size for estimated gestational age is most often normal

D. Abnormal vaginal bleeding is the most common presenting symptom in patients with ectopic pregnancy

4. Regarding threatened miscarriage in the first trimester of pregnancy, which ONE of the following is TRUE?

A. About 90% of patients where embryonic or fetal cardiac activity can be demonstrated on ultrasound, will continue with the pregnancy

B. Embryonic bradycardia is dismissible and does not alter the prognosis

C. Severity of bleeding correlates with the risk of patients proceeding to a complete miscarriage

D. Bed rest is recommended because it may influence the outcome

5. Regarding serial βHCG testing in early pregnancy, which ONE of the following is MOST CORRECT?

A. A rise in βHCG >50% in 48 hours suggests a viable pregnancy

B. A normal doubling time of βHCG in 48 hours on serial testing excludes ectopic pregnancy

C. A very low βHCG <100 mIU/mL excludes an ectopic pregnancy

D. βHCG >1500 mIU/mL is the discriminatory zone above which an IUP can reliably be visualised on transabdominal ultrasound

6. Regarding anti-D prophylaxis during first trimester pregnancy in a Rh negative female, which ONE of the following is the MOST CORRECT?

A. High-level evidence exists to support the use of anti-D for a threatened miscarriage

B. An unruptured ectopic pregnancy in the first trimester is regarded as a sensitising event requiring anti-D

C. Anti-D is not indicated after 72 hours of a sensitising event

D. Anti-D should be given every 3 weeks for ongoing bleeding

7. Regarding administration of anti-D (RhIG) after the first trimester of pregnancy in Rh negative females, which ONE of the following is TRUE?

A. Anti-D is only indicated in blunt abdominal trauma when there is evidence of antepartum haemorrhage or fetal distress

B. Administration of 625 IU is sufficient after all sensitising events

C. The Australian Rh immunoglobin can be administered via the intramuscular (IM) or IV route

D. If a Kleihauer test is performed, maternal venous blood should be collected in an EDTA® tube

8. Regarding preeclampsia in pregnancy, which ONE of the following is TRUE?

A. The diagnostic criteria are hypertension with a blood pressure of ≥140/90 mmHg associated with the presence of proteinuria and pathologic oedema after 20 weeks' gestation

B. Proteinuria 1+ on urine dipstick usually correlates with 300 mg of protein on a 24-hour urine specimen

C. Korotkoff phase IV (muffling of sound) should be used to measure diastolic blood pressure (BP)

D. The use of antihypertensive agents in mild–moderate preeclampsia improves maternal and fetal outcome

9. A 24-year-old female presents to the ED with blurred vision and slight headache. She is 26 weeks pregnant. Her BP is 150/100 mmHg and a urine dipstix shows 1+ protein. Which ONE of the following is the MOST appropriate?

A. She requires conservative management with admission for BP monitoring

B. She is at low risk of developing eclampsia as her BP is not high enough

C. She requires immediate lowering of her BP with intravenous hydralazine

D. Administration of magnesium sulphate will reduce the rate of development of eclampsia by at least 50%

10. A 34-year-old female presents with a new onset generalised tonic–clonic seizure. She is 27 weeks pregnant. Which ONE of the following is TRUE?

A. Magnesium sulphate is more effective in terminating acute convulsions associated with eclampsia than diazepam

B. Eclampsia is excluded in the absence of hypertension or proteinuria

C. A loading dose of magnesium sulphate 1–2 g should be given intravenously, followed by a maintenance infusion, to prevent further seizures

D. Control of BP is essential in preventing further eclamptic seizures

11. A 21–year-old female has been placed on a $MgSO_4$ infusion after she had an eclamptic seizure. Which ONE of the following is TRUE regarding the use of $MgSO_4$ in pregnancy?

A. Serum magnesium levels should be measured and infusion rate adjusted to maintain a therapeutic range for seizure prophylaxis

B. $MgSO_4$ can cause renal insufficiency and therefore hourly urine output should be routinely monitored

C. Brisk reflexes may be an early indicator of toxicity

D. Toxicity follows a dose-response relationship and clinical monitoring is usually adequate to avoid adverse effects

12. Regarding drug use in pregnancy and lactation, which ONE of the following is the MOST appropriate?

A. The combination of paracetamol and ibuprofen can be used for migraine in a female of 18 weeks' gestation

B. The use of gentamicin is regarded as safe in the treatment of pyelonephritis in a female of 22 weeks' gestation

C. Metronidazole 2 g orally as a single dose for the treatment of symptomatic trichomonas is contraindicated in pregnancy

D. Oxycodone should not be given for acute pain relief in a breastfeeding mother

13. Regarding abruptio placentae in pregnancy, which ONE of the following is TRUE?

A. Ultrasound has a sensitivity of 90–95% in detecting abruptio placentae

B. Absence of vaginal bleeding excludes significant placental abruption

C. A fibrinogen level <3 g/L indicates significant consumption of coagulation factors

D. A Couvelaire uterus refers to the uterine atony associated with abruptio after delivery of the fetus

14. Regarding antepartum haemorrhage in the third trimester of pregnancy, which ONE of the following is TRUE?

A. The initial bleed of placenta praevia is usually small and ceases spontaneously

B. Transvaginal ultrasonography is contraindicated when placenta praevia is suspected

C. Vasa praevia is associated with a small amount of bleeding and does not usually cause fetal compromise

D. Careful digital vaginal examination should be performed in the ED if an ultrasound is not available to exclude placenta praevia

15. A 28-year-old female presents in labour. After delivery of the head, you notice the chin retracts tightly into the perineum. Which ONE of the following is the MOST appropriate answer?

A. An episiotomy should always be performed to relieve soft tissue obstruction

B. McRoberts' manoeuvre widens the pelvic diameter and allows for easier delivery of the shoulder

C. Application of fundal pressure in conjunction with McRoberts' manoeuvre may assist in delivery of the anterior shoulder

D. Rubin's manoeuvre is performed by placing pressure on the fetal scapula and rotating the posterior shoulder 180° in a corkscrew fashion

16. A 28-year-old female of 37 weeks' gestation notices dampness on her underwear after coughing. She is uncertain whether it is urine but is concerned that she might have ruptured her membranes. Which ONE of the following statements is MOST appropriate?

A. Premature rupture of membranes refers to the rupture of membranes prior to 37 weeks' gestation

B. Rupture of membranes can be excluded on ultrasound examination

C. A sterile speculum examination should be performed as part of the initial assessment

D. Fetal heart rate should be assessed and, if normal, she should be reassured and asked to return if contractions occur

17. Regarding immediate (primary) postpartum haemorrhage (PPH), which ONE of the following is TRUE?

A. Abruptio placenta is a risk factor for PPH

B. The most common cause of PPH is retained products

C. Passive delivery of the placenta is associated with reduced risk of PPH

D. Oxytocin 20–40 U IV as a bolus is preferred over an infusion to facilitate uterine contractions in the atonic uterus

18. Which ONE of the following is TRUE regarding acute vulvovaginitis?

A. Chlamydiae is the most common infectious cause in symptomatic women

B. A fishy odour on the whiff test usually means bacterial vaginosis is present

C. The presence of clue cells on microscopy is suggestive of trichomonas

D. A positive culture for *Gardnerella* on vaginal discharge confirms vaginitis

19. Regarding pelvic inflammatory disease (PID), which ONE of the following is FALSE?

A. The risk of infection is higher during and shortly after menses

B. Cervical motion tenderness on examination is more sensitive than adnexal tenderness

C. PID is usually polymicrobial and due to sexually acquired pathogens

D. The presence of white blood cells in the vaginal discharge is a sensitive marker for PID

20. A 22-year-old female presents to the ED with lower abdominal pain. She admits to having multiple sex partners. On examination she is well, presenting with a temperature of 37.6°C. The rest of her vital signs are normal. Vaginal examination confirms bilateral adnexal tenderness as well as cervical motion tenderness. Which ONE of the following is TRUE in this setting?

A. Best practice would be to await cervical swab results before commencing antibiotic treatment

B. Amoxycillin+clavulanate 875+125 mg orally, 12-hourly plus doxycycline 100 mg bd orally is an appropriate antibiotic regimen in this scenario

C. Current recommendations for the duration of antibiotic treatment in sexually acquired PID is a 14-day treatment course

D. Azithromycin 1 g orally given as a single dose will be as effective as a course of doxycline for the treatment of *Chlamydia*

21. A 19-year-old female presents to the ED after she has been sexually assaulted the previous day. She does not wish to report the event to the police. Which ONE of the following is TRUE regarding treatment options in this case?

A. A single dose of oral levonorgestrel 1.5 mg is an effective option for emergency contraception

B. The Yuzpe method is a more effective method of emergency contraception and has fewer adverse effects than the progestin-only method

C. Single-dose antibiotic prophylaxis is generally not recommended in preventing sexually transmitted bacterial infections

D. Hepatitis B and HIV prophylaxis should routinely be administered

22. Regarding abdominal pain in a female of reproductive age, which ONE of the following is TRUE?

A. Pelvic pain caused by bleeding into an ovarian cyst usually requires surgical intervention

B. Transvaginal ultrasound can diagnose endometriosis in the majority of cases

C. A normal ultrasound with Doppler reliably excludes ovarian torsion

D. Risk factors for ovarian torsion include pregnancy and chemical induction of ovulation

23. Regarding Fitz-Hugh–Curtis syndrome, which ONE of the following is TRUE?

A. It is a common cause of abdominal and pelvic pain in women

B. Ultrasound is the diagnostic modality of choice to confirm Fitz-Hugh–Curtis syndrome

C. Liver function studies are usually normal

D. Clinical findings of PID are always present

24. A 36-year-old female presents with prolonged vaginal bleeding of one month's duration preceded by a 5-week period of amenorrhoea. She describes it as heavy with clots. She is haemodynamically stable with no organic causes for bleeding found. A pregnancy test is negative. Which ONE of the following statements is MOST appropriate?

A. Her history is consistent with uterine bleeding associated with ovulatory cycles

B. Norethisterone 5 mg orally twice a day for 5 days is most likely to be adequate in stopping the bleeding

C. Medroxyprogesterone acetate 10 mg orally three times daily for 12 days is an appropriate initial treatment regimen

D. She should be admitted for urgent dilation and curettage

25. Regarding dysfunctional uterine bleeding, which ONE of the following is MOST appropriate?

A. Regular periods are always associated with ovulatory-type bleeding

B. Thyroid function should be performed routinely

C. Nonsteroidal anti-inflammatory drugs (NSAIDs) are helpful in the treatment of ovulatory but not anovulatory bleeding

D. Tranexamic acid at a dose of 1 g three times daily for 3 days is useful in ovulatory-type bleeding

Deepak Doshi and Waruna de Alwis

Toxicology

Deepak Doshi and Waruna de Alwis

1. All of the following are techniques of extracorporeal elimination of toxins EXCEPT:

A. Multiple dose activated charcoal (MDAC)

B. Exchange transfusion

C. Continuous veno-venous haemofiltration (CVVH)

D. Haemoperfusion

2. Haemodialysis is LEAST likely to be useful in which ONE of the following toxicities?

A. Carbamazepine toxicity

B. Severe lactic acidosis secondary to metformin toxicity

C. Ethylene glycol toxicity

D. Systemic iron toxicity

3. MDAC is indicated for which ONE of the following overdoses?

A. Sodium valproate

B. Digoxin

C. Lithium

D. Carbamazepine

4. All of the following are complications of urinary alkalinisation EXCEPT:

A. Alkalaemia

B. Hypokalaemia

C. Dehydration

D. Hypocalcaemia

5. Sodium bicarbonate is used for immediate correction of profound life-threatening metabolic acidosis in all of the following EXCEPT:

A. Carbamazepine toxicity

B. Cyanide toxicity

C. Isoniazid toxicity

D. Methanol toxicity

6. Which ONE of the following conditions does NOT cause a wide anion gap (AG) metabolic acidosis?

A. Methanol toxicity

B. Frusemide toxicity

C. Paracetamol toxicity

D. Salicylate toxicity

7. Regarding an increased osmolar gap (OG) in a poisoned patient, which ONE of the following statements is TRUE?

A. It is most likely to be due to ingestion of a toxic alcohol

B. It is specific for toxicological conditions and non-toxicological medical conditions do not cause an increased OG

C. Routine electrolyte results are adequate to calculate the OG

D. In the presence of a high AG metabolic acidosis, an increased OG is not due to a toxin

8. Regarding torsades de pointes occurring in a poisoned patient, all of the following statements are true EXCEPT:

A. It is more likely to occur when the patient is tachycardic

B. It is associated with QT prolongation in the poisoned patients

C. The risk of *occurrence* can be accurately predicted with a nomogram plotted with the patient's QT interval and heart rate (QT nomogram)

D. It can be terminated with $MgSO_4$

9. All of the following medications have a narrow therapeutic to toxic ratio in the presence of diminished renal function EXCEPT:

A. Diazepam

B. Lithium

C. Aspirin

D. Antipsychotics

10. Which ONE of the following drugs or substances is LEAST likely to cause significant toxicity if a 10 kg toddler ingests a small amount?

A. Mercury in a thermometer

B. Two tablets of glibenclamide 5 mg

C. Two tablets of dothiepin 75 mg (tricyclic antidepressant)

D. Two sips of camphor

11. Systemic toxicity from local anaesthetics occurs most commonly by inadvertent intravascular administration. All of the following statements are true EXCEPT:

A. Earliest symptoms of toxicity are neurological including tinnitus, dizziness and perioral numbness

B. Seizures are a feature of severe toxicity

C. Bupivacaine can result in cardiac arrest without a prodrome

D. Incidence of methaemoglobinaemia is dose dependent

12. In which ONE of the following clinical situations may intravenous lipid emulsion (ILE) be a useful antidote?

A. Bupivacaine-induced cardiovascular collapse

B. Sotalol toxicity

C. Systemic toxicity due to iron

D. Metformin toxicity

13. A patient presents to the emergency department (ED) with a history of deliberate ingestion of an unknown medication or substance. He appears agitated and confused with mydriasis, thirst, tachycardia, fever and urinary retention. He is likely to have ingested any of the following EXCEPT:

A. Tricyclic antidepressant

B. Olanzepine

C. Digoxin

D. Antihistamines

14. All of the following electrocardiogram (ECG) changes appear during major tricyclic antidepressant toxicity EXCEPT:

A. Terminal R wave >3 mm in aVR

B. QRS >160 ms with ventricular dysrhythmias

C. Left axis deviation

D. Downsloping ST segment in leads V1–V3

15. When comparing venlafaxine and selective serotonin reuptake inhibitor (SSRI) overdose, which ONE of the following statements is TRUE?

A. Cardiovascular toxicity is common in both situations

B. The incidence of seizures is higher with venlafaxine overdose

C. Severe serotonin syndrome is much more common after an isolated SSRI overdose

D. Both overdoses follow benign courses

16. Which ONE of the following medications is LEAST likely to cause serotonin syndrome in overdosage?

A. Tricyclic antidepressant

B. Levodopa

C. Tramadol

D. Amphetamine

17. Regarding lithium toxicity, which ONE of the following statements is TRUE?

A. Serum lithium levels correlate with clinical severity in chronic toxicity

B. Agitation, tremor, hyperreflexia and ataxia are features of acute toxicity

C. Cardiac monitoring for 24 hours is required in acute toxicity

D. Fluid resuscitation is the mainstay of management in acute toxicity

18. Regarding risk assessment in patients with paracetamol overdose after a single acute ingestion, which ONE of the following statements is TRUE?

A. Survival reaches 100% when N-acetylcysteine (NAC) is commenced within 24 hours

B. In a patient who presents >8 hours from the time of ingestion, elevated hepatic transaminase levels do not indicate hepatotoxicity

C. When a patient presents >24 hours from the time of an acute overdose, a normal paracetamol level and normal liver functions exclude any risk of developing hepatotoxicity

D. A child of <8 years of age who has had an accidental ingestion of 150 mg/kg will typically require decontamination, serum paracetamol level and liver function tests

19. Regarding the use of NAC in paracetamol toxicity, which ONE of the following statements is TRUE?

A. It is contraindicated in pregnancy

B. If biochemical evidence of hepatotoxicity is present, it should be continued beyond 20 hours

C. Anaphylactoid reactions are rare

D. If the anaphylactoid reaction is severe, NAC should be stopped and an alternative therapy should be used

20. Regarding severe toxicity secondary to a large ingestion of aspirin, which ONE of the following statements is TRUE?

A. Rapid complete absorption is typical in large overdoses

B. Bezoar formation in the stomach and intestine is uncommon

C. After intubation, the respiratory alkalosis should be corrected with ventilation

D. Patients should be considered for haemodialysis after intubation

21. Regarding acute digoxin toxicity, which ONE of the following statements is CORRECT?

A. Serum potassium levels do not correlate with prognostic outcome

B. Intravenous calcium gluconate is part of the treatment protocol for severe hyperkalaemia

C. When treated with digoxin immune Fab, digoxin levels should be repeated until levels decrease significantly

D. Therapeutic trial of digoxin immune Fab can be used when the diagnosis is uncertain

22. Which ONE of the following statements regarding the use of digoxin immune Fab (Digibind) is INCORRECT?

A. For patients not in cardiac arrest, it is essential to calculate the accurate immune Fab dose using the serum digoxin level

B. All patients on long-term digoxin therapy should be treated with digoxin immune Fab when presenting with suspected clinical and laboratory features of toxicity

C. An acutely toxic patient who is in a cardiac arrest should be given 20 ampoules

D. The return of normal cardiac conduction and rhythm is an end point of treatment

23. A 4-year-old otherwise healthy child presents with severe toxicity due to accidental overdose of a calcium channel blocker (CCB) drug. Which ONE of the following statements is FALSE?

A. Hyperglycaemia may occur

B. Bradycardia and sustained hypotension may result

C. Verapamil and diltiazem cause most severe negative inotropic and chronotropic features and result in bradycardia, and hypotension

D. Amlodipine and felodipine can cause hypotension and reflex tachycardia

24. Regarding beta-blocker overdose, which ONE of the following statements is TRUE?

A. PR interval prolongation on ECG is an early sign of toxicity

B. In children, ingestion of one or two tablets of sotalol or propranolol is unlikely to cause toxicity

C. All beta-blocker overdoses of more than a few tablets in adults are likely to cause cardiovascular instability

D. Onset of toxicity symptoms occur late in most patients

25. Regarding management of severe toxicity due to a deliberate overdose of sotalol, which ONE of the following statements is TRUE?

A. Atropine should not be used to treat bradycardia

B. $NaHCO_3$ has been proven to be effective to control ventricular arrhythmia

C. Isoprenaline and overdrive pacing should be considered

D. Patients nearly always require intubation and ventilation

26. Regarding the use of high-dose insulin euglycaemic therapy (HIET) for CCB toxicity, which ONE of the following statements is INCORRECT?

A. It should be considered early in the treatment of severe CCB toxicity

B. It improves the metabolic starvation affecting the heart in severe toxicity

C. It is contraindicated when the patient is on inotropes or vasopressors

D. In severe CCB toxicity, hypoglycaemia is less likely to occur as a complication during HIET

27. Regarding intentional overdose with sulphonylurea drugs, which ONE of the following statements is TRUE?

A. Hypoglycaemia is best managed using intermittent bolus doses of 50% glucose supplemented with 5–10% continuous glucose infusion

B. Prophylactic octreotide is indicated only if the dose taken is suspected to be high

C. Early commencement of octreotide to treat hypoglycaemia is recommended

D. Hypoglycaemia tends to be less severe in non-diabetics than in diabetics

28. Regarding thyroxine overdose, which ONE of the following statements is TRUE?

A. Thyroxine levels should be checked every 12 hours for 3 days

B. Immediate cardiac monitoring is essential due to high risk of ventricular arrhythmias

C. The majority of patients experience mild to moderate symptoms 2–7 days later

D. Severe toxicity is more likely to occur in children

29. An elderly woman is brought in by ambulance with a history of intentional ingestion of a presumed large amount of eucalyptus oil within the last 30 minutes. She is fully conscious and has normal vital signs. Which ONE of the following treatments is LEAST likely to be required for this patient in the ED?

A. Activated charcoal

B. Oxygen and bronchodilators

C. Non-invasive ventilation or intubation

D. Seizure control with benzodiazepines

30. Regarding carbon monoxide poisoning, which ONE of the following statements is TRUE?

A. Patients with severe toxicity usually present with focal neurological symptoms

B. The risk for neuropsychological sequelae secondary to acute poisoning is low

C. Ischaemic cardiac injury is common

D. The required duration for normobaric oxygen treatment is well established

31. Accidental cyanide poisoning is a potential hazard in some industrial processes and in house and industrial fires. Which ONE of the following statements is FALSE regarding antidotes used in cyanide toxicity?

A. Dicobalt edetate is the most widely available antidote in Australia

B. Immediate intravenous hydroxycobalamin is recommended as first-line therapy in patients with suspected severe poisoning or in cardiac arrest

C. Dicobalt edetate can cause serious toxicity if administered to a patient without clinical features of definitive cyanide poisoning

D. Sodium thiosulphate is highly effective in severe cyanide toxicity

32. Young children often present to the ED following accidental ingestion of household corrosive substances such as oven cleaners and dishwashing powder. Regarding corrosive ingestion in this age group, which ONE of the following is TRUE?

A. Absence of oral burns is predictive of a good outcome

B. Endoscopy provides the best guide to management and prognosis

C. All children should be kept nil by mouth during an ED stay

D. Dishwashing powder or tablets do not cause serious burns

33. Hydrogen peroxide (H_2O_2) is frequently used in various domestic and industrial products such as disinfectants, bleaches and stain removers. In a patient who has intentionally ingested such products in high concentration, all of the following clinical features may be expected EXCEPT:

A. Seizures

B. Blindness

C. Acute respiratory distress

D. Corrosive injuries to gastrointestinal tract

34. When using atropine in the treatment of organophosphate poisoning, all of the following features are end points of treatment EXCEPT:

A. Resolution of bradycardia

B. Achieving fully dilated pupils

C. Drying of oral and airway secretions

D. Resolution of bronchospasm

35. Regarding cardiac arrest secondary to cardiotoxic drugs, which ONE of the following statements is TRUE?

A. Prolonged resuscitation is generally not effective

B. The clinical effectiveness of antidotes has been verified with high level evidence

C. Cardiac Na^+, K^+ and Ca^{2+} channel blockers and beta-blockers are highly likely to cause cardiac arrest

D. Advanced life support guidelines applied to a poisoned patient are different from that applied to a non-poisoned patient

36. Regarding a toddler presenting with a history of possible ingestion of a button battery, which ONE of the following statements is TRUE?

A. Quantities of metal absorbed are insufficient to cause serious toxicity if the button battery remains in the stomach or intestine for a few days

B. If the battery is lodged in the oesophagus, symptoms always occur within few hours

C. If a chest X-ray (CXR) indicates oesophageal impaction a carbonated drink should be tried first to promote passage of the battery to the stomach

D. Plain films of the chest and abdomen is not indicated in the asymptomatic child

37. A 4-year-old child presents to the ED following an accidental overdose of a liquid iron preparation. He complains of abdominal pain and vomiting. He is awake and alert. He has mild tachycardia but his other vital signs are normal at presentation. When assessing for systemic iron toxicity, which ONE of the following is LEAST important?

A. Serum iron level 4–6 hours from the time of ingestion

B. Total iron binding capacity

C. A high AG metabolic acidosis

D. Venous bicarbonate concentration

38. Regarding drug- or toxin-induced methaemoglobinaemia, which ONE of the following statements is TRUE?

A. The oxygen saturation obtained by a blood gas analyser will produce a falsely elevated result

B. Blood appears initially chocolate-brown in colour and redden on exposure to air or oxygen

C. Pulse oximetry readings are deceptively low

D. NAC is the currently recommended antidote

39. All of the following investigations can be used to investigate 'body packers' EXCEPT:

A. Metal detector

B. Urine toxicology screen

C. Plain abdominal X-ray

D. Contrast CT of the abdomen

40. Which ONE of the following is likely to be the EARLIEST indication of systemic envenoming in a patient who has been bitten by a brown snake?

A. Development of diplopia and ptosis

B. A positive test for brown snake venom with a snake venom detection kit (SVDK)

C. Severe pain in the limb where the bite site is

D. History of early collapse but recovery soon after

41. Brown snake envenoming is the most common cause of death from snake bite in Australia. Severe envenoming results in venom-induced consumptive coagulopathy (VICC). The laboratory characteristics of VICC are all of the following EXCEPT:

A. Elevated or unrecordable international normalised ratio (INR)

B. Thrombocytopenia

C. Undetectable fibrinogen

D. Elevated D-dimer >10 times normal

42. Regarding clinical effects due to envenoming by Australian elapidae snakes, which ONE of the following statements is FALSE?

A. Tiger snake envenoming causes consumptive coagulopathy, neurotoxicity and rhabdomyolysis

B. Rhabdomyolysis and renal failure are the main features of black snake envenoming

C. Paralysis and rhabdomyolysis are uncommon with brown snake envenoming

D. Both red-bellied and blue-bellied black snakes cause features of severe envenoming

43. Regarding the choice of antivenom to be given in the treatment of envenoming due to snake bite, which ONE of the following statements is TRUE?

A. Protein loads given in single doses of polyvalent and monovalent antivenom are equal

B. In severe envenoming polyvalent antivenom should be given without waiting for SVDK results

C. Prophylactic treatment for anaphylaxis is required with polyvalent antivenom because the rate is 20 times higher when compared with monovalent antivenom

D. Serum sickness does not occur following treatment with monovalent antivenom

44. All of the following statements are TRUE regarding redback spider antivenom EXCEPT:

A. Antivenom can be recommended with caution after an acute allergic reaction once control of clinical manifestations has been achieved

B. Antivenom should always be given by intramuscular injection

C. Pregnancy is not a contraindication to give antivenom

D. Antivenom should not be used in patients with unconfirmed diagnosis because of the high risk of allergic reaction

45. Funnel-web spider bite is potentially lethal. All of the following are features of funnel-web spider bite EXCEPT:

 A. Local erythema and swelling

 B. Visible fang marks

 C. Pain at the site of the bite

 D. Sweating

46. Regarding box jellyfish (*Chironex fleckeri*) stings that occur in tropical waters of Australia, which ONE of the following statements is INCORRECT?

 A. Topical application of generous volumes of vinegar is the recommended first aid

 B. Children are at a greater risk of envenoming

 C. If vinegar is not available the stung area should be washed with fresh water

 D. Cardiac arrest can occur within 5 minutes

47. All of the following are used for treatment of Irukandji syndrome EXCEPT:

 A. Fentanyl

 B. Antiemetics

 C. Antivenom

 D. Glyceryl trinitrate

48. All of the following are features of tick paralysis EXCEPT:

 A. It typically occurs in children under 3 years of age

 B. Cranial nerves are frequently involved leading to ptosis and facial paralysis

 C. Search and removal of ticks is important in a patient with tick paralysis

 D. Respiratory muscles are spared

49. Regarding mushroom poisoning due to accidental ingestion in children in Australia and New Zealand, all of the following statements are true EXCEPT:

 A. Diarrhoea and vomiting indicate gastrointestinal toxicity

 B. Cyclopeptide hepatotoxic poisoning is rare in Australasia

 C. Cardiac monitoring should be done for 6 hours

 D. Attention to fluid status is important

50. Regarding acute scombroid poisoning, which ONE of the following statements is TRUE?

 A. It is considered as a severe allergy or anaphylactic reaction

 B. Properly cooking fish prior to consumption reduces the risk of toxicity

 C. It can be diagnosed only when multiple cases are present

 D. Treatment with adrenaline is therapeutic

CHAPTER 20
ENVIRONMENTAL EMERGENCIES

Yolande Weiner

1. Regarding the management of heatstroke, which ONE of the following is TRUE?

A. The end point of cooling techniques is a rectal temperature of 36–38°C

B. Benzodiazepine is an appropriate choice of drug to suppress shivering associated with some cooling techniques

C. Temperature should gradually be reduced over a few hours to reduce shivering

D. Evaporative cooling with ice-cold water is the preferred external cooling technique

2. Regarding heat-related illnesses, which ONE of the following is TRUE?

A. The main distinguishing factor between heat exhaustion and heatstroke is the degree of temperature elevation

B. The presence of profuse sweating excludes the diagnosis of heatstroke

C. Rhabdomyolysis is a common finding in heat exhaustion associated with exercise

D. Antipyretics have no role in the treatment of patients with heat stroke and may be deleterious

3. Regarding Osborne or J waves on the electrocardiogram (ECG) of a patient with severe hypothermia, which ONE of the following is TRUE?

A. Osborne waves are pathognomonic of hypothermia

B. They are best seen in the anterior precordial leads

C. Osborn waves consist of an extra deflection at the end of the QRS complex

D. The development of Osborn waves heralds ventricular fibrillation and is a poor prognostic sign

4. A 32-year-old male developed confusion and dizziness shortly after ascending from a scuba dive. Which ONE of the following is TRUE?

A. The best position to manage him would be at 30–45 degrees with his head up to reduce intracranial pressure

B. Recompression in a hyperbaric chamber is indicated, even if symptoms resolve with normobaric oxygen therapy

C. It is important to distinguish arterial gas embolism (AGE) from decompression sickness (DCS) as the management differs significantly

D. His symptoms can be explained by 'nitrogen narcosis' if the dive was at a depth >50 m

5. Regarding decompression illness, which ONE of the following is FALSE?

A. AGE usually occurs on ascent or soon after surfacing

B. Decompression sickness is mostly associated with prolonged exposure to depths >10 m

C. AGE can occur with ascent from very shallow depths <10 m

D. Boyle's law best explains the uptake of inert gas into tissues when breathing compressed air at depth

6. Regarding submersion events, which ONE of the following statements is TRUE?

A. Significant electrolyte abnormalities are common with saltwater events

B. Drowning is defined as death due to suffocation after submersion in a liquid medium

C. The Conn and Modell classification is a useful neurological classification system and can guide management

D. Current evidence recommends discontinuation of resuscitation efforts if the submersion time was >5 minutes and resuscitation efforts >10 minutes

7. Regarding electrical injuries sustained by household current, which ONE of the following is TRUE?

A. The household current in Australia is low and not capable of causing ventricular fibrillation

B. All patients require 4–6 hours of cardiac monitoring due to the potential for delayed arrhythmia

C. Children who sustain hand wounds from electric outlet injuries should be admitted for 12–24 hours due to potential transthoracic current pathway

D. Severe bleeding from the labial artery, from chewing or biting on electrical cords, is usually delayed for 1–2 weeks

8. Regarding injuries caused by lightning, which ONE of the following is TRUE?

A. Keraunoparalysis is a lightning-induced limb paralysis of transient nature

B. The most common initial rhythm in cardiac arrest is ventricular fibrillation

C. Pathognomonic Lichtenberg figures on the skin are usually associated with deep tissue injury

D. Fixed, dilated pupils seen after resuscitation with return of spontaneous circulation always carry a poor prognosis

9. Regarding altitude-related medical problems, which ONE of the following is TRUE?

A. Acetazolamide is effective in the prevention and treatment of acute mountain sickness (AMS)

B. Headache, dizziness and mild ataxia are typical features of mild AMS

C. Younger age and physical fitness are associated with a decreased susceptibility to development of AMS

D. After oxygen supplementation and descent, dexamethasone is the next most appropriate treatment for high-altitude pulmonary oedema (HAPE)

10. Regarding acute radiation syndrome, which ONE of the following is TRUE?

A. A rapid decline in lymphocytes is one of the best early indicators of the extent of the radiation injury

B. Nausea, vomiting and anorexia seen initially after exposure of ≥2 Gy is due to a direct toxic effect on the intestinal mucosal barrier and carries a poor prognosis

C. Bone marrow suppression with pancytopenia typically occurs within hours of exposure

D. The acuity of onset and duration of the prodromal phase bears no relation to the dose received

Kanchana de Alwis

1. Regarding mental state examination (MSE), which ONE of the following statements is INCORRECT?

A. Diagnosis is an important outcome of MSE

B. MSE starts on commencement of the interview with the patient

C. Command hallucinations in a patient indicate serious illness

D. Restricted affect is commonly found in schizophrenia

2. A 50-year-old female with no previous psychiatric history presents to the emergency department (ED) with symptoms of depression and some vague suicidal ideation. Further assessment reveals her low mood and a containable suicide risk. Which ONE of the following is the MOST appropriate evidence-based treatment for this patient?

A. Referral to the psychiatry emergency team for further assessment, diagnosis and treatment

B. Referral to the psychiatry outpatient team, with a letter informing her primary medical practitioner

C. Admission to the psychiatric ward for further treatment

D. Discharge her with a script for a selective serotonin reuptake inhibitor (SSRI) as it is generally a safe medication to initiate from the ED

3. A 73-year-old man, whose wife died 6 months previously, presents with foot pain from diabetic neuropathy, poor sleep, lack of energy and increasing frustration about his inability to 'keep his diabetes under control'. When being examined, he describes lack of interest in his usual activities, low appetite, and some significant weight loss (about 5 kg) over the past three months. He denies feeling suicidal but feels no desire to continue living, and states that he is better off dead. All of the following statements are correct EXCEPT:

A. Depression in older people is common in women and patients with chronic medical conditions

B. Both depression and grief may present with similar symptoms

C. Older people with clinically significant depression mainly present with associated psychotic symptoms

D. Patients should be assessed by the psychiatry team as inpatients or outpatients mainly present with associated psychotic symptoms

4. Which ONE of the following statements regarding risk factors for completed suicide is INCORRECT?

A. Bisexual or homosexual men are more likely to complete suicide

B. Highly intelligent men are more likely to complete suicide than men with low intelligence

C. A diagnosis of schizophrenia is associated with increased risk for completed suicide

D. Terminal illness increases one's likelihood to complete suicide

5. All of the following statements are true regarding suicidal risk assessment in the ED EXCEPT:

A. The SAD PERSONS scale is a helpful guideline to detect or identify high-risk patients

B. Enquiring about current and previous suicidal ideation and plan in the interview will intensify the risk of subsequent suicide attempts

C. One in 10 previous suicide attempters ultimately kill themselves

D. A patient who has made a suicidal attempt of low lethality generally has inadequate coping styles and therefore needs complete assessment and treatment

6. A 26-year-old woman who is a recurrent presenter to the ED, represents with multiple superficial wrist slashes. She appears very angry and voices suicidal ideation. She demands to be seen by the psychiatry team. Which ONE of the following is the MOST appropriate approach for this patient's management in the ED?

A. Let her wait and calm down first and then be seen by an emergency clinician as a low priority

B. Talk to her about her symptoms and validate the distress she is suffering from

C. Offer a suitable oral benzodiazepine as appropriate and consider behavioural sedation early if further escalation of her behaviour is suspected

D. Liaise with the hospital's emergency psychiatry team and organise a short admission to the psychiatry ward to help her in her situational crisis

7. Borderline personality disorder (BPD) can present with other comorbid psychiatric conditions. All of the following are common presentations to the ED EXCEPT:

A. Mood disorders

B. Alcohol dependence

C. Anorexia nervosa

D. Paranoid schizophrenia

8. A 22-year-old man with bizarre thoughts of 'aliens trying to contact from Mars' is brought in by police to the ED during the night. He has been shouting and being violent in his house, running in and out during the day. The worried neighbours had called the police as they had feared his aggressive behaviour would lead to dangerous behaviour. When he arrives at the ED he is very agitated, looking suspicious and distressed. He keeps shouting and trying to leave the ED, needing the police to physically restrain him. His behaviour is disturbing others around him. The nursing staff urge you to 'do something before he wrecks the place'. Police want to leave because they have more calls to attend to. Regarding this patient's management, all of the following statements are correct EXCEPT:

A. Substance abuse is the most common cause of severe agitation behaviour in young adults

B. Delay in management of agitation leads to violence

C. While the police have physically restrained him he should be treated with rapid tranquilisation using appropriate medications and should be closely monitored in a secure area

D. Attempts at using logical and rational explanations first often work to settle agitation

9. A young woman of Asian origin who is a refugee from a conflict area presents repeatedly to the ED. She is without family and lives in shared accommodation. She often presents at night and often via ambulance with severe abdominal pain. She seems to be in genuine pain and but calms down when a Buscopan® injection is given and some support is offered by the nurses. All investigations done so far to exclude a physical problem have turned out to be negative. Once the pain settles down

she walks to her accommodation, which is only a few metres from the hospital. She has presented 17 times over the past 6 months. Which ONE of the following is the MOST likely diagnosis in this patient?

A. Malingering

B. Adjustment disorder with anxious mood

C. Posttraumatic stress disorder (PTSD)

D. BPD

10. A 17-year-old girl is taken to the ED by worried parents. She has never been obese, but in the past six months she has become determined to reduce her weight. Her weight was 59.1 kg. With a height of 1.7 m, her body mass index (BMI) was 21. She has been extensively dieting and doing exercise. She had lost 14.3 kg and stopped menstruating four months ago. Her current BMI is 15. Her parents found her fainted in the bathroom, which led to her coming to the ED. She denies having problems and is annoyed that her parents, friends, and teachers are concerned. In the ED assessment, which ONE of the following is LEAST important in determining disposition of this patient?

A. Serum K, Na and phosphate levels

B. Body temperature

C. Postural blood pressure (BP)

D. Deep tendon reflexes

11. Which ONE of the following is an important feature of somatisation disorder when differentiating it from conversion disorder, malingering or hypochondriasis?

A. Dysmenorrhea that is recurring over many years

B. Sudden dramatic onset of a single symptom, typically simulating some non-painful neurologic disorder where there is no anatomical explanation

C. Physical symptoms disproportionate to a demonstrable organic disease

D. The illness has a characteristic intentional and conscious simulation or production of disease

12. Which ONE of the following statements is TRUE regarding neuroleptic malignant syndrome?

A. It is caused by antipsychotic medication only

B. It has a low mortality rate

C. It is caused by antipsychotics when given in high doses only

D. Severely ill catatonic patients have an increased risk of developing this condition

13. A young woman is brought in by ambulance to the ED 6 weeks after the birth of her first child. She had called the ambulance service herself, stating her baby was dying and wanted help. Both mother and child were brought to the ED for further assessment. She mentions fears for her baby. She gives a very vague history. She looks tired and rundown. On examination, other than a mild dehydration, the baby appears to be in good health. Which ONE of the following issues is LEAST likely to be involved in this situation?

A. Child abuse and possible child neglect

B. Postnatal depression or psychosis in the mother

C. Lack of social supports to the mother

D. The mother having body image issues

14. Regarding amphetamine-induced psychiatric disorders, all of the following statements are true EXCEPT:

A. Recurrent psychotic episodes frequently occur following re-exposure to even small amounts of amphetamine

B. Amphetamine intoxication is not associated with manic or hypomanic symptoms

C. In the acute stage, delirium can occur with confusion and disorientation

D. Aggression and violence can be secondary to daily heavy use

15. Olanzapine rapid dispersing formulation (wafer) is frequently used in the ED to manage acutely agitated patients with a mental disorder. Which ONE of the following statements is TRUE regarding olanzapine wafer?

A. The risk of extrapyramidal side effects is higher than with haloperidol

B. When placed in the mouth it is considered to be bioequivalent to the olanzapine oral preparation

C. It is useful for an agitated psychotic patient in the ED because it is rapidly effective for both positive and negative symptoms in psychosis

D. Orthostatic hypotension is not a problem with olanzapine wafer as it occurs with haloperidol

Zaahid Pandie

1. Regarding normal physiological changes in the neonate, which ONE of the following is INCORRECT?

A. A neonate will lose approximately 10% of its birth weight in the first week of life

B. Newborns gain approximately 30 g of weight per day for the first 3 months of life

C. If exclusively breastfed, a normal stooling pattern would range from one stool per day to one per week

D. A neonatal heart rate of 200 bpm is indicative of serious pathology

2. When reviewing the leading causes of mortality and morbidity in neonates, which ONE of the following is INCORRECT?

A. The leading causes of neonatal mortality include congenital abnormalities, prematurity and low birth weight

B. A baby who is small for its gestational age has a fourfold increase in mortality risk

C. Group B streptococcus (GBS) colonisation of the cervix of the mother prenatally is associated with an increased risk of severe sepsis in the neonate

D. Transient tachypnoea of the newborn (TTN) often requires mechanical ventilatory support

3. A 10-day-old breastfed boy has been jaundiced for 2 days. No associated symptoms of vomiting or lethargy are present, and the stool pattern is unchanged. Examination reveals a well-looking baby with a weight of 2650 g. The baby was born at 35 weeks' gestational age by spontaneous vertex delivery with a birth weight of 2700 g. Which ONE of the following is INCORRECT?

A. This baby needs a serum bilirubin estimation

B. No significant risk factors for the development of severe hyperbilirubinaemia are present

C. Haemolysis due to ABO incompatibility is an unlikely cause at this age

D. A urinary tract infection (UTI) needs to be excluded

4. Regarding jaundice in the newborn period, which ONE of the following is TRUE?

A. Breastmilk jaundice is a common complication in the first 24–48 hours of neonatal life

B. Criggler-Najjaar syndrome carries a good prognosis

C. Jaundice can occur in the setting of pyloric stenosis

D. Glucose-6-phosphate dehydrogenase deficiency is likely if conjugated bilirubin is elevated

5. Regarding neonatal sepsis and meningitis, which ONE of the following is INCORRECT?

A. Neonatal meningitis is commonly caused by GBS, *Escherichia coli*, *Listeria monocytogenes*, *Streptococcus pneumoniae*, other streptococci and non-typable *Haemophilus influenzae*

B. Neonatal meningoencephalitis may be part of the spectrum of cytomegalovirus (CMV) intrauterine infections

C. 'Redness around umbilicus extending to the skin' and 'not able to feed' are regarded as criteria used in the diagnosis of potential neonatal sepsis

D. Neonatal cerebrospinal fluid (CSF) examination with elevated protein, leukocyte or glucose levels is always Indicative of infection

6. A 10-day-old neonate presents to the emergency department (ED) with cardiorespiratory collapse. Which ONE of the following conditions is unlikely to be the underlying aetiology?

A. Urea cycle disorder

B. Gut malrotation

C. Neonatal withdrawal syndrome

D. Anaemia

7. Which ONE of the following criteria is included in the definition of systemic inflammatory response syndrome (SIRS) in neonates and children?

A. A white cell count (WCC) >12,000/μL or <4,000/μL, or >10% bands

B. A heart rate of more than 90 beats per minute

C. A systolic blood pressure (BP) that is lower than two standard deviations for age

D. In children <1 year old: bradycardia, defined as a mean heart rate <the 10th percentile for the age

8. A 2-month-old immunised, previously well infant has a fever for 1 day. He has no associated symptoms. Clinically there is no obvious focus of infection and the child appears well. Which ONE of the following is CORRECT?

A. The child should be cooled down with tepid sponging if the fever is >38°C

B. Most infants in this age group should have a lumbar puncture (LP) performed to exclude meningitis, if no obvious focus of infection has been found

C. The streptococcal (PCV7) vaccine has significantly lowered the rate of serious bacterial infection in this age group

D. If the urine is positive for a UTI, this most likely represents 'seeding' from bacteremia and not a genuine ascending UTI

9. A 3-month-old previously well child has fever for 2 days without a source. The child appears well and has no evidence of sepsis or toxicity. Urine screening is negative, WCC is 8/mm³, neutrophil count 4/mm³, CSF is normal, chest X-ray (CXR) is normal and blood culture (BC) is pending. Which ONE of the following is CORRECT?

A. Current evidence suggests that this patient cannot be managed as an outpatient

B. Empiric acyclovir is indicated

C. GBS disease does not affect this age demographic

D. Reviewing the band-to-total neutrophil ratio may be of use

10. A 2-year-old fully immunised boy has a 1-day history of fever to 40°C. He appears clinically well with no clear focus of infection. Which ONE of the following is the BEST answer?

A. If investigated, a WCC <15,000 excludes serious bacterial illness

B. This child is at risk of occult bacteremia from pneumococcus and therefore a WCC and BC should be obtained

C. The occult bacteremia rate after introduction of Pneumococcal conjugate vaccine (PCV7) is now estimated <1%

D. In this case the high fever is most likely due to a bacterium rather than a virus

11. Which ONE of the following is TRUE in relation to measuring the body temperature in a child?

A. A tympanic infrared thermometer is equally accurate in children for all ages

B. An axillary thermometer is the gold standard test in neonates

C. A parent's subjective assessment by palpation of the child is inaccurate when assessing temperature and should not be considered in the assessment of potentially febrile children

D. Electronic, chemical and infrared thermometers are equally accurate when used in the axilla

12. Regarding the diagnostic approach to children with fever of 39°C without an obvious focus and who are 'well appearing' and 'non-toxic', which ONE of the following is the BEST answer?

A. Neonates under 1 month should receive ceftriaxone as part of empiric antibiotic treatment

B. A 3-year-old who is unimmunised should receive prophylactic ceftriaxone regardless of the results of screening tests

C. A 1-year-old child who has received pneumococcal vaccination should still be investigated with a WCC and BC

D. CRP testing in children >3 months has limited value and should not be a routine part of investigation in the ED

13. A 10-month-old fully immunised child presents with a high fever of 40°C and no evidence of a focus. The child does not appear toxic but is miserable. Which ONE of the following is the BEST answer?

A. If the child defervesces with paracetamol, it is predictive of a benign process

B. This child should be screened with WCC, LP and BC

C. UTI is the most common potential cause of bacterial infection in this setting

D. Listeria is a common pathogen in this age group

14. A 2-year-old child is referred with fever 39°C, cough and coryza, with tussive vomiting for 1 day. The child is noted to have petechiae. The child appears very well, and is active and alert. Which ONE of the following is the BEST answer?

A. If the distribution of petechiae is restricted to above the nipple line, the cause of petechiae is likely to be benign

B. The incidence of meningococcal disease is 35% in this setting

C. This child should be investigated immediately with WCC, BC and coagulation studies

D. All children with petechiae must receive ceftriaxone

15. A 2-year-old child presents with a fever of 39°C. Regarding the clinical approach to this patient, which ONE of the following is CORRECT?

A. Identifying a source for the fever is the first priority during assessment

B. The first priority in this setting is to exclude signs of overt septic shock

C. If signs of shock are present, rapid infusion of crystalloid up to a total of 20 mL/kg should be commenced, followed by initiation of inotropic support

D. If signs of hypoperfusion are present, a full septic work-up should be performed, including full blood count (FBC), BC, CXR, throat swab, urine and LP

16. A 12-month-old boy presents to the ED with a generalised rash and fever for 6 days. He has been treated for 'tonsillitis' by his general practitioner (GP) with amoxicillin syrup for 3 days with no improvement. Examination reveals a temperature of 39°C, dehydration, dry, fissured lips and injected pharynx. A pink morbilliform rash is present on the trunk, A mild conjunctivitis without exudate is present. Urine microscopy shows 100 leucocytes and no bacteria. Which ONE of the following is the best answer?

A. Measles is the most likely diagnosis

B. Scarlet fever is the most likely cause of the illness

C. Antistreptolysin O titre is likely to be raised

D. Treatment with intravenous immunoglobulin is likely to be required

17. A 2-year-old girl presents with fever, sore throat and coryzal illness for 5 days. She developed a maculopapular pink rash on day 2 of her illness as well as 'pink eyes'. She appears miserable on examination with a temperature of 40°C, bilateral conjunctivitis with exudate, pharyngeal injection and dry, fissured lips. She has painful cervical adenopathy and a profuse pink morbilliform rash on her trunk. Which ONE of the following is INCORRECT?

A. Adenovirus is a potential infective aetiology for this presentation

B. Fever lasting 5 days or more should be investigated further

C. Other causes of infectious mononucleosis (IM) need to be excluded

D. Kawasaki disease (KD) is excluded if an alternative viral cause is found on PCR testing

18. Regarding typical and incomplete (atypical) KD, which ONE of the following is the best option?

A. Children aged 1–4 years have a higher risk of presenting with incomplete KD

B. Cervical adenopathy is the criteria most commonly absent in both typical and incomplete KD

C. Mucous membrane changes were the least consistent finding across the typical and incomplete versions of this illness

D. It is important not to over diagnose incomplete KD because the risk of treatment with aspirin is high in young children

19. Regarding UTI in children, which ONE of the following is CORRECT?

A. A UTI is confirmed on a suprapubic bladder aspirate sample only if a pure growth of >1000 CFU is grown on culture

B. A negative 'urinary bag' sample on dipstick testing is a sensitive test for excluding a UTI

C. Children with a confirmed UTI will need a micturating cystourethrogram (MCUG) to exclude ureteric reflux

D. Children under 4 years with a confirmed first UTI should have a renal ultrasound to exclude obstructive uropathy

20. Regarding meningitis in children, which ONE of the following is CORRECT?

A. A normal blood WCC reliably excludes bacterial meningitis

B. Children with IgG subclass deficiency are at increased risk of infection with *H. influenzae* type b

C. Cochlear implantation increases the risk of *Neisseria meningitidis* meningitis

D. Meningococcal B vaccination is recommended as part of routine childhood immunisation

21. Regarding the clinical manifestation of meningitis in children, which ONE of the following is TRUE?

A. 50% of children with meningitis have focal neurology

B. Papilloedema suggests a severe meningitic process

C. Kernig and Brudzinski signs are reliable in those younger than 18 months

D. Seizures (focal or generalised) occur in 20–30% of patients with meningitis

22. Regarding CSF findings in suspected meningitis in children, which ONE of the following is INCORRECT?

A. Enteroviruses can be diagnosed by viral polymerase chain reaction (PCR) of CSF

B. India ink staining is used to detect fungal meningitis

C. Acid-fast bacilli (AFB) testing for tuberculous meningitis is 95% sensitive

D. Leukaemia may present with blasts in the CSF

23. An 18-month-old girl presents to the ED with a temperature of 39°C and a background history of one previous simple febrile convulsion. Which ONE of the following statements is TRUE?

A. Paracetamol or ibuprofen should be administered to lower her temperature in order to prevent a febrile seizure

B. Indications for admission of febrile seizures include a temperature >39°C, focal seizure or prolonged postictal phase

C. The likelihood of her having a seizure is approximately 20–30%

D. Prophylactic use of a benzodiazepine is indicated to prevent deterioration to a seizure

24. A 3-year-old boy presents to the ED with a simple febrile convulsion following a 1-day history of coryza. Examination reveals a well-looking child with an otitis media as potential source of fever. Which ONE of the following is TRUE?

A. Laboratory studies should be performed to exclude an underlying metabolic disorder if this is his first presentation

B. Laboratory studies are required to exclude an electrolyte abnormality such as hyper- or hyponatraemia

C. Septic work-up including LP to rule out meningitis should be performed

D. Ibuprofen is indicated as treatment for his acute otitis media

25. Which ONE of the following statements is INCORRECT regarding the management of a 4-year-old girl with a known seizure disorder on sodium valproate who presents to the ED with a prolonged seizure of >15 minutes?

A. Buccal and intranasal midazolam are effective for termination of seizures in this setting

B. Phenytoin loading at a reduced dose of 10 mg/kg is indicated if seizures are refractory to benzodiazepines

C. Phenobarbitone loading at 20 mg/kg is indicated if seizures are refractory to phenytoin

D. Intravenous sodium valproate has been shown to be effective in this setting

26. A 3-week-old boy is brought in by his father with a 2-day history of recurrent focal seizures associated with periods of unresponsiveness. On examination he is noted to be drowsy with a distended anterior fontanel and a heart rate of 75 bpm. Which ONE of the following is the MOST appropriate answer?

A. A benzodiazepine for termination of seizures is a good choice in this setting

B. This seizure type is classified as complex partial seizure and the child will most likely benefit from carbamazepine

C. A trial of pyridoxine is indicated as B6 deficiency is a common cause of seizures in this age group

D. The head of the bed should be raised to 30 degrees and mannitol should be available for urgent administration

27. Regarding anti-convulsive therapy for epilepsy syndromes in children, which ONE of the following is TRUE?

A. An anticonvulsive agent should be considered only after a patient has had four documented seizures

B. Carbamazepine is a good agent for the management of absence seizures

C. Ethosuximide is the preferred agent in the management of myoclonic seizures

D. Lamotrigine is indicated in the management of intractable mixed seizures (Lennox-Gastaut syndrome)

28. A 3-day-old neonate presents to the ED with a 1-day history of episodes of abnormal left arm movements associated with perioral cyanosis, 'staring' with eyes deviating to the left and 'lipsmacking'. The episodes last a few minutes in duration. The baby was born at 35 weeks via emergency caesarean section and Apgar scores of 4 and 8, with a birth weight of 2.4 kg. Clinically the child is a sleepy neonate with mild hypotonia, brisk reflexes and normal vital signs with a blood sugar level of 3.1. No evidence of sepsis is present. Which ONE of the following is the BEST answer?

A. The most likely cause of the seizures is meningitis and a full septic screen is indicated

B. The baby is having a combination of subtle seizures and myoclonic seizures, suggesting hypoxic ischaemic encephalopathy as the most likely cause

C. This neonate should be loaded with 15–20 mg/kg of phenytoin immediately as the history is suggestive of status epilepticus in a jittery baby

D. Immediate treatment with 5 mL/kg of 10% dextrose is indicated

29. A 3-day-old neonate presents to the ED with ongoing intermittent episodes of seizures despite an initial dose of buccal midazolam given in the ED. His organic work-up is completely normal and all reversible causes have been excluded. Which ONE of the following is CORRECT regarding his subsequent management?

A. Diazepam is the best first-line agent in this setting

B. Phenytoin should be administered as a second-line agent

C. Lorazepam is a good choice in neonates for termination of seizures

D. Pyridoxine is a good second-line agent in neonates

30. A 2-year old girl presents with a glucose of 25 mmol/L and a history of polydipsia. Her urine shows ketonuria. Her vital signs are: HR 100; RR 42; BP 90/65; saturation 98%; temperature 38° C. Her CRT is 3s and she appears alert but tired. Her mucous membranes and lips appear dry, her eyes are not sunken, she is producing tears and her skin turgor is normal. She has features suggestive of an upper respiratory tract infection (URTI). Which ONE of the following is the BEST answer?

A. The criteria for diagnosing diabetic ketoacidosis (DKA) are satisfied

B. Some features of dehydration are present, which will require slow deficit replacement over 48 hours

C. The child is in hypovolaemic shock and needs immediate bolus management with 20 mL/kg of 0.9% normal saline

D. Urine output is a good indicator of kidney perfusion in the setting of DKA

31. Regarding the development of cerebral oedema in the setting of DKA, which ONE of the following is INCORRECT?

A. Younger age group (<2 years) and first presentation of DKA are protective factors and decrease the risk of cerebral oedema

B. Severe DKA in itself is an independent risk factor for cerebral oedema

C. Administration of sodium bicarbonate has been associated with cerebral oedema

D. The administration of hypotonic fluids such as 5% dextrose or 0.3% normal saline with 3% dextrose is contraindicated in DKA because of the increased risk associated with cerebral oedema

32. Regarding DKA in children, which ONE of the following is FALSE?

A. Olanzapine may precipitate DKA in a child with undiagnosed type 1 diabetes

B. The most common precipitating factor in the development of DKA is infection

C. Administration of insulin should commence concurrently with fluid administration

D. Abdominal pain is common in DKA, and may be due to prostaglandin synthesis in DKA patients

33. Regarding DKA in children, which ONE of the following is TRUE?

A. DKA can present with near normal serum blood sugar levels

B. Leukocytosis is a specific marker of infection

C. Beta-hydroxybutyrate is the most accurate measure of the degree of ketosis and is measurable in the urine

D. Ethylene glycol ingestion may mimic DKA since an anion gap (AG) metabolic acidosis, ketoacidosis, hyperglycemia and hypocalcemia are usually present in both conditions

34. A 6-month-old boy presents with a 2-day history of cough and coryza on the background of four previous episodes of respiratory illness. He was born at 32 weeks' gestation with a birth weight of 2000 g. His current weight is 3000 g. He is sweaty but appears well, is interactive and saturating at 94% on room air. He is apyrexial with mild subcostal recession and diffuse bilateral crepitations and wheeze. HR is 140 and air entry symmetrical. Which ONE of the following is the BEST answer?

A. Lobar bacterial pneumonia is the most likely diagnosis

B. This child has no risk factors to predict a severe course for bronchiolitis

C. Nasal suctioning and nasopharyngeal aspirate are of proven benefit in this setting

D. A CXR is indicated in this child

35. A 7-month-old child presents to the ED with respiratory distress, hypoxia and cardiomegaly on CXR. Regarding the evaluation of suspected congenital heart disease in the ED, which one of the following is INCORRECT?

A. Classification into cyanotic and acyanotic categories is useful

B. Administering the 'hyperoxia test' in this scenario is not useful

C. The CXR is useful in assessing whether the underlying lesion is resulting in increased pulmonary flow or decreased pulmonary flow

D. The electrocardiogram (ECG) is useful in assessing for right or left ventricular (LV) hypertrophy, enabling further narrowing of the differential diagnosis

36. During the examination of a child, to differentiate a pathological murmur from an innocent one, which ONE of the following principles is TRUE?

A. Innocent murmurs can usually occur in diastole or systole

B. The grade of intensity of a flow murmur is usually <4/6

C. Innocent murmurs often radiate to the back and axilla

D. Innocent murmurs are usually not associated with an ejection click

37. A 2-year-old child presents with tachypnoea, respiratory distress and signs of pulmonary oedema. Cardiomegaly is present on the CXR with associated increased vascularity in the lung fields. The child is pink in room air with saturations of 93%. Which ONE of the following is TRUE?

A. Tetralogy of Fallot (TOF) is a likely cause of this presentation

B. Myocarditis is a possible cause of this presentation

C. Eisenmenger syndrome presents in this fashion

D. Ventricular septal defects (VSD) usually present in this age group

38. Regarding the management of an 8-month-old child with moderate severity bronchiolitis and a background history of an allergy to nuts, which ONE of the following is INCORRECT?

A. This child may derive short-term benefit from a salbutamol trial

B. Intravenous hydrocortisone is useful in this setting

C. A transient decrease in saturation is common after commencing salbutamol

D. This child may receive some benefit from a trial of 3% (hypertonic) saline

39. Regarding the management of severe bronchiolitis in a 7-month-old infant, which ONE of the following is TRUE?

A. Adrenaline is effective in preventing the need for intubation

B. High-flow humidified nasal cannula oxygen may be useful in this setting

C. Physiotherapy has been shown to be of clinical benefit in clearing secretions

D. Intravenous fluid administration is the best route for maintaining nutrition in this setting

40. A 4-year-old child presents to the ED with acute asthma. Examination reveals an oxygen saturation of 90% on room air with obvious accessory muscle use and quiet chest. Which ONE of the following is the BEST answer?

A. This patient has moderate to severe asthma and requires continuous nebulised salbutamol therapy

B. Magnesium sulfate is indicated

C. Aminophylline is a first-line therapy in the management of this patient

D. Empiric antibiotics are indicated

41. Regarding an 18-month-old child presenting to the ED with recurrent episodes of mild wheezing and no history of atopy, which ONE of the following is the BEST answer?

A. A trial of salbutamol will prove that the child has asthma

B. If there is a response to salbutamol therapy, steroids are indicated in this situation

C. The likely diagnosis is atypical pneumonia or viral pneumonia causing wheeze

D. This child has transient wheezing of infancy

42. An 8-year-old girl has a history of intermittent wheezing episodes responding to salbutamol as well as a dry cough on most nights of the week. Her growth and development is normal. Which ONE of the following is the most appropriate answer?

A. Cystic fibrosis needs to be excluded by genetic and sweat chloride testing

B. This could represent chronic suppurative lung disease and sputum culture is indicated

C. She needs to commence on a course of inhaled fluticasone proprionate

D. She needs to commence on a course of combined salmeterol and fluticasone therapy

43. A fully immunized 2-year-old child presents to the ED with a chronic cough for 5 weeks following a coryzal illness. The child appears well and clinical examination is unremarkable. Which ONE of the following is the BEST answer?

A. Cough variant asthma is a likely cause for the symptoms and a course of inhaled steroid is indicated

B. This child should be investigated for cystic fibrosis

C. A CXR is indicated because pneumonia is a likely diagnosis

D. A nasopharyngeal aspirate is a useful test in this scenario

44. Regarding pneumonia in children, which ONE of the following is INCORRECT?

A. Bacterial pneumonia usually has a sudden onset with fever >39°C, tachypnoea and cough

B. Mycoplasma usually presents with gradual insidious pneumonia symptoms including fever, malaise and coryza

C. *Staphylococcus aureus* pneumonia is less common than *Streptococcus pneumoniae*, with most cases occurring in younger children

D. Group A *S. pneumoniae* is usually a severe disease with a high case fatality rate

45. Regarding acute pneumonia in children, which ONE of the following is INCORRECT?

A. Viral agents cause 60–90% of pneumonias

B. Bacteria predominate in neonates but are a less common causative agent in toddlers and older children

C. Mixed viral and bacterial infections or concomitant bacterial infections may occur in one-third of pneumonias

D. *Mycoplasma pneumoniae* is one of the most common causes of pneumonia among children younger than 5 years.

46. Regarding the investigation of children with suspected pneumonia, which ONE of the following is INCORRECT?

A. Laboratory and radiographic testing are unwarranted in children with respiratory symptoms who are well-appearing with a fever <39°C and no tachypnoea

B. Viral and atypical pneumonia usually appear as diffuse infiltration on the chest radiograph

C. A WCC that has a marked lymphocytosis is suggestive of a viral pneumonia

D. Sputum cultures are important in the diagnosis of bacterial pathogens

47. An 18-month-old boy presents with severe viral croup. He has an audible stridor on inspiration and expiration and severe respiratory distress. He weighs 11 kg. Which ONE of the following is CORRECT?

A. Prednisone is the best steroid in this setting

B. A very loud stridor is indicative of severe airway obstruction

C. 5 mL of nebulised adrenaline (1:1000) should be given and can be repeated hourly if required

D. Intubation should be delayed until steroids and adrenaline have had a chance to take effect

48. Which ONE of the following is TRUE regarding normal developmental milestones in children?

A. A neonate at 1 month of age is able to fix its gaze on an object and follow to the midline

B. A baby may smile when talked to by 2 weeks of age

C. A baby at 1 month of age is able to roll onto its back

D. Babies usually walk at 9 months of age

49. A 6-month-old boy has a heart rate of 180 bpm, a temperature of 38°C, a CRT of 1 second, a respiratory rate of 28 and normal SaO_2. His mother describes a brief coryzal illness of 1-day duration; the child is comfortable on his mother's lap and is smiling. Which ONE of the following is TRUE?

A. This child has a tachycardia that suggests sepsis

B. The respiratory rate is the most sensitive objective vital sign of serious illness in children

C. This child has a significant tachypnoea

D. BP should be measured with a cuff that covers at least 30% the length of the upper arm

50. Regarding physiological parameters in children and how they may differ from adults, which ONE of the following is CORRECT?

A. Young babies under the age of 1 month often have episodes of apnoea lasting <20 seconds; these are benign and require no further evaluation in the ED

B. Babies who suffer an out-of-hospital cardiac arrest should always be warmed as they have a large surface area-to-weight ratio that may lead to temperature instability

C. Children who are victims of multitrauma are more likely to have cervical spine ligamentous injuries than fractures of the cervical vertebrae

D. Infants over the age of 3 months are obligate nose-breathers and therefore deteriorate rapidly in the setting of bronchiolitis

Larry McGuire

1. Regarding disaster planning, which ONE of the following statements is TRUE?

A. The responsibility for disaster planning in Australia lies with the local government of each region

B. In a nationally agreed standard of specific hazards, Code Black refers to a personal injury threat

C. A major incident may be defined as an incident resulting in harm to more than 100 people

D. Planning processes address four elements – clinical, nursing, pathology services and portering

2. In the event of a mass casualty incident, which ONE of the following statements on site operations is TRUE?

A. Information that must be communicated in an initial alert includes incident location, patient details and services required

B. The Australian Triage Scale (ATS) is used to systematically review patients in order to get the most seriously injured to hospital first

C. Decontamination of unstable patients is most effectively deferred until they can be transported to an emergency department (ED)

D. Communications are a frequent point of poor performance in disaster management, and are the first priority in organising on-site management

3. Regarding preparation or response to an incipient influx of casualties to the ED, which ONE of the following statements is most CORRECT?

A. Surge capacity planning is determined by the number of available or clearable beds in the ED

B. Documentation should clearly distinguish between those patients arriving as part of an incident, and those unrelated patients arriving during the period of the incident

C. Emergency staff should escort as many patients to inpatient areas prior to new patients arriving, to improve capacity

D. Deployment of a surge team including triage and security staff is a key element in the initial phase of ED surge management

4. Regarding roles and responsibilities at a disaster site, which ONE of the following statements is TRUE?

A. The first ambulance officer on site removes the most seriously injured patients to the nearest hospital

B. The senior medical officer on site provides treatment of serious trauma patients

C. Disaster teams are responsible for carrying out resuscitation on patients too unstable or entrapped to be moved to hospital

D. The casualty collection officer is responsible for initial triage, determining who is taken to which area, and in which order

5. Regarding disaster equipment and supplies, which ONE of the following statements is TRUE?

A. Senior medical staff should be identified by name tags to other services

B. Minimum clothing standards include hard-soled shoes and loose, comfortable clothing such as theatre scrubs

C. On-site medical staff are equipped with radio communications tuned to a specific healthcare frequency, to avoid interrupting police and fire communications

D. Opiates supplied by the ED should be transported in a secure, labelled container

6. Regarding health and safety issues at a disaster site, which ONE of the following statements is TRUE?

A. The first priority of healthcare staff is their own safety

B. Chemical decontamination is best achieved by rinsing off under warm shower water

C. Ambulance staff transferring patients to hospital from a contaminated site should wear full personal protective equipment (PPE)

D. Access to the hot zone of an incident is controlled by the ambulance service

7. Regarding biological emergencies, which ONE of the following statements is TRUE?

A. In suspected pulmonary anthrax, patients should be isolated to prevent droplet transmission

B. Pneumonic plague due to *Yersinia pestis* responds rapidly to oral penicillin

C. Smallpox classically presents with a centripetal dense vesicular rash

D. Botulism toxicity induces a lethal spastic paralysis of the respiratory muscles

8. Regarding potential chemical exposures, which ONE of the following statements is TRUE?

A. Symptoms of organophosphate toxicity include muscle fasciculation and late-onset miosis

B. Mustard gas remains actively toxic in the large skin blisters induced

C. In treating severe cyanide toxicity, the drug of choice is pyridoxine (vitamin B1)

D. Sarin gas exposure (isopropyl methylphosphonofluoridate) requires immediate intravenous atropine treatment

9. Regarding a patient experiencing a significant radiation exposure, which ONE of the following statements is TRUE?

A. Patients developing symptoms secondary to gamma irradiation pose an ongoing risk to healthcare staff

B. Bone marrow suppression following a serious exposure develops over 3–5 days

C. Patients developing gastrointestinal symptoms can be expected to recover over 6–8 weeks

D. Potassium iodide blocks the uptake of radioactive material if ingested in the first few hours following exposure

10. In applying a triage sieve to the following patients in a mass casualty incident, which ONE of the following statements is TRUE?

A. A 65-year-old man with respiratory rate 24 and a capillary refill 3s is prioritised P2

B. A 40-year-old pregnant woman with respiratory rate 12 and pulse 100 is prioritised P1

C. A 14-year-old ambulant girl with an open radial fracture is prioritised P3

D. A 22-year-old man who is apnoeic and pulseless is prioritised P1

CHAPTER 24
ED MANAGEMENT AND MEDICOLEGAL ISSUES

QUESTIONS   Larry McGuire

1. Regarding the Australasian College for Emergency Medicine (ACEM) guidelines on emergency department (ED) layout design, which ONE of the following statements is INCORRECT?

A. The total number of treatment areas should be at least 1 per 1,100 yearly admissions

B. Paediatric clinical spaces should be as large as if not larger than those for adults

C. Ambulatory and ambulance entrances are ideally colocated for consistency of triage

D. At least one half of the total number of treatment areas should have physiological monitoring

2. Regarding the ACEM guidelines on equipping an ED, which ONE of the following statements is TRUE?

A. Isolation rooms for potentially infectious patients should have positive ventilation, a dedicated anteroom, and en suite facilities

B. A decontamination room should be accessible directly from the waiting room to prevent the spread of toxic materials to staff and other patients

C. A single central staff area is recommended for staff working in different treatment areas

D. A consultation room adapted for managing ophthalmology conditions should include either a motorised vision screen or a slit lamp

3. Regarding clinical practice guidelines, which ONE of the following statements is TRUE?

A. Implementation of national guidelines require adaptation to individual patients and settings

B. Guidelines are best developed by consensus of established authorities on a particular clinical topic

C. Robust clinical guidelines must be based on evidence from well-designed randomised controlled trials

D. Following development or introduction, a guideline should be reviewed for efficacy at least every 10 years

4. Regarding ED information systems, which ONE of the following statements is NOT TRUE?

A. Manual (paper-based) systems may be more useful than electronic record systems in smaller units

B. Primary concerns in choosing a system include adaptability to the local working environment and practices

C. In financial costing, electronic systems require only an initial outlay for implementation of hardware and software

D. Electronic information technology (IT) systems provide benefits in flexible management of and access to clinical data

5. Regarding performance appraisals, which ONE of the following statements is TRUE?

A. Logbooks are useful in assessing the quality of patient care

B. Appraisals are best performed by a single senior staff member who is responsible for direct supervision of the clinician's work

C. Poor performance of medical staff is most commonly due to lack of motivation

D. Effective positive and negative reinforcement is dependent on understanding the employee's values and goals

6. Regarding rostering of staff in the ED, which ONE of the following statements is TRUE?

A. Rapid rotation through a shift pattern has an adverse impact on health and work/life balance

B. Adaptation of circadian rhythm to night shift usually takes 3–4 days

C. Adverse safety consequences are more frequent in shifts longer than 12 hours

D. Backward rotation (e.g. night, late, morning) shift is better tolerated biologically than forward rotation

7. In considering work-related stress in emergency clinicians, which ONE of the following statements is TRUE?

A. Work-related stressors are usually the main contributor to personal stress

B. Effective strategies include spending more time with family

C. Active time management assists in reducing work stressors

D. Burnout is most commonly seen in female emergency clinicians in the initial years of first consultant posts

8. Regarding complaint management in the ED, which ONE of the following statements is TRUE?

A. Complaints are often most effectively managed in person at the time of the problem

B. Complaints most commonly arise as a result of poor medical performance

C. Apologies should be avoided because they constitute an admission of negligence

D. Most ED complaints are related to issues beyond departmental control

9. Regarding clinical handover, which ONE of the following statements is TRUE?

A. Clinical handover is the transfer of information about individual patients' ongoing care

B. Communication errors between healthcare staff have been found to contribute to over 55% of sentinel adverse events

C. Introducing a standard delivery system, such as ISOBAR, improves reliable transfer of clinical information

D. Bedside handover has an adverse impact on patient satisfaction

10. A 25-year-old man presents to the ED after being assaulted at home late on a Friday night. He has contusions to his scalp and face, Glasgow Coma Scale (GCS) 11/15, and is unable to provide any history. Two hours later, his brother and several friends arrive in the waiting room, demanding to see the patient. When the triage nurse explains that medical staff are all busy, they become verbally abusive, pacing up and down, while one starts smoking next to the desk. Regarding aggression management in this situation, which ONE of the following statements is TRUE?

A. Assigning a member of staff to speak to them in the waiting room will calm the situation

B. Escalation towards violence cannot be predicted in such a situation

C. The brother should be taken to a secluded room to advise him of the patient's condition

D. ED staff should be aware of the location of the relative and communicating doctor

11. You are a staff specialist preparing a business case to purchase an ultrasound scanner for the ED. A senior intensive care unit (ICU) colleague is pushing for the purchase of a different unit, mainly to assist with vascular access. This would be stored in the ICU and made available to the ED on request. The hospital executive will not provide funding for more than one unit. Regarding conflict resolution, which ONE of the following statements is TRUE?

A. Effective negotiating is based on asserting your own priorities over your opponent's

B. Preparing for negotiation includes defining one's own demands clearly

C. Negotiation is best carried out on neutral ground with no advantage to either side

D. Once final agreement in a negotiation is reached, it is important to provide a cooling-off period before formalising the agreement

12. Regarding business planning for the ED, which ONE of the following statements is TRUE?

A. Capital expenditure refers to payments related directly to patient care

B. A budget plan tracks all expenditure over the past year within the ED

C. Activity projections are based on the previous year's casemix and projected changes in demographics

D. Purchases of equipment over $5000 require a business case to be set out for the ED director

13. Regarding continuous quality improvement (CQI), which ONE of the following statements is NOT TRUE?

A. Clinical indicators are structured to identify weak points in the ED care processes

B. A PDSA cycle – Plan-Do-Study-Act – is used to plan quality improvements

C. Assessing CQI processes should involve measuring both desired and undesired outcomes

D. Interactive workshops are more effective than educational lectures by a recognised expert in implementing sustained change

14. Regarding the ED overcrowding, which ONE of the following statements is TRUE?

A. Overcrowding results in loss of capacity in community emergency responses

B. In the event of overcrowding, emergency clinicians have a responsibility to restore a safe working environment

C. Recurrent overcrowding indicates a need to provide more inpatient beds

D. Overcrowding can be prevented by improving community general practitioner (GP) services

15. Regarding access block, which ONE of the following statements is TRUE?

A. Access block is defined as a time > 8 hours from the decision to admit until reaching a bed

B. Access block correlates positively with longer hospital stays

C. Long-term effective strategies in addressing access block include redesigning departmental flow processes

D. Facility planning should aim to reduce access block to 25% or less

16. Regarding short stay units (SSUs), which ONE of the following statements is TRUE?

A. Units are best managed by dedicated staff under the direction of an inpatient clinician

B. SSUs are ideally managed under the care of the general pool of ED nurses

C. SSUs reduce access block by admitting patients until a ward bed is made available

D. Patients admitted overnight awaiting inpatient review become the responsibility of the accepting specialty

17. Regarding observation medicine (OM), which ONE of the following statements is TRUE?

A. Patients with complex medical issues can have their care initiated in a protocol-driven environment

B. Effective OM is dependent on regular daily ward rounds by senior clinicians

C. Observation wards should have preferential access to diagnostic facilities

D. Exclusions should include patients requiring input from multiple allied health workers such as physiotherapy, hospital in the home or community mental health

18. Which ONE of the following patients is appropriate for admission to an SSU?

A. A 32-year-old man recovering from sedation for reduction of a shoulder dislocation

B. A 18-year-old girl with diabetic ketoacidosis

C. A 65-year-old man with an infective exacerbation of chronic obstructive pulmonary disease (COPD)

D. A 22-year-old woman with recurrent pneumothorax post-aspiration

19. Regarding privacy and confidentiality, which ONE of the following statements is TRUE?

A. Emergency clinicians operate under an obligation to provide all requested information to police services

B. Patients have a legal right to access specialist opinions on their care, unless the report states specifically that it is not to be shown to the patient

C. In order to obtain access to personal records, a patient must explain the reason for the request

D. Patient consent is required if transferring health information from Australia to a country without similar privacy or data protection laws

20. Regarding medical errors in the ED, which ONE of the following statements is TRUE?

A. Clinical risk management is a process of identifying underperforming staff in the ED

B. Cognitive errors can be reduced by implementing cognitive forcing strategies

C. The majority of medical errors in the ED are unpredictable, and therefore unpreventable

D. Root cause analysis (RCA) is a systematic process to identify those responsible for errors at each phase of the patient journey

21. A 55-year-old man regularly attends the ED complaining of recurrent abdominal pain, which he relates to episodes of heavy alcohol ingestion. He consistently demands opiate analgesia, discharging himself once treated. One evening, he discharges himself after being refused opiates by a junior doctor, and buys morphine from a dealer. He is found collapsed and hypotensive in the street, and dies from respiratory arrest in the ED. A subsequent autopsy reveals mesenteric infarction. His wife states angrily that the hospital has been negligent and she will sue. Regarding negligence, which ONE of the following statements is TRUE?

A. The junior doctor's duty of care to the patient is established

B. By discharging the patient with a life-threatening condition, the doctor's duty of care has been breached

C. Potential damages considered include the wife's emotional distress

D. The hospital is liable to the charge of negligence if a breach of care is proven

22. A 32-year-old woman with advancing multiple sclerosis (MS) is brought to the ED following a significant paracetamol overdose 12 hours before. She had not informed anyone at the time but had admitted it to her GP on developing vomiting and abdominal pain. She states clearly that she had attempted to kill herself, as she did not wish to end up like her father, now bedbound and in a care facility due to MS. Transaminases are > 2,000 IU. She declines treatment with N-acetyl cysteine infusion. The GP, who accompanies her, insists she should be detained and treated. Regarding consent issues, which ONE of the following statements is TRUE?

A. The presence of a progressive neurological condition is adequate to validate treatment without the need for consent

B. The patient's decision to refuse treatment can be respected if witnessed and documented following explanation of the likely time course and effects of toxicity and treatment

C. Attendance in the ED indicates sufficient implied consent to permit treatment to begin

D. Competence is excluded here by the patient having made a decision contrary to her own best interests

23. In which ONE of the following situations is there NOT a mandatory requirement to report the issue to a relevant authority?

A. A woman presenting with a neck abrasion who admits to being assaulted by her partner

B. A medical practitioner with a concern that a patient with emotional lability post-stroke may be unsafe to possess a firearm

C. A sewage worker with leptospirosis

D. A heavy goods vehicle driver with newly diagnosed epilepsy, who is adamant that he needs his job to support his family

24. Regarding forensic examination in alleged sexual assault, which ONE of the following statements is TRUE?

A. Evidence of sexual contact is required to sustain a charge of sexual assault

B. Forensic examination is mandatory prior to reporting sexual assault

C. Forensic examination is carried out to detect any internal injuries requiring further treatment

D. Evidence collected should be handed directly to police after the exam

25. Regarding preparing medicolegal reports, which ONE of the following statements is TRUE?

A. Provision of a medical report requires the verbal consent of the patient

B. Medical reports should include the opinion of the treating clinician

C. Reports should include comments on subsequent inpatient care if the patient is admitted

D. A medical report should include description of the information on which the report is made

26. Regarding the role of an expert witness, which ONE of the following statements is TRUE?

A. A doctor attending court in response to an allegation of negligence is appearing in the position of an expert witness

B. An expert witness is required to be currently or recently active in their field

C. The expert witness must confine themselves to specific facts of a case

D. The primary duty of an expert witness is to the party engaging their service

27. Regarding a diagnosis of brain death for transplantation purposes, which ONE of the following statements is NOT a requirement?

A. Absence of the cough reflex on endotracheal tube (ETT) suctioning

B. Examination by two doctors, one of whom must be a member of the transplant team

C. Absence of tachycardia in response to atropine

D. Repeat examinations at least 6 hours apart

28. Regarding coronial investigations, which ONE of the following statements is TRUE?

A. A death must be reported to the coroner if it occurs within one week of receiving an anaesthetic agent

B. The coroner may independently institute an inquiry into any death in the community

C. The coroner has exclusive control of the body in a reportable death until deciding it is no longer required for inquest

D. A coronial inquiry may prosecute any individual identified as contributing to a death

29. An 82-year-old woman with severe Parkinson's disease is transferred from a nursing home following an apparent benzodiazepine overdose. You are the senior doctor in the ED, and the attending paramedic informs you on arrival that an advanced healthcare directive at the nursing home states that the patient is not to be resuscitated. In this situation, which ONE of the following statements is TRUE?

A. An advanced healthcare directive is invalid in the case of a suicide attempt

B. Care should be withheld until the directive is present for confirmation

C. Intubation of this patient at this point constitutes assault

D. The nursing home should be telephoned to confirm that the patient is not to be resuscitated

30. A junior trainee contacts the ED before the start of her morning shift, expressing concern that she is still mildly intoxicated following a departmental night out the previous night. A fellow junior notes a history of previous sick days around weekends, following social events. A senior nurse reports that the trainee has been uncharacteristically abrupt with patients over the previous weeks, particularly several with alcohol-related problems. When the nurse had raised this with her, the trainee had become defensive and dismissive. Regarding management of an impaired health practitioner, which ONE of the following statements is TRUE?

A. The doctor's recurrent alcohol-related absences constitute 'notifiable conduct'

B. A doctor failing to report notifiable conduct can face disciplinary action by the Medical Board of Australia

C. The Australian Health Practitioner Regulation Agency (AHPRA) is responsible for providing assistance for health issues affecting a doctor's performance

D. The doctor should be suspended from work while the situation is investigated

ANSWERS

Adult resuscitation

1. Answer: A

The detection of ETCO$_2$ is widely accepted as the most reliable method for verifying tracheal intubation. However, the efficacy of this method can be hindered in situations where insufficient CO$_2$ is exhaled because of reduced pulmonary blood flow, such as during cardiac arrest, which has led to the assumption that the oesophageal detector device (EDD) might be more accurate in cardiac arrest situations. However, conflicting results have been reported regarding the accuracy of EDD in emergency situations, and even less evidence is available for patients with cardiac arrest. Studies of colorimetric ETCO$_2$ detectors, non-waveform ETCO$_2$ capnometers and EDD showed that the accuracy of these devices is similar to the accuracy of clinical assessment for confirming the tracheal position of a tracheal tube in those experiencing cardiac arrest. Two studies of waveform capnography to verify endotracheal tube placement in those experiencing cardiac arrest after intubation demonstrated 100% sensitivity and specificity in identifying correct tracheal tube placement. These studies were reviewed by ILCOR in 2010, which has led to the recommendation that **ETCO$_2$ monitoring with waveform capnography is the most sensitive and specific way to confirm and continuously monitor the position of a tracheal tube in a patient in cardiac arrest and should supplement clinical assessment** (visualisation of the tube through the cords and auscultation).[1-4]

2. Answer: B

Increasing the IPAP increases the pressure support (IPAP–EPAP) provided by the ventilator. Pressure support augments the tidal volume during a spontaneous breath and reduces the work of breathing, resulting in increased alveolar ventilation, and therefore reduced CO$_2$. Increasing the PEEP (also known as EPAP) alone will improve oxygenation due to alveolar recruitment and reduction of intrapulmonary shunting but not ventilation. Increasing PEEP and IPAP proportionally may improve oxygenation but not

ventilation because the pressure support remains unchanged. During S/T mode, the timed ventilations are merely a back-up rate should spontaneous respirations cease and therefore do not influence gas exchange.[5,6]

3. Answer: D

There is high-quality evidence that NIV decreases the need for intubation and induces a more rapid improvement in respiratory distress and metabolic disturbance than does standard oxygen therapy in patients with acute cardiogenic pulmonary oedema. However, there is conflicting evidence regarding the impact of NIV on mortality, with most studies suggesting that it has no effect on short-term mortality.

The optimal mode of NIV (BiPAP versus CPAP) is yet to be established. NIV improves cardiogenic pulmonary oedema by establishing a positive intrathoracic pressure and reducing LV afterload. In patients with acute pulmonary oedema, the application of PEEP can improve haemodynamics by reducing preload and afterload, as positive pressure reduces venous return to the left ventricle. In patients with normal LV function, and hence those sensitive to changes in preload, a subsequent reduction in cardiac output may occur. However, **in patients with impaired LV function, a reduction in preload actually improves cardiac function.** The optimal PEEP remains to be resolved, although 10 cm H$_2$O appears to be safe and effective in the majority of patients. The addition of a differential inspiratory pressure (BiPAP) appears to be as effective as CPAP but does not appear to provide an additional outcome benefit and some concerns have been raised that BiPAP may increase the rate of myocardial infarction.[6-9]

4. Answer: D

BiPAP is particularly indicated in patients with an acute exacerbation of COPD in whom a respiratory acidosis (pH < 7.35) persists despite maximum medical treatment and controlled oxygen therapy. The application of CPAP/PEEP promotes the ability to counteract intrinsic or dynamic PEEP, reducing lung hyperinflation and assisting in passive exhalation. Although no difference in hospital mortality has been demonstrated, patients have a survival advantage that becomes apparent after discharge, at 3 months and 1 year. It is widely accepted to maintain saturation between 88 and 92%. The British Thoracic Society (BTS) recommends even lower levels of 85–90%.[6,8,9]

5. Answer: D

The decision to intubate in acute severe asthma is a clinical decision and should not be based solely on blood gases. Markers of deterioration include rising $PaCO_2$ levels, exhaustion, mental status depression, refractory hypoxaemia and haemodynamic instability. Many patients will present with hypercapnia or hypoxia and will rapidly improve with medical intervention and not require intubation.[10,11]

6. Answer: C

The major concern in commencing mechanical ventilation in acute severe asthma is the risk of worsening lung hyperinflation due to gas trapping, with an increased risk of barotrauma, and inducing or aggravating haemodynamic instability. **Therefore, the focus of mechanical ventilation has moved away from normalising blood gas values to where the primary goal now is to avoid excessive airway pressure and minimising lung hyperinflation, while maintaining adequate gas exchange** (see Table 1.1). As a result, mechanical ventilation strategies are aimed at reducing the likelihood that this complication will occur. To achieve this goal it is often necessary to hypoventilate the patient and therefore to tolerate hypercapnoea, a strategy termed 'controlled hypoventilation' or 'permissive hypercapnoea'.

P_{peak} **is not a reflection of what is happening at the alveolar level.** Subsequently, it is not that useful for assessing lung hyperinflation in asthmatic patients because it depends strongly on the airway resistance and inspiratory flow setting. Higher P_{peak} than usual may be necessary to prevent delivery of inappropriately small tidal volumes. In contrast, P_{plat} is an estimate of the average alveolar pressure at the end of inspiration and is directly proportional to the degree of hyperinflation. This should be maintained at <25–30 cm H_2O in asthma. P_{plat} is associated with VILI, not peak inspiratory pressure (see Table 1.1).

TABLE 1.1 ACCEPTABLE INITIAL VENTILATOR SETTINGS IN THE INTUBATED ASTHMATIC

Ventilatory parameters	Settings
Mode	Volume-controlled ventilation
Minute ventilation	<10 l/min
Tidal volume	6–10 mL/kg ideal body weight
Respiratory rate	10–14 cycles/min
Plateau pressure	<25–30 cm H_2O
Inspiratory flow rate	60–80 l/min
Expiratory time	4–5 sec
PEEP	0–5 cm H_2O
FiO_2	To a SaO_2 of >90%

Both volume- and pressure-controlled ventilation can be used in ventilating asthmatics, but volume-controlled ventilation is usually preferred. Pressure-controlled ventilation entails the risk of variable tidal volume (due to fluctuating high airway resistance and intrinsic PEEP), with sometimes unacceptably low alveolar ventilation.[11–13]

7. Answer: D

The role of NIV in ARDS is still uncertain and not routinely recommended, although it may be considered in certain circumstances. Recommendations for ventilation according to the ARDS Network are:

- tidal volumes (TV) 6–8 mL/kg ideal body weight
- plateau pressures <30 cm H_2O: may require reducing TV as low as 4 mL/kg
- wean FiO_2 to maintain a SaO_2 88–95%
- strategic use of PEEP to permit lower FiO_2 and reduce risk of oxygen toxicity
- rate 20–25 (<30) per minute
- permissive hypercapnoea (pH should be maintained >7.25).[14,15]

8. Answer: B

Continuous $ETCO_2$ monitoring can be used to indicate the quality of CPR, although an optimal target for $ETCO_2$ during CPR has not been established. **An $ETCO_2$ < 10 mmHg is associated with failure to achieve ROSC and may indicate that the quality of chest compressions should be improved.**

Effective external cardiac compressions provide an output of 20–30% of the pre-arrest value. A 2-minute period of CPR before defibrillation has previously been recommended in patients with OHCA. The 2010 ILCOR guidelines recommend that good-quality CPR should be provided while a defibrillator is retrieved, applied and charged, but **the guidelines no longer recommend routine delivery of a specified period of CPR before rhythm analysis and a shock**.

There is insufficient evidence to support or refute the use of a titrated oxygen concentration or constant 21% oxygen (room air) when compared with 100% oxygen during adult cardiac arrest. In the absence of any other data there is no reason to change the current treatment algorithm. However, hyperoxemia may lead to potential harm in patients with ROSC and titrating the inspired oxygen concentration to achieve saturation of 94–98% is recommended in the post-resuscitation phase.[2]

9. Answer: D

When an advanced airway is established, compressions do not have to be paused in order to give ventilation, but ventilations should be timed with compressions and delivered during the relaxation phase of compression without any pause. Ventilations of 6–10 per minute are recommended and can be achieved by giving a timed ventilation after every 15 compressions.

The 2010 ILCOR and ARC guidelines recommend a universal compression ratio of 30:2 (30 compressions followed by two ventilations) regardless of the number of rescuers present. The desired compression point for CPR in adults is over the lower half of the sternum. This location can simply be taught by saying, 'Place the heel of the hand in the centre of the chest'. The use of the internipple line as a landmark for hand placement is not reliable. The depth of compressions should be at least one-third of the depth of the chest or at least 5 cm.[2,16]

10. Answer: D

The default energy level for adults using a biphasic defibrillator should be set at 200 J for all shocks. Other energy levels may be used, providing there is relevant clinical data for a specific defibrillator that suggests that an alternative energy level provides adequate shock success. **ILCOR and the ARC now recommend that chest compressions be continued while the defibrillator is charged if using pads.** This approach appears to be safe and it minimises interruption to chest compressions. CPR should be restarted immediately after delivering a shock, irrespective of apparent electrical success. A pulse check should not be performed. The likelihood of developing a rhythm associated with an output is extremely small in the first minute after a shock has been delivered.

It is now recommended that a **single shock strategy be used in patients with VF/VT arrest with immediate resumption of chest compressions after the shock.** Studies have shown no benefit from a three-stack shock protocol compared with a one-shock protocol. Additionally, there is significantly more hands-off time. However, a sequence of up to 3 stacked shocks can be considered in patients with a perfusing rhythm who develop a shockable rhythm where the setting is:
- a witnessed and monitored setting
- the defibrillator is immediately available (e.g. first shock able to be delivered within 20 seconds
- the time required for rhythm recognition and for recharging the defibrillator is short (i.e. <10 seconds).[16–18]

11. Answer: D

Biphasic waveforms are more effective at terminating ventricular arrhythmias at lower energy levels, have demonstrated greater first-shock efficacy than monophasic waveforms, and have greater first shock efficacy for long duration VF/VT. However, **no randomised studies have demonstrated superiority in terms of neurologically intact survival to hospital discharge.** Biphasic waveforms have been shown to be superior to monophasic waveforms for elective cardioversion of atrial fibrillation, with greater overall success rates, using less cumulative energy and reducing the severity of cutaneous burns, and therefore biphasic is the waveform of choice for this procedure.[16–18]

12. Answer: C

The treatment of VF is defibrillation. The initial shock should be delivered at 200 J followed by 2 minutes of CPR. If the patient remains in VF after 2 minutes of good-quality CPR, a second shock should be delivered. For second and subsequent biphasic shocks the same initial energy level is acceptable but an increased energy level may be used. During CPR, adrenaline should only be given after the second shock and amiodarone after the third shock if VF is resistant to defibrillation. A pulse should only be checked if there is an organised rhythm present on the monitor.[17-20]

13. Answer: A

The aims of resuscitation in patients with cardiac arrest in a non-shockable rhythm are the provision of good-quality CPR and the search for reversible causes. The use of adrenaline has been shown to increase ROSC, but no resuscitation drugs or advanced airway interventions have been shown to increase survival to hospital discharge after cardiac arrest. **Atropine is no longer recommended for routine use during pulseless electrical activity** (PEA). The administration of medication via the tracheal route is also no longer recommended – if IV access cannot be obtained, IO access should be achieved and drugs administered via this route.[19]

14. Answer: D

Two studies (LOE1) reported improvement in ROSC with high-dose adrenaline. However, there are no studies that demonstrate a survival benefit compared with standard dose adrenaline. **Currently, high-dose adrenaline is not recommended in the guidelines due to the lack of survival benefit and potential harmful effects (tachyarrythmias and hypertension after resuscitation).**

There is some evidence to suggest that vasopressors (adrenaline and vasopressin) may improve ROSC and short-term survival. At the same time, there is insufficient evidence to suggest that vasopressors improve survival to hospital discharge and neurological outcome. Current guidelines recommend that the use of vasopressors may be considered in adult cardiac arrest given the observed benefit in short-term outcomes. There is also **insufficient evidence to suggest the optimal dosage of any vasopressor in the treatment of adult cardiac arrest**. ILCOR, as well as ARC, recommend 1 mg of adrenaline, after initial counter shocks have failed (after second shock and then every second cycle).

Three studies (LOE1) and a meta-analysis (LOE1) demonstrated no difference in outcomes (ROSC, survival to discharge, and neurological outcome) with vasopressin compared with adrenaline as first-line

pressor in cardiac arrest and the use of either is acceptable.[19,20]

15. Answer: C

Current resuscitation guidelines acknowledge that research in the area of maternal resuscitation is lacking. Despite this, it is recommended that a perimortem caesarean should be considered early in maternal cardiac arrest if the fetus is of viable age. **Prognosis for the intact survival of infant is best if delivery occurs within 5 minutes of maternal arrest; however, if the 5-minute time frame is exceeded, a caesarean section should still be considered**. One systematic review of perimortem caesarean sections suggested that it may have improved maternal and neonatal outcomes. At older gestational age (30–38 weeks) infant survival was possible even when delivery was after 5 minutes from the onset of maternal cardiac arrest.

There are no RCTs evaluating the effect of specialised obstetric resuscitation versus standard care in post-arrest pregnant women and all recommendations are based on the important physiological changes that occur in pregnancy that may influence treatment recommendations and guidelines for resuscitation of cardiac arrest in pregnancy. **There is no evidence to support that aortacaval decompression improves maternal haemodynamics and fetal wellbeing in pregnant women suffering from cardiac arrest. The evidence is also conflicting in non-arrest literature. Despite the lack of evidence, it should still be considered.** There is some evidence that manual left uterine displacement is as good as or better than left lateral tilt.

There is insufficient evidence to support or refute the use of post cardiac arrest hypothermia. A single case report suggests that post cardiac arrest hypothermia was used safely and effectively in early pregnancy.[19,21]

16. Answer: B

The temperature at which defibrillation should first be attempted and how often it should be tried in the severely hypothermic patient has not been established. **The current recommendation is that rescuers should attempt defibrillation (up to 3 shocks) without regard for core temperature.** It may be impossible to achieve conversion to normal rhythm if <30°C; however, it seems unacceptable to delay defibrillation attempts to assess core temperature. Further care, after initial shocks, is determined by core temperature. If the core temperature is <30°C, withhold defibrillation until it becomes >30°C because the fibrillating myocardium is unlikely to respond at that temperature.

There are concerns that intubation may precipitate VF. Current opinion is that endotracheal intubation is safe in severe hypothermia and early intubation provides effective ventilation with warm, humidified oxygen and isolates the airway to reduce the likelihood of aspiration. **The optimum rewarming technique is still controversial but warming gas and fluids to 40°C is a simple, safe and effective method.**

Drug metabolism is markedly reduced at low temperatures and medications may accumulate to toxic levels if given repeatedly. It is recommended to withhold IV medications if the core temperature is <30°C. Once 30°C has been reached, the intervals between drug doses should be doubled when compared with normothermia intervals. As normothermia is approached (>35°C), standard drug protocols should be used.[1,22]

17. Answer: D

Immediate emergent angiography and PCI is recommended in all patients with ST elevation or new LBBB on ECG following ROSC after an OHCA. It is also recommended in selected patients without ECG changes or prior clinical findings such as chest pain. Coma is a common finding in patients with an OHCA and is not a contraindication to angiography. **Systolic BP should be maintained >100 mmHg and oxygen titrated to achieve a saturation of 94–98%.** Hyperoxaemia may lead to potential harm in patients after ROSC. Insulin infusion should be commenced if the blood sugar level is >10 mmol/l but hypoglycaemia should be avoided.[1,19,23]

18. Answer: B

Several studies have demonstrated improved neurological outcome in comatose patients after out-of-hospital VF cardiac arrest. Recent studies suggest that induced hypothermia might also benefit comatose adult patients with ROSC after an OHCA from a non-shockable rhythm, or after an in-hospital cardiac arrest. **The ILCOR 2010 guideline therefore recommends that comatose adults with ROSC after out-of-hospital VF cardiac arrest should be cooled to 32–34 °C for 12–24 hours and that therapeutic hypothermia should be considered in comatose survivors of an OHCA after all rhythms or after an in-hospital cardiac arrest.** This can be safely initiated with a rapid infusion of 4°C normal saline at 30 mL/kg over 2 hours.[19,24]

19. Answer: B

Regarding prognostication after cardiac arrest:
- In adult patients comatose after cardiac arrest who had not been treated with therapeutic hypothermia:
  - **There are no clinical neurological signs that reliably predict poor outcome <24 hours.**
  - The absence of both pupillary light and corneal reflexes after 72 hours reliably predicts a poor outcome if no confounding factors such as hypotension, sedatives or neuromuscular blockers are present.
  - The absence of vestibulo-ocular reflexes at ≥24 hours and a GCS motor score of ≤2 at >72 hours are less reliable in predicting a poor outcome.
  - **No electrophysiological studies reliably predict a poor outcome in first 24 hours,** but in the absence of confounding circumstances, it is reasonable to use EEG interpretation between 24 and 72 hours to assist in the prediction of a poor outcome.
- In adult patients comatose after cardiac arrest who had been treated with therapeutic hypothermia:
  - There is inadequate evidence to recommend a specific approach to prognosticating a poor outcome.
  - There are no clinical neurological signs, electrophysiological studies, biomarkers or imaging studies that can reliably predict neurological outcome in the first 24 hours after cardiac arrest.
  - Beyond 24 hours, no single parameter for predicting poor neurological outcome is without reported false positives. Potentially reliable prognosticators of a poor outcome include an unreactive EEG background at 36–72 hours and the absence of both corneal and papillary reflexes >72 hours after cardiac arrest.

- A GCS motor score of ≤2 at >72 hours and the presence of status epilepticus are potentially unreliable prognosticators of a poor outcome.[19,23]

20. Answer: A

Emergency transcutaneous pacing (TCP) is indicated in patients with haemodynamic significant bradycardia that is unresponsive to atropine or other chronotropic drugs. **Previously, TCP was recommended in asystolic cardiac arrest, but the 2010 ILCOR and ARC guidelines do not support its routine use anymore**.

Pacing is usually initiated at a rate of 70–80 bpm. The pacing current should be set by starting at the minimum setting and slowly increasing the output until a pacing spike appears on the monitor. Continue increasing the output until *electrical pacing capture* is achieved. Pacing capture is present when each pacing spike is followed by a ventricular depolarisation with visible QRS complex and repolarisation with a T wave. **Each pacer spike that captures the ventricle will produce a wide QRS complex, a consistent ST segment and a broad, slurred T wave that is opposite in polarity (direction) from the QRS complex. Do not mistake the wide, slurred after-potential following an external pacing spike for evidence of ventricular depolarisation associated with ventricular capture.**

Once electrical capture is achieved, the haemodynamic response to pacing also must be confirmed by assessing the patient's arterial pulse and blood pressure (*mechanical capture*) during pacing. The pulse rate obtained should match the pacing rate indicated on the generator monitor. A manual count of the pulse rate should be assessed at the right carotid or right femoral artery to avoid confusion between the jerking muscle contractions caused by the pacer and arterial pulse wave. A significantly lower pulse rate than the pacing rate demonstrated on the pacing unit monitor may indicate failure to capture. Continue pacing at an output 10% higher than the threshold of initial electrical capture (the threshold is the minimal pacemaker output associated with consistent pacing capture).[25,26]

21. Answer: D

Adrenaline can cause hyperlactataemia and its use should be taken into account when interpreting blood lactate measurements.

Lactic acidosis is defined by convention as the combination of an increased blood lactate concentration >5 mmol/L and acidaemia (arterial blood pH < 7.35), whereas hyperlactaemia is defined as a blood lactate level ≥2 mmol/L. Critically ill patients with a lactic acidosis usually have a high mortality, and a blood lactate level >8 mmol/L predicts mortality. **The initial degree to which lactate is elevated has been shown to correspond to the severity of shock. In addition, serial lactate measures can be used as a guide to assess the effectiveness of therapeutic intervention**.

Bicarbonate therapy for lactic acidosis is controversial and its use is generally not recommended regardless of the degree of acidaemia. Cardiac dysfunction in patients is often due to other factors, with cytokines being the major cause in septic shock. There is no evidence to suggest that bicarbonate administration reverses myocardial depression or improves sensitivity to endogenous catecholamines.[27,28]

22. Answer: C

Adequate fluid resuscitation is fundamental in the management of patients with septic shock and should ideally be achieved before the use of vasopressors and inotropes. **The crystalloid–colloid debate is still ongoing and so far there is no conclusive evidence that one is superior to the other**. However, crystalloids are usually preferred as it is much cheaper.

Current recommendations are to maintain a mean arterial pressure (MAP) ≥65 mmHg to achieve minimal perfusion pressure and maintain adequate flow. Vasopressor therapy may be required, in addition to fluids, to achieve this. There is no high-quality evidence to recommend one catecholamine over the other. Animal and human studies suggest some advantages of noradrenaline and dopamine over adrenaline; adrenaline has the potential to cause tachycardia as well as deleterious effects on the splanchnic circulation and hyperlactataemia. However, there is no clinical evidence that adrenaline causes worse outcomes. Subsequently, **the Surviving Sepsis**

Campaign[31] advocates either noradrenaline or dopamine as the initial vasopressor to correct hypotension in septic shock. Adrenaline is recommended as the first chosen vasopressor if septic shock is poorly responsive to noradrenaline or dopamine.

The concept of relative adrenal insufficiency has led to the administration of low doses of hydrocortisone (200 mg/day) and is believed to decrease requirements for vasopressor agents and reduce mortality. However, in a recent multicentre, randomised, double-blind, placebo-controlled trial, hydrocortisone did not improve survival or reversal of septic shock. As a result, the Surviving Sepsis Campaign downgraded their recommendation on the use of steroids and suggests that **intravenous hydrocortisone should be considered for adult septic shock when hypotension remains poorly responsive to adequate fluid resuscitation and vasopressors**. An increased risk of infection and myopathy are known side effects of steroids.[29–32]

23: Answer: C

The *Trendelenburg position* (supine head-down tilt of at least 45°) was originally intended to provide better surgical exposure for abdominal procedures. Over time, the Trendelenburg position has become popular in managing hypotension and shock, the proposed benefit being the shift of intravascular volume from the lower extremities and abdomen to the heart and brain therefore improving perfusion to these vital organs. **However, current evidence does not support the use of the Trendelenburg position or head-down tilt in hypotensive patients because it does not appear to have any improvement in blood pressure or cardiac index**. In addition, it may also have untoward effects on lung ventilatory mechanics and pulmonary gas exchange and is likely to increase intracranial pressure due to the effect on increased central venous pressure.

Passive leg raising (PLR) has been shown to be useful in predicting fluid responsiveness as it transiently increases venous return and causes an increase in cardiac output in patients who are preload responsive. It mimics an approximate equivalent of 300 mL blood bolus that persists for 2–3 minutes before resulting in intravascular volume redistribution. Furthermore, it has the advantage that this effect is reversible and can be used in the spontaneously breathing patient. The best way to perform a PLR manoeuvre is to elevate the lower limbs to 45° while at the same time placing the patient in the supine from a 45° semirecumbent position. Starting the PLR manoeuvre from a total horizontal position may induce an insufficient venous blood shift to elevate significantly cardiac preload. By contrast, starting PLR from a semirecumbent position induces a larger increase in cardiac preload because it induces the shift of venous blood not only from both the legs but also from the abdominal compartment.

Variations in arterial blood pressure can be observed during positive pressure mechanical ventilation as a result of changes in intrathoracic pressure and lung volumes. A large number of studies have demonstrated that the *pulse pressure variation* (PPV), derived from analysis of the arterial waveform, and the *stroke volume variation* (SVV), derived from pulse contour analysis, are accurate predictors of cardiac preload and highly predictive of fluid responsiveness. However, **respiratory variability of haemodynamic signals cannot be used for predicting volume responsiveness in spontaneously breathing patients**.[33–36]

24. Answer: C

Goal-directed resuscitation within the first 6 hours has been associated with decreased mortality rates in sepsis. It is aimed at restoring systemic perfusion and vital organ function. Patients are resuscitated to predefined physiological end points, which includes:

- urine output >0.5 mL/kg/hr
- CVP 8–12 mmHg
- MAP 65–90 mmHg
- central venous oxygen saturation (ScvO$_2$) ≥70% or mixed venous oxygen saturation (SmvO$_2$) ≥65%.[30,31]

25. Answer: D

As Table 1.2 shows, *dopamine*'s actions are complex and dose-dependent (Table 1.2). At low doses (<5 μg/kg/min) dopamine causes vasodilation at vascular D1 receptors in renal, mesenteric and coronary beds. **Dopamine might produce a diuresis but does not reduce the likelihood of renal failure.** Therefore, the use of low-dose or 'renal-dose' dopamine to protect the kidneys is now discouraged and should not be used. At doses of 5–10 µg/kg/min, dopamine demonstrates activity at cardiac β1 receptors producing inotrope, whereas at higher doses (>10 µg/kg/min) it acts predominantly as an α-agonist, with a profile increasingly more like noradrenaline as the dose increases.

Noradrenaline is a potent α-agonist with significant activity at β1 receptors and minimal or no activity at β2 receptors. Due to the relative absence of β2 effect, noradrenaline causes an increase in both systolic and diastolic pressures. However, its effect on heart rate and cardiac output might be variable despite its positive inotropic and chronotropic actions as there is often a vagal mediated reduction in heart rate at low doses. Subsequently, despite the rise in MAP, cardiac output may remain the same or even fall.

Metaraminol has an indirect effect by stimulating release of noradrenaline from sympathetic nerve terminals and is therefore a potent and selective α-agonist. Its duration of action is about 20 minutes; subsequently it is often administered peripherally as a bolus for the short-term treatment of hypotension. **However, metaraminol may induce a reflex bradycardia and increased ventricular afterload, which might be harmful in patients with cardiogenic shock or decompensated mitral regurgitation.**

Isoprenaline is a synthetic non-selective β-agonist with β1 and β2 activities. The peripheral vasodilation due to β2 stimulation produces a marked reduction in peripheral vascular resistance with subsequent fall in diastolic and MAP, limiting its clinical utility.[37–39]

26. Answer: B

Metaraminol is a potent and selective α-agonist and therefore does not exhibit any positive inotropic

effects. This makes it a useful agent for managing hypotension in patients with severe aortic stenosis or hypertrophic cardiomyopathy.

Although administration of dobutamine via the central route is preferred, it can safely be infused via the peripheral route. Infusion of adrenaline and noradrenaline should be restricted to the central route.

Due to the absence of β2 effects, noradrenaline causes no or minimal vasodilation in skeletal muscle vasculature. Therefore, it causes an increase in systolic as well as diastolic BP. Even though noradrenaline is currently the recommended first-line vasopressor agent in septic shock, this has mainly been based on pathophysiological principles and to date there is no evidence that adrenaline is any worse than other vasoactive agents in terms of mortality outcome.[37–39]

27. Answer: B

Hypertonic saline has been shown to reliably decrease intracranial pressure (ICP) in patients with traumatic brain injury (TBI) (LOE II) and it is at least as effective as mannitol. However, no studies so far have demonstrated improved cerebral blood flow; neither is there good evidence showing an outcome benefit. Despite the potential benefits in reducing ICP in patients with TBI, there is currently no evidence to recommend hypertonic saline over isotonic saline for fluid resuscitation and restoration of the intravascular volume.[40]

28. Answer: A

Fluid resuscitation in trauma remains a controversial topic. However, **hypotensive resuscitation, also known as 'permissive hypotension' or 'small**

TABLE 1.2 ACTIONS OF VASOPRESSORS AND INOTROPES

	α_1 Positive inotropy vasoconstriction	α_2 Positive inotropy vasoconstriction	β_1 Positive inotropy dromotropy chronotropy	β_2 Positive inotropy vasodilation	DA_1 Splanchnic vasodilation natriuresis
Adrenaline	++	+	++++	+++	–
Noradrenaline	++++	+	++	+	–
Dobutamine	+	++++	++++	++	–
Dopamine	>10 µg/kg/min	–	5–10 µg/kg/min	5–10 µg/kg/min	<5 µg/kg/min
Isoprenaline	–	–	++++	+++	–

Adapted from: Senz A, Nunnink L. Inotrope and vasopressor use in the emergency department. EMA 2009;21:342–351.

volume resuscitation', is advocated in patients with a strong potential for ongoing internal haemorrhage (uncontrolled bleeding) until rapid surgical control of bleeding can be achieved. Most studies supporting deliberate hypotension were performed on patients with penetrating thoraco-abdominal trauma, and the most significant results were observed in cases in which distinct vascular injuries were the main source of haemorrhage. This approach still remains controversial in the setting of multisite blunt trauma and severe head injury. Traditional fluid resuscitation is recommended for patients with controllable haemorrhage, isolated extremity injuries and isolated traumatic brain injury.[37,39,41]

29. Answer: A

Resuscitative thoracotomy is a dramatic intervention performed outside of the operating room and usually in the absence of trained cardiothoracic surgeons. The role of resuscitative thoracotomy is more established in penetrating trauma, especially in cardiac stab wounds, and best results are obtained for pericardial tamponade. Better survival has been reported with the penetrating mechanism, with a survival rate of >40% reported in traumatic arrest, specifically precordial stab wounds. Survival was dependant on thoracotomy performed within 10 minutes of arrest and the presence of an organised cardiac activity. **Unresponsive hypotension with a systolic blood pressure <70 and a FAST positive for pericardial tamponade is a consensus-based indication for immediate resuscitative thoracotomy.** The usual trauma resuscitation principles are valid in penetrating injuries to the thorax. A tension pneumothorax can present in a similar way (distended neck veins, hypotension and tachycardia) and should be excluded prior to embarking on resuscitative thoracotomy as a less dramatic intervention such as decompression needle thoracostomy or open thoracostomy can be performed. The role of resuscitative thoracotomy in blunt trauma is more controversial, with a relatively low survival rate of <3%.[42,43]

30. Answer: B

TRALI presents abruptly, usually within 6 hours of transfusion of plasma containing blood products (FFP, packed cells, platelets, cryoprecipitate). It results from the transfusion of white blood cell antibodies (leukoagglutinins) that react with the recipient's leucocytes. Clinically, TRALI is indistinguishable from ARDS. The patient has acute respiratory distress, diffuse bilateral alveolar and interstitial infiltrates on chest X-ray, and varying degree of hypoxaemia. The overall prognosis is better than what would be expected with many other causes of ALI.[44]

31. Answer: B

Fluid resuscitation should not be withheld in patients with PE presenting with persistent hypotension or shock; however, fluid loading should generally not exceed 1 L unless coexistent dehydration or hypovolaemia is suspected. The reason is that in massive PE the right ventricle is already pressure overloaded and failing and excessive fluids might overstretch an already failing ventricle (Starling's law). Persistent hypotension will require inotropic support.

In the International Cooperative Pulmonary Embolism Registry, the death rate from PE is nearly 58% among haemodynamically unstable patients and about 15% among haemodynamically stable patients. Mortality can be as high as 60% in untreated patients and can be reduced to <30% with prompt treatment.

It is acceptable to proceed to immediate thrombolysis without a **CT pulmonary angiogram** (CTPA) in haemodynamically unstable patients with clinically suspected PE in which a bedside echocardiography has shown unequivocal signs of RV overload. The optimum thrombolytic agent and regime are yet to be studied in patients with acute pulmonary emboli. tPA is the only approved drug so far for this indication and short infusion times (≤2 hours) are recommended over prolonged infusion times. Infusions of 100 mg over 2 hours have been used successfully. Tenecteplase should be just as effective and easier to use, although it has not been properly studied in PE and does not have Therapeutic Goods Administration (TGA) approval for this indication.[45,46]

32. Answer: D

Most emergency clinicians have been taught the subxiphoid approach for pericardiocentesis. However, one large review looked at 1127 pericardiocentesis procedures, and found that the optimal placement of the needle was where the distance to the effusion was the least and the effusion size was maximal.[49]

The apical position at the point of maximal impulse on the left lateral chest wall was chosen in 80% of these procedures, based on these variables. The subxiphoid approach was only chosen in 20% of these procedures, as the investigators recognised the large distance the needle had to travel through the liver to enter the pericardial sac.

A phased array probe with a median frequency of 3.5 MHz (2.5–5 MHz) has good penetration and is the most appropriate to examine cardiac structures. High-frequency probes have poor penetration but very detailed superficial images and are mainly used for superficial structures like nerves.

Effusions can be categorised by maximal width of the echogenic pericardial stripe. One classification system divides effusions into small (<10 mm), moderate (10–15 mm) and large (>15 mm). **However, cardiac tamponade is not dependant on the amount of fluid in the pericardial sac but rather on the rate of fluid collection.** Because the pericardium is a relatively thick and fibrous structure, acute pericardial effusions may result in cardiac tamponade despite only small amounts of fluid. When cardiac effusion develops acutely, tamponade can occur with as little as 150 mL of fluid. In contrast, chronic effusions can grow to a large volume without haemodynamic instability. Ultrasonographic signs of tamponade include the presence of a pericardial effusion with:

- associated right atrial (RA) collapse during ventricular systole
- RV diastolic collapse
- lack of respiratory variation in inferior vena cava (IVC) and hepatic veins

Compression of the right side of the heart occurs first as it is under relatively less pressure compared with the left side due to the lower pressure within the pulmonary vascular circuit. Therefore, most echocardiographers define tamponade as compression of the right side of the heart. High pressure within the pericardial sac keeps the chamber from fully expanding during the relaxation phase of the cardiac cycle and therefore it is best recognised during diastole. As the effusion may affect either chamber, both the right atrium and right ventricle should be closely inspected for diastolic collapse.[47,48]

References

1. Nolan JP, Soar J, Zideman DA, et al. European resuscitation council guidelines for resuscitation. Resuscitation 2010;81(10):1219–452.
2. Nolan JP, Hazinski MF, Billi JE, et al. 2010 International consensus on cardiopulmonary resuscitation and emergency care science with treatment recommendations. Resuscitation 2010;81(1) suppl1:e1–e332.
3. Australian Resuscitation Council, New Zealand Resuscitation Council. Equipment and techniques in adult advanced life support. ARC and NZRC guideline 2010. Emerg Med Austr 2011;23(3):286–91.
4. Tanigawa K, Takeda T, Goto E, et al. The efficacy of esophageal detector devices in verifying tracheal tube placement: A randomized cross-over study of out-of-hospital cardiac arrest patients. Anesth Analg 2001;92:375–8.
5. Anderson ML, Younger JG. Mechanical ventilation and noninvasive ventilatory support. In: Marx JA, Hockberger RS, Walls RM, et al, editors. Rosen's emergency medicine: concepts and clinical practice. 7th ed. Philadelphia: Elsevier; 2009. p. 23–8.
6. Hostetler MA. Use of non-invasive positive-pressure ventilation in the emergency department. Emerg Med Clin N Am 2008;26:929–39.
7. Gray A, Goodacre S, Newby DE, et al. Noninvasive ventilation in acute cardiogenic pulmonary edema. N Engl J Med 2008;359(2):142–51.
8. Keenan SP, Kernerman PD, Cook DJ, et al. Effect of noninvasive positive pressure ventilation on mortality in patients admitted with acute respiratory failure: a metanalysis. Critical Care Medicine 1997;25(10): 1685–92.
9. Baudouin S, Blumenthal S, Cooper B, et al. Non-invasive ventilation in acute respiratory failure. Thorax 2002;57:192–211.
10. Tuxen DV, Naughton MT. Acute severe asthma. In: Berston AD, Soni N, editors. Oh's intensive care manual. 6th ed. Philadelphia: Elsevier; 2009. p. 399–413.
11. Oddo M, Feihl F, Schaller M, et al. Management of mechanical ventilation in acute severe asthma: practical aspects. Intensive Care Med 2006;32:501–10.
12. Stather DR, Stewart TE. Clinical review: mechanical ventilation in severe asthma. Critical Care Medicine 2005;9:581–7.
13. Marik PE, Varon J, Fromm Jr R. The management of acute severe asthma. The Journal of Emergency Medicine 2002;23(3):257–68.
14. The Acute Respiratory Distress Syndrome Network. Ventilation with lower tidal volumes as compared with traditional tidal volumes for acute lung injury and the acute respiratory distress syndrome. N Engl J Med 2000;342:1301–8.
15. Berston AD. The acute respiratory distress syndrome (ARDS). In: Berston AD, Soni N, editors. Oh's intensive

care manual. 6th ed. Philadelphia: Elsevier; 2009. p. 375–85.

16. Australian Resuscitation Council, New Zealand Resuscitation Council. Cardiopulmonary resuscitation for advanced life support providers. ARC and NZRC guideline 2010. Emerg Med Austr 2011;23(3):286–91.

17. Sunde K, Jacobs I, Deakin CD, et al. Part 6: Defibrillation. 2010 International consensus on cardiopulmonary resuscitation and emergency care science with treatment recommendations. Resuscitation 2010;81(1) suppl1:e71–e85.

18. Australian Resuscitation Council, New Zealand Resuscitation Council. Electrical therapy for adult advanced life support. ARC and NZRC guideline 2010. Emerg Med Austr 2011;23(3):277–81.

19. Deakin CD, Morrison LJ, Morley PT, et al. Part 8: Advanced life support. 2010 International consensus on cardiopulmonary resuscitation and emergency cardiovascular care science with treatment recommendations. Resuscitation 2010;815:e93–e174.

20. Australian Resuscitation Council, New Zealand Resuscitation Council. Medications in adult cardiac arrest. ARC and NZRC guideline 2010. Emerg Med Austr 2011;23(3):282–5.

21. Datner EM, Promes SB. Resuscitation issues in pregnancy. In: Tintinalli JE, Stapczynski JS, Ma OJ, editors.Emergency medicine: a comprehensive study guide. 7th ed. New York: McGraw-Hill; 2011. p. 91–6.

22. Rogers I. Hypothermia. In: Cameron P, Jelinek G, Kelly A, et al, editors.Textbook of adult emergency medicine. 3rd ed. Edinburgh: Elsevier; 2009. p. 852–5.

23. Australian Resuscitation Council, New Zealand Resuscitation Council. Post-resuscitation therapy in adult advanced life support. ARC and NZRC guideline 2010. Emerg Med Austr 2011;23(3):292–6.

24. Australian Resuscitation Council, New Zealand Resuscitation Council. Therapeutic hypothermia after cardiac arrest. ARC and NZRC guideline 2010. Emerg Med Austr 2011;23(3):297–8.

25. Craig K. How to provide transcutaneous pacing. Nursing 2005;35(10):52–3.

26. Bessman ES. Emergency cardiac pacing. In: Roberts JR, Hedges JR, editors. Clinical procedures in emergency medicine. 5th ed. Philadelphia: Elsevier; 2009. p. 269–86.

27. Cooper DJ, Nichol AD. Lactic acidosis. In: Berston AD, Soni N, editors. Oh's intensive care manual. 6th ed. Philadelphia: Elsevier; 2009. p. 145–51.

28. McLuckie A. Shock – an overview. In: Berston AD, Soni N, editors. Oh's intensive care manual. 6th ed. Philadelphia: Elsevier; 2009. p. 97–104.

29. Sprung CL, Annane D, Keh D, et al. Hydrocortisone therapy for patients with septic shock. NEJM 2008;358:111–24.

30. Nguyen BN, Rivers EP, Abraham FM, et al. Severe sepsis and septic shock: review of the literature and emergency department management guidelines. Ann Emerg Medicine 2006;48:1–54.

31. Dellinger RP, Levy M, Carlet J. Surviving Sepsis Campaign: international guidelines for management of severe sepsis and septic shock. Intens Care Med 2008;34:17–60.

32. Holdgate A. Sepsis and septic shock. In: Cameron P, Jelinek G, Kelly A, et al, editors.Textbook of adult emergency medicine. 3rd ed. Edinburgh: Elsevier; 2009. p. 57–60.

33. Schroeder RA, Barbeito A, Bar-Yosef S, et al. Cardiovascular monitoring. In: Miller RD, Eriksson LI, Fleisher LE, et al, editors. Miller's anesthesia. 7th ed. Elsevier; 2009. p. 1267–328.

34. Marik PE, Monnet X, Teboul J. Hemodynamic parameters to guide fluid therapy. Annals of Intensive Care 2011;1:1. Online. Available: http://www.annalsofintensivecare.com/content/1/1/1; 9 Dec 2011.

35. Casserly B, Read R, Levy MM. Hemodynamic monitoring in sepsis. Crit Care Clin 2009;25:803–23.

36. Makic MBF, VonRueden KT, Rauen CA. Evidence-based practice habits: putting more sacred cows out to pasture. Crit Care Nurse 2011;31(2):38–62.

37. Senz A, Nunnink L. Inotrope and vasopressor use in the emergency department. EMA 2009;21:342–51.

38. Miller BA, Clements EA. Pharmacology of vasopressor agents. In: Tintinalli JE, Stapczynski JS, Ma OJ, editors.Emergency medicine: a comprehensive study guide. 7th ed. New York: McGraw-Hill; 2011. p. 162–5.

39. Garret P. Shock overview. In: Cameron P, Jelinek G, Kelly A, et al, editors.Textbook of adult emergency medicine. 3rd ed. Edinburgh: Elsevier; 2009. p. 45–56.

40. Banks CJ, Furyk JS. Review article: Hypertonic saline use in the emergency department. EMA 2008;20:294–305.

41. Roppolo LP, Wigginton JG, Pepe PE. Intravenous fluid resuscitation for the trauma patient. Current Opinion in Critical Care 2010;16:283–8.

42. Fitzgerald M, Gocentas R. Chest trauma. In: Cameron P, Jelinek G, Kelly A, et al, editors.Textbook of adult emergency medicine. 3rd ed. Edinburgh: Elsevier; 2009. p. 104–9.

43. Boczar ME, Rivers E. Resuscitative thoracotomy. In: Roberts JR, Hedges JR, editors. Clinical procedures in emergency medicine. 5th ed. Philadelphia: Elsevier; 2009. p. 312–24.

44. Emery M. Blood and blood components. In: Marx JA, Hockberger RS, Walls RM, et al, editors.Rosen's emergency medicine: concepts and clinical practice. 7th ed. Philadelphia: Elsevier; 2009. p. 42–6.

45. Mountain DM, Cameron P. Pulmonary embolism. In: Cameron P, Jelinek G, Kelly A, et al, editors.Textbook of adult emergency medicine. 3rd ed. Edinburgh: Elsevier; 2009. p. 232–8.

46. Agnelli G, Becattini C. Current concepts: acute pulmonary embolism. N Engl J Med 2010;363:266–74.

47. Reardon RF, Joing SA. Cardiac. In: Ma JO, Mateer JR, Blaivas M, editors. Emergency ultrasound. 2nd ed. New York: McGraw Hill; 2008. p. 109–48.

48. Perera P, Mailhot T, Riley D. et al. The RUSH exam: rapid ultrasound in shock in the evaluation of the critically ill. Emerg Med Clin N Am 2010;28:29–56.

49. Tsang T, Enriquez-Sarano M, Freeman WK. Consecutive 1127 therapeutic echocardiographically guided pericardiocenteses: clinical profile, practice patterns and outcomes spanning 21 years. Mayo Clin Proc 2002;77:429–36.

Paediatric resuscitation

1. Answer: C

The ILCOR Neonatal Task Force recommends a compression-ventilation ratio of 3:1 for resuscitating newborns *in the delivery room*, with a pause for ventilation whether or not the infant has an advanced airway. It is **unknown what the optimal compression-ventilation ratio is during CPR for all infants in the first month of life** *beyond the delivery room*. If the aetiology of the arrest is cardiac, a 15:2 ratio (two rescuers) may be more effective than a 3:1 ratio. If it is suspected to be asphyxial or respiratory in nature, then 3:1 provides more effective ventilation, at the expense of interrupted CPR. The level of evidence (LOE) is poor at best (level 5). Generally, all infants beyond the immediate perinatal period should be managed according to paediatric guidelines. The Pediatric Task Force recommends a 15:2 compression-ventilation ratio with a pause for ventilation in infants without an advanced airway, and continuous compressions without a pause for ventilation for infants with an advanced airway.

Traditionally, the initial mode of providing assisted positive pressure ventilation in critically unwell children has been via a BVM ventilation device. When definitive airway protection and invasive ventilation has been deemed necessary, endotracheal intubation using an endotracheal tube has been the next logical step. The laryngeal mask airway (LMA) has in recent years become a useful rescue airway technique, in whom intubation has proved difficult. No studies have directly compared BVM with the use of supraglottic airway devices during paediatric resuscitation other than for the newborns in the delivery room. Nine LOE 5 case reports demonstrated the effectiveness of supraglottic airway devices, primarily the LMA, for airway rescue of children with airway abnormalities. Unfortunately, in anaesthetic-based studies, complication rates with LMAs increase with decreasing patient age and size. In the intensive care unit (ICU) setting, time to effective ventilation was shorter and tidal volumes were greater with BVM. **The ILCOR guidelines treatment recommendation on this issue is that BVM remains the preferred technique for emergency ventilation during the initial steps of paediatric resuscitation.** In infants and children for whom BVM is unsuccessful, use of the LMA may be considered for either airway rescue or support of ventilation.

LMAs should not be used in semiconscious patients or when the gag reflex is present. They are subject to dislodgment during transport. Their use should not replace mastery of BVM ventilation. Children older than 9 years of age may be managed according to adult resuscitation guidelines, although clinical judgement should be exercised in considering the child's weight, height and developmental age.[1-3]

2. Answer: C

Prevention of illness in children is a cardinal paediatric principle. **Cardiorespiratory arrest in children is often preceded by a period of recognisable deteriorating respiratory function, and is usually respiratory or asphyxial in nature. This deterioration can readily be detected if systems are in place to recognise and treat this warning phase, therefore preventing cardiorespiratory arrest.** METs have been shown to be effective in preventing respiratory and cardiac arrests in selected paediatric inpatient settings, although the LOE for MET teams is level III at best. The Australian Resuscitation Council recommends that all institutions that manage childhood illnesses should have a system enabling staff at the bedside to quickly summon expert help if needed (Recommendation Class A). One LOE I randomised controlled trial in children with severe sepsis or fluid refractory septic shock showed that protocol-driven therapy targeting a superior vena caval oxygen saturation of 70%, coupled with treating clinical signs of shock (prolonged capillary refill, reduced urine output and reduced blood pressure), improved patient survival to hospital discharge in comparison with standard treatment aimed at clinical signs alone. There are insufficient data regarding the use of lactate and pH to guide management of shock in children.[1,2]

3. Answer: B

Cardiorespiratory arrest occurs in a wide variety of conditions among infants and children. The majority is caused by hypoxaemia, hypotension, or both. Examples are trauma, drowning, septicaemia, SIDS, asthma, upper airway obstruction and congenital anomalies of the heart and lung. The initial cardiac rhythm discovered during early electrocardiographic monitoring is often severe bradycardia or asystole. VF is much less common in children than in adults, with an incidence of primary VF in children of 10%. The optimal effective and safe dose of electricity to be used is unknown. The incidence of primary VF in children is 10%.[4,5]

Seven LOE 3 studies showed that mutations causing channelopathies occurred in 2–10% of infants with SIDS, while one LOE 3 and two LOE 4 studies showed 14–20% of young adults with sudden death had genetic mutations causing channelopathies.[2]

4. Answer: D

Healthcare providers commonly assess pulse status inaccurately; they mistakenly palpate a pulse when it is non-existent or fail to detect a pulse when it is present. Additionally, pulse assessment often takes longer than 10 seconds. As a result, **ILCOR suggests that palpation of a pulse (or its absence) is not reliable as the sole determinant of cardiac arrest and therefore decided to deemphasize but not eliminate the pulse check as part of the healthcare provider assessment.** Current recommendations are that if the victim is unresponsive, not breathing normally, and there are no signs of life, lay rescuers should begin CPR. Healthcare providers should begin CPR unless they can definitely palpate a pulse within 10 seconds. CPR should be commenced promptly if doubt exists. The circulation may be assessed by palpation of a carotid, brachial or femoral pulse (Class B; Expert Consensus Opinion).

To be effective, chest compressions must be deep. The Australian Resuscitation Council recommends a chest compression depth of at least one-third of the anterior–posterior dimension of the chest or approximately 5 cm in children and approximately 4 cm in infants (Class A; Expert Consensus Opinion).

The optimal method of chest compression, two-thumb or two-finger, is yet to be determined and either technique may be performed (Class A; LOE IV). However, the two-thumb technique is the strongly preferred technique for healthcare rescuers (Class A; Expert Consensus Opinion).

Approximately 50% of a compression cycle should be devoted to compression of the chest and 50% to relaxation to enable recoil of the chest wall.[6,7]

5. Answer: D

Intraosseous (IO) access in the setting of paediatric and adult resuscitative care is an old intervention that has found its way back into modern critical care. It provides faster and more reliable access than traditional peripheral routes when practitioners are trained in their use. The newer drill devices have not been prospectively shown to actually improve outcomes in paediatric resuscitation, but this question is posed as an area for future research in the ILCOR guidelines.

All resuscitative drugs and fluids may be given via the IV or IO route but only adrenaline, atropine and lignocaine are absorbed when given via ETT.

It is generally accepted that **bone marrow may be reliably used for venous biochemical and haematological analysis but not for venous blood gas analysis.** Most of the laboratory studies looking at IO samples have been done in animal settings. Recent data, however, suggests that white cell counts in IO samples are higher, and CO_2 and platelet levels are lower, while most other analytes are similar.[1,2,3,8]

6. Answer: C

An LMA cannot offer airway protection. Definitive airway protection requires insertion of an endotracheal tube, cuffed or uncuffed. No studies have proven that an ETT is better than BVM in the prehospital setting. Studies of resuscitation at out-of-hospital paediatric arrest either favour BVM or show no advantage of endotracheal intubation. One LOE I study compared paramedic out-of-hospital BVM with intubation for children with cardiac arrest, respiratory arrest or respiratory failure and found equivalent rates of survival to hospital discharge and neurologic outcome. One LOE I systematic review that included this study also reached the same conclusion.

A nasopharyngeal airway of appropriate length is the equivalent distance from the tip of the nose to the tragus of the ear.

Differences in the anatomy of the airway of the child compared with adults include a more anterior and cephalad larynx, a long floppy epiglottis and a shorter trachea.[1, 2,7,9]

7. Answer: D

Adequate inflation of the lungs is often possible with BVM ventilation, but this is a difficult technique for the non-expert. BVM ventilation is an acceptable technique if the lungs can be inflated adequately (Class B). BVM ventilation was associated with fewer complications than endotracheal intubation in out-of-hospital prospective controlled studies when transport times to hospital were short (LOE II). BVM ventilation was no less appropriate than endotracheal intubation during cardiac arrest or trauma in retrospective studies (LOE III-2).

Cricoid pressure has not been shown to decrease aspiration risk. One LOE 5 study in adults has shown that cricoid pressure or laryngeal manipulation aids in intubation in some patients, but is a hindrance in others. The ILCOR treatment recommendation is that if cricoid pressure is used during emergency intubations in infants and children it should be discontinued if it impedes ventilation or interferes with the speed or ease of intubation.

Both cuffed and uncuffed tracheal tubes are acceptable for infants and children undergoing emergency intubation. Current ILCOR and ARC recommendations for endotracheal tube size, based on the internal diameter, consist of the following:

- Uncuffed tubes:
  - Term newborn of 2000–3000 g birth weight: size 3.0 mm
  - Term newborn of >3000 g: size 3.5 mm
  - Infants ≤6 months of age: 3.5–4 mm
  - Infants 7–12 months of age: 4 mm
  - Children over 1 year: size (mm) = age (years)/4 + 4
- Cuffed tubes:
  - Newborn ≥3 kg and ≤1 year of age: 3mm
  - Children 1–2 years of age: 3.5mm
  - Children >2 years of age: size (mm) = age (years)/4 + 3.5

If the tracheal tube meets resistance during insertion, a tube with an internal diameter (ID) of 0.5 mm smaller should be used. If there is no leak around the tube with the cuff deflated, reintubation with a tube ID 0.5 mm smaller may be beneficial when the patient is stable.

The Khine formula of estimating the appropriate cuffed tracheal tube size is: ID (mm) = (age/4) + 3. It is used in young children, from full-term newborns to children aged 8 years. However, recent evidence suggests that this formula underestimates the optimal tube size by 0.5 mm.[2,7]

8. Answer: D

Children generally suffer cardiopulmonary arrest after a respiratory insult, therefore in an unwitnessed arrest attention is given to airway and breathing management – hence CPR first, then call for help. **A single rescuer encountering an *unwitnessed* collapse of an infant or child should start CPR immediately and then obtain assistance. A rescuer *witnessing* a sudden collapse should obtain help immediately and then start CPR**.

A variable dose manual defibrillator is preferred in children. A semi-automated external defibrillator may be used for infants and children (Class A) but its safety has not been proven. If a manual defibrillator is not available for infants and small children (aged 1–8 years), use of an adult AED with dose attenuation (e.g. delivering 50 J) is acceptable. If that is not available, an adult AED dose machine should be used. For children older than 8 years, a standard AED machine (for adults) may be used.[1–3,7]

9. Answer: D

TABLE 1.3 SUMMARY OF RATES AND RATIOS[7]

	BLS	ALS	
Ratio	30:2	15:2	
Ventilation	Mouth-to-mouth	BVM/LMA	ETT
Cycles	5 in 2 min	5 in 1 min	Continuous
Cardiac compressions	75/min	75/min	100/min
Breaths	5/min	10/min	12–14

Based on: Australian Resuscitation Council. Guideline 12.2. Advanced life support for infants and children, diagnosis and initial management. December 2010. Online. Available: www.resus.org.au; 5 Jan 2011.

10. Answer: C

Weight estimation is very important in paediatric resuscitation. Some evidence has shown that current estimation formulae underestimate children's weights.

The doses of drugs and volume of fluid therapy are based on body weight, which in non-obese patients is estimated according to age or height. **In obese patients, initial doses, except selected drugs such as suxamethonium, should be based on ideal weight estimated from height.**

Approximate weights according to age are:

- newborn – I year : 3.5–10 kg or (age x 2) plus 8 kg
- ≤9 years: [2 (age +4)]
- ≥10 years: age x 3.3 kg

Alternatively, weight can be estimated using a standard chart of children's height and using the 50th percentile to estimate weight.[1,2,7,10–12]

11. Answer: C

The optimal dose for safe and effective cardioversion or defibrillation in children is unknown. **The new recommended initial dose of 2–4 J/kg reflects LOE III/IV showing lower success in termination of VF in children with 2 J/kg.** Adult data clearly shows that long pauses in chest compressions required for stacked shocks are associated with worse resuscitation outcomes and so the recommendation for single shock followed by prompt resumption of CPR is emphasised.

The dose in VF arrest and pulseless VT is unsynchronised. Synchronised cardioversion for unstable VT, that is, VT with hypotension or evidence of poor perfusion, is the current recommended first therapeutic approach in children.

The safety of AEDs in infants <1 year is unknown but case reports have documented successful defibrillation using AEDs in infants. Many AED devices can safely and accurately distinguish between shockable and non-shockable rhythms in infants and adults. A manual defibrillator or an AED with paediatric attenuation capabilities is preferred for use in infants and small children. If a manual defibrillator is not available, an adult AED with dose attenuation to 50 J may be used in infants (≤1 year old) and children 1–8 years of age. If neither a manual defibrillator nor an adult AED with an attenuated energy level is available, an AED with an adult preset dose may be used. Children aged over 8 years may be treated with adult AED preset energy levels.[1–3,13]

12. Answer: D

The optimal timing for intubation of children in shock remains unclear. Individual case reports of children and adults with septic shock suggest potential beneficial effects of early intubation.

There are no studies specifically investigating the role of intubation and assisted ventilation before the onset of respiratory failure in infants and children with shock. The decision to initially stabilise the patient according to a sepsis protocol, which may include early use of inotropes, is a case-by-case decision. Early intubation and mechanical ventilation will decrease the work of breathing and lessen metabolic demand, as well as decrease afterload. However, intubation of a critically unwell child always has the potential for precipitating critical hypotension with cardiac arrest.

Parasympathetic cardiac blockade with atropine may be indicated if bradycardia is caused by vagal stimulation or cholinergic drug toxicity. The IV or IO dose is 20 mcg/kg (Class A; Expert Consensus Opinion) and the ETT dose 30 mcg/kg. **Bradycardia caused by hypoxaemia should be treated with ventilation and oxygen but, if unresponsive, should be treated with adrenaline.** Severe bradycardia and/ or bradycardia with hypotension should be treated with adrenaline, not atropine.[2,13]

13. Answer: C

IO insertion has a complication rate of <1%. IO insertion has been rigorously studied in preterm babies and its use is effective and safe. Multiple studies have shown there is no risk to bone growth, damage to the epiphyseal plate is not a common complication, and growth failure is not reported solely on the basis of IO use.[14,15]

14. Answer: C

Newborn infants who are born at term with clear amniotic fluid, who are breathing or crying with good tone, must be dried and kept warm and do not require resuscitation. Any deviation from this normal state requires careful, staged assessment to determine whether the following actions are needed in sequence:

1. initial steps in stabilisation (clearing the airway, positioning, stimulating with drying)
2. ventilation
3. chest compressions
4. medications or volume expansion

Progression from one stage to the next is based on simultaneous assessment of three vital signs: respirations, heart rate and colour. Thirty seconds is allotted to complete one stage successfully, reevaluate, and decide whether to progress to the next. After the initial steps in stabilisation have been performed and assessment of the heart rate reveals a rate below 100 bpm, positive pressure ventilation is required.

Full-term babies who are depressed in terms of crying, breathing or tone immediately after birth should have their airway cleared, be stimulated and dried, then reassessed before commencing with formal resuscitative steps. Additionally, the ILCOR guidelines clearly state that if resuscitation is required: 'There is currently insufficient evidence to specify the concentration of oxygen to be used at initiation of resuscitation.'[16] The reason for this is that there is conflicting evidence on whether room air is better than 100% oxygen, and there is evidence that providing oxygen in this setting may cause tissue damage from free oxygen radicals.

There is no indication to suction a newborn who is showing vigorous signs of life, and who is crying and breathing spontaneously.

Auscultation of the heart is the most accurate clinical measure, with palpation of the umbilical cord less so. However, both are relatively insensitive. Several studies have addressed the accuracy of pulse oximetry in measuring heart rate in the delivery room. Pulse oximetry (SpO_2) and heart rate can be measured reliably after 90 seconds from birth with a pulse oximeter designed to reduce movement artifact and a neonatal probe (LOE 4).[16]

15. Answer: C

The need for resuscitation is determined by repeated and staged assessment of heart rate, respiration and colour in 30-second stages. Apgar scores are measured at 1 and 5 minutes and therefore are useless as a resuscitation assessment tool. The use of the Apgar score is limited to reviewing a neonate's response to initial successful resuscitation. The probe should be attached to the right hand or wrist.

Heart rate should remain the primary vital sign by which to judge the need for and efficacy of resuscitation. Auscultation of the precordium should remain the primary means of assessing heart rate. There is a high likelihood of underestimating heart rate with palpation of the umbilical pulse, but this is preferable to other palpation locations. For babies who require ongoing resuscitation or respiratory support or both, the goal should be to use pulse oximetry. The sensor should be placed on the baby's right hand or wrist before connecting the probe to the instrument. Because of concerns about the ability to

consistently obtain accurate measurements, pulse oximetry should be used in conjunction with and should not replace clinical assessment of heart rate during newborn resuscitation. Furthermore, saturation monitoring is inconsistent in the first 90 seconds after birth – precisely the period during which heart rate assessment is needed to determine the need for resuscitation.[16]

16. Answer: D

When babies have meconium-stained amniotic fluid, they are at risk of developing meconium aspiration syndrome (MAS) – upon taking their first breath they inhale thick meconium that may cause a form of pneumonitis. In the past these babies would be suctioned intrapartum on the perineum – this is no longer recommended. Tracheal intubation and suctioning of meconium-stained but vigorous infants at birth does not reduce the incidence of MAS. Similarly, there are no systematic studies to address the benefit or complications of tracheal suctioning in meconium-stained, depressed infants. With meconium-stained depressed infants, ILCOR therefore still recommends the current traditional management of tracheal suctioning via an endotracheal tube, immediately after birth and before stimulation (to prevent meconium inhalation with the first breaths). If meconium is retrieved on this initial suctioning, further intubations and repeat suctioning is needed until the airway is clear of meconium. Review of the need for ventilation, compressions or adrenaline can then take place according to the standard neonatal resuscitation protocol. Positive pressure ventilation is inappropriate in this setting until it is certain that meconium has been cleared from the airway. Tracheal suctioning is not necessary for babies with meconium-stained fluid who are vigorous.

Air is the initial choice during newborn resuscitation. In full-term infants receiving resuscitation at birth with positive pressure ventilation, it is best to begin with air rather than 100% oxygen. If despite effective ventilation there is no increase in heart rate or if oxygenation (guided by oximetry) remains unacceptable, use of a higher concentration of oxygen should be considered.[16]

17. Answer: A

There is currently no evidence to support the use of inflation pressures higher than those that are necessary to achieve improvement in heart rate or chest expansion. This can usually be achieved in term infants with an inflation pressure of 30 cm H_2O (LOE 4) and in preterm infants with pressures of 20–25 cm H_2O (LOE 4). Occasionally, higher pressures are required (LOE 4). If positive-pressure ventilation is required, an initial inflation pressure of 20–25 cm H_2O is adequate for most preterm infants. If prompt improvement in heart rate or chest movement is not obtained, then higher pressures to achieve effective ventilation may be needed. PEEP is likely to be beneficial during initial stabilisation of apnoeic preterm infants who require positive-pressure ventilation and should be used if suitable equipment is available.

For spontaneously breathing preterm infants at ≥25 weeks' gestation who have signs of respiratory distress, there is no significant difference between starting CPAP or intubation and mechanical ventilation in the delivery room when considering death or oxygen requirement at 36 weeks postmenstrual age. In spontaneously breathing infants at 25–28 weeks' gestation, CPAP compared with intubation reduced the rates of mechanical ventilation from 100% to 46% and surfactant use from 77% to 38% (LOE 14).[16]

18. Answer: C

In the initial stages of cardiac arrest due to an asphyxial cause (which is most common in children),

the $ETCO_2$ is usually elevated. Level 4 evidence from adult and paediatric case series suggest that $ETCO_2$ readings rise with interventions that increase cardiac output, and may be useful in assessing the quality of interventions such as good chest compression. **As an estimate, if the $ETCO_2$ is consistently <15 mmHg, it may indicate the quality of chest compressions is poor or excessive ventilation is decreasing the CO_2 level.** The $ETCO_2$ must be interpreted with caution for 1–2 minutes after administration of adrenaline or other vasoconstrictive medications because these medications may decrease the $ETCO_2$.

In one LOE 4 and two LOE 5 adult case series an abrupt and sustained rise in $ETCO_2$ often preceded identification of ROSC. Two LOE 4 paediatric cases series showed that a low $ETCO_2$ (10–15 mmHg) despite 15–20 minutes of advanced life support is strongly associated with failure to achieve ROSC. The data is insufficient to recommend this as a threshold for terminating resuscitation measures.

There is insufficient evidence (small case series, level 4 or 5 evidence) to recommend for or against the routine use of echocardiography during paediatric cardiac arrest. Clearly, however, in the hands of trained personnel, echo may be useful in identifying a case for arrest such as tamponade. The use of echo must be weighed against the obvious deleterious effect of delayed or interrupted CPR.[1]

References

1. Australian Resuscitation Council. Guideline12.1. Introduction to paediatric advanced life support. December 2010. Online. Available: www.resus.org.au; 5 Jan 2011.
2. De Caen AR, Kleinman ME, Chameides L, et al. Part 10: Paediatric basic and advanced life support. International consensus on cardiopulmonary resuscitation and emergency cardiovascular care science with treatment recommendations. Resuscitation 2010;81:e213–e259.
3. Australian Resuscitation Council. Guideline 12.6: Techniques in paediatric advanced life support. December 2010. Online. Available: www.resus.org.au; 5 Jan 2011.
4. Nadkarni VM, Larkin GL, Peberdy MA, et al. First documented rhythm and clinical outcome from in-hospital cardiac arrest among children and adults. JAMA 2006;295:50–7.
5. Kleinman ME, De Caen AR, Chameides L, et al. Part 10: Paediatric basic and advanced life support: International consensus on cardiopulmonary resuscitation and emergency cardiovascular care science with treatment recommendations. Circulation 2010;122(suppl 2):S466–S515.
6. Tibballs J, Russell P. Reliability of pulse palpation by healthcare personnel to diagnose paediatric cardiac arrest. Resuscitation 2009;80:61–4.
7. Australian Resuscitation Council. Guideline 12.2. Advanced life support for infants and children, diagnosis and initial management. December 2010. Online. Available: www.resus.org.au; 5 Jan 2011.
8. Miller LJ, Philbeck TE, Montez D, et al. A new study of intraosseous blood for laboratory analysis. Arch Pathol Lab Med 2010;134(9):1253–60.

9. Gausche M, Lewis RJ, Stratton SJ, et al. Effect of out-of-hospital pediatric endotracheal intubation on survival and neurological outcome: a controlled clinical trial. JAMA 2000;283:783–90.

10. Luscombe MD, Owens BD, Burke D. Weight estimation in paediatrics: a comparison of the APLS formula and the formula 'Weight=3(age)+7'. Emerg Med J 2011;28: 590–593.

11. Lubitz SL, Seidel JS, Chameides L, et al. A rapid method for estimating weight and resuscitation drug dosages from length in the paediatric age group. Ann Emerg Med 1988;17:576–581.

12. Australian Resuscitation Council. Guideline 12. 4 Mediactions and fluids in paediatric advanced life support. December 2010. Online. Available: www.resus.org.au; 5 Jan 2011.

13. Tibballs J, Carter B, Kiraly NJ, et al. Biphasic DC shock cardioverting doses for paediatric atrial dysrhythmias. Resuscitation 2010;81:1101–4.

14. Fiser RT, Walker WM, Seibert JJ, et al. Tibial length following intraosseous infusion: a prospective, radiographic analysis. Pediatr Emerg Care 1997;13:186–8.

15. LaRocco BG, Wang HE. Intraosseous infusion. Prehosp Emerg Care 2003;7:280–5.

16. Perlman JM, Wyllie J, Kattwinkel J, et al. Part 11: Neonatal resuscitation: 2010 International consensus on cardiopulmonary resuscitation and emergency cardiovascular care science with treatment recommendations. Circulation 2010;122 (suppl 2):S516–S538.

1. Answer: A

A detailed history obtained from the patient regarding the nature of chest pain is important for the diagnosis and risk stratification. The positive likelihood ratios (LRs) have been determined for various descriptions of chest pain. **The positive LR for pain radiating to the right arm or shoulder as an indicator of myocardial infarction is 4.7 compared with LR of 2.3 for pain radiating to left arm.** The positive LR for pain radiating to both arms and shoulders is 4.1. Burning or indigestion pain can be associated with ACS (LR 2.8), while pain reproducible by palpation and described as pleuritic, sharp or positional does not exclude ACS or AMI.[1,2]

2. Answer: C

Approximately half of the patients with AMI will have an initial ECG showing a new ST segment elevation ≥1 mm in two contiguous leads. Its positive predictive value for diagnosis of AMI has been described as >90%.

Patients with an elevated troponin have a worse 2- and 28-day prognosis compared with patients without an elevated troponin.

Compared with conventional troponin assays, with the use of new high-sensitive troponin assays (both TnT and TnI), troponin can be detected at much lower levels. Consequently, these superior performing high-sensitivity assays have increased sensitivity in early detection of AMI. However, these increased sensitivities have been achieved at the expense of reduced specificities (see Table 2.1).

In the absence of ischaemic heart disease, troponin can be elevated in a range of non-ischaemic pathologies. This should be considered when interpreting troponin results. Troponin can be elevated in the following non-ischaemic conditions including:

- sepsis and critically unwell patients
- PE
- renal failure
- myocarditis, myopericarditis and myocardial extension of endocarditis
- stroke and subarachnoid haemorrhage
- aortic dissection
- congestive cardiac failure – both acute and chronic
- cardiac contusion
- pacing, ablation, cardiac surgery
- tachyarrhythmias, bradiarrhythmias and heart block
- respiratory failure.

Exercise stress testing is a functional test that is prognostically useful in predicting adverse events for coronary artery disease (CAD) despite its limited sensitivity and specificity in diagnosing CAD. It is useful for risk stratifying low to intermediate risk patients.[1–4]

3. Answer: A

TIMI score has been validated as a predictor of adverse outcomes (subsequent myocardial infarction, mortality, arrhythmia) and the need for early invasive management for NSTEAC syndrome. TIMI refers to the name of the research organisation that conducted the trials.

Age, diabetes and previous aspirin use are all variables that need to be considered in risk stratification of NSTEACS. Patients with a low TIMI score still have considerable risk for adverse events, with a score of 0–1 having a risk of up to 4.7%.

TIMI score calculations (1 point for each factor present)

- Age 65 years or over
- At least 3 risk factors for CAD (hypertension ≥140/90 or on antihypertensives, cigarette smoking, HDL < 40, diabetes, family history of CAD (CAD in male first-degree relative, or in father when <55 years of age, female first-degree relative or mother <65 years of age)
- Aspirin use in the past 7 days
- At least 2 angina episodes within last 24 hours
- Known coronary artery disease (coronary stenosis 50% or more)
- ST changes of at least 0.5 mm on ECG
- Elevated serum cardiac biomarkers

Table 2.2 shows the percentage of risk at 14 days of mortality due to all causes, new or recurrent MI or severe recurrent ischaemia requiring urgent revascularisation.[5–7]

Duration since presentation with chest pain	30 min	2 hours	3 hours
Cumulative sensitivity	93%	98%	100%
Specificity	N/A	57%	54%

TABLE 2.2 TIMI SCORE INTERPRETATION

TIMI score	% of risk
0–1	4.7
2	8.3
3	13.2
4	19.9
5	26.2
6–7	40.9

4. Answer: B

ST elevation in leads II, III and aVF suggests an inferior infarction that may involve the right coronary or circumflex arteries, as can posterior infarctions. Posterior infarction may also be caused by occlusion of the circumflex artery in patients with dominant left-sided circulation. Inferior and posterior AMI may be associated with RV infarction. Posterior AMI are associated with ST segment depression in V1 and V2 and ST segment elevation in posteriorly placed leads. One of the earliest markers of an inferior AMI may be ST depression in lead aVL.[1,8,9]

5. Answer: A

ST segment elevation in aVR in a patient with ischaemic-sounding chest pain is a marker for proximal left system disease, which has a mortality of up to 70%, and should not be treated as a non-STEMI.

Posterior STEMI is often difficult to diagnose. It is characterised by:
- ST depression in the anterior chest leads
- tall/wide R waves in V1–V2
- R/S ratio >1 in V1–V2 without right axis deviation
- upright T waves in V1–V2
- ST segment elevation when leads V7–9 are performed

Wellen's syndrome is characterised by abnormal T wave inversion or biphasic T waves, especially in leads V2–4. These changes may be a marker of proximal left main disease, particularly in patients with ischaemic-sounding chest pain.

ECG criteria for reperfusion are:
- ST segment elevation of ≥1 mm in two or more contiguous limb leads, or
- ST segment elevation of ≥2 mm in two or more contiguous chest leads, or
- new LBBB.[5,10,11]

6. Answer: C

The ECG is the only investigation required to select a patient for emergency reperfusion. An echocardiogram may assist in decision making in difficult or less clear cut cases, looking for wall motion abnormalities in the area suggested by ECG changes. A negative troponin excludes a myocardial infarction but does not exclude an ACS, although does reduce the risk, especially in a patient with a normal ECG who is aged <40 years and has no cardiac risk factors. Troponin takes 6–12 hours after the onset of pain to become positive. Consequently, an early troponin may be a false negative. The CXR adds little to most patients in the assessment of ACS, although it may be potentially useful where aortic dissection is a possibility. CXR cannot exclude thoracic aortic dissection and CT angiogram of the aorta is required for that purpose.[5,6]

7. Answer: B

There are multiple mimics of STEMI including:
- bundle branch block
- pacemaker
- cardiomyopathy
- pericarditis
- myocarditis
- preexcitation
- hyperkalaemia
- benign early repolarisation
- ventricular hypertrophy
- PE
- subarachnoid haemorrhage.

Up to 50% of AMI have normal or non-diagnostic ECGs. A clinical decision rule developed by Sgarbossa et al.[12] attempts to predict the likelihood of AMI in a patient presenting with ischaemic symptoms and LBBB. This rule consists of a scoring system based on:

- ST segment elevation ≥1 mm concordant with the QRS complex
- ST segment depression ≥1 mm in V1, V2 or V3
- ST elevation ≥5 mm discordant with the QRS complex.

Only 1–2% of patients presenting with ischaemic symptoms to the ED have a new or presumed new (not known to be old) LBBB. **The first Sgarbossa criterion, ST segment elevation ≥1 mm that is *concordant* with the QRS complex, if present, seems to be the most specific in diagnosing AMI in those patients.** However, the Sgarbossa criteria have a limited sensitivity in diagnosing AMI in patients with LBBB. In clinical practice, because of their low sensitivity, these criteria may not be helpful (any diagnostic test/criteria should be highly sensitive to diagnose a critical condition such as AMI).

Patients presenting with ischaemic-sounding chest pain and ST segment elevation of ≥2 mm in 2 or more contiguous chest leads and ≥1 mm in the limb leads meet reperfusion criteria.[5,8,9,12–14]

8. Answer: D

Posterior myocardial infarction is rarely isolated, and is usually associated with inferior or lateral wall infarction. It can be subtle and presents as ST segment depression in V1–V4. It is associated with RV infarction and failure. **Anterior or anterior septal infarction is associated with ST elevation in V1–V4 and is the most common STEMI, with the worst prognosis.** Lateral infarction is associated with ST elevation in leads 1, aVL and V5 and V6, and is due to occlusion of the left anterior descending (LAD) or circumflex arteries, while inferior AMI is manifested by ST segment elevation in leads II, III and aVF and is less common than anterior or anteroseptal AMI (see Table 2.3).[5,9]

TABLE 2.3 LOCALISATION OF MYOCARDIAL INFARCTION USING THE ECG

Infarct area	ECG changes
Inferior wall	ST elevation II, III, aVF
Lateral wall	ST elevation I, aVL, V5, V6
Anterior, anteroseptal wall	ST elevation V1–V4
Posterior myocardial infarction	ST depression V1–V4
Right ventricle	ST elevation V4R

9. Answer: D

Chest pain with new neurology suggests aortic dissection, which is an absolute contraindication to thrombolysis. Absolute contraindications include those illnesses that increase bleeding risk and those conditions that increase the risk of intracranial haemorrhage. Some authors and manufacturers of tenecteplase do not differentiate between absolute and relative contraindications.

Absolute contraindications include:
- any previous intracranial bleeding and haemorrhagic stroke
- ischaemic stroke within the past 3 months
- a known structural vascular lesion in the brain (e.g. cerebral aneurysm, arteriovenous malformation)
- a known intracranial neoplasm
- active internal bleeding (except menstrual period)
- suspicion for aortic dissection or pericarditis

Relative contraindications include:
- a previous stroke of unknown origin
- a previous ischaemic stroke >3 months ago
- severe uncontrolled hypertension (BP > 180/100)
- recent trauma including trauma associated with current AMI (within the past 2 weeks)
- prolonged CPR (>10 min)
- major surgery (within the past 3 weeks)
- recent biopsy of a parenchymal organ
- recent non-compressible vascular punctures (including subclavian and internal jugular lines)
- recent internal bleeding (within the past 4 weeks)
- a known arterial aneurysm or arterovenous malformation
- current anticoagulant use
- known bleeding diathesis
- known subacute bacterial endocarditis
- current acute pancreatitis
- severe hepatic dysfunction
- neoplasm with increased bleeding risk
- pregnancy
- other conditions likely to increase bleeding risk.[5,6,8]

10. Answer: A

The CAPTIM trial, conducted in France, has suggested that prehospital thrombolysis given within 2 hours of symptom onset has better outcomes than percutaneous coronary intervention (PCI) and had equivalent outcomes with PCI if given within 4 hours.

PCI is the reperfusion treatment of choice for cardiogenic shock associated with AMI.

Tenecteplase has a higher risk of intracranial haemorrhage than streptokinase. Thrombolysis has a higher risk of bleeding-related adverse effects in females (because they generally weigh less), the elderly and patients with hypertension.

The number needed to treat (NNT) to save a life for inferior STEMI is approximately 100–120.[11,15]

11. Answer: D

Aspirin alone has up to 25% relative risk reduction in mortality.

Large trials have not shown any benefit in the early use of beta-blocker therapy in patients with STEMI. Recognising this, the 2007 focused update to the American College of Cardiology / American Heart Association guidelines for managing patients with ST-segment elevation myocardial infarction now recommends *oral (not intravenous) beta-blocker therapy* to be initiated during the first 24 hours of care of STEMI patients who have none of the following:

- signs of heart failure
- evidence of a low cardiac output state
- increased risk for cardiogenic shock, cumulatively:
  - age ≥70 years
  - systolic BP ≥120 mmHg
  - sinus tachycardia ≥110 beats/min or bradycardia ≤ 60 beats/min
  - longer duration of STEMI symptoms before diagnosis and treatment
- standard relative contraindications to beta-blockade.

Intravenous beta-blockers may be used with caution in patients with tachycardia, hypertension or both and patients with ongoing chest pain resistant to nitrates and none of the above-mentioned contraindications.

The CLARITY-TIMI 28 trial and COMMIT trials outlined the efficacy of clopidogrel in combination with aspirin for non-STEMI patients. Neither study incorporated a loading dose in patients older than 75 years of age.

ExTRACT-TIMI 25 identified the benefits of enoxaparin over unfractionated heparin for STEMI patients treated with thrombolysis (RRR of 17%) at the expense of increased major bleeds (2.1%) and no increased ICH.[16,17]

12. Answer: B

Although at least 50% of patients with heart failure have a low ejection fraction of 40% or less on echocardiography, approximately one-third of all patients have a normal or near normal ejection fraction. **Features such as orthopnoea, paroxysmal nocturnal dyspnoea, raised JVP and third heart sound have a 70–90% specificity for diagnosis when present**. However, the sensitivity of those features is low. Diastolic dysfunction defined as abnormalities in diastolic distensibility, filling or relaxation of the left ventricle may cause heart failure with pulmonary venous congestion and oedema in the presence of a normal left ventricular (LV) ejection fraction and in the absence of any valvular abnormalities. Many conditions promote fluid retention with precipitation of heart failure and these include uncontrolled hypertension, AF, myocardial ischaemia, renal failure and use of NSAIDs.[18,19]

13. Answer: B

Systolic heart failure is the most common, caused by a range of diseases such as AMI, valvular pathology, cardiomyopathy, anaemia, toxicological causes, arrhythmias, diet, fluid overload, medications (negative inotropes or noncompliance), myocarditis, or progression of disease. Most normotensive/hypertensive patients are not fluid overloaded – may in fact be globally underfilled. Hence, the mainstay of management is no longer diuretics, but vasodilators and non-invasive ventilation to decrease preload, systemic vascular resistance and un-load the heart. The value of BNP remains controversial, and mostly unhelpful. Most values fall between 100–500 pg/mL, which is regarded as non-diagnostic. Values <100 make a diagnosis of acute heart failure less likely, whereas values >500 makes the diagnosis more likely. BNP has not been shown to be better than the clinical judgement of an experienced emergency clinician.[20,21]

14. Answer: D

Myocardial infarction is the most common cause of cardiogenic shock, with shock complicating about 6–7% of cases of AMI. Other causes include arrhythmia, valvular pathology, cardiomyopathy, toxicological causes, and ventriculoseptal defect (VSD). Older patients with anterior AMI, previous infarction, diabetes and known congestive cardiac failure are at higher risk of cardiogenic shock. Early revascularisation with PCI or coronary artery bypass graft (CABG) has a mortality benefit, with vasopressors, inotropes and intra-aortic balloon pump being useful as a bridge to reperfusion. PCI or CABG is preferable to thrombolysis. Thrombolysis is only really indicated if timely transfer to a facility with PCI or CABG is not available.[22]

15. Answer: B

Inotropes alone do not alter outcome but may temporise until definitive treatment is arranged. The overall mortality for cardiogenic shock complicating AMI sits at about 80% and depends on the age and comorbidities. However, long-term survival is improved in those patients with AMI who receive urgent revascularisation. Indeed, those patients with LAD occlusion have an almost 100% mortality unless urgent reperfusion is obtained. Intra-aortic balloon counterpulsation is only useful if combined with revascularisation.[22,23]

16. Answer: B

The medical treatment of acute mitral regurgitation aims to increase forward flow. This can be achieved by using an inotrope to improve cardiac contractility and a vasodilator to decrease afterload.

IV fluids are a first-line treatment for cardiogenic shock caused by RV failure. In this situation, an increase in preload will improve RV output.

Endotracheal intubation will nearly always exacerbate hypotension in cardiogenic shock by decreasing preload. Cardiac arrest is common post intubation in these patients.

Intra-aortic balloon pump counter pulsation will increase cardiac output by timed inflation during diastole and deflation during systole. Therefore, diastolic BP is increased (and coronary artery flow improved) and afterload reduced when the balloon deflates in systole.[20]

17. Answer: C

Hypertensive encephalopathy is characterised by neurological dysfunction resulting from severe hypertension. Common symptoms are decreased level of consciousness, headache, vomiting, seizures and visual disturbances. The symptoms are acute in onset and reversible. Treatment should aim to reduce the mean arterial pressure (MAP) by about 25% over 1–2 hours. Malignant hypertension is not characterised by a BP reading alone but requires end-organ dysfunction for diagnosis.

There is no evidence for reduction of blood pressure in ischaemic stroke. Indeed, hypertension is often required for adequate cerebral perfusion of neighbouring viable brain tissue.[24,25]

18. Answer: B

Hydralazine is a direct arteriolar vasodilating agent. It is usually given in 5 mg boluses. Reflex tachycardia is common.

The treatment of aortic dissection requires reduction of shearing forces on the torn intima of the aorta. Initial treatment with vasodilators will actually increase shearing forces by predominantly reducing diastolic pressure (thereby increasing pulse pressure and hence flow). Reflex tachycardia resulting from vasodilation also increases the shear forces per unit of time. Hence, initial treatment of aortic dissection should be with rate control and systolic BP reduction. Beta-blockers are ideal.

Sodium nitroprusside has a rapid onset and short duration of onset, and therefore is given via infusion.

GTN predominantly reduces preload by reducing venous tone.[26,27]

19. Answer: B

It is often difficult to differentiate pericarditis from AMI and benign early repolarisation (BER) on the ECG. Consequently, the diagnosis is primarily clinical. ECG changes associated with pericarditis include ST segment elevation and PR depression (stage 1) which are present in 60% of initial ECGs, followed by normalisation, followed by T wave inversion and then normalisation. The ST segment elevation is concave and is not associated with reciprocal changes. Changes occur over more than one anatomical area compared with BER, which typically occurs in the precordial leads only. Tall-tented T waves are characteristic of hyperkalaemia, or hyperacute infarction.[28–30]

20. Answer: D

PR segment depression is suggestive of pericarditis, and is not present in AMI.

ECG may be useful in the diagnosis of cardiac tamponade. Electrical alternans, where the QRS axis alternates between beats, and low voltage complexes may suggest the diagnosis of tamponade.

ECG findings may be present for several months following acute pericarditis. Generally the ECG will follow four stages:

1. (hours to days) concave upwards ST elevation and PR depression
2. normalisation of the PR and ST segments
3. (days to weeks) T wave inversion
4. (up to 3 months) normalisation of ECG.

Q waves suggest full wall thickness myocardial infarction.[28]

21. Answer: C

Patients with cardiac tamponade usually display tachycardia, low systolic BP and a narrow pulse pressure. Malignancy is the cause of about 40% of non-traumatic cases of pericardial tamponade. Idiopathic, uraemic and infective causes are the next most common. CXR lacks both sensitivity and specificity in this diagnosis. Pulsus paradoxus is not peculiar to pericardial tamponade. Other cardiopulmonary diseases, such as acute asthma, may cause this finding.[31]

22. Answer: B

Three major pathogens account for more than 80% of cases – *Streptococcus* species, *Staphylococcus aureus* and *Enterococcus* species. A single blood culture may not help in identifying the causative organism, especially when the patient is partially treated with antibiotics. The aortic valve is involved in 20% of intravenous drug use (IVDU)-related endocarditis. The Duke criteria has the following major and minor components (Box 2.1).[28,32]

Box 2.1 DUKE criteria for infective endocarditis

MAJOR CRITERIA

Positive blood culture for infective endocarditis (IE)

- Typical microorganism consistent with IE from two separate blood cultures, as noted below:
  - viridans streptococci, *Streptococcus bovis*, or HACEK group, or
  - community-acquired *Staphylococcus aureus* or enterococci, in the absence of a primary focus, or
- Microorganisms consistent with IE from persistently positive blood cultures defined as:
  - two positive cultures of blood samples drawn >12 hours apart, or
  - all of three or a majority of four separate cultures of blood (with first and last sample drawn 1 hour apart)

Evidence of endocardial involvement

- Positive echocardiogram for IE defined as:
  - oscillating intracardiac mass on valve or supporting structures, in the path of regurgitant jets, or on implanted material in the absence of an alternative anatomic explanation, or
  - abscess, or
  - new partial dehiscence of prosthetic valve
- New valvular regurgitation (worsening or changing of pre-existing murmur not sufficient)

MINOR CRITERIA

- Predisposition: predisposing heart condition or intravenous drug use
- Fever: temperature >38.0°C
- Vascular phenomena: major arterial emboli, septic pulmonary infarcts, mycotic aneurysm, intracranial haemorrhage, conjunctival haemorrhages, and Janeway lesions
- Immunologic phenomena: glomerulonephritis, Osler's nodes, Roth spots and rheumatoid factor
- Microbiological evidence: positive blood culture but does not meet a major criterion as noted above or serological evidence of active infection with organism consistent with IE
- Echocardiographic findings: consistent with IE but do not meet a major criterion as noted above

Clinical criteria for IE requires:

- two major criteria, or
- one major and three minor criteria, or
- five minor criteria

23. Answer: C

Multiple sets of blood cultures prior to antibiotic treatment will yield a microbiological diagnosis in at least 95% of cases. In the toxic patient, empirical antibiotic treatment should be given after three sets of blood cultures from different sites. Otherwise antibiotics should be delayed until blood cultures are positive.

With respect to right-sided endocarditis in intravenous drug users, the most common valve involved is the tricuspid valve (tricuspid 45%, mitral 30% and aortic 20%), and *Staphylococcus aureus* is responsible for about three-quarters of cases. Coagulase negative *Staphylococcus* is less common.

Overall mortality of both native and prosthetic valve endocarditis is 20–25%.[33,34]

24. Answer: A

Clinical examination is the most useful part of diagnosis in patients with syncope. Up to 45% of patients will be diagnosed on clinical examination alone. Further tests are generally of low yield. This includes ECG, which although clearly important, is not often diagnostic in this group. Up to 50% of patients with syncope will not have a clear diagnosis after ED evaluation.

The San Francisco syncope rule is a tool for identifying patients at high risk of adverse outcomes in the following 7 days.

Five criteria are included:
- abnormal ECG
- shortness of breath
- systolic BP <90 mmHg
- haematocrit <30%
- congestive cardiac failure.[35,36]

25. Answer: D

Unexplained syncope (up to 50% of ED presentations with syncope) requires further investigation. Inpatient investigation is warranted for those at high risk of cardiac events. Most syncope risk stratification tools are developed for this purpose.

The diagnosis of orthostatic hypotension requires a suggestive history and demonstration of systolic BP reduction of >20 mmHg upon standing. It does not confer any change in mortality.

CT scan of the brain is a very low yield test in this patient population and should only be used for patients with abnormal neurological examination, with historical features suggestive of a neurological cause, or with complication of the syncopal event.[37]

26. Answer: D

Third-degree heart block complicating AMI confers an increased mortality, even when rate is controlled with pacing. In particular, anterior myocardial infarction with third-degree heart block implies extensive anterior infarction and poor prognosis.

First-degree heart block will display a PR interval of >200 ms.

Mobitz type I second-degree heart block is where the PR interval progressively lengthens, eventually resulting in a non-conducted or 'missed' atrial complex. Mobitz type II second-degree heart block displays a constant PR interval with intermittent failure of P wave conduction. Often the ratio of conducted to non-conducted beats is constant.

Third-degree heart block is a complete failure of conduction between atria and ventricles. The escape rhythm is generated either at the AV node (which will be evident by a narrow QRS complex) or at an infranodal level (where the QRS will be prolonged).[38,39]

27. Answer: C

The location of the block in Mobitz type I is at or above the AV node. Mobitz type II is characterised by conduction abnormality below the AV node in the bundle of His, hence the QRS complex is usually widened. The block in third-degree heart block may be at or below the AV node. If the block is at the AV node then the escape rhythm may be narrow complex, otherwise the escape rhythm will be broad (ventricular). The most frequent block in AMI is Wenckebach (Mobitz type I) at 15%. Complete heart block is the most common unstable rhythm complicating AMI at 8–10%, particularly inferior AMI.[38,40]

28. Answer: B

AV dissociation is the hallmark of VT, but occurs infrequently in up to 25% of cases. A north-west QRS axis (−90 to +180) is the only QRS axis that is specific for VT. Other ECG findings suggestive of VT include:
- a QRS complex wider than 140 ms if RBBB morphology and 160 ms if LBBB morphology
- a generally regular rate of 140–200 beats per minute

- fusion beats
- capture beats
- concordance of the QRS axis across the precordial leads.

RBBB morphology is more likely to be SVT with aberrancy, although an rSR morphology suggests VT. VT may be slower than 140 beats per minute in patients taking cardioactive medications (e.g. amiodarone).[38,40]

29. Answer: A

Cannon A waves result from dissociation between atrial and ventricular activity and in this setting indicate that VT is the likely diagnosis. In the ED, VT is responsible for about 80% of broad-complex tachycardias. Retrograde P waves on ECG can be found with either VT or SVT. Cardiac ischaemia is occasionally the cause of torsades de pointes. More common causes are drug toxicity, electrolyte abnormalities and congenital prolonged QT syndrome.[38]

30. Answer: C

Age >35 years makes VT the more likely diagnosis. A preceding P wave indicates a supraventricular origin to the tachycardia. Care must be taken, however, to make sure it is not mistaken for a retrograde P wave, which can occur in both VT and SVT. Carotid sinus massage will have no effect on VT but may slow the AV nodal rate of an SVT. An rSR pattern in lead V1 is typical of an RBBB pattern, and therefore would be more common in SVT with aberrancy.[39]

31. Answer: A

Drugs that block potassium channels will prolong the QT interval and therefore predispose to torsades de pointes. Likewise, electrolyte abnormalities (hypomagnesemia, hypokalaemia and hypocalcemia) that cause long QT will also predispose. Benzodiazepines have no effect on the QT interval.[38]

32. Answer: B

Recurrent torsades de pointes, refractory to magnesium therapy, can be effectively managed with overdrive pacing. This can be achieved electrically, or pharmacologically with an agent such as isoprenaline. Class III agents, such as sotalol, will further prolong the QT interval and exacerbate the problem.

Lignocaine is a class 1b antiarrhythmic. Class 1 agents block the sodium channel, therefore reducing the slope of phase zero of the action potential. They are further subclassified based on their effect of the action potential duration: 1a prolong the AP duration, 1b decrease the AP duration and 1c have no effect.

The dose of adenosine may need to be increased in those patients taking methylxanthines, such as theophylline, which are competitive antagonists at adenosine receptors.[38,41]

33. Answer: D

Brugada syndrome is a recognised cause of syncope and sudden cardiac death in young patients (especially in Asian males) with structurally normal hearts. It is inherited in an autosomal dominant manner and is associated with defects in the sodium channel. It is associated with an incomplete RBBB pattern and the ST segment elevation in the right precordial leads that is either convex and downsloping with T wave inversion or saddle shaped or concave. Patients with syncope who are suspected of having Brugada syndrome should be admitted to a monitored bed. Management is with an implantable defibrillator – there is no place for class la and lc or sodium channel blocking agents.[38,42]

34. Answer: C

Isoprenaline causes beta-adrenergic receptor stimulation and has a potential antiarrythmic effect in patients with Brugada syndrome. All other drugs have the potential to block sodium channels and precipitate arrhythmias.[41]

35. Answer: C

Adenosine is the first-line therapy for the treatment of stable SVT in both adults and children because of its short half-life (<60 seconds) and safety profile. Its overall efficacy in converting SVT to sinus rhythm (SR) is over 90%. However, because of its short half-life, approximately one-third of the patients who are converted to SR can be expected to be reversed to SVT again within a few minutes. It has also been shown that efficacy of adenosine increases with faster heart rates. Adenosine is far superior to magnesium in reversing SVT. Reversion rate for magnesium is approximately 16%.[43]

36. Answer: D

Tachycardia associated with Wolff-Parkinson-White syndrome (WPW) can be:

- reentrant tachycardia with orthodromic/antegrade conduction down the AV node, resulting in a concealed pathway and narrow complex tachycardia – the most common reentrant tachycardia of WPW
- reentrant tachycardia with antidromic conduction down the accessory pathway, resulting in a wide complex QRS
- rapid conduction of atrial tachycardia through the accessory pathway.

Verapamil, digoxin, adenosine and beta-blockers are only absolutely contraindicated in AF with preexcitation as they enhance conduction through the accessory pathway. The may also unmask a concealed pathway when given in SVT and WPW. Amiodarone and flecalnide are the drugs of choice in AF with preexcitation, and cardioversion is required in unstable patients.[38,44]

37. Answer: D

Most (about 60%) of reentrant SVT have their reentry within the AV node as described in the previous question. About 20% have reentry involving a bypass tract (accessory pathway) and the remainder have reentry elsewhere.

In WPW syndrome, 85% of reentrant SVT are orthodromic (pass through the AV node in the usual direction) and hence have a narrow QRS on ECG. Antidromic conduction will produce a broad complex QRS on the ECG.

Adenosine will revert about 90% of reentrant SVTs.[39]

38. Answer: D

Only 1–2% of patients with WPW present with arrhythmias. The approximate breakdown of different types of arrhythmias in WPW are:

- 80%: AV reentrant tachycardia
- 15–30%: AF
- 5%: atrial flutter.

Characteristic ECG features of WPW are a triad of:

- short PR interval (<0.12 seconds)
- slightly prolonged QRS complex (>0.1 seconds)
- slurring of the upstroke of the R wave (delta wave).

Additionally, WPW may also produce a tall R wave in V1, which may be misdiagnosed as a posterior myocardial infarction.[45,46]

39. Answer: A

Amiodarone or digoxin are recommended as IV agents to control heart rate in the acute care setting in patients with AF and heart failure, who do not have an accessory pathway.

Dihydropyridine calcium channel blockers do not reduce heart rate (indeed, they may result in reflex tachycardia). Nondihydropyridine calcium channel blockers and beta-blockers are recommended in the acute care setting for rate control in AF, taking care in patients with hypotension and heart failure.

Cardioversion is not recommended after 48 hours due to the increased risk of thromboembolism.

Digoxin and nondihydropyridine sodium-channel blockers are contraindicated in preexcitation syndromes, where ventricular rate may be paradoxically accelerated.[47]

40. Answer. D

About 90% of 'lone fibrillators' will spontaneously revert with no treatment in the subsequent 48 hours.

More than 60% of patents with AF will cardiovert with 100 J DC shock. When the patient is unstable due to rapid ventricular rate, immediate cardioversion should be attempted. It is important to exclude underlying illness, such as haemorrhage or sepsis, as the cause of the rapid ventricular rate prior to attempting cardioversion.

In the patient with chronic AF, rate control is the priority. Indeed, these patients carry a significant risk of embolic events if cardioverted without the necessary period of anticoagulation before and after cardioversion.[38,39]

41. Answer: D

In AF, the conducted QRS complexes are usually narrow except in patients where AF is associated with a bundle branch block or an accessory pathway.

In WPW, when the accessory pathway exhibits a very short antegrade refractory period, very rapid conduction from atria to ventricles may occur. AF in this situation can be a dangerous arrhythmia. Conduction across the accessory pathway during AF in patients with WPW can result in very rapid ventricular rates. In this broad QRS complex

(>0.12 second) AF, the heart rate can be higher than 250/min. **This rapid ventricular response can degenerate into ventricular fibrillation (VF) and lead to potential death.**

In AF not related to preexcitation syndromes, the relatively long refractory period in the AV node protects the ventricle from achieving very high rates, therefore preventing AF degenerating into VF.

Calcium channel blockers, beta-blockers and digoxin prolong the refractory period in AV node and this slows down AV nodal conduction. The resultant increase in the impulse transmission through the accessory pathway causes a rapid ventricular rate. **Although calcium channel blockers, beta-blockers and digoxin are beneficial in the treatment of non-WPW AF, they should not be used in WPW AF because of the risk of precipitating VF.**

Treating a stable patient with broad-complex AF known or suspected to be caused by WPW should be aimed at prolonging the refractory period of the accessory pathway for antegrade conduction and this will allow impulses to traverse through the AV node, slowing down the ventricular rate. Amiodarone and procainamide appear to be the drugs of choice. An unstable patient with very rapid ventricular rates should be cardioverted.[45,48]

42. Answer: A

Identification of atrial flutter on a 12-lead ECG can be challenging. In atrial flutter, the atrial complexes (flutter waves) are precisely regular. There should not be any variability. The rate of the atrial complexes are between 215 and 350/min and in adults it will not exceed >350/min. There is absolutely no flat or isoelectric segment between atrial complexes (flutter waves) and therefore they have a saw-tooth appearance. Usually these waves are visible in one lead system only – mainly in limb leads but can appear in a single other lead. There is a unique appearance at the junction between a flutter wave (atrial complex) and the QRS complex. Here the two waves always intersect above the baseline. Flutter waves disappear into the QRS complex and reappear on the other side of the complex, maintaining the precise regularity.[39]

43. Answer: C

'T' stands for triggered, and indicates that pacing is triggered in response to sensed cardiac activity.

The first letter refers to the chamber paced, the second letter refers to the chamber sensed, the third letter to the response to sensing, the fourth letter to programmability and the fifth letter, if present, to the antiarrhythmic function (pacing, shock or dual).

'R' in the fourth position refers to the ability of the pacemaker to modulate its response to sensing depending on rate.[39]

44. Answer: D

In a patient with a pacemaker, failure to pace may be due to a lack of pacemaker output or failure to capture.

There are a few reasons that can contribute to failure to capture. If the energy in the pacemaker is insufficient to generate an adequate impulse to successfully depolarise the myocardium this may lead to failure to capture myocardium electrically and mechanically. This can happen in pacemaker battery failure. A local inflammatory reaction in the initial few weeks following the insertion of pacemaker, can cause a local fibrosis in the myocardium to occur. This can increase the resistance at the electrode–myocardial interface, leading to failure to capture. Lead problems such as lead fracture or dislodgement, cardiac perforation and faulty connections of leads can cause failure to capture. High levels of antiarrhythmic drugs can cause failure to capture. Flecainide is known to cause failure to capture at therapeutic levels.

As expected, a prolonged refractory period of the myocardium causes failure to capture. Electrolyte abnormalities may be a cause for a prolonged refractory period of myocardium.[39,49]

45. Answer: C

Oversensing, therefore inappropriate inhibition of the pacemaker, may cause failure of pacemaker output. Oversensing of P and T waves and skeletal muscle activity by the pacemaker can occur, causing failure of output. The depolarising muscle relaxant suxamethonium causes muscular fasciculation during rapid sequence induction, hence it may cause pacemaker failure during this time.

When pacemaker output fails, a pacemaker-dependent patient should exhibit signs of hypoperfusion. There will be no pacemaker spikes visible in the ECG and on the monitor. Unipolar electrodes are more likely to oversense normal electrical and muscle activity than modern bipolar electrodes.[39]

46. Answer: B

Tetralogy of Fallot results in right heart outflow obstruction, causing right to left shunting and cyanosis. Treatment aims to decrease right to left shunting.

The ideal position for these children is the 'squatting' position where afterload is increased, therefore decreasing shunt size. For the same reason, vasoconstrictors such as metaraminol can be used. Crying will increase pulmonary pressures and hence increase right to left shunting. Children with 'tet' spells should be kept as calm as possible, usually with parental help. A small fluid bolus will increase RV preload and decrease functional obstruction.[50]

47. Answer: C

Paroxysmal supraventricular tachycardia represents 90% of tachyarrhythmias in children. The mechanism is due to either an accessory pathway (AV reciprocating tachycardia) or AV nodal reentry; however, accessory pathway is a more common mechanism in children. Some of these children with an accessory pathway may have WPW. These infants usually present to the ED early as they may appear unwell and lethargic. In a stable child vagal manoeuvres may be attempted first. In this age group the vagal manoeuvre commonly used is intermittent placement of a bag filled with ice and some water. If vagal manoeuvres fail adenosine as an intravenous bolus is used. If this fails other options such as beta-blockers and amiodarone should only be used with caution. Verapamil can cause cardiovascular collapse and death in this age group and therefore should be avoided. If the child is unstable, synchronised cardioversion is the treatment of choice.[51,52]

48. Answer: B

A neonate in the first few weeks of life who presents with undifferentiated shock should be presumed as having a duct-dependent congenital heart lesion until proven otherwise while considering all possible other causes of shock in that age group. Duct dependency means the neonate had been dependent on a patent ductus arteriosus to supply partially oxygenated blood to the systemic circulation and the closure of the duct has caused the cardiovascular collapse and shock. This presentation is most common in the first week and rare after 4 weeks of age.

The cyanotic lesions which may be ductal dependent are tetralogy of Fallot, tricuspid atresia and Ebstein's anomaly, hypoplastic left heart syndrome, interrupted aortic arch and transposition of great arteries without a mixing lesion (e.g. ventricular septal defect, or VSD). Acyanotic lesions that may be ductal dependent are pulmonary stenosis and severe coarctation of the aorta.

Coarctation of the aorta presents with hypertension in the older child. In infancy it may present with congestive cardiac failure.

The mainstay treatment for ductal-dependent shock is prostaglandin E1 (PGE1) infusion. Neonates may present with signs of congestive cardiac failure, however, this is not common.

Early soft systolic murmur may indicate a benign murmur, which is common in children. It is believed that significant murmurs in children do not belong to diastolic, late systolic or pansystolic categories.[50,53,54]

49. Answer: A

The hyperoxia test is an important test that should be considered if immediate echocardiography is not available for a neonate who presents to the ED with features of suspected congenital heart disease. Pulse oxymetry alone may be unreliable during this test and arterial blood gas (ABG) sampling is advised. PaO_2 is obtained first with the neonate on room air (if not tolerated with a low tolerable amount of supplemental oxygen). PaO_2 is then assessed after 100% oxygen supplement for 15 minutes. If PaO_2 is >250 mmHg ('passed hyperoxia test') on the second ABG it usually excludes hypoxia secondary to congenital heart disease. Another cause for the child's hypoxia should be sought. PaO_2 < 100 mmHg ('failed hyperoxia test') is considered to be caused by a right to left shunt due to a cyanotic congenital heart lesion. PaO_2 100–250 mmHg range may be due to intracardiac mixing as a result of a structural heart lesion. A neonate with a failed hyperoxia test needs urgent evaluation for an anatomical diagnosis and should immediately be treated with prostaglandin E1.[54]

50. Answer: A

Childhood hypertension is defined as either systolic or diastolic BP ≥95th percentile of the normal values for the age and the height and BP between 90–95th percentile is defined as prehypertension. Although hypertension is an infrequent finding in children presenting to an ED it requires thorough assessment to identify and treat a secondary cause. The aetiology depends on the age. Renal parenchymal disease such as glomerulonephritis is rare in early infancy but it is an important cause in both young and older children. In the neonate, renal vascular thrombosis or stenosis and coarctation of the aorta are important causes. In the older child, once secondary causes are excluded, essential hypertension is considered as the most common cause. Hyperthyroidism and hypercortisol states can be life threatening if unrecognised.[55]

References

1. Goodcare S. Chest pain. In: Cameron P, Jelinek G, Kelly A, et al, editors. Textbook of adult emergency medicine. 3rd ed. Edinburgh: Churchill Livingston Elsevier; 2009. p. 202–7.

2. Green G, Hill P. Chest pain: cardiac or not. In: Tintinalli J, Stapczynski J, Ma O, et al, editors. Tintinalli's emergency medicine: a comprehensive study guide. 7th ed. New York: McGraw Hill Medical; 2011:361–7.

3. Loten C, Isbister G, Jamcotchian M, et al. Adverse outcomes following emergency department discharge of patients with possible acute coronary syndrome. Emerg Med Austral 2009;21:455–64.

4. Chew D, Aroney C, Aylward P, et al. Addendum to the National Heart Foundation of Australia/Cardiac Society of Australia and New Zealand guidelines for the management of acute coronary syndromes (ACS) 2006. Heart Lung Circ 2011;8:487–502.

5. Goodcare S, Kelly A. Acute coronary syndromes. In: Cameron P, Jelinek G, Kelly A, et al, editors. Textbook of adult emergency medicine. 3rd ed. Edinburgh: Churchill Livingston Elsevier; 2009. p. 208–14.

6. Brady W, Harrigan R, Chan T. Acute coronary syndrome. In: Marx J, Hockberger R, Walls R, et al, editors. Rosen's emergency medicine: concepts and clinical practice. 7th ed. Mosby Elsevier; 2009. p. 947–83.

7. Antman E, Cohen M, Bernink P. The TIMI risk score for unstable angina/non-ST elevation MI. JAMA 2000;284(7):835–42.

8. Hollander J, Diercks D. Acute coronary syndromes, acute myocardial infarctionand unstable angina. In: Tintinalli J, Stapczynski J, Ma O, et al, editors. Tintinalli's emergency medicine: a comprehensive study guide. 7th ed. New York: McGraw Hill Medical; 2011. p. 367–85.

9. Janz T, Hamilton G. Acute coronary syndromes: regional issues. In: Chan C, Brady W, Harrigan R, et al, editors. ECG in emergency medicine and acute care. Philadelphia: Elsevier Mosby 2005. p. 173–81.

10. Brady W. T wave. In: Chan C, Brady W, Harrigan R, et al, editors. ECG in emergency medicine and acute care. Philadelphia: Elsevier Mosby; 2005. p. 66–9.

11. Dunn R, Dilley S. Acute coronary syndromes (ACS) In: Dunn R, Dilley S, Brookes J, et al, editors. Manual of emergency medicine. Adelaide: Venom Publishing; 2010. p. 407–38.

12. Sgarbossa E, Pinski S, Barbagelata A. Electrocardiographic diagnosis of evolving acute myocardial infarction in the presence of left bundle-branch block. N Engl J Med 1996;334:481–7.

13. Jain S, Ting H, Bell M. Utility of left bundle branch block as a diagnostic criterion for acute myocardial infarction. Am J Cardiol 2011;107:1111–16.

14. Tabas J, Rodriguez R, Seligman H, et al. Electrocardiographic criteria for detecting acute myocardial infarction in patients with left bundle branch block: a meta-analysis. Ann Emerg Med 2008;52:329–36.

15. Bonnefoy E, Steg PG, Boutite F, et al. Comparison of primary angioplasty and prehospital fibrinolysis in acute myocardial infarction (CAPTIM) trial: a 5-year follow-up. Eur Heart J 2009;30:1598–606.

16. Pollack C, Antman E, Hollander J. 2007 Focused update to the ACC/AHA guidelines for the management of patients with ST-segment elevation myocardial infarction: implications for emergency department practice. Annals of Emergency Medicine 2008;52(4):344–55.

17. Sinert R, Newman D, Brandler E, et al. Immediate B-blockade in patients with myocardial infarctions: Is there evidence of benefit? Ann Emerg Med 2010;56: 571–7.

18. McMurray J. Systolic heart failure. N Engl J Med 2010;362:228–38.

19. Aurigemma G, Gaasch W. Diatolic Heart Failure. N Engl J Med 2004;351:1097–105.

20. Dunn R. Cardiac failure. In: Dunn R, Dilley S, Brookes J, et al, editors. Manual of emergency medicine. Adelaide: Venom Publishing; 2010. p. 439–45.

21. Lightfoot D. Assessment and management of acute pulmonary oedema. In: Cameron P, Jelinek G, Kelly A, et al, editors. Textbook of adult emergency medicine. 3rd ed. Edinburgh: Churchill Livingston Elsevier; 2009. p. 215–19.

22. Garrett P. Shock overview. In: Cameron P, Jelinek G, Kelly A, et al, editors. Textbook of adult emergency medicine. 3rd ed. Edinburgh: Churchill Livingston Elsevier; 2009. p. 45–56.

23. Weber J, Peacock W. Cardiogenic shock. In: Tintinalli J, Stapczynski J, Ma O, et al, editors. Tintinalli's emergency medicine: a comprehensive study guide. 7th ed. New York: McGraw Hill Medical; 2011. p. 385–9.

24. Lee M. Hypertension. In: Cameron P, Jelinek G, Kelly A, et al, editors. Textbook of adult emergency medicine. 3rd ed. Edinburgh: Churchill Livingston Elsevier; 2009. p. 259–62.

25. Gray R. Hypertension. In: Marx J, Hockberger R, Walls R, et al, editors. Rosen's emergency medicine: concepts and clinical practice. 7th ed. Mosby Elsevier; 2009. p. 1076–87.

26. Coman M. Aortic dissection. In: Cameron P, Jelinek G, Kelly A, et al, editors. Textbook of adult emergency medicine. 3rd ed. Edinburgh: Churchill Livingston Elsevier; 2009. p. 263–8.

27. Ankel F. Aortic dissection. In: Marx J, Hockberger R, Walls R, et al, editors. Rosen's emergency medicine: concepts and clinical practice. 7th ed. Mosby Elsevier; 2009. p. 1088–92.

28. Hayes J, Kelly A. Pericarditis, cardiac tamponade and myocarditis. In: Cameron P, Jelinek G, Kelly A, et al, editors. Textbook of adult emergency medicine. 3rd ed. Edinburgh: Churchill Livingston Elsevier; 2009. p. 239–45.

29. Dunn R, Dilley S, Brookes J. Non ACS chest pain. In: Dunn R, Dilley S, Brookes J, et al, editors. Manual of emergency medicine. Adelaide: Venom Publishing; 2010. p. 387–406.

30. Brady W. ST segment. In: Chan C, Brady W, Harrigan R, et al, editors. ECG in emergency medicine and acute care. Philadelphia: Elsevier Mosby; 2005. p. 60–5.

31. Niemann J. The cardiomyopathies, myocarditis and pericardial disease. In: Tintinalli J, Stapczynski J, Ma O, et al, editors. Tintinalli's emergency medicine: a comprehensive study guide. 7th ed. New York: McGraw Hill Medical; 2011. p. 423–30.

32. Dunn R. Structural heart disease. In: Dunn R, Dilley S, Brookes J, et al, editors. Manual of emergency medicine. Adelaide: Venom Publishing; 2010. p. 446–71.

33. Lee M. Heart valve emergencies. In: Cameron P, Jelinek G, Kelly A, et al, editors. Textbook of adult emergency medicine. 3rd ed. Edinburgh: Churchill Livingston Elsevier; 2009. p. 246–53.

34. Rothman R, Yang S, Marco C. Infective endocarditis. In: Tintinalli J, Stapczynski J, Ma O, et al, editors. Tintinalli's emergency medicine: a comprehensive study guide. 7th ed. New York: McGraw Hill Medical; 2011. p. 1042–7.

35. De Lorenzo R. Syncope. In: Marx J, Hockberger R, Walls R, et al, editors. Rosen's emergency medicine: concepts and clinical practice. 7th ed. Mosby Elsevier; 2009. p. 142–8.

36. Quinn J, Stiell I, McDermott D. Derivation of the San Francisco syncope rule to predict patients with short-term serious outcomes. Ann Emerg Med 2004;43(2):224–32.

37. Quinn J. Syncope. In: Tintinalli J, Stapczynski J, Ma O, et al, editors. Tintinalli's emergency medicine: a comprehensive study guide. 7th ed. New York: McGraw Hill Medical; 2011. p. 399–405.

38. Ong M, Lim S, Teo W. Arrhythmias. In: Cameron P, Jelinek G, Kelly A, et al, editors. Textbook of adult emergency medicine. 3rd ed. Edinburgh: Churchill Livingston Elsevier; 2009. p. 219–31.

39. Piktel J. Cardiac rhythm disturbances. In: Tintinalli J, Stapczynski J, Ma O, et al, editors. Tintinalli's emergency medicine: a comprehensive study guide. 7th ed. New York: McGraw Hill Medical; 2011. p. 129–54.

40. Brady W, Harrigan R. Atrioventricular block. In: Chan C, Brady W, Harrigan R, et al, editors. ECG in emergency medicine and acute care. Philadelphia: Elsevier Mosby; 2005. p. 85–8.

41. Miller B, Clements E. Pharmacology of antiarrhythmics. In: Tintinalli J, Stapczynski J, Ma O, et al, editors. Tintinalli's emergency medicine: a comprehensive study guide. 7th ed. New York: McGraw Hill Medical; 2011. p. 154–62.

42. Jensen S, Stahmer S. Ventricular tachycardia and ventricular fibrillation. In: Chan C, Brady W, Harrigan R, et al, editors. ECG in emergency medicine and acute care. Philadelphia: Elsevier Mosby; 2005. p. 118–28.

43. Innes JA. Adenosine use in the emergency department. Emerg Med Austral 2008;20:209–15.

44. Lindberg J, Brady W. Preexcitation syndromes. In: Chan C, Brady W, Harrigan R, et al, editors. ECG in emergency medicine and acute care. Philadelphia: Elsevier Mosby; 2005. p. 112–17.

45. Chew HC, Lim SH. Broad complex atrial fibrillation. Am J Emerg Med 2007;25:459–63.

46. Mattu A, Brady W. Part 2: 12-lead ECG (intermediate level). In: Mattu A, Brady W, editors. ECGs for the emergency physician 2. Malden: Blackwell Publishing; 2008. p. 29–115.

47. Australian Resuscitation Council. Guideline 11.9: Managing acute dysrhythmias. November 2009. Online. Available: www.resus.org.au.

48. Fuster V, Ryden L, Cannom D, et al. 2011 ACCF/AHA/HRS focussed updates incorporated into the ACC/AHA/ESC 2006 guidelines for the management of patients with atrial fibrillation. J Am Coll Cardiol 2011;57(11):e101–98.

49. McMullan J, Valento M, Attari M, et al. Care of the pacemaker/implantable cardioverter defibrillator patient in the ED. Am J Emerg Med 2007;25:812–22

50. Choong R. Cyanotic heart disease and tetralogy of Fallot spells. In: Cameron P, Jelinek G, Everitt I, et al, editors. Textbook of paediatric emergency medicine. 2nd ed. Edinburgh: Churchill Livingston Elsevier; 2006. p. 105–7.

51. Sharieff G, Donige S. Dysrhythmias in children. In: Strange G, Ahrens W, Schafermeyer R, et al, editors. Pediatric emergency medicine. 3rd ed. New York: McGraw Hill Medical; 2009. p. 445–53.

52. Williams G. Paediatric arrhythmias. In: Cameron P, Jelinek G, Everitt I, et al, editors. Textbook of paediatric emergency medicine. Edinburgh: Churchill Livingston Elsevier; 2006. p. 127–34.

53. O'Meara M. Congenital heart disease. In: Cameron P, Jelinek G, Everitt I, et al, editors. Textbook of paediatric emergency medicine. 2nd ed. Edinburgh: Churchill Livingston Elsevier; 2006. p. 113–19.

54. Horeczko T, Young K. Congenital heart disease. In: Strange G, Ahrens W, Schafermeyer R, et al, editors. Pediatric emergency medicine. 3rd ed. New York: McGraw Hill Medical; 2009. p. 413–30.

55. MacNeill E. Pediatric hypertension. In: Strange G, Ahrens W, Schafermeyer R, et al, editors. Pediatric emergency medicine. 3rd ed. New York: McGraw Hill Medical; 2009. p. 456–60.

1. Answer: D

Differentiating the cause for dyspnoea in a patient presenting to the ED can be challenging because both congestive cardiac failure and pulmonary conditions such as COPD may coexist, especially in the elderly population. Contrary to popular belief, symptoms such as dyspnoea on exertion, orthopnoea, paroxysmal nocturnal dyspnoea and leg oedema have a low positive likelihood ratio (LR) for the diagnosis of congestive cardiac failure (CCF). Previous history of coronary artery disease raises our suspicion but does not help in the diagnosis. **In contrast, third heart sound (gallop) found on examination, pulmonary venous congestion and interstitial oedema found on the CXR have high positive LRs therefore strongly support the diagnosis of CCF.** Furthermore, clinical gestalt, raised jugular venous pressure (JVP) or hepatojugular reflex on examination, and presence of alveolar oedema on CXR are helpful in the diagnosis. Cardiomegaly found on the CXR may not be helpful.

Hypercapnoea (defined as $PaCO_2$ >45 mm Hg) is the result of pulmonary hypoventilation due to a variety of causes. Hypercapnoea, both in its acute and chronic states, is associated with increased HCO_3 production albeit due to different mechanisms. However, in the acute state the serum HCO_3 level is normal, and in the chronic state, which starts after the first 6–12 hours of hypercapnoea the HCO_3 level is often raised. **In acute respiratory acidosis caused by hypercapnoea, the H^+ ions are buffered by the intracellular proteins. The HCO_3 produced in this process raises the serum HCO_3 by 1 mmol/L for every 10 mm Hg rise in $PaCO_2$ level in hypercapnoea (1:10 rise).** In other words, this serum HCO_3 rise is minimal in acute respiratory acidosis. **In contrast, in chronic respiratory acidosis due to chronic hypercapnoea, as a means of buffering acid, renal retention of HCO_3 occurs. In this process serum HCO_3 raises by 3.5 mmol/L for every 10 mm Hg rise in $PaCO_2$ (3.5:10 rise).** These figures can be used to differentiate acute from chronic hypercapnoea and to identify acute-on-chronic hypercapnoea in clinical practice.[1,2]

2. Answer: C

Blood gas analysis is performed in the ED mainly to assess:
- metabolic (acid–base) status: pH, HCO_3, base excess
- respiratory function: PCO_2, pH, pO_2.

ABG sampling is notorious for producing significant pain to the patient and repeat sampling requires repeated needle punctures or insertion of an arterial line. Arterial sampling is not without serious complications – occasionally arterial injury and thrombosis may occur. In contrast, venous sampling is much easier to perform and has other technical advantages.

Currently available evidence suggests venous pH, HCO_3 level and base excess to have sufficient agreement with the same arterial parameters in patients in most clinical situations such as diabetic ketoacidosis. However, there is no data to confirm that this level of agreement is maintained in shock states, cardiac arrest and mixed acid–base disorders and therefore VBG should not be used in these states.

The mean difference between venous and arterial pH varies between 0.02 and 0.035 pH units.

Currently available evidence shows that the agreement between the venous and arterial PCO_2 to be poor. **Venous PCO_2 is not a substitute for arterial PCO_2 in clinical situations such as acute exacerbations of COPD and asthma.** An ABG should be done in these patients to detect hypercapnoeic respiratory failure.[3]

3. Answer: D

A patient with a newly diagnosed pleural effusion should be carefully assessed to determine the cause of the effusion. As a first step in the ED, a careful history, physical examination and investigations should be performed to deferentiate pleural effusion into one of either exudate or transudate.

Transudative causes include:
- congestive cardiac failure or left ventricular (LV) failure

- cirrhosis
- nephrotic syndrome
- superior vena cava obstruction
- myxoedema.

Exudative causes include:

- parapneumonic effusions – bacterial pneumonia, bronchiectasis, lung abscess
- malignancy – 75% are due to lung carcinoma, breast carcinoma and lymphoma
- other infective causes – tuberculosis, viral, fungal and parasitic infections
- PE
- collagen vascular disease.

A diagnostic thoracocentesis should be performed and pleural fluid should be tested for protein and LDH levels. **Exudative pleural fluid will fulfil at least one of the following *Light's criteria*. The vast majority of the transudative effusions will not fulfil any of these criteria.**

- Pleural fluid protein/serum protein >0.5
- Pleural fluid LDH/serum LDH >0.6
- Pleural fluid LDH is >2/3 the upper normal range of serum LDH

The presence of transudative effusion will usually mean the patient requires treatment of the underlying condition, but exudative pleural fluid should be tested further for white cell count and differential, glucose level, microscopy, culture/sensitivity and cytology to establish the underlying cause.

Overall, the most common cause of pleural effusion is heart failure in which isolated right-sided effusions are more common than left-sided effusions. Often the effusions are bilateral. When effusions are not bilateral, when there is a significant difference in effusion sizes and when heart failure diagnosis is unclear, diagnostic thoracocentesis should be considered to rule out other potential causes.

Empyema is a grossly purulent effusion and it is often loculated and pleuraly based. This is visible in the CXR as a pleuraly based collection.

PE is often overlooked as a cause of an effusion. During patient assessment this should be carefully considered, especially in patients with small pleural effusions.[4,5]

4. Answer: D

Haemoptysis can originate from both bronchial vessels (systemic circulation) and from alveolar capillaries (pulmonary circulation). About 90% of massive haemoptysis originate from bronchial arteries. Rapid and large haemorrhage caused by the systemic arterial pressure can drown the patient before any chance of clearance of the airway. **Therefore, the cause of death in massive haemorrhage is usually due to asphyxia rather than exsanguination.** Although some practitioners will position the patient with the bleeding side down to prevent blood from going in to the non-bleeding lung, this can be detrimental to the patient as it worsens ventilation perfusion mismatch. **Usually, the *non-bleeding lung* is intubated to prevent blood entering in to that lung.** Selective intubation of a non-bleeding right lung can be easily attempted in the ED by advancing the ETT to the right main bronchus. This will occlude the bronchus to the right upper lobe and ventilate the right middle and lower lobes. Successful selective intubation of the left lung may require considerable skills. A 90-degree rotational method using a size 7 mm endotracheal tube (ETT) after passing through the cords can be tried in the ED to enter either the right or left side. The success rate is described at 94% for the right side and 72% for left side. Double lumen tubes require fibre optic method.[6]

5. Answer: C

CXR abnormalities can be identified in the majority of patients who present with haemoptysis due to lung malignancy. **PE is a common cause of haemoptysis; however, it usually does not cause severe haemoptysis.** The chance of identifying the bleeding lesion is highest if the bronchoscopy is performed within the first 48 hours. **When associated with right upper lobe collapse, it is usually due to a lung malignancy.**[6,7]

6. Answer: D

Pertussis is a highly contagious respiratory illness that is transmitted by droplet infection and has approximately an 80% attack rate for susceptible contacts. Humans are the only reservoir and the incubation period is approximately 7–10 days.

Morbidity and mortality (0.5–1%) is highest in infants under 6 months of age. Despite vigorous

immunisation schedules this subset of patients **is not protected, as three or more injections are required to confer protection.** The current Australian immunisation schedule recommends vaccination against pertussis at 2, 4 and 6 months of age, with a booster at 4 years. Furthermore, maternal antibodies do not guarantee protection of the neonate against developing pertussis and it is recommended that women in the last trimester of pregnancy who have been exposed to pertussis should receive chemoprophylaxis.

The *laboratory diagnosis* of pertussis, irrespective of the technique used, is challenging and unfortunately not a very sensitive tool. **While a positive result is useful, a negative result doesn't exclude pertussis.** Commonly used tests for pertussis include culture, PCR, and serology.

Culture of pertussis from nasopharyngeal specimens has traditionally been regarded as the 'gold standard' for laboratory diagnosis but, unfortunately, has sensitivity as low as 0–67%. It is important to only collect specimens from the nasopharynx (aspirate rather than a swab) as *Bordetella pertussis* is found in areas with ciliated epithelium and specimens from the anterior nose, throat and sputum are of little value. **PCR is the most sensitive and specific of all investigations and unlike culture specimens can be performed on throat swabs.** Furthermore, it is not as readily affected by prior antibiotic therapy and remains positive for longer than cultures. Only IgG and IgA are used in *serological testing* to make a diagnosis of pertussis. While a raised IgG can occur with both natural infection and vaccination, IgA is only produced after natural infection. For patients presenting early (within the first 3 weeks) and before the start of antibiotic therapy, PCR, immunofluorescence and culture may be useful. For patients who present later, serological testing – which is reliant on an immune response – is often more helpful.

A macrolide antibiotic is the treatment of choice. However, antibiotic therapy will render the patient noninfectious but will be unlikely to alter the course of their illness. The patient will only become noninfectious after 5 days of antibiotic therapy and should therefore be excluded from school/work for this period.[8–11]

7. Answer: B

CAP severity assessment in the ED should be based on the emergency clinician's clinical judgement based on the history, examination and investigation findings as well as the use of at least one severity scoring system. There are a number of severity scoring systems available, some are more validated than others. The PSI seems to be the most validated but it has a number of disadvantages. **Currently, the Australian Therapeutic Guidelines Antibiotic Expert Group recommends the use of SMART-COP score** (Table 3.1) **and CORB score** (Table 3.2) **as severity assessment tools.** A significant advantage of using SMART-COP score is its ability to identify the patient who will require intensive respiratory and vasopressor support (IRVS). CORB score may predict the need for IRVS, whereas the PSI is good at predicting the mortality risk but may not identify patients who will clinically deteriorate and require IRVS.

Severity of CAP does not identify the aetiology; neither do the findings on the history, examination and CXR.

TABLE 3.1 SMART-COP SCORE

	Parameter	Points
S	Systolic BP < 90 mm Hg	2
M	Multilobar infiltrates on CXR	1
A	Albumin < 35 g/L	1
R	Respiratory rate Age ≤ 50 years: RR ≥ 25/min Age > 50 years: RR ≥ 30/min	1
T	Tachycardia (> 125/min)	1
C	Confusion	1
O	Oxygen Age ≤ 50 years: PaO_2 < 70 mm Hg, or SpO_2 93% or less, or PaO_2/FiO_2 < 333 Age > 50 years: PaO_2 < 60 mm Hg, or SpO_2 90% or less, or PaO_2/FiO_2 < 250	2
P	Arterial pH < 7.35	2

0–2 points: low risk for IRVS
3–4 points: moderate risk for IRVS (1 in 8)
5–6 points: high risk for IRVS (1 in 3)
7 or more points: very high risk of IRVS (1 in 2)

TABLE 3.2 CORB SCORE

	Parameter	Points
C	Confusion (new)	1
O	Oxygen saturation 90% or less	1
R	Respiratory rate 30/min or more	1
B	BP – systolic < 90 mm Hg or diastolic < 60 mm Hg	1

Patients with 2 or more points is considered as having severe CAP and a high risk of needing IRVS.[12,13]

8. Answer: D

The evidence suggests that routine use of blood cultures to diagnose the aetiological agent in a patient who is likely to have CAP is of low value. In admitted patients only up to 16% of the blood cultures become positive. However, when positive this can confirm the aetiological agent of CAP. **As a result, blood cultures are recommended in the following selected subgroups of patients with CAP including**:

- patients requiring an ICU admission
- immunocompromised patients (including leukopenic and asplenic patients)
- patients with a pleural effusion
- patients with cavitary lesions in the lung
- patients with severe liver disease
- patients who abuse alcohol.

There is a moderate level of evidence to support blood cultures in the above subgroups.

When empiric antibiotic treatment is initiated in the ED for CAP according to the locally accepted therapeutic guidelines, the subsequent results of the blood culture rarely result in a change of the initial antibiotic therapy.[12,14]

9. Answer: A

It is difficult to predict the causative organism associated with pneumonia with the CXR findings as the changes are often non-specific. However, some radiological changes are more likely to be associated with a specific group of organisms. These include:

- area of segmental or subsegmental infiltration, lobar consolidation, appearance of air bronchograms – bacterial pneumonia
- interstitial pattern – mycoplasma, viruses
- cavitation – S. aureus, anaerobes, aerobic gram-negative bacilli, tuberculosis (TB), fungal

- pleural effusions – many types of bacterial pneumonia, atypical organisms such as viruses and Chlamydia, Legionella and TB
- abscess – S. aureus, Klebsiella
- empyema – S. aureus, Pseudomonas, anaerobic organisms.

Sputum culture results are not likely to change the antibiotic treatment. However, when correctly collected (i.e. prior to initiation of antibiotic therapy) and when the specimen is not heavily contaminated with squamous epithelial cells, the chance of identifying a causative organism increases up to 40%. The results of the sputum specimens collected after the commencement of antibiotics can be misleading. Similarly, the yield from blood cultures is relatively low. In general, blood culture may yield a 5–10% positive result in admitted patients with CAP. In Streptococcus pneumonia the blood culture yield is said to be 15–30%. The yield of blood cultures increases with increasing severity of pneumonia.

In patients with suspected Streptococcus pneumonia, Streptococcal urinary antigen assay can be performed on routinely collected urine and this can be done even after the commencement of antibiotics. Similarly Legionella pneumophila serotype 1 can be identified with Legionella urinary antigen assay. This test is indicated in patients requiring intensive care admission, alcoholics and in a recently returned traveller.

Testing for nucleic acid with polymerase chain reaction (PCR) in nose and throat swabs is usually helpful to identify a respiratory viral and influenza aetiology of pneumonia. For identification of atypical organisms often antibody testing on a set of acute and convalescent sera is used.[13–15]

10. Answer: B

Pneumonia caused by S. aureus may originate both as a community-acquired and hospital-acquired infection. It may account for up to 25% of pneumonia occurring in nursing home residents. It is also more common in intravenous drug users. During influenza epidemics, S. aureus pneumonia may occur as a secondary infection in otherwise healthy adults. Radiological findings on the CXR vary and empyema and cavity formation may be present, but these finding are not common. **A S. aureus infection tends to cause comparatively severe pneumonia and** hence associated with higher incidence of septic shock and mortality.[12,14]

11. Answer: D

Virulent strains of community-associated methicillin-resistant *S. aureus* (CA-MRSA) are increasingly becoming more prevalent in many parts of Australia including Queensland, NSW and the ACT. These strains can cause severe skin infections such as furunculosis, as well as rapidly fatal severe CAP. **This severe pneumonia usually occurs in previously healthy children and young adults with a history of furunculosis or folliculitis.** Please note that this is entirely a community-acquired infection. Usually, there is a history of family members affected by the same skin infection. These virulent strains produce a potent necrotising toxin. **Rapidly progressive septic shock is common**. The mortality rate has been described as 37% within 48 hours from presentation. To maximise the survival an early high index of suspicion, early treatment with appropriate antibiotics and rapid interventions for correction of shock are essential. **The current national recommendations for empirically treating suspected MRSA pneumonia are intravenous vancomycin and a beta lactam antibiotic (flu/dicloxacillin or cephalothin).**[14,16]

12. Answer: B

Aspiration pneumonitis is a chemical pneumonitis due to aspiration of sterile gastric contents with gastric acid. This causes direct lung injury and non-cardiogenic pulmonary oedema. This may lead to progressively worsening respiratory symptoms and subsequently acute respiratory distress syndrome (ARDS). **Aspiration pneumonitis is the most severe form of pulmonary aspiration** (see next answer). **Most patients present early (within a few hours) and the initial CXR is usually abnormal**. Patient may develop ARDS and respiratory failure within 2–5 hours after aspiration. The pneumonitis is not due to infection; however, secondary bacterial infection can occur later.[12,14]

13. Answer: B

Clinical features of pulmonary aspiration are due to three mechanisms:

- aspiration of gastric acid causing pulmonary pneumonia

- aspiration of contaminated oropharyngeal secretions and gastric contents
- aspiration of particulate matter.

Routine use of antibiotic therapy after suspected aspiration is controversial. If the suspected aspiration is of a minor degree, patients can be observed without initial antibiotic treatment. Aspiration pneumonia due to secondary bacterial infection can be diagnosed when the patient has typical symptoms of pneumonia, with radiological changes indicating that process. The CXR changes tend to occur in the dependent segments of the lung; in a supine patient, posterior segments of the upper lobes and superior segments of the lower lobes and, if erect, in the basal segments. The changes may appear as a bronchopneumonia or, in case of delayed presentation, may show as a lung abscess (i.e. cavitory lesion with an air fluid level).

The indications for antibiotic therapy in suspected aspiration are:

- failure to improve despite initial symptomatic treatment
- clinical deterioration
- CXR suggesting aspiration pneumonia
- aspiration of contaminated fluid such as in a patient with bowel obstruction.

Rigid bronchoscopy is indicated when aspiration of particulate matter (in gastric content, vegetable matter, teeth, etc.). The patient may present with small airway obstruction and resultant distal atelectasis and hypoxia. **There is no evidence to suggest that steroids are beneficial in pulmonary aspiration.** Most elderly patients require observation in hospital (even if asymptomatic) to detect any deterioration with development of bronchospasm, respiratory distress, hypoxia and fever.[12,14]

14. Answer: A

Bronchiectasis is described as an abnormal and permanent dilatation of bronchi and is most often due to an infectious process causing inflammation and destruction of the bronchial walls. This usually affects older patients and can be focal or diffuse. Typical offending organisms include viruses, mainly adenovirus and influenza, and bacteria such as *S. aureus*, *Klebsiella*, anaerobes, tuberculosis and *Bordetella pertussis*. Many other causes have been described including alpha 1 antitrypsin deficiency. As a result of reduced host defence mechanisms (due to destruction of air passages), a perpetual cycle of recurrent infections and further inflammation, obstruction and destruction occurs. Secretions accumulate and bacteria colonise obstructed air passages. The organisms found most typically include *Haemophilus* species and *Pseudomonas* species. These organisms can cause ongoing damage and episodic infectious exacerbations.

The reason for ED presentations is often acute exacerbations due to respiratory tract infections; **antibiotic therapy is the mainstay of management in acute exacerbations**. Sputum cultures done when the patient is stable and, ideally not taking antibiotics, can be used to guide the management of their next exacerbation. As the respiratory tract is often colonised with *Pseudomonas aeruginosa* a review of microbiology results of previous sputum cultures is important and empiric antibiotic treatment should be based on the previous culture results. Infection with *Pseudomonas aeruginosa* is associated with the greatest rate of lung function deterioration and the worst quality of life. Bronchial hyperreactivity and reversible obstruction is relatively common in bronchiectasis patients and **bronchodilator therapy may be helpful to relieve the reversible obstruction and also may aid in the clearance of secretions.** Improved clearance of tracheobronchial secretions should be attempted with chest physiotherapy using a variety of methods. The use of mucolytic agents to thin secretions has not been proven to be beneficial. However, nebulised hypertonic saline and inhaled mannitol appear promising in assisting sputum clearance.

Patients with bronchiectasis are at high risk for haemoptysis, sometimes massive, due to hypertrophied bronchial arteries.[17,18]

15. Answer: D

Cessation of cigarette smoking has been shown to reduce the risk of recurrence of a pneumothorax. About 20–30% of the primary spontaneous and 40–50% of the secondary spontaneous pneumothoraces recur. Resolution of a pneumothorax or the rate of reexpansion of the lung has no bearing on recurrence. The recurrence is prevented by definitive treatment. **Definitive treatment is usually indicated after the first recurrence, but for any** **patient in whom it is critical to prevent a recurrence (e.g. airline pilots) it should be offered following the first pneumothorax.**[19]

16. Answer: C

It is often difficult to identify a pneumothorax on a supine CXR. ED patients who are ventilated may develop pneumothoraces due to barotrauma, as well as due to attempted central line insertion. In the supine position in a patient with pneumothorax, the air in the pleural cavity collects anterior to the lung, therefore the collapsed lung edge is not often visible in this position. This is true even for a pneumothorax under tension. **Furthermore, the presence of a presumed well-positioned intercostal catheter (ICC) alone is not helpful in excluding a tension pneumothorax in a similar patient. Tension can develop even in a patient with an ICC.**

A number of features have been described to help identify a pneumothorax in a supine patient including:[19,20]

- deep sulcus sign – shown as a deep lateral costophrenic angle due to the air in that position
- pericardial fat tag sign – a sharp outline of the pericardial fat due to air in the lower part of the pleural cavity
- lucency due to air over the upper abdomen – often visible over the liver
- pleural air, which may cause a sharp appearance of the mediastinal and diaphragmatic borders
- subcutaneous emphysema without direct evidence of a pneumothorax.

17. Answer: B

Both inspiratory and expiratory posteroanterior (PA) films are equally sensitive (sensitivity only 83%) in the diagnosis of a pneumothorax. However, in COPD patients often the issue is to differentiate bullae from a spontaneous pneumothorax. **On a CXR a bulla appears with a concave inner margin (lung edge) and rounded edges, but a pneumothorax has a convex lung edge.** CT has a higher sensitivity in detection of a pneumothorax, as well as in the differentiation of a bulla from a pneumothorax in a COPD patient. This is very significant as, if a chest tube is inadvertently inserted into a bullous, it may cause a large pneumothorax and a resultant bronchopulmonary fistula and associated sequelae.[19]

18. Answer: C

In a supine patient, including trauma patient, bedside ultrasound can be used to detect or exclude an anteriorly placed pneumothorax. Some of these pneumothoraces are not visualised on a supine chest radiograph. In a trauma patient, the low-frequency curvilinear probe can be used in an extended FAST (eFAST) to look for a pneumothorax. In others, either high-frequency linear probe or curvilinear probe can be used. **In the absence of pleural adhesions in the normal lung the parietal and visceral pleurae are opposed and slide on each other during respiration. When there is no air sitting between the two pleural surfaces (i.e. when there is no pneumothorax), this lung sliding can be seen between the shadows of two anterior ribs with ultrasound.** The probe should be placed on the anterior chest wall perpendicular to the ribs. Two to three intercostal spaces should be scanned usually in the midclavicular line.

Signs in a normal lung when there is no pneumothorax

- Lung sliding sign: The pleural line can be identified and the lung sliding should be seen with the curvilinear or linear probe.

M-mode (motion mode) can be used as an adjunct to confirm the above finding. The following sign can be identified with M-mode.

- Seashore sign: A linear laminar pattern superficial to the pleural line and a granular pattern deep to the pleural line. It indicates normal lung sliding.

B-mode (brightness mode) may show comet-tail artefacts.

- Comet-tail artefacts: Reverberation artefacts that arise from interlobular septae under the visceral pleura. These are vertical and project to the depth of the ultrasound image. The comet-tail artefacts are only visible when both pleura are opposed to each other.

Signs indicating presence of a pneumothorax

- No lung sliding.
- Stratosphere sign (barcode sign): On M-mode ultrasound in the absence of lung sliding. This is a linear laminar pattern superficial to the pleural line as well as deep to the pleural line.
- Lung point sign: Visible on B-mode. The 'lung point' sign is an intermediate sign, which is visualised when the lung intermittently contacts the parietal pleura during inspiration, therefore alternating between the seashore (normal lung sliding) and stratosphere sign (pneumothorax). It is a dynamic point and can be seen at various locations. In small pneumothoraces it can be located anteriorly and in large pneumothoraces more laterally. The detection of lung point can be difficult but when detected it is 100% specific for the diagnosis.[21–23]

19. Answer: B

The aim of providing supplemental oxygen to patients with spontaneous pneumothoraces is to accelerate the rate of absorption of air from the pleural cavity. 100% oxygen as a treatment should be provided to patients with small primary pneumothoraces who are admitted to hospital for observation alone. **Supplemental oxygen reduces the alveolar partial pressure of nitrogen creating a nitrogen gradient between the pleural space and the alveoli. This increases the air absorption from the pneumothorax into the alveoli.** By providing 100% oxygen, the usual 1–2% per day of air absorption can be increased by fourfold. Oxygen has no effect in preventing the rare complication of reexpansion pulmonary oedema.

For small primary pneumothoraces chest tube drainage is not necessary. Even for large primary pneumothoraces it has not shown to be more effective than aspiration. Success rate for aspiration is said to be 45–71%. The success rate of aspiration reduces:

- in patients over 50 years of age
- when the volume of air aspirated is >2.5 L (means large air leak).[5,19]

20. Answer: A

The intercostal catheter or tube size should be determined on the basis of the anticipated amount of air leak from the lung. If a large air leak is anticipated a relatively larger catheter or tube should be used to prevent development of a tension pneumothorax. Tension may develop in spite of the presence of a catheter/tube that is inadequate comparative to the amount of air leak. Aspiration of >4 L of air suggests a large air leak from the lung. A large air leak can also be expected from a secondary spontaneous pneumothorax and from a patient who is going to be mechanically ventilated. The following catheter sizes are generally acceptable.

- For a small pneumothorax, a small size catheter/tube (10F–14F).
- For a large pneumothorax, a medium size tube (16F–22F).

Between 2 and 7% of spontaneous pneumothoraces have associated blood in the thoracic cavity (haemopneumothorax). If this is expected or visible on imaging, a large tube (24F–36F) should be used. French tube size represents the diameter of the tube. 1 French means a diameter of one-third of a millimetre (1/3 mm). For example, 24F = a diameter of 8 mm.[19]

21. Answer: A

Reexpansion pulmonary oedema is an infrequent but important complication that may occur following insertion of a chest tube for a large pneumothorax, especially when a patient presents late (after 72 hours from the onset). It is often described as occurring following rapid reexpansion due to application of suction, but it may occur without suction. Patients are usually younger patients. **Clinical presentation is dyspnoea and hypoxaemia after the insertion of a chest tube and pulmonary oedema will be evident on the side of the penumothorax on a CXR.** Unlike in cardiogenic pulmonary oedema, aggressive fluid resuscitation is part of the management. A severely hypoxaemic patient with florid pulmonary oedema who does not respond to oxygen therapy may require intubation and ventilation.[19]

22. Answer: D

A life-threatening admission with asthma in the previous 12 months predicts the risk of another near-fatal episode. In one study, two-thirds of patients who had an admission with life-threatening asthma had a further near-fatal or fatal attack within 12 months. Severe asthma is not usually associated with marked arterial desaturation. Arterial desaturation occurs late and indicates a life-threatening situation. Severe asthma is associated with an increased respiratory rate and resultant hypocarbia on blood gas analysis. **As the patient tires and respiratory failure sets in, $PaCO_2$ normalises. This should be considered a danger sign that requires aggressive management.** Current corticosteroid use increases

the potential for the patient to respond less to the acute treatment for a severe episode. However, it is the least valuable predictor of a near-fatal episode.[24]

23. Answer: C

In severe asthma, the current recommendation is to use inhaled salbutamol delivered either via an MDI with a large spacer or wet nebulisation. The onset of action is 5 minutes and duration is 6 hours. However, 'back to back' nebulisation, as opposed to intermittent nebulisation, is routinely used in the ED because drug delivery to the bronchiolar site depends on the patient's respiratory rate and the tidal volume. **The patient inhales approximately only 33% of the dose placed in the nebuliser chamber and only 20% reaches the bronchioles because patients with severe asthma usually take small tidal volume breaths due to tachypnoea.** Current evidence shows that intravenous bronchodilator therapy (as a bolus dose or as an infusion) with salbutamol does not offer additional clinical benefit over that offered by inhaled bronchodilator therapy. However, it is unclear whether there would be additional benefits in ventilated patients and the paediatric population. Intravenous salbutamol therapy should be considered when the critically unwell patient is unable to take inhaled therapy effectively, such as intolerance of inhaled therapy, but without indications for intubation. **If inhaled therapy is not effective and there are indications for intubation it is prudent to intubate and ventilate the patient early.** In ventilated patients inhaled salbutamol can be used with a nebulisation port or an MDI port in the circuit. Nebulisation with high oxygen/air flows in to the circuit may contribute to dynamic hyperinflation of the lungs in an asthmatic patient.

Although adrenaline infusion is used in severe asthma, especially in ventilated patients, currently there are no recommendations for its use. One advantage adrenaline has over salbutamol is its ability to reduce airway oedema because of its α-agonist effects. When severe asthma is complicated by hypotension (this should not be due to dynamic hyperinflation), adrenaline seems to be a reasonable option as a rescue agent. Continuous use of both salbutamol and adrenaline contributes to lactic acidosis in asthma patients.[12,24]

24. Answer: A

A single dose of intravenous magnesium sulphate is an effective adjunct in the treatment of severe asthma. The usual recommended dose in adults is 1.2–2 g and 50 mg/kg in children, given slowly via IV over 20–30 minutes. **There is evidence to suggest that the response from the drug is greatest in patients with most severe airflow obstruction due to bronchospasm on presentation to the ED.** Therefore, it is not recommended for routine use in mild to moderate asthma episodes. Even in severe asthma it does not reduce the rate of hospital admission, but it is associated with a significant improvement in lung function. Current evidence fails to show any clear benefit for use of nebulised magnesium sulphate in all age groups, whereas **intravenous magnesium sulphate can be used in patients in all age groups with severe asthma.**[12,24]

25. Answer: B

Intubation of a patient with severe or life-threatening asthma is a challenging situation. It requires carefully considering many factors and involving the most experienced airway operators. The absolute indications for intubation are:

- deteriorating consciousness
- severe exhaustion
- cardiopulmonary arrest.

In the presence of severe hypercapnoea and acidosis in a patient with normal level of consciousness and who is not exhausted, further aggressive bronchodilator therapy should be continued prior to reconsidering intubation.

These severely unwell patients are often volume depleted because of fluid losses through respiration and reduced intake. Induction agents may cause vasodilatation and loss of sympathetic tone, therefore causing severe hypotension at induction. Fluid resuscitation and careful adjustment of induction dose is therefore required. **In the ED, ketamine at a dose of 1–2 mg/kg is considered by many as the induction agent of choice because it has sympathomimetic and bronchodilating properties.** It should be used with a paralytic agent such as suxamethonium to facilitate the easy passage of the tube. Brisk repeated bagging should be avoided because it results in increased intrinsic positive end-expiratory pressure (PEEP) due to dynamic hyperinflation of the lung that can contribute to hypotension.[24,25]

26. Answer: D

Dynamic hyperinflation in a patient with severe asthma can cause barotruma to the lung and severely compromise venous return to the heart. As a result marked hypotension may develop. Hence, after intubation, the patient should be carefully manually ventilated with a slow breath rate not exceeding 6–8/min. This allows adequate time for exhalation of air from the lungs. **Patients should be clinically assessed to determine the degree of bronchospasm, the time taken for full expiration and the degree of gas trapping. Once the above are determined the patient can be connected to the ventilator circuit with carefully selected ventilator settings.** Generally a ventilator rate of 6–8 breaths/min and a tidal volume of 5–6 mL/kg are recommended. A long expiratory time should be set with an I:E ratio > 1:2. **Full expiration before the next breath should be confirmed clinically by observing the patient's chest rise and fall. In addition, this should be confirmed on the ventilator graph.** Moderate hypercarbia and acidosis is well tolerated but hypercarbia may be detrimental in patients with myocardial depression. During pressure-controlled ventilation, tidal volume may fluctuate and this may cause significant hypoventilation. Therefore, pressure-controlled ventilation may not be the ideal mode and volume-controlled ventilation is usually preferred.[24,26]

27. Answer: A

The principles of ventilation include small tidal volumes, a long expiratory time and a slow respiratory rate. The high-inspiratory flow rate is an important component of allowing long expiratory times. The peak inspiratory pressure (PIP) is likely to be high with these settings, but there does not appear to be a correlation between high PIPs and barotrauma in ventilated patients with asthma. Dynamic hyperinflation can be assessed by measuring the plateau airway pressure by occluding the expiratory valve at the end of inspiration and recording the pressure after a 5-second pause. This is the most easily measured estimate of alveolar pressure at the end of inspiration and is affected by the degree of hyperinflation. Ideally this should be maintained at <25 cm H_2O.

There is a paucity of randomised trial data regarding the use of NIV in asthma. Some case series suggest benefit. There are as yet no clear guidelines for the use of NIV in severe asthma. A trial of NIV is reasonable once patients are screened for contraindications and are willing to cooperate.

Similarly, there is a paucity of good evidence regarding the use of IV salbutamol. However, IV β-agonists should be considered if there is no response to nebulised bronchodilator therapy. Increasing airway obstruction may prevent nebulised drug delivery and some studies have demonstrated improved response when intravenous β-agonist is used. Salbutamol (e.g. 250 mcg) may also be given IV to non-intubated patients with severe asthma.[27]

28. Answer: D

Emergency clinicians should be vigilant about the possibility of desaturation after intubation. This is a complication that may occur in the severe asthmatic. The 'DOPE' mnemonic describes the practical drill that should be adopted during such a scenario (it does not describe the order of the drill).

DOPE

Displacement of ETT – check ETT position.

Obstruction of ETT – check tube kink by passing a suction catheter through the tube. Also suction the ETT to remove mucus plugs if any.

Pneumothorax – check for a pneumothorax clinically and obtain a CXR immediately.

Equipment – disconnect from the ventilator. Commence bagging patient with 100% oxygen and obtain assistance in checking the ventilator, circuit and oxygen supply.

Although a supine CXR may occasionally miss a pneumothorax, in most situations in a ventilated patient a pneumothorax that is significant enough to cause hypoxaemia can be detected by a supine CXR. Dynamic hyperinflation of the lungs may be contributory to desaturation due to hypoxaemia. Mucus plugging is a major concern and this may be due to drying and thickening of secretions. A mucus plug may cause collapse of one or more segments of the lung, causing severe desaturation. To dislodge the mucus plug adequate suctioning through

the ETT with assistance from physiotherapy is required and sometimes may need to proceed to bronchoscopic lavage. Adequate humidification of inspired gas is recommended to prevent mucus plugging in ventilated asthmatics.[12,24]

29. Answer: B

Salbutamol is commonly used for bronchodilator therapy in acute asthma. Evidence suggests that salbutamol administration via MDI and spacer is not only more effective but is also associated with fewer side effects such as tachycardia, vomiting and hypoxia, as compared with administration via nebuliser. However, in a life-threatening exacerbation of asthma, continuous nebulised salbutamol should be used. If the initial response to nebulised salbutamol is inadequate, salbutamol can be administered via the intravenous route at a dose of 15 mcg/kg over 10 minutes followed by a maintenance infusion of 1 mcg/kg/min. However, the role of intravenous bronchodilators in addition to nebulised treatment remains unclear. The referenced guidelines vary in their recommendations.

Aminophyllin can be considered in children with severe and life-threatening attacks unresponsive to maximal other therapies. It has been shown to have an effect on the outcome (intubation). Recommendations in guidelines vary, however, and it remains a controversial area.

There is a paucity of evidence to clarify the role of NIV in acute severe paediatric asthma. NIV has had some success in adults with restrictive lung conditions and it has been used in acute adult asthma. None of the current paediatric guidelines recommend the use of NIV.

In select patients, NIV may avoid the need for intubation. For a child who is alert and cooperative and who does not have increased airway secretions, NIV may be considered in the following situations at experienced hands:

- hypoxaemic child despite high-flow oxygen and/or has hypercarbia
- while awaiting maximal therapeutic effects of corticosteroids and bronchodilators to ease the child's work of breathing
- a child who is progressing towards respiratory muscle fatigue.[28,29,30]

30. Answer: B

Spirometry is indicated in all patients presenting with acute exacerbations of COPD except rare occasions of altered level of consciousness. FEV 1.0 manoeuvre can be performed by even unwell COPD patients with a normal conscious state. When FEV 1.0 is <1 L or <40% predicated, it usually indicates a severe exacerbation in a patient with mild to moderate disease.

In a patient with advanced disease (severe COPD), worsening hypoxaemia, acute hypercapnoea, acute/chronic hypercapnoea or acidosis indicates severe exacerbation. **ABG should be obtained in all patients with severe exacerbations of COPD and with suspected respiratory failure or cor pulmonale.** Hypercapnoea may occur during acute exacerbations in both patients with normal CO_2 levels and chronically elevated CO_2 levels. Excessive oxygen administration may worsen this hypercapnoea. Several mechanisms promote CO_2 retention including reduced ventilation due to reduced hypoxic drive and increased ventilation–perfusion mismatch due to hypoxic pulmonary vasoconstriction. **Early identification of a patient who is in hypercapnoeic respiratory failure will alert against excessive oxygen administration.** Excessive oxygen administration has been shown to increase length of hospital stay, increased rate of admission to the high dependency unit (HDU) and increased use of NIV. Excessive oxygen administration is rarely required to treat hypoxia in COPD and ideally should be treated with Venturi mask at 24% or 28%. Although nasal prongs provide variable amounts of oxygen, at a rate of 0.5–2 L/min is less likely to cause CO_2 retention. Oxygen saturation (SpO_2) should be maintained at 88–92%. SpO_2 >92% does not provide additional advantages. Between 8 and 10 puffs of a 100 mcg MDI salbutamol provides an equivalent dose to 5 mg nebulised salbutamol and may be used in patients with acute exacerbations.[31,32]

31. Answer: D

COPD patients in acute respiratory failure belong to one of two distinct clinical categories:
- patients with normocapnic respiratory failure ($PaCO_2$ 35–45 mm Hg)
- patients with hypercapnic respiratory failure ($PaCO_2$ >45 mm Hg).

It is important to identify the patients who have a high risk of developing hypercapnic respiratory failure on presentation to the ED so as to prevent further deterioration of the condition with too aggressive oxygen therapy. In such patients, oxygen therapy should be continued in a controlled manner as clinically appropriate (e.g. up to 2 L/min via nasal prongs or via Venturi mask) and all nebulised bronchodilator therapy should be delivered using medical air.

Generally, COPD patients with chronic bronchitis tend to present with hypercapnic respiratory failure more than those with emphysema. Obese patients and those with obstructive sleep apnoea are more likely to develop hypercapnoea. Patients using central nervous system depressants such as sedatives and alcohol have a high risk of developing hypercapnic respiratory failure.

Patients with emphysema, thin physique, hyperinflated lungs and those exhibiting accessory muscle use and pursed-lip breathing are more likely to be normocapnic. Both categories of patients can have right heart failure (RHF) but hypercapnic patients are likely to develop RHF early.[33]

32. Answer: B

In asthma, there is a significant reversible component of airways obstruction. In contrast, in COPD exacerbation, major reductions in peak flow and FEV1 measurements can be seen only in some patients. Because of the high negative predictive value of a very low BNP, acutely dyspnoeic patients with very low BNP values despite a moderate degree of clinical suspicion for congestive heart failure (CHF) should be considered to have COPD. Ultimately it is appropriate to perform chest CT when clinical suggestion of a pneumothorax remains and results of plain films and ultrasound are non-diagnostic. The presence of COPD may result in false-positives using bedside USS and the data in this setting are limited. A sufficiently sensitive D-dimer is suitable to exclude PE in patients with COPD who do not have a high clinical probability of PE. **Patients with COPD have an elevated risk of venous thromboembolism and PE should be considered when an acute exacerbation is considered, especially if deterioration occurs rapidly with no other apparent cause.**[34]

33. Answer: A

The use of NIV in patients presenting with an acute exacerbation of COPD, in addition to usual medical care, is associated with reductions in mortality, need for intubation and treatment failure. NIV should be considered early in the course of respiratory failure before severe acidosis ensues (in line with global and Australasian guidelines). This may reflect the benefit of starting earlier in the process when respiratory muscles are less fatigued.

Indications for NIV include:
- moderate to severe dyspnoea with the use of accessory muscles and paradoxical abdominal motion
- moderate to severe acidosis (pH< 7.35) and hypercapnia (PaCO$_2$ >45 mm Hg)
- respiratory rate >25 breaths/min.

There are no definite clinical predictors to identify which patients with respiratory failure will benefit from NIV. Patients with a pH between 7.25 and 7.30 appear to receive the greatest benefit.[34,35]

34. Answer: C

Although it is common practice to use anticholinergic and beta-sympathomimetic bronchodilator agents in combination for their synergistic effects, a recent review found that there was no significant difference between the agents, and the combination did not appear to increase the effect on FEV1 over either agent alone. However, the duration of action of anticholinergic agents is longer than short-acting β-agonists and they have a lower adverse effect profile. **Depending on the clinical situation either types of agents can be used alone or in combination.**

Bacteria play a role in approximately 50% of exacerbations. **The presence of increased dyspnoea, increased sputum purulence or volume, leucocytosis or fever is a reasonable trigger for commencing antibiotics.** Patients with more severe exacerbations are more likely to benefit from antibiotic treatment than those with less severe exacerbations. Antibiotics should be chosen to cover *Strep. pneumoniae*, *H. influenzae*, and *Moraxella catarrharis*. *Mycoplasma* and *Chlamydia pneumoniae* are possible infections in some patients.

Systemic steroids hasten recovery as well as reduce hospital stay and early treatment failure in patients with acute exacerbations of COPD. The effects of inhaled corticosteroids on the course of an exacerbation are uncertain. The inpatient mortality is 17–30%, with the best predictors of successful weaning from ventilator being pre-existing functional status and FEV1.[34, 35]

35. Answer: C

The International Cooperative Pulmonary Embolism Registry demonstrates a death rate of 15% for haemodynamically stable patients with PE and 58% for haemodynamically unstable patients. Among haemodynamically stable patients with PE, several factors have been shown to be associated with increased rate of death. **A meta-analysis of several studies has shown that increased troponin levels (as a marker of myocardial dysfunction or injury) in haemodynamically stable patients with PE increases both short-term mortality risk and risk of death by PE by a factor of 5.2 and 9.4 respectively.** Right ventricular (RV) dysfunction on echocardiography is another important factor associated with increased rate of death in these patients. In these patients RV hypokinesis and dilatataion are shown to be independent predictors of 30-day mortality. In addition, RV septal bowing has been shown to be a predictor of death in a large retrospective study. However, application of these findings to the clinical setting in the ED is controversial because RV assessments were done using computerised reformatted images and hence not available to bedside echocardiography. However, RV dysfunction as visualised on CTPA has been suggested as an independent predictor of 30-day mortality. The subgroup of patients who have both RV dysfunction on echocardiography and elevated troponin levels seem to have a significantly higher risk of death. Other factors that have been shown to be associated with increased mortality in haemodynamically stable patients are:
- age >75 years
- presence of cardiac or respiratory disease
- cancer
- immobilisation because of neurologic disease.

There is no clear evidence for increased risk of death in pregnancy but they may be more prone to have other adverse outcomes directly related to PE or anticoagulation.[36]

36. Answer: B

Venous thromboembolism (DVT and/or PE) occurs in 0.1% of pregnancies. At least in 50% of these cases it is associated with an inherited or acquired thrombophilia (a disorder of haemostasis that predisposes an individual to thrombotic events). However, thrombophilia screening done in pregnant patients with DVT or PE will add minimal value in the treatment of these patients during the current pregnancy. The results obtained during the pregnancy can be unreliable as pregnancy and the treatment of DVT or PE both can alter the circulating levels of coagulation factors. **Thrombophilia screening should be done after the delivery and especially when the treatment with anticoagulants is ceased and the results may be useful for managing future pregnancies.**

Between 70 and 90% of the cases of DVT during pregnancy occur in the left leg because the left iliac vein is compressed by the right iliac artery. The incidence of iliac vein thrombosis may be higher in pregnant patients than in non-pregnant women. **The diagnosis of iliac vein thrombosis is generally difficult with compression ultrasonography. MRDTI seems to have a high sensitivity and specificity of this diagnosis and can be safely used in pregnancy.**[37]

37. Answer: C

Diagnosis of PE in a pregnant woman is one of the challenging areas in relation to PE. Furthermore, the inclusion or exclusion of this diagnosis in a patient presents with suspicious symptoms is of great importance becuase PE is described as the leading cause of maternal death in developed countries. **Pretest probability scores cannot be directly applied in the diagnostic process in this situation, because they have not been validated in pregnancy.** During pregnancy there is a significant ongoing haemostatic processes and this reflects the increasing presence of D-dimer. D-dimer levels increase as the pregnancy advances. **Additionally, a negative D-dimer alone may not be helpful to rule out the diagnosis of PE irrespective of the stage of pregnancy.**

As delays in treatment are associated with increased risk of maternal death associated with PE, it is reasonable to treat these patients with low molecular weight heparin (LMWH) on suspicion unless contraindications exist. **Compression ultrasonography is recommended as the first-line investigation. If USS confirms DVT and the patient is stable, further lung imaging may not add value and will deliver radiation for both the fetus and the mother.** When USS is negative further lung imaging is required. CXR is of value to exclude alternative diagnoses.

Either CTPA or V/Q scan is selected depending on the age of gestation, presence of lung diseases such as asthma, availability, local practices and preference. The following facts should be carefully considered when selecting further imaging.

- V/Q scan delivers a higher dose of radiation to the fetus than CTPA.
- V/Q scan causes a slightly higher risk of development of childhood cancer than CTPA (1 in 280,000 vs < 1 in one million).
- The dose of radiation delivered in the V/Q scan can be reduced by the use of perfusion scan alone initially. The ventilation scan should subsequently be peformed only if the perfusion scan is positive.
- CTPA delivers a higher radiation dose to the mother than V/Q scan.
- The risk of developing breast cancer will be 13% higher in the mother with CTPA than from a V/Q scan.[37]

38. Answer: A

The testing threshold (TT) is the pretest probability on clinical grounds below which a clinician may defer a diagnostic test. In other words, this indicates an acceptable missed diagnosis rate in clinical practice. **This is important because below the testing threshold even a simple investigation such as D-dimer test has the potential to cause more harm than benefit to the patient.** For example, an inappropriately ordered D-dimer test can become positive due to myriad other reasons in a clinically low-risk patient for PE, which in turn leads to further testing of the patient with CTPA. CTPA is associated with an increase in lifetime cancer risk, anaphylaxis to contrast and risk of contrast-induced nephropathy. In contrast, patients falling above the acceptable testing threshold should have further diagnostic investigations.

The authors of PERC estimated that this testing threshold for further testing to be 1.8% and the PERC is based on this assumption. In other words, a missed rate of 1.8% is acceptable to defer diagnostic testing that may cause more harm than the disease itself. In a recent study this testing threshold was found to be 1.4%. **However, PERC can be applied only to patients with a suspected PE with a low pretest probability according to the clinician's overall clinical impression or clinical gestalt. All eight criteria must be met in these low-probability patients to defer further diagnostic testing.** These criteria include:[38–41]

- age <50
- heart rate <100/min
- oxygen saturation on room air >94%
- no prior history of DVT/PE
- no recent history of trauma or surgery
- no hemoptysis
- no exogenous oestrogen
- no clinical signs suggesting DVT.

39. Answer: C

LMWH is the appropriate initial treatment in most patients with haemodynamically stable PE, including pregnant patients. This choice is based on its ease of use. The efficacy and the safety of LMWH has been shown to be similar to intravenous unfractionated heparin. Intravenous unfractionated heparin is indicated and should be considered in the following circumstances:

- creatinine clearance <30 L/min; LMWH is renally excreted
- in the morbidly obese patient; absorption of subcutaneously injected LMWH may be erratic and unreliable

Warfarin should be commenced preferably at the commencement of the heparin treatment. Heparin can be ceased when the target international normalised ratio (INR) of 2.0–3.0 is reached and warfarin should be continued for at least 3 months. **Extended warfarin treatment is indicated in patients with a high risk for recurrence.** Risk factors for recurrence include:

- being male
- advanced age

- PE in the absence of identifiable risk factors (this is up to 50% of PEs)
- presence of a malignancy.

Risk of recurrence of a pulmonary embolism is <1% per year during the treatment with anticoagulant therapy. This increases to 2–10% per year after the discontinuation of the anticoagulation therapy. Long-term LMWH is indicated for patients with PE provoked by malignancy because the recurrence rate is high.

During pregnancy, LMWH should be continued at least until delivery because warfarin is contraindicated. Warfarin crosses the placenta and may cause teratogenesis in the early part of pregnancy and fetal intracranial haemorrhage in late pregnancy. Both unfractionated heparin and LMWH do not cross the placenta, therefore teratogenesis or fetal haemorrhage will not occur.[37]

40. Answer: A

DVT can affect the upper extremity veins and in the majority of the cases it affects the axillary and subclavian veins. About 10% of all DVTs are said to involve the upper extremities and 80% of these cases are due to secondary causes including catheter-associated thrombosis (associated with central venous lines, port and catheter for treatment of cancers, pacemaker or defibrillator leads), cancer, surgery or trauma to the upper extremity. **DVT of the upper extremity is more likely to be associated with malignancies than DVT of the legs.** In comparison, it is less likely to be due to thrombophilia than DVT of the legs. One of the primary causes of DVT in the upper extremity that is worth noting is strenuous exercise involving usually the dominant arm in a young male patient causing DVT in that arm.

D-dimer testing, even in the presence of a low pretest probability, is unreliable in suspected cases of DVT of the upper extremity because these patients have many associated secondary conditions that may result in a positive D-dimer. Therefore it is not recommended as a screening test.

The recurrence rate and rate of post-thrombotic syndrome are less than that occurring with DVT of the legs. PE is an important complication; however, again, the rate is less than that occurring in DVT of the legs (6% vs 15–32%).[42]

References

1. Sarko J, Stapczynski J. Respiratory distress. In: Tintinalli J, Stapczynski J, Ma O, et al, editors. Tintinalli's emergency medicine: a comprehensive study guide. 7th ed. New York: McGraw Hill Medical; 2011. p. 465–73.

2. Collings J. Acid–base disorders. In: Marx J, Hockberger R, Walls R, et al, editors. Rosen's emergency medicine: concepts and clinical practice. 7th ed. Philadelphia: Mosby Elsevier; 2010. p. 1640–14.

3. Kelly A. Review article: Can venous blood gas analysis replace arterial in emergency medical care? Emerg Med Austral 2010;22(6):493–8.

4. Light Richard W. Chapter 257. Disorders of the pleura and mediastinum. Fauci AS, Braunwald E, Kasper DL, et al, editors. Harrison's principles of internal medicine, 17th ed. 2008. Online. Available: http://www.accessmedicine.com/content.aspx?aID=2861952.

5. Kosowsky J. Pleural disease. In: Marx J, Hockberger R, Walls R, et al, editors. Rosen's emergency medicine: concepts and clinical practice. 7th ed. Philadelphia: Mosby Elsevier; 2010. p. 939–46.

6. Young W. Hemoptysis. In: Tintinalli J, Stapczynski J, Ma O, et al, editors. Tintinalli's emergency medicine: a comprehensive study guide. 7th ed. New York: McGraw Hill Medical; 2011. p. 473–6.

7. Airway and lung collapse: right upper lobe collapse. Online. Available: http://radiologymasterclass.co.uk/gallery/chest/airways/airways_i.html; 4 Dec 2011.

8. Therapeutic Guidelines Limited Antibiotic Expert Group. Respiratory tract infections: other. Therapeutic guidelines: antibiotic Version 14. Melbourne: Therapeutic Guidelines Limited; 2010.

9. The Royal Children's Hospital Melbourne. Clinical practice guidelines. Whooping cough (pertussis). Online. Available: http://www.rch.org.au/clinicalguide/cpg.cfm?doc_id=5236; 12 Jun 2011.

10. Senanayake S. Pertussis in Australia today. A disease of adolescents and adults that can kill infants. Australian Family Physician 2007;36(1/2):51–5. Online. Available: www.racgp.org.au/afp/200701/20070129senayake.pdf; 23 May 2011.

11. Marchant J. Managing pertussis in adults. Aust Prescr 2009;32:36–8.

12. Brookes J, Dunn R. Respiratory disease. In: Dunn R, Dilley S, Leach D, et al, editors. The emergency medicine manual. 5th ed. Tennyson: Venom Publishing; 2010. p. 500–33.

13. Therapeutic Guidelines Limited Antibiotic Expert Group. Respiratory tract infections: pneumonia. Therapeutic guidelines: antibiotic Version 14. Melbourne: Therapeutic Guidelines Limited; 2010.

14. Emerman C, Anderson E, Cline D. Community-acquired pneumonia, aspiration pneumonia, and noninfectious pulmonary infiltrates. In: Tintinalli J, Stapczynski J, Ma O, et al, editors. Tintinalli's emergency medicine: a comprehensive study guide. 7th ed. New York: McGraw Hill Medical; 2011. p. 479–91.

15. Moran G, Talan D. Pneumonia. In: Marx J, Hockberger R, Walls R, et al, editors. Rosen's emergency medicine: concepts and clinical practice. 7th ed. Philadelphia: Mosby Elsevier; 2010. p. 927–38.

16. Risson D, O'Connor E, Guard R, et al. A fatal case of necrotising pneumonia due to community-associated methicillin-resistant Staphylococcus aureus. Med J Aust 2007;186(9):479–80.

17. Tino G, Weinberger S. Bronchiectasis and lung abscess. In: Fauci A, Braunwald E, Kasper D, et al, Harrison's principles of internal medicine. 17th ed. 2008. Online. Available: http://www.accessmedicine.com/content.aspx?aID=2869490.

18. McLean A. Bronchiectasis: a new look at an old adversary. Australian Prescriber 2008;31(3):77–9.

19. Humphries R, Young W. Spontaneous and iatrogenic pneumothorax. In: Tintinalli J, Stapczynski J, Ma O, et al, editors. Tintinalli's emergency medicine: a comprehensive study guide. 7th ed. New York: McGraw Hill Medical; 2011. p. 500–4.

20. Joyce C, Saad N, Kruger P, et al. Chapter 1: Chest. Diagnostic imaging in critical care: a problem based approach. Sydney: Churchill Livingston Elsevier; 2010. p. 37.

21. Ma O J, Mateer J R, Kirkpatrick A W. Trauma. In: Ma JO, Mateer JR, Blaivas M, editors. Emergency ultrasound. 2nd ed. New York: McGraw-Hill; 2007. p. 77–108.

22. Nagdev A. Focus on: ultrasound detection of traumatic anterior pneumothorax. ACEP News December 2008. Online. Available: www.acep.org.

23. Ma J, Reardon R, Sabbaj A. Emergency ultrasonography. In: Tintinalli J, Stapczynski J, Ma O, et al, editor. Tintinalli's emergency medicine: a comprehensive study guide. 7th ed. New York: McGraw Hill Medical; 2011. p. e146–63.

24. Holley A, Boots R. Review article: Management of acute severe and near-fatal asthma. Emerg Med Austral 2009;21:259–68.

25. Nowak R, Takarsi G. Asthma. In: Marx J, Hockberger R, Walls R, et al, editors. Rosen's emergency medicine: concepts and clinical practice. 7th ed. Philadelphia: Mosby Elsevier; 2010. p. 888–903.

26. Cydulka R. Acute asthma in adults. In: Tintinalli J, Stapczynski J, Ma O, et al, editors. Tintinalli's emergency medicine: a comprehensive study guide. 7th ed. New York: McGraw Hill Medical; 2011. p. 504–11.

27. Tuxen D, Naughton M. Acute severe asthma. In: Bersten A, Soni N, editors. Oh's intensive care manual. 6th ed. London: Butterworth-Heinemann Elsevier; 2009. p. 399–413.

28. Wolters Kluwer Health. Acute severe asthma exacerbations in children: intensive care unit management. Online. Available: www.uptodate.com.

29. Powell C. Acute asthma. In: Cameron P, Jelinek G, Everitt I, et al, editors. Textbook of paediatric emergency medicine. 2nd ed. Edinburgh: Churchill Livingston Elsevier; 2012. p. 128–33.

30. National Asthma Council Australia. Asthma management handbook 2006. Online. Available: www.nationalasthma.org.au.

31. Joosten S, Koh M, Bu X, et al. The effects of oxygen therapy in patients presenting to an emergency department with exacerbation of chronic obstructive pulmonary disease. MJA 2007;186:235–8.

32. Abramson M, Brown J, Crockett A, et al. COPD-X plan: Australian and New Zealand guidelines for management of chronic obstructive pulmonary disease. Online. Available: www.copdx.org.au; 25 May 2011.

33. Naughton M, Tuxen D. Acute respiratory failure in chronic obstructive pulmonary disease. In: Bersten A, Soni N, editors. Oh's intensive care manual. 6th ed. London: Butterworth-Heinemann Elsevier; 2009. p. 343–54.

34. Swadron S, Mandavia, D. Chronic obstructive pulmonary disease. In: Marx J, Hockberger R, Walls R, et al, editors. Rosen's emergency medicine: concepts and clinical practice. 7th ed. Philadelphia: Mosby Elsevier; 2010. p. 904–12.

35. Leung J, Duffy M. Chronic obstructive pulmonary disease. In: Cameron P, Jelinek G, Kelly A, editors. Textbook of adult emergency medicine. 3rd ed. Edinburgh: Churchill Livingstone Elsevier; 2012. p. 298–303.

36. Agnelli G, Becattini C. Current concepts: acute pulmonary embolism. N Engl J Med 2010;363:266–74.

37. Marik P, Plante L. Venous thromboembolic disease and pregnancy. N Engl J Med 2008;359:2025–33.

38. Kline J, Mitchell A, Kabrhel C, et al. Clinical criteria to prevent unnecessary diagnostic testing in emergency department patients with suspected pulmonary embolism. J Thromb Haemost 2004;2:1247.

39. Kline J. Thromboembolism. In: Tintinalli J, Stapczynski J, Ma O, et al, editors. Tintinalli's emergency medicine: a comprehensive study guide. 7th ed. New York: McGraw Hill Medical; 2011. 430–41.

40. Lessler A, Isserman J, Agarwal R, et al. Testing low-risk patients for suspected pulmonary embolism: a decision analysis. Ann Emerg Med 2010;55:316–26.

41. Newman D, Schriger D. Rethinking testing for pulmonary embolism: less is more. Ann Emerg Med 2011;57(6):622–7.

42. Kucher N. Deep-vein thrombosis of the upper extremities. N Engl J Med 2011;364:861–9.

1. Answer: D

Migraine headache can be associated with two types of symptoms:

- prodromal symptoms
- symptoms of aura.

The usual prodromal symptoms are lethargy, yawning, hyperactivity and food craving. These symptoms start many hours before the onset of headache.

The majority of migraine headaches are not associated with an aura. When associated with aura, it can precede or accompany the headache. Aura does not usually last more than 60 minutes. **A variety of neurological symptoms can occur during aura. The most common of these symptoms are visual (dark spots and flashing lights etc.). Other symptoms may include hemiparaesthesia, hemiparesis and speech deficits.** The headache in migraine can be unilateral or bilateral and pulsating or non-pulsating. **External ocular muscle palsy can be associated with migraine.** This occurs in ophthalmoplegic migraine, which is a less common type of migraine. In this type the headache is associated with cranial nerve palsies involving III, IV and VI. **When a patient presents with ophthalmoplegia associated with a headache for the first time other causes for focal neurological deficit should be carefully excluded before diagnosing migraine.** Migraine is a diagnosis of exclusion in these patients.[1]

2. Answer: B

The primary causes of headache (migraine, tension-type headaches and cluster headaches) are more common than secondary causes, even in patients over 50 years of age. However, careful consideration should be given to exclude life-threatening and other secondary-type headaches. The most common location of a SAH headache is the occipitonuchal location but other intracranial pathology may also cause headaches in this location. **Although the location of the headache needs to be considered seriously, its PPV for diagnosis of a serious pathology is relatively low.** About 25% of the SAH are associated with an exertional onset.

Patients over 50 years of age who present with new onset unilateral headache should be carefully assessed to exclude temporal arteritis. The most significant complication associated with temporal arteritis is sudden visual loss secondary to ischaemic optic neuritis. Irregularity, tenderness or loss of pulsation over the temporal artery and an erythrocyte sedimentation rate (ESR) >50 mm are some of the other features of this condition.[1,2]

3. Answer: B

The risk of cerebral venous thrombosis increases in hypercoagulability states such as:

- when using the oral contraceptive pill
- during pregnancy
- postpartum periods
- in postoperative period.

This diagnosis should be considered in all pregnant patients who present to the ED with headache. In cerebral venous thrombosis neurological findings may not correspond to any anatomical region and they may fluctuate. In the majority of patients, pregnancy improves the migraine symptoms. Therefore, before attributing headache to migraine in a pregnant patient, other serious causes should be considered.

At the initial presentation, the majority of patients with a brain tumour do not have abnormal neurological findings. **Hypertension can cause headache and higher diastolic pressures have been found to cause more severe headaches.** Usually headache related to hypertension resolves when blood pressure (BP) is adequately controlled. Only 2% of all ischaemic strokes are secondary to spontaneous dissection of cervical arteries. However, this is a very important cause of ischaemic stroke in the young and middle-aged population, responsible for 10–25% of all ischaemic strokes. Although it affects all age groups including children, the peak incidence is in the fifth decade of life.[1,3,4]

4. Answer: B

Temporal arteritis is a steroid-responsive large-vessel vasculitis with both local arteritic and non-specific systemic inflammatory features. This condition itself is relatively rare.

Local arteritic features include:

- temporal artery abnormalities such as
  - beading
  - irregularity
  - tenderness
  - pulselessness
- jaw claudication (34% of patients have this symptom)
- visual loss and ischaemic optic neuropathy
- scalp and tongue necrosis
- diplopia.

Systemic features include (these are non-specific):

- polymyalgica rheumatica (PMR) – up to 40% of patients with temporal arteritis have concomitant PMR, hence this diagnosis should be considered in patients with PMR
- fever
- anorexia
- fatigue
- elevated ESR in the absence of other causes.

Temporal arteritis is almost exclusively limited to the over-50 age group and the patient's classic presentation is a severe throbbing frontotemporal headache in the area of the temporal artery, which may often be a new onset headache (65–75% of patients). However, some patients do not present with headache. In these patients jaw claudication may be a prominent feature. Ischaemic optic neuropathy is the cause of loss of vision in this condition and, once established, the visual loss is permanent. The most important feature associated with the *least* chance of having a positive temporal artery biopsy (therefore able to rule out this disease), is the absence of an elevated ESR > 50 mm/h (negative likelihood ratio of 0.2). Once clinically suspected, temporal artery biopsy should be arranged to establish or rule out the diagnosis. The sensitivity of unilateral biopsy is approximately 90% and bilateral biopsy is slightly higher. Considering all clinical features and judgement when the pretest probability is high for a diagnosis of temporal arteritis, corticosteroid therapy should be commenced while waiting for an urgent biopsy. In the absence of a well-established optimal dose and route of administration, the common practice is to give prednisolone at 1 mg/kg.[1,5]

5. Answer: A

A non-contrast CT may help to predict the site of the rupture of an aneurysm, especially involving the anterior cerebral artery and anterior communicating artery. Only 20% of the patients with SAH have another aneurysm in addition to the one that ruptured. However, this is important to identify for intervention. In the absence of trauma, subhyaloid haemorrhage is pathognomonic, but this is seen only in <25% of the patients presenting with SAH. SAH does not present with syncope as a sole symptom and usually there are associated symptoms, mainly headache, prior to or after the syncopal event.[6,7]

6. Answer: A

When performed within 12 hours of the onset of symptoms, the sensitivity of non-contrast CT in detecting subarachnoid blood is up to 98%. MRI is not as sensitive as non-contrast CT in detecting acute blood in the brain. It is generally believed that a reducing number of RBCs in CSF tubes 1–4 would indicate a traumatic tap. This has not been proven. It has been reported that there could be a 25% reduction in the RBC count in successive tubes in patients with SAH. Consequently, a reducing RBC count in tubes should be interpreted with caution. Xanthochromia from a traumatic tap can develop as early as 2 hours. Otherwise, xanthochromia from SAH may take 6–12 hours to develop. Xanthochromia is due to the presence of bilirubin. Bilirubin degradation can occur when a CSF sample is exposed to light, hence less xanthochromia. It has a negative predictive value – when CT is normal, negative xanthochromia and up to a few RBCs (0–5) reliably excludes SAH.

Currently, there is inadequate evidence to suggest the use of CTA as a first-line investigation for the diagnosis of SAH as there are only a few studies comparing CTA with non-contrast CT and LP for the diagnosis. CTA may detect an unruptured aneurysm and a systematic review found the risk of rupture of such an aneurysm in patients symptomatic with headache to be 8.3%.[6,8]

7. Answer: C

Cerebral vasospasm is most common in 2 days to 3 weeks. There is moderate protective benefit with nimodipine, and this should be started within 96 hours. The need for seizure prophylaxis is controversial. One in 5 patients with SAH will have at least one seizure. Delayed cerebral ischaemia is known to be associated with hyperglycaemia, hypothermia and hyperthermia. Rebleeding can be reduced by adequate BP control. Ideal target BP is unsure. Premorbid BP or MAP < 130 mmHg may be reasonable targets. Antiemetics, analgesia or IV titratable antihypertensives may be needed.[6]

8. Answer: A

Usually the maximal headache in SAH occurs within a few hours (approximately 2 hours) after the onset of headache. If headache maximises after 6 hours it is less likely to be SAH. Often the opening pressures at LP is high but normal pressure does not exclude SAH. White cells may be present if red cell count is high (1 WBC for every 500 RBC). Homogenously bloody CSF in successive tubes is more likely to occur in SAH.[6,9]

9. Answer: D

Careful selection of investigations and interpretation of results to rule out a SAH is important in a patient with a suspicious headache who presents late. The sensitivity of the CT scan to detect subarachnoid blood reduces to 50% by day 7 from the onset of symptoms. By 2 weeks most blood is reabsorbed. During this period when the initial non-contrast CT is negative it should be followed with an LP to detect xanthochromia in the CSF. Xanthochromia can result from the presence of bilirubin and oxyhaemoglobin in the CSF due to the haemoglobin degradation. Bilirubin is formed in vivo only but oxyhaemoglobin can be formed in the CSF both in vivo and in vitro. Red cells due to a traumatic tap can produce oxyhaemoglobin in vitro in case of a prolonged storage. This can be reduced by prompt transportation and centrifugation in the laboratory. This prevents the contribution of in-vitro formed oxyhaemoglobin towards xanthochromia. Traumatic taps occur in up to 15% of all LPs. Progressive reduction of RBC count in successively collected tubes (e.g. tubes 1–4) alone is not sufficient to rule out a traumatic tap because this

has been shown to occur in some cases of SAH. Current opinion is when xanthochromia is negative and CSF RBC count is <5, it is sufficient to rule out SAH. When RBC count is >5, even though the xanthochromia is negative, the patient will require further evaluation to rule out SAH. CT angiography should be the next step.[10–12]

10. Answer: C

Embolic stroke is the result of obstruction of a cerebral arterial branch by material originating from a remote intravascular site. The common causes include: mural thrombus associated with a previous myocardial infarction, atrial fibrillation, dislodgement of fragments from valvular vegetations and atherosclerotic plaques in major arteries. Also, paradoxical embolisation may occur through a patent foramen ovale. In intravenous drug users, embolic stroke may occur as a result of embolisation of foreign material injected intravenously or a result of septic emboli. The symptom onset in embolic stroke is usually sudden. In thrombotic stroke, the symptoms are often of gradual onset and fluctuation of symptom severity may occur. Previous transient neurological deficits involving more than one vascular area suggests an embolic cause.[13,14]

11. Answer: A

The NIHSS is an easy-to-use tool for assessing and documenting neurological deficits in a patient with a stroke. It can be repeated during the course of the hospital stay and later (e.g. at 90 days) to assess the progression and the extent of recovery and functional outcome. It has been shown to have a high interrater reliability. A score over 22 is considered a severe stroke because the score correlates well with infarct volume. However, it gives more weight to the symptoms and signs of anterior circulation than posterior circulation. A score of 0 does not exclude a stroke.[13,14]

12. Answer: D

The majority of ischaemic strokes involve the middle cerebral artery territory. The typical clinical features of MCA occlusion are contralateral hemiplegia affecting the face, arms and legs (arms are more affected than legs – compare this with anterior cerebral artery occlusion where the lower extremity is more affected with sparing of the hand and face), contralateral hemisensory loss, homonymous hemianopia and gaze preference towards the side of the infarct. If the dominant hemisphere is affected (left in right-handed people and 80% of left-handed), aphasia or dysphasia (receptive, expressive or both) can be expected. Inattention, neglect, constructional apraxia and dysarthria (without aphasia) may occur if the non-dominant hemisphere is affected. In the absence of other exclusion criteria, to be eligible for thrombolytic therapy, the patient's non-contrast head CT should rule out any haemorrhage and should show no evidence or very minimal evidence of a recent stroke. The stroke is considered severe and/or of delayed presentation if the CT shows involvement of more than one-third of the middle cerebral artery (MCA) territory. The aim of thrombolysis is to salvage the potentially salvageable ischaemic penumbra surrounding the infarcted brain tissue. The hyperdense sign, which can be seen on non-contrast CT, is occasionally due to the presence of a thrombus at that site. This, in itself, is not an eligibility criterion for thrombolysis.[13–16]

13. Answer: B

The most common symptom of a posterior circulation stroke is an occipital headache. Symptoms can be unilateral or bilateral, depending on the extent of involvement in the brainstem, cerebellum, thalamus, medial temporal and occipital lobes. Unilateral or bilateral weakness, or sensory disturbance, may occur. Homonymous hemianopia may be due to posterior cerebral artery occlusion or middle cerebral artery occlusion. In posterior cerebral artery occlusion this is usually associated with macular sparing as this area is supplied by the middle cerebral artery. In any type of stroke, the significant altered level of consciousness is due to direct involvement of the medulla, as in posterior circulation stroke, or indirect involvement of the medulla due to mass effect and/or increased intracranial pressure from ischaemic or haemorrhagic stroke involving other parts of the brain. This can also occur with extensive involvement of cerebral hemispheres.[14,15]

14. Answer: A

Patients with TIAs have substantial overall short-term risks of developing ischaemic strokes. Overall 2-day

stroke risk is 3.9%, 7-day risk is 5.5% and 90-day risk is 9.2%. The $ABCD^2$ risk assessment tool has been validated to predict short-term risk at 2, 7 and 90 days. The $ABCD^2$ score is useful to determine which patients need to be admitted for observation and, above all, for arrangement of urgent investigations such as head CT and imaging of the carotid arteries. In these patients, antiplatelet and statin therapy can be started early. As the 2- and 7-day stroke risk is substantial, these investigations should be done as early as practical. Early carotid endarterectomy reduces high stroke risk in symptomatic patients with significant stenosis. The finding of an infarct on imaging in a patient who otherwise had transient symptoms and now is asymptomatic (as in a TIA), puts them in the category of minor stroke. This predicts an increased short-term risk of further strokes. There is an increased chance of finding a new infarct on imaging in patients with diabetes who have transient neurological symptoms.[13,14,17,18]

$ABCD^2$ score
- Age:
  - <60 years: 0 points
  - ≥60 years: 1 point
- BP:
  - ≥140/90 at initial evaluation: 1 point
- Clinical features:
  - Speech disturbance without weakness: 1 point
  - Unilateral weakness: 2 points
- Duration:
  - <10 min: 0 points
  - 10–59 min: 1 point
  - >59 min: 2 points

Presence of diabetes: 1 point

Interpretation of $ABCD^2$ score
- Score 1–3: low risk
  - 2-day risk: 1.0%
  - 7-day risk: 1.2%
- Score 4–5: moderate risk
  - 2-day risk: 4.1%
  - 7-day risk: 5.9%
- Score 6–7: high risk
  - 2-day risk: 8.1%
  - 7-day risk: 11.7%

15. Answer: B

Both very high blood pressures and too aggressive reduction of blood pressure are associated with poor outcomes in ischaemic stroke. However, there is no consensus about an ideal BP during the treatment of ischaemic stroke. According to the National Institute of Neurological Disorders and Stroke (NINDS) eligibility criteria for thrombolysis in stroke, a BP over 185/110 is a contraindication for thrombolysis and a reduction in BP below this level should be carefully attempted, using titratable intravenous agents. BP should also be maintained during and after thrombolysis to reduce the chance of haemorrhagic transformation of the ischaemic stroke. In a patient who is not a candidate for thrombolysis, too aggressive attempts at BP control may cause poor outcomes because this reduces perfusion to the already vulnerable ischaemic penumbra. Therefore, in this situation, BP reduction is not advised unless the BP is over 220/120 and there is no evidence of other end-organ damage. Dehydration is known to result in poor outcomes. Consequently, adequate hydration of the patient in the ED is essential. Routine oxygen administration has not shown to improve the outcome in stroke patients.[13]

16. Answer: D

The yearly incidence of ischaemic stroke increases with age. It is slightly more frequent in young females than males aged 20–30 years, as well as in males than females in those over 35 years. The traditional stroke risk factors such as diabetes, hypertension and other vascular risk factors are less frequently associated in young adults. The important stroke risk factors in young adults include:
- smoking
- recreational drug use: especially intravenous drugs and sympathomimetics (amphetamines, cocaine)
- migraine with aura (migraine without aura does not seem to increase the risk)
- pregnancy, especially in the late third trimester and 6 weeks postpartum.

Cardioembolism and cervical artery dissection are the most common causes of ischaemic stroke in this age group and each contributes to approximately 20% of cases. The sources of embolism include mitral stenosis, endocarditis, dilated cardiomyopathy, intracardiac thrombi, cardiac tumours (e.g. atrial myxoma) and prosthetic valves. Although patent foramen ovale (found in up to 25% of the normal population) is often attributed as a cause of

paradoxical embolisation causing ischaemic stroke in young people, its direct association with stroke is uncertain. The causes of ischaemic stroke in young adults can be summarised as:
- intracranial and extracranial large vessel arterial disease
  - occlusion – for example, carotid stenosis
  - extracranial arterial dissection – carotid and vertebral arterial dissection
  - intracranial arterial dissection – basilar artery
- cardioembolism
- small vessel disease – causes hemispherical or brainstem lacunar infarcts
- infections – tuberculous meningitis, syphilis, varicella zoster infection, patients with HIV (HIV patients have increased risk for both ischaemic and haemorrhagic stroke)
- systemic lupus erythematosus (SLE)
- antiphospholipid syndrome
- haematological disorders – sickle cell anaemia, leukaemias, intravascular lymphoma, thrombotic thrombocytopenic purpura.[13,14,19]

CT angiography demonstrates a very high sensitivity in detecting both carotid and vertebral artery dissections. See Table 4.1 regarding sensitivities of other diagnostic modalities.

TABLE 4.1 DIAGNOSIS OF CERVICAL ARTERIAL DISSECTION

Imaging modality	Sensitivity	Comments
Ultrasound	80–96%	Slightly better to detect carotid dissection than vertebral dissection Low sensitivity when only local signs present
CT angiography	92–100%	Better than MRA for vertebral arteries Can obtain more details of dissection
MRI and MRA	87–100%	Better for carotid dissection
Catheter angiography		Use when non-invasive results are inconclusive, for endovascular repair

17. Answer: C

In both internal carotid artery and vertebral artery dissection the symptoms and signs can be transient initially and more devastating neurological consequences may occur later. The incidence of cervical arterial dissection peaks in the fifth decade of life. A variety of risk factors have been identified and those include major neck trauma, trivial neck manipulations, migraine and connective tissue disorders. Atherosclerosis and hypertension are not considered risk factors. Typical early symptoms are unilateral headache, neck pain and facial pain for internal carotid artery dissection and both unilateral or bilateral occipital headache and posterior neck pain for vertebral artery dissection. Later, other neurological symptoms and signs may appear (depending on the areas of cerebral ischaemia) and this may take from a few hours to up to 2 weeks.[13]

18. Answer: D

Cerebral amyloid angiopathy follows hypertension as the second most important risk factor for intracerebral haemorrhage in the elderly. The haemorrhage is due to the rupture of small and medium-sized arteries secondary to deposition of beta amyloid protein. It causes lobar haemorrhage in patients older than 70 years of age. One-quarter to one-half of the patients with spontaneous intracerebral haemorrhage die within 6 months. A low Glasgow Coma Scale (GCS), large haematoma volume and presence of intraventricular blood on the initial CT are consistently associated with a high mortality rate. Ventricular blood may cause obstructive hydrocephalus or direct mass effect, both causing cerebral hypoperfusion. If the patient is on warfarin, the treatment of the coagulopathy is necessary and therefore any higher level of INR should be normalised.[13,20]

19. Answer: C

A non-contrast CT of the head is the investigation of choice in most instances for diagnosising intracerebral haemorrhage. However, contrast CT, CTA and MRI may show evidence of intracranial aneurysms, neoplasms, arteriovenous malformations and dural venous sinus thrombosis as an underlying cause. Conventional cerebral angiography is indicated in a select group of patients to identify the cause of haemorrhage. This group of patients includes all patients with no clear cause for the haemorrhage and who are candidates for surgery, as well as young patients (<45 years) who do not have hypertension. Decompression of supratentorial haemorrhages with open craniotomy have shown higher rates of death and dependency at 6 months. However, urgent neurosurgical consultation for possible surgical evacuation is necessary for cerebellar haemorrhage. There is a very high and unpredictable rate of neurological deterioration in these patients due to compression of the brainstem caused by haematoma. Early decompression of a cerebellar haemorrhage reduces morbidity and mortality, especially when the haemotoma is >3 cm and GCS is <14. Routine use of mannitol to reduce mass effect secondary to haematoma volume, oedema surrounding the haematoma and obstructive hydrocephalus is not recommended. Intravenous mannitol should be given and other measures to reduce the increased intracranial pressure should be applied to patients with severe mass effect with impending transtentorial herniation or brainstem compression.[13,20]

20. Answer: B

In Ménière's disease and viral or bacterial labyrinthitis, there is a sudden onset of vertigo of peripheral origin with associated nausea and vomiting. In Ménière's disease tinnitus and reduced hearing may occur but the middle ear examination is usually normal. In acute labyrinthitis, in contrast, an associated otitis media may be present as an origin or sequelae of labyrinthitis. Meningitis is a serious complication of acute bacterial labyrinthitis. In Ramsay Hunt syndrome, grouped vesicles are visible in the external auditory canal and vertigo may be a symptom.[21]

21. Answer: B

Vertebrobasilar insufficiency causes a 'positional vertigo' of central origin. It may or may not cause neurological deficits such as diplopia, dysarthria and bilateral long tract signs. The transient ischaemia to the brainstem that occur in this condition may present as a posterior circulation TIA. If the reticular activating system is sufficiently affected, presyncope or syncope may occur.

In 85% of the patients with BPPV, the posterior semicircular canal is affected unilaterally with free-floating particles (canalolithiasis hypothesis). In these patients Dix-Hallpike manoeuvre will be positive. The horizontal semicircular canal is affected in approximately 15% of patients in BPPV. In these patients Dix-Hallpike manoeuvre is negative and diagnosis can be made with a supine roll test. Although hearing loss and tinnitus is associated with conditions causing a peripheral type of vertigo such as Ménière's disease, vestibular neuronitis, or viral or bacterial labyrinthitis, in BPPV these symptoms are not present. In BPPV examination of the middle ear is usually normal; alternatively, in labyrinthitis changes in the middle ear due to otitis media is a significant finding.[21]

22. Answer: A

Generalised convulsive status epilepticus has been traditionally defined as a seizure lasting more than 30 minutes or two or more seizures without full recovery of consciousness between seizures. This traditional definition has been questioned by some authors and Lowenstein and Cloyd[24] suggest 5 minutes of continuous seizure activity to be taken as status because it is less likely for the seizure to terminate spontaneously and more likely for neuronal damage to occur after this duration.

Generalised convulsive status epilepticus is more common in children in whom over 50% of the cases occur. In children, it is most common in those younger than 2 years. In adults, the incidence is proportionately higher in the elderly in whom cerebrovascular disease is often the cause.

As the duration of seizures progresses, permanent neurological damage becomes more common. Brain compensatory mechanisms remain intact during the early phases of seizures. However, they begin to fail as the duration prolongs despite attempts at adequate delivery of oxygen and nutrients during resuscitation. The brain injury is exacerbated by the contributory hypoglycaemia, hypotension, hypoxia and hypercarbia due to failing brain mechanisms. **The longer the seizure duration, the less refractory it becomes to treatment.** Mortality increases from <5% when the status epilepticus lasts <1 hour to over 30% when seizures continue beyond 1 hour.[22–25]

23. Answer: B

Phenytoin is generally effective in seizure control in a dose of 15–20 mg/kg body weight given as an intravenous infusion. **One of the important limitations with phenytoin is the safe rate of delivery, which is 50 mg/min. This should be reduced to 25 g/min in the elderly and patients with significant cardiovascular disease.** At faster rates it is known to cause cardiac arrhythmias secondary to prolonged QT interval as a result of sodium channel blocking effect and hypotension due

to the diluent (propylene glycol) used in the phenytoin preparation. The dose of 1 g intravenously is not adequate in controlling seizure in most adults and correct dosage calculated according to actual or approximate body weight should be infused (usually no more than 1.5 g).

The adverse effects associated with a full loading dose are thought to be minimal in a patient with status epilepticus who is on regular oral phenytoin. In these patients, the drug levels are often subtherapeutic. Therefore, full loading dose is indicated.[23]

24. Answer: C

Both minor and major alcohol withdrawal can cause alcohol-related seizures in a patient with or without previous seizure history. However, delirium tremens occurs at least 3 days after abstinence and it is uncommon (5% of the patients). Patients who continue to have seizure activity with a reduced level of consciousness often require intubation and ventilation. During rapid sequence intubation a suitable muscle relaxant such as suxamethonium or rocuronium can be used; however, **further use of paralytic agents should be avoided because ongoing seizure activity cannot be recognised without electroencephalogram (EEG) if paralytic agents are given. Patients' ventilation should be facilitated with adequate use of sedation.** The diagnosis of **non-convulsive status** is usually made by the EEG during the suspicious activity. These patients often present with a prolonged unconsciousness or postictal period following a convulsive seizure. The subsequent course is typically with a fluctuating level of consciousness, subtle motor signs such as eye deviations and blinking without obvious seizure activity.[23,26,27]

25. Answer: C

Absence seizures are generalised seizures that typically occur in childhood and resolve as the child matures into adulthood (similar seizures in adults are complex partial seizures). Sudden loss of consciousness is a feature but the patient does not fall to the ground (there is no loss of postural tone). The patient suddenly stops the activity he/she is performing at that time and will appear to be not focusing (inattention). There is no response to voice or other stimuli, no motor activity (except blinking of the eyes), no urinary incontinence and no tongue biting during the episodes. The seizure activity terminates abruptly and there is no postictal phase. Absence seizures can occur many times a day and can go unrecognised. These seizures can occur in patients presenting to the ED with other types of seizures or they can occur alone.

Intact consciousness and mentation is a hallmark of simple partial seizures where seizure activity remains localised.[22]

26. Answer: C

A true generalised seizure may cause a high AG metabolic acidosis (lactic acidosis). In pseudoseizures this acidosis is not usually present. Serum prolactin level may be elevated in a true seizure up to 60 minutes from the time of cessation of seizure activity, but this is not a feature in a pseudoseizure. Abrupt onset and termination is a feature of true seizures, but in pseudo seizures the onset may be gradual over several minutes and the seizures happen in the presence of witnesses only. Unlike in generalised seizures the seizure activity in the limbs may be asymmetrical and alternating from one limb to the other.[22]

27. Answer: B

In the majority of HIV-infected patients who present with a seizure a cause cannot be identified. In the others the most common causes of seizures are:
- mass lesion in the brain (secondary to toxoplasmosis or lymphoma)
- HIV encephalopathy
- meningitis – can be cryptococcal or bacterial.

Other causes include:
- encephalitis due to herpes zoster or cytomegalovirus (CMV)
- progressive multifocal leukoencephalopathy
- central nervous system (CNS) tuberculosis
- cysticercosis
- neurosyphilis.

Once raised intracranial pressure is ruled out with clinical examination and with a head CT, an LP should be performed. **A contrast head CT or MRI should be done because a non-contrast CT may miss a small mass lesion due to cerebral toxoplasmosis or tumour in these patients.**[22]

28. Answer: B

Guillain-Barré syndrome (GBS) is a rare presentation to the ED, but diagnosis is important because it can lead to life-threatening respiratory failure in one-third of patients. The typical features are progressive, relative symmetrical and global (both proximal and distal) weakness. Loss of deep tendon reflexes is usually an early part of the illness. However, in one variant (acute motor axonal neuropathy) reflexes may be retained. At least three variants of the disease have been described. In the Miller Fisher variant, there is areflexia with no or less severe weakness, ataxia and ophthalmoplegia. Assessment for respiratory failure is important in the ED as this is not usually associated with dyspnoea. Measurement of vital capacity is essential to determine the time for intubation. About 75% of patients have a preceding respiratory and gastrointestinal infection. Established associated infections are *Campylobacter jejuni*, Epstein-Barr virus (EBV), CMV, mycoplasma and HIV. One-third of the patients have antibodies for *C. jejuni*, and therefore serological testing for *C. jejuni* can confirm the diagnosis in a suspected case. CSF examination with a lumbar puncture in patients with GBS typically shows a high protein but $<10 \times 10^6$/L cells, and these are mainly mononuclear cells. When the cell count is more than 50×10^6/L GBS is unlikely and other diagnoses should be considered.[28–30]

29. Answer: D

The most common complication of CSF shunts (including common ventriculoperitoneal shunts) is shunt malfunction. This can be due to: proximal or distal obstruction of the shunt; mechanical causes such as fracture or disconnection of the tubing, migration and misplacement of the end of the tubing; overdrainage of the CSF; non-drainable CSF loculations in the ventricles; and pseudocyst formation at the drainage site in the abdomen. Although the valve chamber or reservoir can be located and compressed to assess its filling to determine the potential obstruction, this is known to be unreliable to exclude shunt obstruction, therefore further imaging is indicated. Although shunt series X-rays may detect the abovementioned mechanical causes, even in combination with a head CT, shunt malfunction cannot safely be ruled out in the ED. Therefore input from neurosurgery will be required. Shunt infection may coexist with features for shunt obstruction. Fever and meningism may not be present and lumbar puncture findings are unreliable for diagnosis. Neurosurgical referral for shunt tap for microbiological testing is indicated.[31]

30. Answer: B

Infant botulism is a rare presentation but has been reported in Australasian hospitals. Because of the rarity of the condition and the less overt nature of clinical features, the diagnosis is often delayed. Infant botulism results from systemic absorption of *Clostridium botulinum* toxin released from the spores of bacteria colonising the intestinal tract. It has been reported that infants who live close to construction sites (where soil contains spores) or who are given contaminated honey are more at risk of developing this illness. There is no associated fever or altered level of consciousness in these infants who usually present during 6 weeks to 9 months of age. The presentation is a descending paralysis with poor sucking, poor swallowing, ptosis and lack of facial expression. Infants may be hypotonic and may progress to symmetrical paralysis with respiratory failure.[29,32]

References

1. Denny C, Schull M. Headache and facial pain. In: Tintinalli J, Stapczynski J, Ma O, et al, editors. Tintinalli's emergency medicine: a comprehensive study guide. 7th ed. New York: McGraw Hill Medical; 2011. p. 1113–18.
2. Swadron S. Pitfalls in the management of headache in the emergency department. Emerg Med Clin N Am 2010;28:127–47.
3. Acheson J, Malik A. Cerebral venous sinus thrombosis presenting in the peuperium. Emerg Med J 2006;23:e44. Online. Available: http://www.emjonline.com/cgi/content/full/23/7/e44; 21 Jan 2011.
4. Schievink W. Spontaneous dissection of the carotid and vertebral arteries. N Engl J Med 2001;344(12):898–906.
5. Shmerling R. An 81-year-old woman with temporal arteritis. JAMA 2006;295(21):2525–34.
6. Hackman J, Johnson M, Ma O. Spontaneous subarachnoid and intracerebral hemorrhage. In: Tintinalli J, Stapczynski J, Ma O, et al, editors. Tintinalli's emergency medicine: a comprehensive study guide. 7th ed. New York: McGraw Hill Medical; 2011. p. 1118–22.
7. Suarez J, Tarr R, Selmann W. Aneurysmal subarachnoid hemorrhage. New Engl J Med 2006;354:387–96.
8. Sen A. Bet 4: Computed tomographic angiography for detection of subarachnoid haemorrhage. Emerg Med J 2008;25:290–1.
9. Lee C, Chang Y. Images in emergency medicine. Ann Emerg Med 2010;56:701–707.
10. Edlow J, Malek A, Ogilvy C. Aneurysmal subarachnoid hemorrhage: Update for emergency physicians. J Emerg Med 2008;34:237–51.
11. Al-Shahi R, White P, Devenport R, et al. Subarachnoid haemorrhage. BMJ 2006;333:235–40.
12. Cruickshank A, Beetham R, Halbrook I, et al. Spectrophotometry of cerebrospinal fluid in suspected subarachnoid haemorrhage. BMJ 2005;330:138.
13. Go S, Worman D. Stroke, transient ischemic attack and cervical artery dissection. In: Tintinalli J, Stapczynski J, Ma O, et al, editors. Tintinalli's emergency medicine: a comprehensive study guide. 7th ed. New York: McGraw Hill Medical; 2011. p. 1122–35.
14. Alpin P. Stroke and transient ischaemic attacks. In: Cameron P, Jelinek G, Kelly A, et al, editors. Textbook of adult emergency medicine. 3rd ed. Edinburgh: Churchill Livingston Elsevier; 2009. p. 372–81.
15. Cubuk R, Tasali N, Sahin S. Hyperdense middle cerebral artery sign: an early radiological finding in acute ischaemic stroke. Emerg Med J 2011;28:344.
16. Carpenter C, Keim S, Milne W. Thrombolytic therapy for acute ischemic stroke beyond three hours. J Emerg Med 2011;40(1):82–92.
17. Johnston S, Rothwell P, Nguyen-Huynh N, et al. Validation and refinement of scores to predict very early stroke risk after transient ischemic attack. Lancet 2007;369:283–92.
18. Stead L, Suravaram S, Bellolio F, et al. An assessment of the incremental value of the ABCD² score in the emergency department evaluation of transient ischemic attack. Ann Emerg Med 2011;1:46–51.
19. Ferro J, Massaro A, Mas J. Aetiological diagnosis of ischaemic stroke in young adults. Lancet Neurol 2010;9:1085–96.
20. Qureshi A, Tuhrim S, Broderick J, et al. Spontaneous intracerebral hemorrhage. New Engl J Med 2001;344:1450–60.
21. Goldman B. Vertigo and dizziness. In: Tintinalli J, Stapczynski J, Ma O, et al, editors. Tintinalli's emergency medicine: a comprehensive study guide. 7th ed. New York: McGraw Hill Medical; 2011. p. 1144–52.
22. Lung D, Catlett C, Tintinalli J. Seizure and status epilepticus in adults. In: Tintinalli J, Stapczynski J, Ma O, et al, editors. Tintinalli's emergency medicine: a comprehensive study guide. 7th ed. New York: McGraw Hill Medical; 2011. p. 1153–59.
23. Wilkes G. Seizures. In: Cameron P, Jelinek G, Kelly A, et al, editors. Textbook of adult emergency medicine. 3rd ed. Edinburgh: Churchill Livingston Elsevier; 2009. p. 392–7.

24. Lowenstein DH, Cloyd J. Out-of-hospital treatment of status epilepticus and prolonged seizures. Epilepsia 2007;48(Suppl. 8):96–8.

25. Shearer P, Riviello J. Generalised convulsive status epilepticus in aduls and children: treatment guidelines and protocols. Emerg Med Clin N Am 2011;29:51–64.

26. Chang A, Shinnar S. Nonconvulsive status epilepticus. Emerg Med Clin N Am 2011;29:65–72.

27. McMicken D, Liss J. Alcohol-related seizures. Emerg Med Clin N Am 2011; 29:117–24.

28. Andrus P, Jagoda A. Acute peripheral neurologic lesions. In: Tintinalli J, Stapczynski J, Ma O, et al, editors. Tintinalli's emergency medicine: a comprehensive study guide. 7th ed. New York: McGraw Hill Medical; 2011. p. 1159–66.

29. Lennon R. Acute weakness. In: Cameron P, Jelinek G, Everitt I, et al, editors. Textbook of paediatric emergency medicine. 3rd ed. Edinburgh: Churchill Livingston Elsevier; 2006. p. 233–24.

30. Winer J. Guillain-Barré syndrome. BMJ 2008;337:227–31.

31. Ladde J. Central nervous system procedures and devices. In: Tintinalli J, Stapczynski J, Ma O, et al, editors. Tintinalli's emergency medicine: a comprehensive study guide. 7th edn. New York: McGraw Hill Medical; 2011. p. 1178–85.

32. Fuchs S. Weakness. In: Strange G, Ahrens W, Schafermeyer R, et al, editors. Pediatric emergency medicine. 3rd ed. New York: McGraw Hill Medical; 2009. p. 481–87.

1. Answer: D

Ulcer development in the feet of people with diabetes is promoted by peripheral neuropathy, impaired circulation in macrovascular and microvascular beds, plantar pressure, recurrent trauma and delayed wound healing. **Unlike those due to venous or vascular insufficiency, diabetes-related ulcers occur particularly in pressure-bearing areas such as the sole of the foot.**

Diabetic peripheral neuropathy consists of a number of heterogenous nerve dysfunction syndromes, which include chronic sensorimotor distal symmetrical polyneuropathy, autonomic neuropathy, mononeuropathies and proximal motor neuropathy. The distal symmetrical polyneuropathy and autonomic neuropathies are more common. **Only half of these patients develop symptoms and many are diagnosed only by physical examination.**

In chronic sensorimotor distal symmetrical polyneuropathy, glove-and-stocking loss of peripheral sensations occurs but is more marked in lower than upper limbs. These sensations include light touch, pain, temperature, position and vibration, and loss of tendon reflexes. Neuropathic arthropathy (Charcot's joint) occurs due to loss of pain and position sense. The subsequent damage is irreversible; therefore, management must focus on prevention by improved glycaemic control. Pretibial myxoedema is seen on the shins of patients with Graves' disease, whereas diabetic patients may develop yellow-brown plaques of necrobiosis lipoidica due to necrosis of subdermal tissue.[1,2]

2. Answer: B

Ocular haemorrhage is uncommon in patients who have been treated with thrombolytic therapy for acute myocardial infarction. Considering the potential benefits of thrombolysis in a patient with diabetes with ST segment elevation myocardial infarction (STEMI), confirmed or suspected diabetic retinopathy is no longer considered a contraindication for thrombolysis.

In advanced proliferative retinopathy, retinal detachment may occur due to traction from fibrous tissue associated with neovascularisation. Both closed- and open-angle glaucoma are more common in people with diabetes. Measurement of intraocular pressure along with visual acuity and fundoscopy should therefore be part of the assessment in people with diabetes presenting with visual complaints.[1,2]

3. Answer: B

In the Somogyi effect, nocturnal insulin may reduce blood glucose levels overnight. If prolonged, this can stimulate the release of glucagon and catecholamines, resulting in hyperglycaemia.

Strict glycaemic control has been shown to slow the development of long-term diabetic complications such as neuropathy, nephropathy and vascular problems. It is also important in the short term because of the more obvious risks of immediate complications. It has not, however, been shown to reverse vascular disease.

Acarbose is effective in reducing post-prandial blood glucose rise by selectively inhibiting disaccharidases, therefore decreasing carbohydrate absorption from the gut.

The most common cause of unstable blood sugar levels is underlying infection, which should be carefully sought because the site may appear relatively minor. Other precipitants include changes in oral hypoglycaemic drugs, and poor compliance. Recurrent episodes of hypoglycaemia or DKA should prompt a careful drug history and review to detect patterns such as diurnal variations. Medication use should be reviewed with the patient for their education. Considerations of safety should ensure the patient is not only euglycaemic but is returning to a stable environment before planning discharge.[1]

4. Answer: C

Oral glucose preparations will raise blood glucose to normal in minutes but require subsequent slower release carbohydrates to maintain the rise. Glucagon functions by increasing glycogenolysis and gluconeogenesis, and peak effect is of slower onset. **Glucagon usually takes 7–10 minutes for** normalisation when a patient has an altered mental status due to hypoglycaemia. Due to its mechanism of action, it is less effective in patients with low glycogen stores such as chronic alcoholics or children.

The critical level for a patient to develop symptomatic hypoglycaemia varies between individuals, but symptoms start usually below 5 mmol/L. The adrenergic response to hypoglycaemia may be prevented by the use of β-receptor antagonists, but not by calcium channel blockers.[1]

5. Answer: B

Sulfonylurea-induced hypoglycaemia in a patient with type 2 diabetes is more challenging to manage in the ED than insulin-induced hypoglycaemia. Often hypoglycaemia persists and recurs despite initial treatment, and therefore requires admission for treatment and close monitoring of blood glucose levels. In a previously stable patient with diabetes who has been on a regular dose of sulfonylurea, sudden development of hypoglycaemia is usually associated with an underlying precipitating factor. This may include an increased drug level due to interactions, reduced metabolism and excretion. Vigilance is also required to detect underlying precipitating factors such as sepsis or acute adrenal insufficiency.

In the management, the initial treatment would be oral or intravenous glucose as for any other type of hypoglycaemia; however, blood glucose maintenance is more important in this situation. Generally this may be achieved with intravenous infusion of 10% glucose titrated against the blood glucose level. **If the blood glucose is difficult to be maintained with the above, octreotide should be considered. Octreotide is a potent inhibitor of pancreatic insulin release, and has been shown to be effective in preventing recurrences in sulfonylurea-induced hypoglycaemia.** Dose recommendations vary but octreotide can be give as an intravenous infusion.[2]

6. Answer: B

The standard urine ward test using test strips detects only acetoacetate as ketones but not beta-hydroxybutyrate. Blood or serum should be tested to detect both types of ketones. This can be performed at the bedside using special test strips or in the laboratory. Measuring both types of ketones is important for monitoring the response to insulin therapy in DKA. **Insulin infusion should be continued until ketones are completely cleared from blood and the AG is normalised.** The majority of DKA patients present with metabolic acidosis with a wide AG due to ketonaemia. However, some patients may present with compensatory metabolic alkalosis with normal or high HCO_3 levels. In these patients a wide AG is still present due to ketonaemia.

Kussmaul hyperventilation is a compensatory respiratory reflex induced by severe metabolic acidosis. In DKA, there are increased renal losses of important electrolytes (sodium, chloride, potassium, calcium, magnesium and phosphate) due to the high osmotic load provided by hyperglycaemia. Acidaemia increases renal losses of potassium ion (K^+), further depleting the total body K^+. **However, acidaemia pushes intracellular potassium to the extracellular space, which can result in initial normal or high serum K^+ level. When volume depletion is corrected and acidaemia improved with treatment, hypokalaemia develops unless potassium is adequately replaced.**[1,3]

7. Answer: B

The main priority in the treatment of DKA is to replace the total body water deficit, which averages 5–10 L (100 mL/kg) in an average adult. It is recommended that 50% of this volume is replaced within the first 12 hours and the rest during the next 12 hours.

A loading dose of insulin is not recommended for use in children and is optional in adults. In the majority of patients, initial serum K^+ level is either normal or elevated despite the gross depletion of total body potassium. This is mainly due to total body water depletion and movement of potassium ions to the extracellular space secondary to acidosis. **Consequently, initial hypokalaemia means there is a severe depletion of total body potassium, and acidosis and water depletion have not been able to increase the serum K^+ concentration.** Initial hypokalaemia < 3.5–4.0 mmol/l should be aggressively corrected before commencement of insulin therapy. **Initial hypokalaemia does not indicate less severe disease process.**

Correction of the metabolic problem will normally correct the associated acid–base disorder. Sodium bicarbonate is not recommended to correct acidosis except in a limited subset of patients including patients who are critically unwell with arterial pH < 6.9 (severe acidaemia).[1,3]

8. Answer: C

Cerebral oedema is a serious complication that occurs (especially in children) during treatment of DKA. It has a mortality risk of 70% once developed, with 10% of survivors having permanent neurological sequelae. Cerebral oedema usually develops when it appears to be having clinical and biochemical improvement in the child. However, at that point the child develops mainly neurological signs and symptoms. These include:

- altered level of consciousness
- headache
- seizures
- focal deficits.

Cerebral oedema is a clinical diagnosis. Immediate treatment with intravenous mannitol is indicated to prevent potential serious consequences.

Intubation and ventilation are required to control rising intracerebral pressure. A head CT can be performed once mannitol is given. Specific risk factors associated with the development of cerebral oedema include:

- young age (more common in <5 years)
- severe hyperosmolarity
- persistent hyponatraemia
- severe acidosis.

There is no evidence to suggest increased volume replacement, sodium-containing fluids, or rate of fall of blood glucose cause cerebral oedema.

Rapid volume expansion during treatment improves glomerular filtration rate (GFR) and urine output. In the kidneys, this increases ketone excretion with an increase in chloride reabsorption (as HCO_3 is low). This may cause hyperchloraemic acidosis with a normal AG, and hypophosphataemia. As described in answer 7, correction of fluid depletion and acidaemia without adequate supplementation may also cause rapid development of severe hypokalaemia.[1,3,4]

9. Answer: A

HHS presents most commonly in elderly, poorly controlled or undiagnosed type 2 diabetes patients. It often develops insidiously over days or weeks after a variety of serious illnesses. These patients often have multiple comorbidities and lack capacity to communicate. They may have limited ability to access water intake freely. All these factors may contribute to the higher mortality seen in HHS. **In HHS, blood glucose levels are often much higher than seen in DKA, often >60 mmol/L.**

There is severe total body water (TBW) contraction secondary to losses caused by osmotic diuresis due to severe hyperglycaemia in the face of severely restricted access to free water intake. **TBW loss may reach 8–10 L in an average adult (compared with 5–6 L in DKA).** Therefore calculated serum osmolality is often >315 mmol/L. Arterial pH usually remains >7.3, although wide AG metabolic acidosis may develop during the course of disease. This is mainly due to hypoperfusion of tissues and may be contributed by starvation ketosis. The ketone bodies remain small in amount and do not significantly contribute to acidosis.[1,5]

10. Answer: D

HHS patients are significantly dehydrated and poorly mobile, and may develop disseminated intravascular coagulation. Thromboembolic risk is therefore high, and so heparin prophylaxis should be initiated at an early point.

These patients are usually sensitive to insulin, with insulin resistance being quite uncommon. Higher doses are usually not required. Insulin therapy should be started only after adequate volume repletion and correction of hypokalaemia. Adequate volume replacement prior to administration of insulin in HHS prevents cardiovascular collapse, caused by a sudden intracellular fluid shift that accompanies the intracellular glucose movement induced by insulin. Insulin should therefore be administered cautiously to produce a slow fall in blood glucose. **While total body potassium deficits are significant, the initial serum level may be normal in the face of severe volume contraction.** Insulin therapy will result in the intracellular movement of potassium causing hypokalaemia, so replacement will generally be required at an early stage.

In HHS there is a total body sodium deficit. However, initial corrected serum sodium may be low, normal or high, depending on the degree of volume depletion. **Hypernatraemia along with very high serum osmolality, are poor prognostic factors and correspond to severe volume depletion.** Fluid replacement, guided by central venous pressure (CVP) monitoring if necessary, should aim first to correct hypotension, then to slowly replace water deficit over a period of several days.[1,5]

11. Answer: D

The diagnosis of underlying osteomyelitis associated with a diabetic foot ulcer can be difficult. **A diabetic foot ulcer extending deep down to the bone is highly likely to be associated with underlying osteomyelitis.** This can be determined with sterile surgical probing of the ulcer, if necessary under an appropriate anaesthetic.

Wound swabs taken from diabetic foot ulcers usually grow colonising organisms only. **It may not be possible to identify deep-seated infection purely from wound swabs, and collection of purulent material from the depth of the ulcer is usually required.** It has also been found that there is a relatively high positive likelihood ratio for the diagnosis of osteomyelitis when the foot ulcer is >2 cm.[2] There is no direct association between Charcot's arthropathy and osteomyelitis.[2]

12. Answer: D

Lower extremity infections in diabetics often start as an ulcer, due either to skin breakdown in pressure areas of the foot, or to minor injury. They have the potential to spread rapidly to limb-threatening or life-threatening infections, and therefore demand careful assessment and initiation of appropriate treatment.

Any ulcer with the following features should be considered as limb-threatening:
- a deep ulcer
- ulcer associated with >2 cm of surrounding cellulitis
- ulcer associated with lymphangitis
- presence of purulent or malodorous discharge
- presence of necrotic or gangrenous tissue
- associated limb ischaemia with no palpable pulses.

If not treated promptly and aggressively these infections often become life threatening with sepsis and septic shock. Intravenous antibiotics should be given without delay on presentation.

Broad-spectrum antibiotics should be used to cover staphylococci and streptococci, gram-negative and anaerobic bacteria.

Uncomplicated ulcers are not limb-threatening, and can be managed in the community. If the ulcer is longstanding and is not infected (no surrounding cellulitis or discharge), it does not require antibiotic treatment. When peripheral pulses are not palpable, urgent vascular assessment is needed and revascularisation should be considered.[2]

13. Answer: C

Alcoholic ketoacidosis typically presents in patients with a history of chronic alcohol abuse. These patients usually present with vomiting and abdominal pain 1–3 days after termination of an alcoholic binge. Prolonged vomiting results in severe dehydration and contraction of the extracellular fluid compartment. This is associated with depletion of carbohydrate stores. While ethanol may have initially functioned as a carbohydrate source for gluconeogenesis, the patient is likely to have been abstinent for several days by the time of the presentation, and most chronic alcoholics have poor glycogen stores.

Unlike in DKA, Glasgow Coma Scale (GCS) is usually normal despite metabolic disturbance; confusion or altered level of consciousness should prompt investigation for other pathology. In severe acidosis, ketone bodies exist largely as beta-hydoxybutyrate, which is not detected by Ketostix testing.[6]

14. Answer: B

While the patient is significantly fluid depleted due to prolonged vomiting, intravenous glucose provides a metabolic substrate, halting ketogenesis and returning the patient to normal.

In contrast, while intravenous saline reduces lactate levels, it may result in elevated beta-hydroxybutyrate levels, paradoxically worsening acidosis. Insulin does not affect resolution. Thiamine (vitamin B1) prevents Wernicke's encephalopathy and is a cofactor in pyruvate metabolism to glucose.[6]

15. Answer: B

Vitiligo is an autoimmune disorder, commonly associated with other organ-specific autoimmune disorders including primary adrenal insufficiency (Addison's disease).

Hyperpigmentation occurs in the presence of primary adrenal failure when adrenocorticotropic hormone (ACTH) levels are elevated in the absence of negative feedback. Elevated ACTH levels stimulate melanin production in skin and mucosa. **The most common cause of secondary adrenal insufficiency is chronic glucocorticoid therapy inhibiting ACTH production, and so suppressing primary adrenal function.** A careful drug history should be taken, and any recent illness or stress noted. Other sources of hypothalamic–pituitary dysfunction – including pituitary or hypothalamic tumours, infiltrative disorders, severe head trauma and pituitary necrosis or bleeding – may cause secondary adrenal insufficiency. Cushingoid features are usually not found in a patient with Addison's disease but may be present in a patient who has been on long-term glucocorticoid therapy.[7,8]

16. Answer: C

Adrenal crisis is a life-threatening emergency that occurs in patients with primary as well as secondary adrenal insufficiency. Features include:
- unexplained hypotension
- circulatory shock (which can be refractory to treatment including vasopressors)
- weakness
- lethargy
- delirium
- hyponatraemia
- hyperkalaemia.

In adrenal crisis there is a severe exacerbation of adrenal insufficiency due to increased physiological demand or decreased supply of cortisol. In vulnerable patients any major stress such as intercurrent illness, sepsis, surgery, major trauma, acute myocardial infarction or acute complete/partial withdrawal of long-term steroids may provoke the crisis. Profound hypoglycaemia is not normally a significant issue in this condition.[7,8]

17. Answer: A

In suspected adrenal crisis, intravenous fluid resuscitation should be commenced rapidly to correct fluid loss and hypotension. **Both intravenous hydrocortisone and dexamethasone will provide effective steroid replacement, and hydrocortisone**

is considered the drug of choice because it has both glucocorticoid and mineralocorticoid actions. However, hydrocortisone interferes with cortisol assay in the ACTH stimulation test (short synacthen test) and therefore intravenous dexamethasone may be used for initial treatment if diagnostic testing is planned. Fluid resuscitation should be commenced immediately. Crystalloid containing both normal saline and 5% dextrose is recommended to treat associated hyponatraemia and hypoglycaemia. Specific mineralocorticoid (fludrocortisone) therapy is not usually required if adequate fluid and sodium replacement is delivered, and the patient receives hydrocortisone. Patients unresponsive to fluid resuscitation may require vasopressor treatment to normalise their haemodynamic status.[7,8]

18. Answer: D

This patient has been treated with long-term steroids and hence there is a high risk of developing adrenal crisis as a result of stress caused by sepsis. As the patient is in septic shock with hypotension, intravenous hydrocortisone may not be adequate to provide adequate mineralocorticoid activity, although it provides adequate glucocorticoid activity. **Until shock resolves, both hydrocortisone and fludrocortisone is recommended to prevent adrenal crisis.** If the patient is not in shock, intravenous hydrocortisone alone is adequate to provide both glucocorticoid and mineralocorticoid cover. In non-shock situations, intravenous dexamethasone, which mainly provides glucocorticoid cover, can also be used.[8]

19. Answer: C

Lid lag, lid retraction and proptosis (exophthalmos) are part of thyroid ophthalmopathy and all seen in Graves' autoimmune thyroid disease. Lid lag (von Graefe's sign) is a delay in downward movement of the upper eyelid following the downward-moving iris on directing gaze inferiorly, exposing the sclera above the iris. It may resolve with treatment of the underlying endocrine disorder. Lid retraction (hyperthyroid stare or Dalrymple's sign) is due to retraction of the upper eyelid more than normal, exposing the globe above the iris. Proptosis due to chronic inflammation and swelling of retro-orbital tissues may precede or succeed the appearance of thyroid dysfunction. Lid retraction and proptosis may both continue to deteriorate despite correcting the hormone imbalance. Tarsorrhaphy may be indicated in thyroid ophthalmopathy to protect the cornea from drying and ulceration.[7]

20. Answer: B

Patients may present acutely with thyrotoxic periodic paralysis. Hypokalaemia is generally present during these attacks, which may be recurrent. The condition is distinct from familial periodic paralysis, a group of inherited disorders.

Graves' disease is due to a type 2 hypersensitivity reaction, in which IgG antibodies stimulate thyroid cells to produce and release thyroxine. Thyroid ophthalmopathy is due to IgG antibodies provoking a chronic inflammatory cell infiltrate of extraocular muscles. It may predate the onset of clinical hyperthyroidism by several years, or may develop or deteriorate despite successful treatment of the thyroid disorder itself. The development of pretibial myxoedema (pinkish-brown plaques on the shins) is likewise independent of thyroid status.[7]

21. Answers: B

Beta-blockers (IV propranolol or esmolol) reduce cardiovascular effects by antagonising effects of thyroid hormones, reducing sensitivity to catecholamines, and inhibiting peripheral conversion of T_4 to T_3.

In thyrotoxic crisis, propylthiouracil is given to reduce the synthesis of new hormone in the thyroid gland. It also inhibits the peripheral conversion of T_4 to T_3, but does not inhibit the release of stored hormone from the thyroid. **At least 1 hour after PTU is given, iodine (e.g. Lugol's iodine, potassium iodide) can be given to stop the release of stored hormone.** It decreases iodide transport and oxidation in the follicular cells.

Glucocorticoids (hydrocortisone or dexamethasone) should be given to prevent the peripheral conversion of T_4 to T_3, and also to manage the risk of relative adrenal insufficiency.

Salicylates are contraindicated because they displace T_4 peripherally, exacerbating the crisis.[7,10]

22. Answer: C

In a patient with previously diagnosed hyperthyroidism, thyroid storm is a clinical diagnosis. A patient presenting to the ED without this background diagnosis but with highly suspicious clinical features of thyroid storm should be given careful consideration for a number of important differential diagnoses. These include:

- sepsis
- sympathomimetic abuse such as amphetamine or cocaine
- malignant neuroleptic syndrome
- alcohol withdrawal – delirium tremens
- heat stroke
- hypothalamic stroke
- malignant hyperthermia.

In acute salicylate overdose, the clinical features depend mainly on the dose of ingestion. The typical presentation is with tinnitus, hearing loss, sweating, nausea and vomiting and these occur with mild toxicity. In severe toxicity, altered level of consciousness, tachypnoea, hyperpyrexia and seizures may occur but the overall clinical picture may be different to thyroid storm.[5,10]

23. Answer: A

Myxoedema crisis is a clinical diagnosis and is precipitated mainly in elderly patients with previously untreated hypothyroidism. **Precipitating conditions include underlying infection or sepsis, acute myocardial infarction, heart failure, cerebrovascular accident (CVA), seasonal exposure to cold environments, post-surgery or multitrauma. Sedative and anaesthetic use may precipitate the condition as well.** The main clinical features are due to reduced metabolic rate:

- hypothermia
- bradycardia
- hypotension
- hypoventilation
- altered mental status leading to coma.

Up to 75% of patients with myxoedema crisis present with hypothermia, and if their temperature is normal, an underlying infection may be contributory to the normal temperature. Due to hypoventilation and respiratory failure, CO_2 narcosis may occur. Due to fluid retention and oedema, hyponatraemia is a common finding.[7,9,11]

24. Answer: D

Myxoedema coma is a severe manifestation of hypothyroidism, with all of the typical features of hypothyroidism plus those of a reduced metabolic rate. Patients are often elderly and frail, and may have associated comorbidities. For these reasons, the patient must be intensively monitored.

Supportive care includes:
- attention to airway, breathing and circulation
- treatment of hypoglycaemia and hyponatraemia
- vasopressor support for hypotension
- treatment of associated adrenal insufficiency with intravenous hydrocortisone
- treatment of the underlying infection with intravenous antibiotics.

These should be performed along with careful hormone replacement therapy. The treatment should be started after blood collection for thyroid function tests and serum cortisol levels and it should not be delayed until confirmation of the diagnosis.

It has been suggested that active rewarming may provoke further cooling of core temperature due to an increased return of cool peripheral circulation. Due to peripheral vasodilatation active rewarming may cause hypotension. Rewarming should be carried out passively using blankets. **Intravenous hydrocortisone is recommended because acute adrenal insufficiency is commonly associated with myxoedema crisis.** This is especially important if the patient is hypotensive. A hypotensive patient in severe crisis may not respond to vasopressors without steroid support and thyroid hormone replacement.

Thyroid hormone replacement can be initiated with intravenous T4 (levothyroxine) alone or a combination of T_4 and T_3 or T_3 (liothyronine) alone[7,9,11] – see also answer 25.

25. Answer: A

Rapid correction of thyroid hormone deficiency can precipitate cardiac arrhythmias and myocardial ischaemia due to a sudden increase in myocardial oxygen consumption. Therefore, in an elderly hypothyroid patient thyroid hormone replacement should be commenced with no more than half the recommended dose. T4 (levothyroxine) is given in a single daily dose, starting low (e.g. 25 mcg). T4 may be less prone than T_3 to precipitate cardiac arrhythmias. It is reasonable to avoid T_3 in elderly patients. When treating hypothyroidism it is not essential to initiate treatment intravenously and it is preferred to initiate via the oral route. However, in myxoedema crisis the oral absorption is often affected

by gastric stasis and paralytic ileus, so intravenous hormone replacement should be continued until the patient is alert and able to tolerate oral therapy.[7,11]

26. Answer: A

Over 95% of cases of hypopituitarism in adults are caused by pituitary adenomas. Other causes include intrasellar and parasellar tumours, inflammatory/infectious distruction, radiation-induced destruction, traumatic brain injury, subarachnoid haemorrhage and postpartum pituitary necrosis (Sheehan's syndrome).

In hypopituitarism, patients usually have a combination of pituitary hormonal deficiencies (ACTH, TSH, FSH, LH, GH, prolactin, ADH and oxytocin); however, all hormones are rarely involved. Patients may develop a striking pallor, with loss of melanocyte stimulating hormone (MSH) activity caused by reduced ACTH secretion. These patients often have secondary adrenal insufficiency. Unlike in patients with primary adrenal insufficiency, these patients do not present with marked hyperkalaemia or hyponatraemia. The patient usually has a normal serum potassium or mild hyperkalaemia. Aldosterone secretion is normal as well.

Patients with a diagnosis of hypopituitarism may present to the ED appearing unwell, with acute decompensation secondary to an acute stress such as infection, noncompliance with hormone replacement, emotional stress and trauma.

The priorities in the ED intervention for such patients are:
- resuscitation
- *emergent* glucocorticoid replacement (hydrocortisone is the drug of choice)
- thyroxine replacement is second most important (intravenous levothyroxine is preferred)
- treatment of stressors such as antibiotics
- treatment of the cardiovascular and electrolyte effects of hormone deficiencies.[7,12]

27. Answer: B

Elevated aldosterone levels induce sodium retention and potassium excretion in the urine. The resulting proton shift at cell membrane level results in a metabolic alkalosis with an elevated serum bicarbonate level.

Primary hyperaldosteronism is most commonly due to an adrenal adenoma, less commonly to bilateral adrenal hyperplasia. Excess aldosterone induces elevated blood pressure, which is invariable at presentation. Patients may present with muscle weakness due to hypokalaemia, or polyuria due to nephrogenic diabetes insipidus related to renal tubular damage.[7]

28. Answer: A

In 80–90% of cases causes of hypercalcaemia in patients presenting to the ED include:
- **primary hyperparathyroidism**
  - parathyroid adenoma (most common)
  - parathyroid hyperplasia
  - parathyroid carcinoma
  - as a part of multiple endocrine neoplasia (MEN) type 1 and type 2A)
- **malignancy** (most patients seen in the ED with hypercalcaemia)
  - metastases
  - multiple myeloma
  - haematological malignancy.

Other less common causes include:
- thiazide diuretic use
- sarcoidosis
- hyperthyroidism
- renal osteodystrophy with tertiary hyperparathyroidsm
- primary adrenal insufficiency
- vitamin D toxicity
- milk–alkali syndrome.

Hypercalcaemia induces vomiting and polyuria, often resulting in a total body deficit of several litres of water by the time of presentation. Polyuria secondary to hypercalciuria continues while the serum calcium level is elevated. Deterioration of renal function further increases the serum calcium level.

Parathyroid adenomas are not palpable because they arise from the posterior surface of the thyroid gland.

ECG manifestations of hypercalcaemia include:
- a shortened QT interval (common)
- a shortened PR interval
- at higher calcium levels
  - widened QRS
  - T wave flattening or inversion
  - variable degrees of heart block
  - increased digoxin effects.

Management of hypercalcaemia includes the following steps.

1. Rehydration
   - Reduces serum calcium level but it does not normalise.
   - Administer 4–6 L of normal saline over 24 hours.
   - Rapid fluid resuscitation may be required.
2. Intravenous bisphosphonate
   - The indication is severe hypercalcaemia with inadequate response to fluid therapy.
   - Reduce calcium levels over several days by inhibiting bone osteoclastic activity.
   - Pamidronate or zoledronic acid may be used.
3. In acute life-threatening hypercalcaemia
   - Prescribe intravenous or intramuscular calcitonin.
   - This can be used in addition to bisphonates to rapidly lower calcium level.
4. IV hydrocortisone
   - In patients with refractory hypercalcaemia in malignancy, sarcoidosis or vitamin D toxicity.[7,13–15]

29. Answer: B

Phaeochromocytoma is a catecholamine-producing neuroendocrine tumour. Approximately 80–85% arise from the adrenal medulla and 15–20% from extra adrenal chromaffin tissue. The prevalence of phaeochromocytoma in outpatients with hypertension is 0.1–0.6%. This condition is described as a 'great mimic' because similar clinical features are produced by many other clinical conditions. Usually there is a delay of about 3 years between the initial appearance of symptoms and the final diagnosis. Most of the clinical features are produced by the direct actions of catecholamines secreted by the tumours. The following important presentations to the ED may raise the suspicion for a pheochromocytoma:[7,16]

- **episodic headache, palpitations and sweating (although these are non-specific when all three symptoms present together the specificity reaches >90%)**
- **Hypertension, which is often paroxysmal (between paroxysms BP may be normal or remain elevated)**
- unexplained orthostatic hypotension on a background of hypertension
- unexplained hypotension or shock (mainly in adrenal secreting tumours, also in tumour necrosis)

- cardiovascular complications of hypertension (hypertensive crisis, myocardial infarction, aortic dissection, cardiac arrhythmias, heart failure, cardiomyopathy, pulmonary oedema, **CVA**).

30. Answer: D

Patients with type 1 and type 2 diabetes who are on insulin treatment commonly present to the ED with uncomplicated hyperglycaemia for stabilisation. These patients routinely are on one of the following insulin regimes:

- *basal insulin* only (once-daily long-acting insulin dose or twice-daily intermediate-acting insulin dose)
- *basal insulin* plus *mealtime (prandial)* dose of rapid/short-acting insulin 5–30 minutes before a meal
- mixed insulin in 2 doses/day.

The regimes belong to two categories:

- non-intensive insulin treatment – these patients receive 1–2 injections per day: basal insulin only or mixed insulin
- intensive insulin treatment – they receive more than two injections per day, usually basal plus prandial insulin doses.

As a general rule, patients who are eating normally and are not unwell do not require intravenous insulin infusions. The hyperglycaemia can be managed with stat and supplemental subcutaneous insulin, as well as appropriate increases in routine basal and mealtime insulin doses. **The initial stat dose and the supplemental doses can be given using either rapid-acting or short-acting (regular) insulin.** The rapid-acting preparations are insulin analogues such as insulin lispro (e.g. Humalog), aspart (e.g. NovoRapid) and glulisine, which have many advantages over regular short-acting insulin. They act more like naturally occurring insulin. An example of short-acting insulin is actrapid (see Table 5.1). Because of the rapid onset of action of rapid-acting insulin, they can be accurately and easily timed with food intake. They cause fewer episodes of hypoglycaemia. The duration of action of short-acting regular insulins becomes prolonged with increasing dose. The initial stat and supplemental dose of subcutaneous rapid or short-acting insulin should be determined using the **patient's blood glucose level** as well as his/her **previous total daily insulin dose.**[17,18]

TABLE 5.1 ACTION TIME OF RAPID- AND SHORT-ACTING INSULIN

	Onset	Peak action	Duration
Rapid-acting insulin	5–15 min	1–3 hours	3–6 hours
Short-acting insulin	Over 30 min	2.5–5.0 hours	6–10 hours

References

1. MacLean A, Dunn R. Diabetic emergencies. In: Dunn R, Dilley S, Leach D, et al, editors. The emergency medicine manual. 5th ed. Tennyson: Venom Publishing; 2010. p. 701–9.
2. Jalili M. Type 2 diabetes mellitus. In: Tintinalli J, Stapczynski J, Ma O, et al, editors. Tintinalli's emergency medicine: a comprehensive study guide. 7th ed. New York: McGraw Hill Medical; 2011. p. 1419–32.
3. Chansky M, Lubkin C. Diabetic ketoacidosis. In: Tintinalli J, Stapczynski J, Ma O, et al, editors. Tintinalli's emergency medicine: a comprehensive study guide. 7th ed. New York: McGraw Hill Medical; 2011. p. 1432–8.
4. Vella A. The child with diabetes. In: Tintinalli J, Stapczynski J, Ma O, et al, editors. Tintinalli's emergency medicine: a comprehensive study guide. 7th ed. New York: McGraw Hill Medical; 2011. p. 958–62.
5. Graffeo C. Hyperosmolar hyperglycemic state. In: Tintinalli J, Stapczynski J, Ma O, et al, editors. Tintinalli's emergency medicine: a comprehensive study guide. 7th ed. New York: McGraw Hill Medical; 2011. p. 1440–4.
6. McGuire L, Cruickshank A, Munro P. Alcoholic ketoacidosis: diagnosis & management. Emergency Medicine Journal 2006. p. 23:417–20.
7. Maclean A, Dunn R. Other endocrine disorders. In: Dunn R, Dilley S, Leach D, et al, editors. The emergency medicine manual. 5th ed. Tennyson: Venom Publishing; 2010. p. 710–21.
8. Idrose A. Adrenal insufficiency and adrenal crisis. In: Tintinalli J, Stapczynski J, Ma O, et al, editors. Tintinalli's emergency medicine: a comprehensive study guide. 7th ed. New York: McGraw Hill Medical; 2011. p. 1453–6.
9. MacLean A, Rosengartan P. Thyroid and adrenal emergencies. In: Cameron P, Jelinek G, Kelly A, et al, editors. Textbook of Adult Emergency Medicine. 3rd ed. Sydney: Churchill Livingstone Elsevier, 2009. p. 497–507.
10. Idrose A. Thyroid disorders: hyperthyroidism and thyroid storm. In: Tintinalli J, Stapczynski J, Ma O, et al, editors. Tintinalli's emergency medicine: a comprehensive study guide. 7th ed. New York: McGraw Hill Medical; 2011. p. 1447–52.

11. Idrose A. Thyroid disorders: hypothyroidism and myxedema crisis. In: Tintinalli J, Stapczynski J, Ma O, et al, editors. Tintinalli's emergency medicine: a comprehensive study guide. 7th ed. New York: McGraw Hill Medical; 2011. p. 1444–7.

12. Mills L. Emergent management of acute symptoms of hypopituitarism. Medscape Reference: drugs, diseases and procedures. Jun 17, 2011. WebMD LLC. Online. Available: http://emedicine.medscape.com.

13. Pasco, J. Electrolyte disturbances. In: Cameron P, Jelinek G and Kelly A, et al, editors. Textbook of adult emergency medicine. 3rd ed. Sydney: Churchill Livingstone Elsevier; 2009. p. 497–507.

14. Therapeutic Guidelines Limited. Hypercalcaemia. eTG35. Therapeutic Guidelines Ltd. 2011. Online. Available: www.tg.org.au.

15. Hemphill R. Hypercalcemia in emergency medicine. Medscape reference: drugs, diseases and procedures. WebMD LLC. Online. Available: http://emedicine.medscape.com.

16. Lenders J, Eisenhofer G, Mannelli M, et al. Phaeochromocytoma. Lancet 2005;366:665–75.

17. Goyal N, Schlichting A. Type 1 diabetes mellitus. In: Tintinalli J, Stapczynski J, Ma O, et al, editors. Tintinalli's emergency medicine: a comprehensive study guide. 7th ed. New York: McGraw Hill Medical; 2011. p. 1415–9.

18. Nau K, Lorenzetti R, Cucuzzella M, et al. Glycemic control in hospitalized patient not in intensive care: beyond sliding-scale insulin. Am Fam Physician 2010;81(9):1130–5.

1. Answer: C

A recent systematic review showed that prolonged capillary refill time, abnormal skin turgor and abnormal respiratory pattern were the three best clinical signs for identifying dehydration, whereas laboratory tests were often unhelpful and non-specific.

Historically, in the 1990s, the severity of dehydration was classified as 1) *mild* (3–5%), 2) *moderate* (6–9%) and 3) *severe* (>10%). However, increasing evidence shows that signs of dehydration can be imprecise and incorrect, making clinicians unable to predict the exact degree of dehydration, with the severity of dehydration frequently being under- or overestimated. Where it may be easy to recognise the patient at the extremes of the spectrum, that is, not dehydrated (<5%) or severely dehydrated/shocked (>10%), it is not that easy to distinguish between mild–moderate (5–10%) dehydration. **This has led to the adoption of a new classification system for severity assessment in the early 2000s that divides patients into:**

1) *no signs* of dehydration

2) *some signs* of dehydration, and

3) *severe* dehydration

This estimate is employed to determine the initial need for therapy and the type of therapy to be administered.

In 2009 the National Collaborating Centre for Women's and Children's Health reviewed the available evidence and adopted a new and even simpler clinical assessment scheme.[6] Patients would be classified as 1) *no clinically detectable dehydration*, 2) *clinical dehydration*, and 3) *clinical shock* (suspected or confirmed). **This classification system was adopted by the National Institute for Health and Clinical Excellence (NICE) in 2009.** This simplified scheme does not imply that the degree of dehydration is uniform but rather acknowledges the difficulty clinicians face in accurately assessing the degree of dehydration with the severity of dehydration frequently being under- or overestimated. At the same time, it further helps to:

- determine conservatively which patients can safely be *sent home* for therapy and which ones should

remain for observation during therapy (*no dehydration*)

- provide us with a *starting point* for treatment (*clinical signs of dehydration*)

- determine which ones should *immediately* receive more intensive therapy (*clinical shock suspected or confirmed*).[1–6]

2. Answer: D

This child has evidence of clinical dehydration (5–10%) without any features of poor perfusion or shock. **Enteral (oral or nasogastric) rehydration is the treatment of choice in patients with clinical dehydration (LOE 1, A).** It has been shown to be as effective as intravenous rehydration with the additional benefit that it has fewer complications, is more cost-effective, decreases admission rates, and has a shorter hospital stay and quicker return to normal diet and fluids. Children who are able to receive enteral rehydration therapy should not be given intravenous fluids (LOE 1, A). **Intravenous therapy is reserved for those with evidence of poor peripheral perfusion or shock where an initial bolus of 10–20 mL/kg IV is indicated, as well as in children with clinical evidence of deterioration despite oral rehydration therapy.** Furthermore, deficit can be safely replaced over 4 hours in most children and this 'rapid rehydration' is recommended. A slower rate is recommended in children with significant comorbidities such as renal failure, diuretic therapy and diabetes.

Hypotonic oral rehydration solutions (approximately 240 mOsm/L, sodium 60–90 mEq/L, carbohydrate : sodium ratio ~1 : 1, potassium ~20 mEq/L,) is the rehydration solution of choice as the properties of oral rehydration salts (ORS) promote its effective absorption (LOE 1, A). Commercially available solutions in Australia include Gastrolyte, Hydralyte, Pedialyte and Repalyte.

There are no published trials comparing clear fluids (water, carbonated drinks, fruit drinks) with glucose–electrolyte solutions for treating dehydration. **However, physiological studies have shown that these drinks, which are low in sodium and** potassium and have a high sugar content and high osmolarity, may exacerbate diarrhoea and dehydration and cause electrolyte disturbance. Therefore, their use is not recommended in children with evidence of dehydration.[3-12]

3. Answer: D

Traditionally, a period of fasting has been recommended. **However, current recommendations suggest early introduction of an age-appropriate diet with the early reintroduction of cow's milk, milk formula or solid food as soon as the child is rehydrated.** Early refeeding improves weight gain without increasing diarrhoea or vomiting and may shorten the duration of the diarrhoeal illness.

Historically, a common practice in formula-fed infants has been to give diluted milk (half or quarter strength) and then gradually increase the concentration to full strength (graded feeding). **However, the available evidence shows no benefit from diluted or graded feeding and giving full-strength formula is likely to be beneficial in terms of nutrition and weight gain (LOE 1, A).**

Furthermore, **the routine use of a lactose-free diet is not recommended** because the vast majority of young children with AGE can safely continue to receive lactose-containing milk formula. The number of treatment failures is negligible versus children with acute diarrhoea on a lactose-free diet (LOE 1, A). Temporary lactose intolerance may develop in some children with acute gastroenteritis due to damage to the small intestinal mucosa by pathogens. In a child with prolonged watery diarrhoea (>7 days) associated with perianal excoriation, carbohydrate malabsorption should be excluded by testing the stool for reducing substances and, if confirmed, lactose-free feeds may be indicated.

Weaned children should be fed whatever they eat normally. Full feeding of appropriate-for-age foods are well tolerated and are definitely better than the practice of withholding food (better weight gain without increasing complication rates or treatment failures). The BRAT diet of bread, rice, apples and toast is a limited diet low in energy density, protein and fat that was formerly empirically recommended, although no studies have ever evaluated its safety or efficacy. It is recommended though that fatty foods or foods high in simple sugars should be avoided.[4-6]

4. Answer: C

Bloody diarrhoea in children usually results from toxigenic and invasive intestinal bacterial infections. Other non-infective conditions are rarer but should always be considered because they can be serious and even life threatening. These include:
- IBD
- intussusception
- malrotation
- volvulus
- systemic vasculitis
- necrotising enterocolitis
- Hirschsprung's disease

Potential pathogens of invasive bacterial enterocolitis include:
- *Shigella*
- *Salmonella*
- *Campylobacter*
- *Yersinia*
- *Vibrio parahaemolyticus*
- *E. coli* O157:H7

The most likely causative agents in Australia are *Salmonella* and *Campylobacter*. In the developing world, shigella and parasitic infections with *Entamoeba histolitica* (amoebic dysentery) are important and should be considered in patients who have recently travelled overseas.

Bacterial gastroenteritis is usually self-limiting and antibiotics are needed only in selected cases. Empirical antibiotic treatment for bloody diarrhoea should be approached with caution, especially in children, as it may increase the risk of haemolytic uremic syndrome. **Empiric antibiotics should, however, be considered in all children presenting with symptoms of systemic infection (high fever, tachycardia).** The choice of antimicrobial agent depends on local prevalence and resistance pattern. **Parenteral antibiotics are preferred in patients with toxic appearance, underlying immune deficiency and febrile infants <3 months.** A blood culture should be performed before administration of antibiotics and a stool sample should be collected.

Children with acute (<7 days' duration) and mild–moderate disease (<6 stools per day) who are systemically well may be managed as an outpatient after stool has been collected for microscopy, culture and sensitivity (MCS) including *E. coli* O157:H7, pending results.

Alternatively, the patient can be admitted for observation. All children with severe disease (≥ 6 stools per day), who are systemically unwell (fever, tachycardia) or with abdominal complications, should be admitted. Children with persistent (>7 days) of bloody diarrhoea should be referred for further investigation of other causes, including IBD.[13–15]

5. Answer: A

The causes of travellers' diarrhoea depend on the destination, setting and season.

- Enteric bacteria are most commonly implicated and include:
  - strains of enterotoxigenic *Escherichia coli* (ETEC)
  - *Salmonella*
  - *Campylobacter*: this, along with *Salmonella*, appear to be increasing in importance in Asia.
- Norovirus infection is the predominant cause on cruise ships.
- Parasites are less common causes of travellers' diarrhoea:
  - Protozoa, *Giardia intestinalis* and *Cryptosporidium* are most commonly identified.
  - *Entamoeba histolytica* is a less common cause and typically associated with long-term travel.

Despite the fact that antibiotic prophylaxis seems to be effective in preventing travellers' diarrhoea, it is not currently recommended for healthy travellers, including children. There are several reasons for this including the lack of data on the safety and efficacy of antibiotics given for >2 weeks. **In addition, early self-treatment of travellers' diarrhoea is highly efficacious.** Chemoprophylaxis can be considered for travellers with underlying conditions that make progression to severe and/or complicated diarrhoea more likely (e.g. immunodeficiency, type 1 diabetes, active IBD, cardiac or renal failure). Expert opinion supports the use of prophylactic antibiotics when a trip is vitally important or the consequences of watery diarrhoea would be difficult to manage (e.g. after colostomy or ileostomy). In this scenario, prophylactic antibiotics might therefore be considered as she has an important business trip coming up.

As traveller's diarrhoea is usually self-limiting, antibiotic treatment is not indicated in mild cases. **For moderate to severe disease, antibiotics have been**

shown to be effective and may be combined with loperamide in adults. Antimotility drugs should be avoided in children or where fever or bloody diarrhoea is present. A single large dose of antibiotics is usually effective. Recommended regimens include azithromycin orally, as a single dose *or* norfloxacin orally, as a single dose. The rapid emergence of quinolone resistance in gram-negative pathogens, particularly in South Asia, is likely to reduce the effectiveness of norfloxacin and ciprofloxacin.[16,17]

6. Answer: D

Antibiotic-associated diarrhoea is defined as otherwise unexplained diarrhoea that occurs in association with the administration of antibiotics.

Infection with *C. difficile* causes a toxin-mediated enteric disease that can result in:

- mild to severe diarrhoea (usually watery)
- colitis (fever, cramps, faecal leucocytes)
- toxic megacolon
- intestinal perforation
- death

Although infection with *C. difficile* accounts for only 10–20% of the cases of antibiotic-associated diarrhoea, it accounts for the majority of cases of *colitis* associated with antibiotic therapy.

Antibiotic-associated enterocolitis caused by *C. difficile* is unique in that the organism is normally present in the colon and it causes illness primarily during or after the administration of antimicrobial agents. Symptoms may appear during the course of antimicrobial therapy or commonly up to 3–4 weeks after discontinuation of antibiotics.

Clindamycin, cephalosporins, and penicillins are the antibiotics most frequently associated with *C. difficile* diarrhoea, although they also cause diarrhoea that is unrelated to this organism. The rates of diarrhoea associated with parenterally administered antibiotics are similar to rates associated with orally administered agents.

Spontaneous resolution usually occurs within 48–72 hours after discontinuing the offending antibiotic. If not, treatment should be commenced with metronidazole or vancomycin. The usual duration of therapy is 10 days. Indications for oral vancomycin, as opposed to metronidazole, are pregnancy, lactation, intolerance of metronidazole, or failure to respond to metronidazole after 3–5 days of treatment.

Ideally, all antibiotic treatment should be oral since C. difficile is restricted to the lumen of the colon. If intravenous treatment is required, only metronidazole (and not vancomycin) is effective, since this approach will still result in moderate concentrations of the drug in the colon. Intravenous vancomycin generally is not effective because it does not reach effective intraluminal concentrations.[14,18,19]

7. Answer: C

Both *Staphylococcus* and *Bacillus cereus (B. cereus)* produce preformed toxins and therefore the onset of symptoms will occur early, within 1–6 hours, after ingestion of contaminated food. However, *Staphylococcus* food poisoning is associated with the consumption of protein-rich food, including eggs, potato salad and mayonnaise, whereas *B. cereus* food poisoning is commonly caused by the ingestion of fried rice.

B. cereus foodborne illness is mostly due to improper holding temperatures for cooked food. The heat-resistant spores survive boiling and then germinate when boiled foods such as fried rice are left unrefrigerated, producing the toxin. Flash-frying or brief rewarming of the food before serving often is not sufficient to destroy the preformed, heat-stable emetic toxin.

Food contamination with *Staphylococcus* is extremely common and the organism can be isolated from the hands of about 50% of the population. The bacterium itself is killed by high cooking temperatures but the enterotoxin is heat-stable. Therefore, once it is present in food, reheating or even boiling will not prevent illness.

Clostridium perfringens (C. perfringens) and *Vibrio* produces toxins only after colonisation and therefore symptoms usually occur after a longer period (6–24 hours). Illness with *C. perfringens* is caused by the ingestion of meat or poultry heavily contaminated with *C. perfringens.* Typically, the food is cooked more than 24 hours before consumption, allowed to cool slowly at room temperature, and then served either cool or rewarmed. During this period of incubation, spores that survived cooking germinate, and clostridia multiply to reach sufficient numbers to constitute an infectious inoculum. Ingestion of live organisms is required to produce disease, but illness is not caused by infection; rather, it is from an enterotoxin produced by sporulation of the organism in the GIT. Symptoms usually start after an incubation period of 6–24 hours and is characterised by acute onset abdominal cramps and watery diarrhoea.

Vibrio is associated with the ingestion of seafood, particularly raw shell fish. Symptoms start after 24–48 hours with diarrhoea and abdominal cramps.[14,20]

8. Answer: C

Diarrhoea is a frequent complaint in patients with IBD. **Bloody diarrhoea, mucus, tenesmus and rectal complaints are more common in UC.** The symptoms of CD are more heterogenous and include abdominal pain, diarrhoea and weight loss. Additionally, systemic symptoms of malaise, anorexia or fever are more common with CD.

***Extraintestinal manifestations* occur in both CD and UC, although they are more common in CD.** Nearly half of patients with CD will have extraintestinal manifestations. Extraintestinal manifestations often involve the musculoskeletal system, skin and eyes:

1. Musculoskeletal
   - Peripheral arthritis
   - Sacroiliitis
   - Ankylosing spondylitis
   - Osteoporosis
2. Skin
   - Erythema nodosum
   - Pyoderma gangrenosum
   - Aphthous stomatitis
3. Eyes
   - Uveitis
   - Scleritis
   - Episcleritis

Similarly, *fistulae and abscesses* occur in both UC and CD but are much more common in CD. Both CD and UC are associated with an equivalent increased risk of colonic carcinoma.[21–23]

9. Answer: A

Patients with IBD presenting to the ED should be assessed to determine the activity/severity of the disease as well as the presence of complications. **The Truelove and Witts' classification is commonly**

Activity	Mild	Moderate	Severe
Number of bloody stools per day	<4	4–6	>6
Temperature	Afebrile	Intermediate	>37.8
Heart rate (beats per minute)	Normal	Intermediate	>90
Haemoglobin (g/dl)	>11	10.5–11	<10.5
ESR (mm/h)	<20	20–30	>30

used to establish disease severity in patients with ulcerative colitis (see Table 6.1).

The Crohn's Disease Activity Index is a useful score in determining the disease severity of CD and uses the following parameters in the assessment:

- stool frequency
- abdominal pain
- general wellbeing and opiate use
- presence of complications
- abdominal masses
- anaemia
- weight loss

Plain abdominal and chest radiographs are essential to detect free gas with perforation, dilated bowel loops and air-fluid levels with obstruction, or dilated transverse colon >6 cm with toxic megacolon. A dilated transverse colon >12 cm indicates imminent perforation, causing peritonitis and septicaemia with subsequent high mortality rate.

The effect of NSAIDs in exacerbating IBD is still unclear. However, it seems like non-selective NSAIDs may exacerbate IBD, whereas non-selective NSAIDs most likely do not exacerbate IBD. NSAIDs should therefore be avoided if possible.

Stool microscopy, culture and C. difficile toxin assay should be performed as part of the initial assessment because pseudomembranous colitis can complicate or mimic severe ulcerative colitis. C. difficile has a higher prevalence in patients with IBD through unknown mechanisms and is associated with increased mortality.[21-24]

10. Answer: B

A focused ED ultrasound of the gallbladder is useful to confirm the presence or absence of:

- gall stones
- cholecystitis
- bile duct obstruction

Finding both gallstones and a sonographic Murphy's on bedside ultrasound has a 92.2% positive predictive value (PPV) for diagnosing cholecysitis, whereas the absence of both these signs have an NPV of 95.2%. A sonographic Murphy's sign refers to pain on compression of the fundus of the gallbladder with the probe tip and is probably the most specific sign of inflammation.

Other common sonographic findings include gallbladder wall thickening and pericholecystic fluid. The anterior wall of the gallbladder should be measured, as the acoustic enhancement artifact will obscure an accurate picture of the posterior wall. Gallbladder wall thickness >3 mm is regarded as abnormal.

A dilated common bile duct (CBD) demonstrates obstruction. A normal CBD typically measures <6 mm in the transverse diameter and should be measured from inner wall to inner wall. The CBD diameter can increase with age but, in general, a diameter >8 mm is regarded as abnormal (in the absence of previous cholecystectomy).[25]

11. Answer: A

The most common cause of PUD is infection with H. pylori, accounting for 70–90% of ulcers. It is the major cause, or at least a cofactor, in the development of PUD, with 90–95% of patients with duodenal ulcers and 70% of those with gastric ulcers infected with H. pylori. Although H. pylori is commonly present in the mucosa of many people, only 10–20% of infected patients will develop PUD. Interestingly, the prevalence of H. pylori is lower in patients with complicated duodenal ulcers (bleeding or perforation) than in those with uncomplicated disease.

The second most common cause of PUD is NSAIDs, including low-dose aspirin. While H. pylori is most commonly associated with duodenal ulceration, NSAIDs are more commonly associated with gastric ulceration.[27,28]

12. Answer: B

As the majority of PUD is caused by H. pylori, it is tempting to eradicate all patients with suspected PUD. However, testing for H. pylori is easily done and the absence of *H. pylori* may have prognostic implications. **H. pylori-negative ulcers appear to have a significantly worse outcome, especially if treated empirically for infection.**

Various non-invasive techniques are available. The urea breath test is one such test that is highly sensitive and specific and is also useful in assessing eradication. *H. pylori* tests cannot demonstrate the presence of PUD but a negative test in patients *not taking NSAIDs* makes the likelihood of PUD low. **Testing does not need to be done in the ED but treatment can appropriately be started in the ED with a PPI. The patient can then be referred to their primary care provider for further testing and, if positive, eradication therapy commenced.**

PPI is most effective when taken with or shortly before meals, as the acidic compartments within the stimulated parietal cell are essential for activation. PPI works poorly in fasting patients as well as when given simultaneously with other antisecretory agents (H_2 receptor blockers).

Not all patients with dyspepsia require endoscopy but those with alarm features do, as they raise the index of suspicion for gastric or oesophageal cancer. 'Alarm features' suggesting the need for endoscope referral include:

- age > 55 years
- unexplained weight loss
- early satiety
- persistent vomiting
- dysphagia
- anaemia or GI bleeding
- abdmonial mass
- persistent anorexia
- jaundice[26-28]

13. Answer: A

Upper gastrointestinal bleeding (UGIB) is regarded as bleeding originating from a site proximal to the ligament of Treitz. The ligament of Treitz is a fold of peritoneum that suspends the fourth part of the duodenum.

Peptic ulcer disease (gastric, duodenal, oesophageal and stomal ulcers) **is the most common cause of upper gastrointestinal bleeding**, accounting for 35–50% of all cases. Erosive gastritis, oesophagitis and duodenitis are responsible for about 15%, whereas oesophageal and gastric varices

account for about 10% of cases. Mallory-Weiss tears (longitudinal mucosal lacerations at the gastroesophageal junction or gastric cardia) account for a further 5–15%. It is classically associated with repeated retching or vomiting; however, repeated vomiting is only present in one-third of cases. The remaining cases include rare causes like angiodysplasia and aortoenteric fistulae.

Aortoenteric fistulae usually develop secondary to a pre-existing graft. The initial bleed is usually not significant and self-limited ('herald bleed') and the diagnosis is confirmed with an abdominal CT, not endoscopy. One should have a high index of suspicion in patients with previous abdominal vascular surgery, as a herald bleed precedes massive haemorrhage, which is difficult to control and often fatal.[29-32]

14. Answer: D

Although most patients with upper GIT bleeding present with a chief complaint of haematemesis or blood in the stool, this is not always the case. **Upper GIT bleeding can present subtly with hypotension, tachycardia, dizziness, angina, confusion or syncope without any melena or haematemesis and clinical suspicion for GIT bleeding must remain high in these patients.**

The presence of haematemesis is highly suggestive of bleeding from the upper GIT tract. Although placement of a nasogastric tube in the ED to assess aspirate is no longer routinely recommended, it may still have diagnostic and therapeutic benefits. In patients presenting with haematemesis, it may help to assess the presence of ongoing bleeding as well as prepare the patient for endoscopy. In patients presenting without haematemesis, a positive aspirate provides strong evidence for an upper GIT source. **However, a negative aspirate does not exclude an upper GIT source and may result from intermittent bleeding, pyloric spasm or oedema preventing reflux of duodenal blood.**

Melena usually represent bleeding from an upper GIT source (70%) but can rarely be due to a lower GIT source (20–30%). The black, tarry stool is produced as result of bacterial degradation of haemoglobin in the gut. At least 150–200 mL of blood that has spent at least 8 hours in the intestines is necessary to produce melena. **Melena of itself is not** associated with poorer outcomes in upper GIT bleeds but haematochezia is associated with a three times higher risk of death.

Haematochezia is the passage of bright red or maroon-coloured blood per rectum and suggests a source distal to the ligament of Treitz. Approximately 14% of bleeds presenting with hematochezia are caused by a brisk upper source with rapid transit. Haematochezia due to an upper tract source of bleeding has been associated with a higher transfusion requirement, need for surgery and mortality rate.[29-32]

15. Answer: C

A routine CXR is of limited value in patients with an upper GIT bleed and not needed in the absence of specific clinical indications. Additionally, it has not been found to alter clinical outcomes or management decisions in the absence of pulmonary examination findings or known pulmonary disease. A CXR is indicated in the following cases:

- suspected aspiration
- suspected perforation
- in the elderly
- cardiopulmonary comorbidities

Perforation associated with significant upper GIT bleed is rare. CXR is only 70–80% sensitive for picking up a perforated peptic ulcer. Therefore, a negative CXR for free air under the diaphragm does not exclude perforation and an abdominal CT should be performed if in doubt.

The initial haemoglobin level often will not reflect the actual amount of blood loss, as 24–48 hours is required for intravascular volume to equilibrate. Normal haemoglobin levels therefore do not exclude a large bleed. A haemoglobin level of <100 g/L has been associated with increased rebleeding and mortality rates.

An elevated urea level relative to creatinine is more indicative of an upper rather than lower GIT source, as there is a combination of increased protein load in the gut and intravascular volume depletion.[26,28,31,32]

16. Answer: C

Bleeding from an upper GIT source stops spontaneously in most cases and requires no further intervention. It would therefore be useful if we could reliably identify patients at low risk for rebleeding and death, as these patients are unlikely to require endoscopic intervention and could potentially be managed as outpatients. Current recommendations advise admission for all patients and endoscopy within 24 hours as the sensitivity of endoscopy is optimised if performed within 12–24 hours of presentation. Early endoscopy allows the prediction of likelihood of rebleeding and mortality, according to the nature and location of lesion and stigmata of recent haemorrhage.

Risk stratification using a combination of clinical and endoscopic findings has been well validated as a means of predicting the risk of rebleeding and in-hospital mortality. The *Rockall score* is an example of such a scoring tool and frequently used for risk stratification. However, only a small number of studies looked at risk stratifying patients solely on clinical features without including endoscopy findings. These studies suggest that a subset of low-risk patients may be discharged safely with an upper GIT bleed. Characteristics of these low-risk patients included:

- <60 years of age with follow-up care
- no significant comorbid conditions
- no signs of shock
- no history of liver disease or varices
- no severe anaemia
- no frequent haematemesis or melena

The *Glasgow-Blatchford bleeding score* is a scoring tool based solely on clinical and laboratory criteria. It has been suggested that selected patients can be safely discharged and managed as outpatients without early endoscopy as they are unlikely to need treatment and therefore may not require admission if they satisfy the following criteria:

- urea < 6.5 mmo/l,
- haemoglobin > 130 g/L (men) or 120 g/L (women),
- SBP > 110 mmHg
- pulse < 100 bpm
- absence of melena
- absence of syncope
- no cardiac or liver disease

Interestingly, it does not include age despite the fact that age >65 years has been associated with an increased risk of rebleeding and death. Although promising, clinical predictive scores are not yet widely accepted and still need further validation to make a graded recommendation.

Peptic ulcer disease may be painless, especially in the elderly and particularly in those taking NSAIDs or steroids. Rectal examination and faecal occult blood testing should be performed in all patients with suspected upper GIT bleeding. A positive test requires at least 8 mg of haemoglobin per gram of stool. **A positive guaiac test is dependant on the time of onset of the bleeding in relation to gastrointestinal transit time. It is therefore possible that in some acute bleeds, the blood may not have traversed the bowel by the time testing is done.** False-positive guaiac tests can be caused by certain bacterial and vegetable peroxidases, such as bananas and horseradish. Therapeutic iron intake is commonly believed to cause false-positive guaiac testing. Most studies in vivo, however, have shown that this is not a common cause of false-positive testing.[29–37]

17. Answer: C

Traditionally, *gastric lavage* was thought to decrease bleeding or rebleeding, particularly if cold water was used, but the evidence does not support this. Cold water may indeed exacerbate bleeding. Gastric lavage is now mainly used to allow better visualisation during endoscopy and room-temperature water is recommended.

PPIs are recommended before endoscopy, as they reduce the likelihood of bleeding or need for intervention during endoscopy. It also significantly reduces the risk of rebleeding and blood transfusions. A recent metanalysis showed no change in mortality though.

Octreotide reduces splancnic blood flow and portal venous pressure while preserving cardiac output and SBP. It is therefore useful for upper GIT bleeds of variceal origin. **However, octreotide has also been shown to decrease the risk for persistent bleeding and rebleeding in patients with PUD, although the results are conflicting, and may be considered in patients awaiting endoscopy.**

Concerns that *NGT* placement may provoke bleeding in patients with varices are unwarranted and NGT can safely be used in these patients.[29–31]

18. Answer: B

Variceal bleeding may be catastrophic, with 30% mortality for a first bleed. Early control of bleeding should be achieved. Significant advances in the treatment of acute variceal bleeding have been made since the era of balloon tamponade with the Sengstaken-Blakemore tube. This is now rarely used due to significant complications and rebleeding upon balloon deflation but should still be considered as a temporising measure if bleeding is uncontrolled and pharmacological options and endoscopy are not immediately available. After insertion of the tube, the gastric balloon is inflated first with air and the tube pulled until resistance is felt, at which point the balloon is tamponading the gastro-oesophageal junction. If bleeding continues despite inflation of the gastric balloon, the oesophageal balloon should be inflated, taking care not to overinflate the oesophageal balloon as it may cause oesophageal necrosis or rupture.

Advances include endoscopic techniques, mainly sclerotherapy or band ligation, and vasoactive pharmacological options like octreotide. Sclerotherapy was the first available endoscopic therapy for bleeding varices. It is effective in controlling bleeding and reduces rebleeding and the need for blood transfusion. It is, however, associated with significant complications including deep oesophageal ulcerations, strictures, mediastinitis, pleural effusions, sepsis and death. Endoscopic band ligation appears to be more effective and associated with fewer complications and is the preferred endoscopic treatment in most cases.

Pharmacological therapy with octreotide is comparable to injection sclerotherapy in terms of bleeding control and with the advantage of fewer side effects. Additionally, combination endoscopic and pharmacological therapy improves initial haemostasis and early rebleeding rates. **It is therefore imperative that octreotide infusion be initiated as soon as possible to all patients with suspected varices.**

Up to 01% of patients with known varices have an alternative bleeding site. Intravenous PPI, such as esomeprazole, should therefore be initiated early for presumed PUD, oesophagitis, gastritis or duodenitis.

Infection occurs in 35–66% of patients with cirrhosis and gastrointestinal bleeding. Not only does it carry the risk of sepsis but concurrent infection also impairs coagulation, thereby increasing the risk or rebleeding. **Several studies have shown that antibiotic** prophylaxis in cirrhotic patients with gastrointestinal bleeding improves mortality and reduces the risk of further bleeding. Gram-negative bacteria have been most commonly isolated in these patients. Fluoroquinolones have been traditionally used in the past but recent resistance patterns have encouraged the use of third-generation cephalosporins.[30,31]

19. Answer: D

A normal liver span usually measures 8–13 cm in the midclavicular line. **Percussion is the only clinical method to measure the span of the liver. Measurement of the liver span is more important than the presence of a palpable liver edge to detect hepatomegaly, as 80% of people have some palpable extension of the liver beyond the costal margin.** Palpation of the liver edge may be normal, due to enlargement or due to lung hyperinflation. Extension of the liver >2 cm beyond the rib margin is, however, most likely due to hepatomegaly.

The presence of ascites is suspected in patients with abdominal distension, bulging flanks, flank dullness to percussion, shifting dullness to percussion, and/or a fluid thrill. **Bulging flanks are 80% sensitive in the detection of ascites but only 50% specific, whereas a fluid thrill is only 60% sensitive but 90% specific.**

Spider naevi is usually found in the superior vena cava (SVC) distribution. They may occur on normal individuals but the presence of >5 are abnormal and chronic liver disease should be suspected.[38]

20. Answer: A

The accuracy of physical findings to detect ascites is variable and depends in part upon the amount of fluid present, the technique used to examine the patient, and the clinical setting. Approximately 1500 mL of fluid has to be present for flank dullness to be detected; therefore, lesser degrees of ascites can be missed. If no flank dullness is present, the patient has a 10% chance of having ascites. Ultrasonography can be helpful when the physical examination is not definitive.

Ascitic fluid had been classified as an exudate if the total protein concentration is ≥ 30 g/L and a transudate, if it is <30 g/L. **However, the exudate/**transudate system of ascitic fluid classification has been replaced by the SAAG, which is a more useful measure for determining whether portal hypertension is present.** SAAG has been proved in many prospective studies to categorize ascites better than the total protein-based exudate/transudate concept. Calculating the SAAG involves measuring the albumin concentration of serum and ascitic fluid specimens obtained on the same day and subtracting the ascitic fluid value from the serum value:

- If the SAAG is ≥11 g/L, the patient has portal hypertension with approximately 97% accuracy. Other causes for high SAAG include congestive cardiac failure (CCF), Budd-Chiari syndrome and portal vein thrombosis and 'mixed' ascites.
- If the SAAG is <11 g/L, peritoneal carcinomatosis, tuberculous peritonitis, pancreatic ascites, biliary ascites and nephrotic syndrome should be considered.

A cell count and differential should be performed in all patients undergoing abdominal paracentesis. Cirrhotic ascites should generally contain <250 WBCs/µL. **Up to 500 WBC/mm³ is acceptable in uncomplicated cirrhosis. Lymphocytes should predominate, and clinical signs or symptoms of peritoneal infection should be absent.**[39,40]

21. Answer: D

In a cirrhotic patient, ascites is caused by a combination of portal hypertension, hypoalbuminaemia, and poor renal management of sodium and water. These patients are usually responsive to salt restriction and diuretics and therefore **the mainstay of treatment of patients with cirrhosis and ascites includes education regarding dietary sodium restriction and oral diuretics.** Fluid restriction is not necessary in treating most patients with cirrhosis and ascites. Similarly, it is sodium restriction, not fluid restriction, that results in weight loss as fluid follows sodium passively. However, severe hyponatraemia does warrant fluid restriction and a reasonable threshold for fluid restriction is a serum sodium <120–125 mmol/L.

The usual diuretic regimen consists of a combination of a single morning dose of oral spironolactone and frusemide, beginning with 100 mg of the former and 40 mg of the latter. The doses of both oral diuretics can be increased simultaneously every 3–5 days (maintaining the 100 mg: 40 mg ratio) if weight loss and natriuresis are inadequate. Usual maximum doses are 400 mg/day of spironolactone and 160 mg/day of furosemide. Spironolactone can be used as a single agent; however, hyperkalaemia and its long half-life limit its use. As a result, it is mainly reserved for patients with minimal fluid overload. Single-agent furosemide has been shown to be less efficacious than spironolactone. Starting with both drugs appears to be the preferred approach in achieving rapid natriuresis and maintainig normokalemia. **In the largest, multicentre, randomised controlled trial performed in patients with ascites, dietary sodium restriction and a dual diuretic regimen has been shown to be effective in more than 90% of patients in achieving reduction in the volume of ascites to acceptable levels.** Serial paracentesis remains an alternative for patients refractory to medical therapy.

Outpatient treatment can be attempted initially if no precipitants are identified. However, some patients with cirrhosis and ascites also have gastrointestinal haemorrhage, hepatic encephalopathy, bacterial infection, and/or hepatocellular carcinoma, and may require hospitalisation for definitive diagnosis and management of their liver disease as well as management of their fluid overload.[39]

22. Answer: A

Various sites are suitable for abdominal paracentesis. One site is approximately 2 cm below the umbilicus in the midline where the fasciae of the rectus abdominis join to form the fibrous, thin, avascular linea alba. Large collateral veins may occasionally be present and should be avoided. Another site is the left lower quadrant (LLQ). The abdominal wall in the LLQ, 3 cm cephalad and medial to the anterior superior iliac spine, has been shown to be thinner and with a larger pool of fluid than the midline and is usually a good ohoice for needle Insertion for performance of therapeutic paracentesis. This is also the preferred site by many clinicians as abdominal obesity increases the midline thickness. The right lower quadrant (RLQ) may be a suboptimal choice in the setting of a dilated cecum (due to lactulose) or an appendectomy scar. **It is important to remain lateral to the rectus sheath at all times to avoid the inferior epigastric arteries;** these vessels are located midway between the pubis

and anterior superior iliac spines and then run cephalad in the rectus sheath.

The removal of up to 5–6 L of ascitic fluid is regarded as routine and is well tolerated, and for therapeutic purposes, at least this volume should be removed. Up to 10 L may be safely removed in most patients with chronic ascites. One controversial issue regarding therapeutic paracentesis is the role of colloid replacement. So far, studies have failed to show more clinical morbidity and mortality in patients not receiving colloids. However, there has been no study large enough to demonstrate decrease survival in patients who are given no plasma expander compared with patients given albumin. Current recommendations do not recommend colloid replacement for a single paracentesis of <5 L, but it remains optional, due to lack of evidence, if larger volumes are removed. The recommended infusion is 6–8 g of intravenous albumin per litre of ascitic fluid removed.

As many as two-thirds to three-quarters of patients undergoing paracentesis will have a coagulopathy. However, the only prospective study to evaluate the complications of paracentesis determined that transfusion-requiring abdominal haematomas occurred in <1% of cases despite the fact that 71% of patients had an abnormal prothrombin time (PT). Because transfusion-requiring haematoma is so unlikely, even in this population, prophylactic administration of fresh frozen plasma or platelets is not standard and is associated with considerable cost, in addition to the risk of transfusion-related complications, with little net gain. Furthermore, routine tests of coagulation do not reflect the bleeding risk in patients with cirrhosis. **Therefore, for patients undergoing repeated therapeutic paracentesis, in the absence of prior problems or obvious clotting issues, obtaining preprocedure platelet count and INR is not routine.**

Serial paracentesis should preferably be reserved for the 10% of patients who truly fail medical therapy. It is therefore important that the patient's compliance with dietary sodium restriction be reviewed and appropriate adjustment of oral diuretics should occur before discharge.[39,40]

23. Answer: B

A standard 3.8-cm (1.5-inch) metal needle can be used in most cases and can safely be left in the abdomen during a therapeutic tap for intervals of an hour or more without injury. An 18-gauge needle is preferred for large-volume therapeutic paracenteses because this permits expeditious outflow, whereas a smaller-gauge (20- to 22-gauge) needle may be sufficient for diagnostic taps and lessen the likelihood of post-procedural ascitic fluid leak through the wound site. Plastic sheath cannulas tend to kink and run the risk of being sheared off into the peritoneal cavity. The needle should be inserted slowly in 5-mm increments to detect undesired entry of a vessel and to help prevent unnecessary puncture of the small bowel. **Continuous manual aspiration should be avoided because it may attract bowel or omentum to the end of the paracentesis needle with resultant occlusion.**

Despite concerns regarding haemorrhagic complications (abdominal wall haematomas and haemoperitoneum) in patients with ascites, it is sufficiently rare, regardless of the PT. In a study of 1100 large-volume paracentesis, there were no haemorrhagic complications despite platelet counts as low as 19,000 cells/mm³ and INRs as high as 8.7 (75% >1.5 and 26.5% > 2). The risks and cost of prophylactic blood products may exceed the benefit. Traditional recommendations suggest the administration of platelets to patients with levels <50,000/mm³ and to give fresh frozen plasma to those with a PT exceeding 20 seconds (1.5 times the therapeutic level). **However, this practice is not evidence supported and current recommendations are to reserve the use of FFP and platelets for clinically evident hyperfibrinolysis (three-dimensional ecchymosis/haematoma) and disseminated intravascular coagulation.**

Clinical assessment for detection of spontaneous bacterial peritonitis by emergency clinicians is only 75% sensitive. Furthermore, 5% of patients are asymptomatic. Although it is common in cirrhotic patients, SBP is difficult to diagnose because signs of abdominal pain and fever are not always present, and physical examination does not always demonstrate abdominal tenderness. Patients who are diagnosed with ascites for the first time, or who have ascites and develop fever, abdominal pain, GI bleeding or encephalopathy, should undergo paracentesis to check for SBP. Ascitic fluid infection is sufficiently common (12% in a recent series) at the

time of admission that it is recommended that all patients with ascites admitted to hospital should undergo abdominal paracentesis.[39,42]

24. Answer: A

The diagnosis of SBP is made when there is a positive ascitic fluid bacterial culture and an elevated ascitic fluid absolute PMN count ≥ 250 cells/mm³ (0.25 x 10⁹/L) without an evident intraabdominal, surgically treatable source of infection.

However, treatment should commence immediately and one should not wait until the ascitic fluid culture grows bacteria as it may result in the death of the patient from overwhelming infection. Microscopy is usually available before culture results. While patients with ascitic polymorphonuclear (PMN) counts ≥ 250 cells/mm³ is presumed to have bacterial peritonitis and should receive empirical antibiotic, infection can also be present in some patients before there is a neutrophil response (i.e. <250 cells/mm³). **Therefore, in a clinical setting compatible with ascitic fluid infection (fever, abdominal pain or unexplained encephalopathy), all patients should receive empiric antibiotic therapy awaiting culture results.**

Clinical examination is not helpful in separating patients who need surgical intervention (secondary peritonitis) from those who have SBP and need only antibiotic treatment. **In contrast, the initial ascitic fluid analysis can assist in distinguishing between spontaneous and secondary peritonitis and it is useful to order an ascitic fluid gram stain, culture, total protein, LDH and glucose in patients with ascitic fluid PMN count ≥ 250 cells/mm³.** The characteristic analysis in the setting of free perforation is PMN ≥ 250 cells/mm³ (usually thousands), multiple organisms on gram stain and culture, as well as at least two of the following criteria:

- total protein >10 g/L
- LDH > upper limit of normal for serum
- glucose < 5 g/L

However, these criteria are only 50% sensitive in detecting non-perforation secondary peritonitis.

When ascitic fluid is collected in a syringe or tube, positive cultures are obtained in about 50% of cases compared with 80% if inoculated into a blood culture bottle prior to administration of antibiotics. Gram-negative enteric organisms, primarily *E. coli*, are the most frequently identified organisms in SBP.

Polymicrobial and anaerobic infections have been reported but are not common. A third-generation cephalosporin, such as cefotaxime, is usually sufficient in treating SBP. Anaerobic coverage should be added if secondary peritonitis is suspected.[39,41–43]

25. Answer: C

Lactulose, a nonabsorbable disaccharide, is the first-line treatment in patients with hepatic encephalopathy. It is effective via various mechanisms:

- It reduces the intestinal production and absorption of ammonia, which is achieved through a laxative effect.
- It facilitates movement of ammonia from the portal circulation into the colon.
- It causes interference with the uptake of glutamine by the intestinal mucosa and its subsequent metabolism to ammonia.

Lactulose should be given at 30 mL orally, 1–2-hourly initially to induce a rapid laxative effect. Once a laxative effect has been achieved, the dosage should be reduced to lactulose 30 mL orally, 3–4 times daily. In unconscious patients or patients who cannot swallow, lactulose may be given by nasogastric tube or mixed with water and given rectally as a retention enema.

Antibiotics such as neomycin reduce intestinal ammonia production by acting against urease-producing bacteria. However, its efficacy has never been demonstrated, and there is significant risk of ototoxicity and nephrotoxicity with long-term use. Neomycin is currently not recommended. However, a nonabsorbable oral antibiotic, rifaximin, has been shown to reduce repeated episodes of hepatic encephalopathy, even in patients taking lactulose regularly. Rifaximin is not registered for use in Australia but is available via the Special Access Scheme.

If no precipitant of acute encephalopathy is readily identifiable, the patient should be started on empirical treatment for infection while waiting for the results of a septic work-up. One gram of intravenous ceftriaxone daily or 1g of cefotaxime 8-hourly are suggested regimens. When culture results become available, modify the antibiotic therapy appropriately. Continue therapy until the clinical signs of infection have resolved (usually for 5–10 days). Antibiotics can be stopped earlier if an alternative precipitant is identified.

Contrary to previous practice, protein restriction is not recommended in patients with acute encephalopathy. However, oral and nasogastric feeding should be suspended in patients with severe encephalopathy who do not have airway protection.[44,45]

26. Answer: B

This man has contracted hepatitis A. Transmission is usually by the faecal–oral route and incubation period is 2–6 weeks. **He will be infectious approximately 2 weeks before the onset of jaundice until 1 week after the onset of jaundice.**

NHIG should be given as a single intramuscular injection to close contacts of hepatitis A cases to prevent secondary cases. NHIG should be administered to close contacts within 2 weeks of the last exposure to the case. NHIG may not be effective if given >2 weeks after the exposure. 'Close contacts' are those who have had contact with a case during the 2 weeks before, up until 1 week after the onset of jaundice, and usually include only household and/or sexual contacts (but in some circumstances may include close occupational exposure).

Although one study suggests that hepatitis A vaccine may be effective in preventing secondary cases of hepatitis A in close contacts, there is currently insufficient evidence to be able to recommend it for this purpose.[46]

27. Answer: C

An increase in *conjugated bilirubin* indicates obstruction, preventing the secretion of conjugated bilirubin produced by normally functioning hepatocytes. It is due to either:

- hepatocellular damage – sarcoidosis, lymphoma, toxins
- impaired excretion of conjugates – Dubin-Johnson and Rotor's syndrome
- biliary epithelial damage – hepatitis, cirrhosis, intrahepatic cholestasis, drugs, sepsis
- extrahepatic obstruction – gallstones, carcinoma, biliary atresia

The *transaminases* (AST and ALT) are commonly used to detect acute hepatocyte injury. They are intracellular hepatic enzymes and are released into the circulation with hepatocyte injury. AST, however, is not specific to hepatocytes and also occurs in other cells, for example, the heart, smooth muscle, kidney and brain. Therefore, **ALT is a more specific marker of hepatocyte injury than AST.**

- Alcohol stimulates AST production. Subsequently, an AST:ALT ratio >2 is common in alcoholic hepatitis.
- With viral hepatitis, AST and ALT levels increase over 1–2 weeks to levels in the thousands, and return to normal within 6 weeks in uncomplicated cases.
- In cholestatic disorders, AST increases before ALT, and the levels usually do not exceed a fivefold increase.

ALP elevation **is associated with biliary obstruction and cholestasis. Mild to moderate elevations accompany virtually all hepatobiliary disease, whereas elevations >4 times normally strongly suggests cholestasis.** Again, ALP is a non-specific marker as it is also derived from bone, placenta, intestines kidneys and leucocytes. Therefore, in the absence of elevated gamma-glutamyl transpeptidase (GGT), causes other than cholestasis should be considered. GGT is slightly more sensitive than ALP in obstructive liver disease. It is also elevated by drugs inducing hepatic microsomal enzyme activity, such as warfarin, phenytoin and baribiturates. There may be an isolated elevation in chronic ethanol ingestion or chronic barbiturate or phenytoin therapy.

Urine bilirubin and urobilinogen are sometimes used as screening tests for liver disease in the ED. The sensitivities of these urine assays are 70–74% for identifying elevated serum bilirubin. For correlation with other liver enzyme tests, their sensitivity is in the 43–53% range. Specificity for showing either bilirubin or transaminase abnormality is 77–87%. Blood-tinged urine will give a false positive urobilinogen on urine dipstix. Taken together, these statistics do not support screening for liver disease with urine dipstick testing.[42,47,48]

28. Answer: D

The tube insertion length should be estimated prior to insertion of a NGT to prevent placement of the tip of the tube in the oesophagus and to ensure intragastric positioning without excess coiling. The distance should be measured from the tip of the xiphoid to the earlobe. Add the distance from the earlobe to the tip of the nose. Then add another 15 cm. Typically, a 16- or 18-Fr sump tube is used in adults for aspiration/drainage. Sizes are available up to size 20.

Vasoconstrictors and topical anaesthetics should always be used whenever the time and clinical situation permit. **The nares, nasopharynx and oropharynx should all be anaesthetised at least 5 minutes before the procedure.** Gagging is reduced if the pharynx is anaesthetised as well as the nose. Lignocaine 1% or 4% nebulised through a face mask (≤4 mg/kg; not to exceed 200 mg per dose in adults) is an option and seems to be superior to lignocaine spray to reduce gagging and vomiting and to increase the chance of successful passage. Alternatively, lubrication and anaesthesia of the nares can be facilitated by using a syringe filled with 5 mL of anaesthetic lubricant, such as 2% lignocaine gel. Simply putting anesthetic jelly on the tube before insertion will not provide any anesthesia.

Successful tube placement can most accurately be confirmed with X-ray; however, it is not the standard to routinely obtain X-ray confirmation. Aspiration of stomach contents, especially if pH tested, is more reliable than insufflation of air to confirm placement in the stomach. If the pH is <4, there is an approximately 95% chance that the tube is in the stomach and nonrespiratory placement is almost guaranteed.[40]

29. Answer: A

Fever is the most common reason for a transplant recipient to present to the ED. Factors other than infection such as rejection, drug effects, hypersensitivity reaction or malignancy can also cause fever and are sometimes indistinguishable from infection. **Furthermore, it is often difficult to differentiate infection from rejection and they may also occur simultaneously. For this reason, treatment for rejection and infection are often started at the same time.** Consultation with the transplant team should occur early to direct the most appropriate treatment regime.

The timing of infection after transplant can be separated into three periods, which is helpful in determining the aetiological agent:

1. <1 month

   Fever is usually due to complications of surgery and hospitalisation. Nosocomial pathogens are prominent.

2. 1–6 months

   a) immunomodulating viral infections including cytomegalovirus (CMV), hepatitis B and C, and Epstein-Barr virus (EBV)
   b) opportunistic infections including *Pneumocystis*, *Listeria*, and fungal species

3. >6 months

   Infections are further divided into three groups relative to infection susceptibility:
   a) healthy transplant – community-acquired infections
   b) chronic viral infection – progressive disease due to immunomodulating viral infections
   c) chronic rejection – opportunistic infection predominate

   NSAIDs should generally be avoided as many transplant patients will have recurrent bouts of thrombocytopenia from chemotherapy or renal insufficiency as a side effect of immunosuppresive drugs. Some patients will be on anticoagulants due to deep venous thrombosis (DVT) or other reasons, whereas others will have unexpected episodes of bleeding due to transplant complication or graft-versus-host disease.[49,50]

30. Answer: A

Transfusion-associated graft-versus-host disease (TA-GvHD) is a rare, but almost universally fatal, iatrogenic complication of transfusion. It occurs when immunocompetent T-lymphocytes engraft in an immune-suppressed patient. Irradiation of cellular blood components (whole blood, red cells, platelets and granulocytes) is the mainstay of TA-GvHD prevention. Frozen blood components, such as fresh frozen plasma and cryoprecipitate, and fractionated products, such as albumin, factor concentrates and intravenous immunoglobulin, do not require irradiation before administration. Unlike most transfusion-related reactions, TA-GvHD usually presents after only a few days, with a median onset of 10 days.

In comparison with patients who have received haematopoietic stem cell transplants, solid-organ transplant recipients are generally less immunocompromised and are subsequently more capable of abrogating the effect of donor lymphocytes and preventing engraftment. For this reason, the **Australian and New Zealand Society of Blood Transfusion does not recommend the routine irradiation of cellular blood components for solid organ transplant recipients.**[50,51]

References

1. Gorelick MH, Shaw KN, Murphy KO. Validity and reliability of clinical signs in the diagnosis of dehydration in children. Pediatrics 1997;99;e6.

2. Steiner MJ, DeWalt DA, Byerley JS. Is this child dehydrated? JAMA 2004;291(22):2746–54.

3. World Health Organization. The treatment of diarrhoea: A manual for physicians and other senior health workers. Geneva: World Health Organization. Online. Available: http://whqlibdoc.who.int/publications/2005/9241593180.pdf, 2011.

4. European Society for Paediatric Gastroenterology, Hepatology, and Nutrition / European Society for Paediatric Infectious Diseases. Evidence-based guidelines for the management of acute gastroenteritis in children in Europe. Journal of Pediatric Gastroenterology and Nutrition 2008;46:S81–4.

5. Elliott EJ, Dalby-Payne JR. Acute infectious diarrhoea and dehydration in children. MJA 2004;181:565–70.

6. National Collaborating Centre for Women's and Children's Health. Diarrhoea and vomiting caused by gastroenteritis: Diagnosis, assessment and management in children younger than 5 years. Online. Available: http://www.nice.org.uk/nicemedia/pdf/CG84FullGuideline.pdf; 2011.

7. Spandorfer PR, Alessandrini EA, Joffe MD, et al. Oral versus intravenous rehydration of moderately dehydrated children. Pediatrics 2005;115(2):295–301.

8. Nager AL, Wang VJ. Comparison of nasogastric and intravenous methods of rehydration in pediatric patients with acute dehydration. Pediatrics 2002;109(4):566–72.

9. Atherley-John YC, Cunningham SJ, Crain EF. A randomized trial of oral versus intravenous rehydration in a pediatric emergency department. Arch Ped Adol Med 2002;156(12):1240–3.

10. Fonseca BK, Holdgate A, Craig JC. Enteral versus intravenous rehydration therapy for children with gastroenteritis. Arch Ped Adol Med 2004;158(5):483.

11. CHOICE. Multicentre randomized double blind clinical trial to evaluate the efficacy and safety of a reduced osmolarity oral rehydration salt solution in children with acute watery diarrhoea. Pediatrics 2001;107(4):613–8.

12. Centre for Disease Control and Prevention. Managing acute gastroenteritis among children: Oral rehydration, maintenance, and nutritional therapy. Centre for Disease Control and Prevention. Online. Available: http://www.cdc.gov/mmwr/preview/mmwrhtml/rr5216a1.htm; 2011.

13. Murphy MS. Clincal review. Management of bloody diarrhoea in children in primary care. BMJ 2008;336:1010–5.

14. Craig SA, Zich DK. Gastroenteritis. In: Marx JA, Hockberger RS, Walls RM, editors. Rosen's emergency medicine: concepts and clinical practice. 7th ed. Philadelphia: Elsevier; 2009. p. 1200–27.

15. Freedman SB. Thull JD. Vomiting, diarrhea and dehydration in children. In: Tintinalli JE, Stapczynski JS, Ma OJ, editors. Emergency medicine: a comprehensive study guide. 7th ed. New York: McGraw-Hill; 2011. p. 830–9.

16. Therapeutic Guidelines Limited. Infectious diarrhoea: bacterial infections (revised 2008). In: eTG complete. Online: Available: www.tg.org.au.

17. Hill DR, Ryan ET. Management of travellers' diarrhoea. BMJ 2008;337:863–7.

18. Bartlett GB. Antibiotic-associated diarrhoea. N Engl J Med 2002; 346(5):334–9.

19. Cheng AC, Ferguson JK, Richards MJ, et al. Australasian Society for Infectious Diseases guidelines for the diagnosis and treatment of Clostridium difficile infection. MJA 2011;194:353–8.

20. McGauly PL, Mahler SA. Foodborne and waterborne diseases. In: Tintinalli JE, Stapczynski JS, Ma OJ, editors. Emergency medicine: A comprehensive study guide. 7th ed. New York: McGraw-Hill; 2011. p. 1062–70.

21. Mowat C, Cole A, Windsor A, et al. Guidelines for the management of inflammatory bowel disease in adults. Gut 2011;60:571–607.

22. Kman NE, Werman HA. Disorders presenting primarily with diarrhea. In: Tintinalli JE, Stapczynski JS, Ma OJ, editors. Emergency medicine: a comprehensive study guide. 7th ed. New York: McGraw-Hill; 2011. p. 531–40.

23. Yates K. Inflammatory bowel disease. In: Cameron P, Jelinek G, Kelly A, et al, editors. Textbook of adult emergency medicine. 3rd ed. Edinburgh: Elsevier; 2009. p. 353–6.

24. Jakobovits SL, Travis SPL. Management of acute severe colitis. British Medical Bulletin 2006;75–76:131–44. Online. Available: http://bmb.oxfordjournals.org; 2011.

25. Noble VE, Nelson BP. Gallbladder ultrasound. In: Noble VE, Nelson BP, editors. Manual of emergency and critical care ultrasound. 2nd ed. Cambridge: Cambridge University Press; 2011. p. 151–71.

26. Ooi S, Dilley S. Peptic ulcer disease and gastritis. In: Cameron P, Jelinek G, Kelly A, et al, editors. Textbook of adult emergency medicine. 3rd ed. Edinburgh: Elsevier; 2009. p. 339–43.

27. Gratton MC. Peptic ulcer disease and gastritis. In: Tintinalli JE, Stapczynski JS, Ma OJ, editors. Emergency medicine: a comprehensive study guide. 7th ed. New York: McGraw-Hill; 2011. p. 554–7.

28. Therapeutic Guidelines Limited. Helicobacter pylori: effects of infection and indications for eradication (revised 2011). In: eTG complete. Online: Available: www.tg.org.au.

29. Kumar R, Mills AM. Gastrointestinal emergencies. Emerg Med Clin North Am 2011;29(2):159–468.

30. Perera TB, Carron J. Upper gastrointestinal bleeding. Emergency medicine reports 2007;28(8):81–92.

31. Graham C. Haematemesis and melaena. In: Cameron P, Jelinek G, Kelly A, et al, editors. Textbook of adult emergency medicine. 3rd ed. Edinburgh: Elsevier; 2009. p. 334–9.

32. Overton DT. Upper gastrointestinal bleeding. In: Tintinalli JE, Stapczynski JS, Ma OJ, editors. Emergency medicine: A comprehensive study guide. 7th ed. New York: McGraw-Hill; 2011. p. 543–5.

33. Westhoff JL, Holt KR. Gastrointestinal bleeding: An evidence-based approach to risk stratification. Emergency Medicine Practice 2004;6(3):1–20. Online. Available: http://www.ebmedicine.net/topics.php?paction=showTopicSeg&topic_id=75&seg_id=1505.

34. Worthley DL, Fraser RJ. Management of acute bleeding in the upper gastrointestinal tract. Australian Prescriber 2005;28(3):62–6.

35. Courtney AE, Mitchell RMS, Rocke L, et al. Proposed risk stratification in upper gastrointestinal haemorrhage: Is hospitalisation essential? Emerg Med J 2004;21:39–40.

36. Barkun AN, Bardou M, Kuipers EJ, et al. International consensus recommendations on the management of patients with nonvariceal upper gastrointestinal bleeding. Ann Intern Med 2010;152:101–13.

37. Henneman PL. Gastrointestinal bleeding. In: Marx JA, Hockberger RS, Walls RM, editors. Rosen's emergency medicine: concepts and clinical practice. 7th ed. Philadelphia: Elsevier; 2010. p. 170–5.

38. Dunn R, Maclean A. General gastroenterology. In: Dunn R, Dilley S. Brookes J, editors. The emergency medicine manual. 5th ed. Adelaide: Venom Publishing; 2010. p. 547–9.

39. Runyon BA. Management of adult patients with ascites due to cirrhosis: an update. Hepatology 2009;49(6):2087–103.

40. Runyon MS, Marx JA. Peritoneal procedures. In: Roberts JR, Hedges JR, editors. Clinical procedures in emergency medicine, 5th ed. Philadelphia: Elsevier; 2009. p. 773–89.

41. Dunn R, Maclean A. Liver disease. In: Dunn R, Dilley S. Brookes J, editors. The emergency medicine manual. 5th ed. Adelaide: Venom Publishing; 2010. p. 588–90.

42. O'Mara SR, Gebreyes K. Hepatic disorders, jaundice, and hepatic failure. In: Tintinalli JE, Stapczynski JS, Ma OJ, editors. Emergency medicine: a comprehensive study guide. 7th ed. New York: McGraw-Hill; 2011. p. 566–74.

43. Guss DA, Oyama LC. Disorders of the liver and biliary tract. In: Marx JA, Hockberger RS, Walls RM, editors. Rosen's emergency medicine: concepts and clinical practice. 7th ed. Philadelphia: Elsevier; 2010. p. 1153–71.

44. Therapeutic Guidelines Limited. Hepatic encephalopathy (revised 2011). In: eTG complete. Online: Available: www.tg.org.au.

45. Sundaram V, Shaikh OS. Hepatic encephalopathy: pathophysiology and emerging therapies. Med Clin N Am 2009;93:819–36.

46. National Health and Medical Research Council. Hepatitis A. In: The Australian immunisation handbook. 9th ed. 2008. p. 139–48: Online. Available: http://www.health.gov.au/internet/immunise/publishing.nsf/content/handbook-home.

47. Dunn R. Clinical biochemistry. In: Dunn R, Dilley S, Brookes J, editors. The emergency medicine manual. 5th ed. Adelaide: Venom Publishing; 2010. p. 251–86.

48. Privette Jr TW, Carlisle MC, Palma JK. Emergencies of the liver, gallbladder and pancreas. Emerg Med Clin N Am 2011;29:293–317.

49. Keadey MT. The solid organ transplant patient. In: Marx JA, Hockberger RS, Walls RM, editors. Rosen's emergency medicine: concepts and clinical practice. 7th ed. Philadelphia: Elsevier; 2010. p. 2365–74.

50. Fish RM, Massad MG. The transplant patient. In: Tintinalli JE, Stapczynski JS, Ma OJ, editors. Emergency medicine: A comprehensive study guide. 7th ed. New York: McGraw-Hill; 2011. p. 1997–2012.

51. Australian and New Zealand Society of Blood Transfusion. Guidelines for prevention of transfusion-associated graft-versus-host disease (TA-GVHD). 1st ed. Online. Available: http://www.anzsbt.org.au/publications/PreventionofTA-GVHD.pdf.pdf; 2011.

1. Answer: C

ARF itself is usually asymptomatic until severe uraemia has developed. More commonly, patients will present with symptoms of the underlying cause.

Papillary necrosis results from ischaemia of the renal medullary pyramids and papillae. This is usually associated with diabetes mellitus, analgesic use, pyelonephritis and urinary obstruction. Presenting symptoms in the acute form include fever and chills, flank or abdominal pain and haematuria. It may also manifest as episodes of pyelonephritis and hydronephrosis, and mimics nephrolithiasis. Acute *renal artery occlusion* is usually marked by flank pain, whereas gradual stenosis is asymptomatic. Fever, arthralgia and rash are common with acute *interstitial nephritis*. The presence of fever usually suggests an *autoimmune* or infectious cause.[1]

2. Answer: C

Prerenal causes are responsible for 70% of community-acquired and 20% of hospital-acquired ARF, whereas intrinsic causes are responsible for 20% of community-acquired and 70% of hospital-acquired ARF. The incidence of postrenal causes is 10% and is similar in both community and hospital-acquired ARF. **Up to 90% of community-acquired cases have a potentially reversible cause as volume depletion is responsible for the majority of community-acquired ARF.**

Intrinsic renal failure is subdivided into four categories: tubular, glomerular, interstitial and small-vessel disease. Ischaemic ARF, typically acute tubular necrosis (ATN), is the most common cause of intrinsic renal failure. Acute interstitial nephritis is usually due to a drug reaction but may also be caused by autoimmune disease, infection or infiltrative disease.[1]

3. Answer: B

The mortality for ARF has not improved over many decades in spite of the introduction of dialysis, primarily because affected patients are now older and have more comorbid conditions. **Infection is the most common cause of death associated with ARF, accounting for 75% of deaths.**

Cardiorespiratory complications are the second most common cause of death.

Surprisingly, patients aged over 80 years with ARF have mortality rates similar to those of young adults. ARF in children has a different set of causes and mortality rates average 25%.[1,2]

4. Answer: D

NSAIDs, ACE-I and angiotensin-receptor blockers (ARBs) usually cause a gradual and asymptomatic decrease in glomerular filtration rate (GFR) but can cause acute kidney injury.

ACE inhibitors may precipitate renal failure, most likely due to impairment of renal autoregulation. Renal autoregulation and maintenance of GFR mainly depends on a combination of preglomerular arteriolar vasodilatation, mediated by prostaglandins, and postglomerular arteriolar vasoconstriction, mediated by angiotensin II. Reduced angiotensin II levels may cause efferent arteriolar vasodilation and subsequently decrease GFR. This is particularly relevant in patients with bilateral renal artery stenosis and renal hypoperfusion (caused by volume depletion or decreased 'effective' circulating volume as in oedematous states) because maintenance of GFR is dependant on postglomerular arterial vasoconstriction. **ACE inhibitors may cause hyperkalaemia but through a different mechanism than renal impairment as described above.** Suppression of angiotensin II leads to a decrease in aldosterone levels. Aldosterone is responsible for increasing the excretion of potassium; therefore, ACE inhibitors ultimately can cause retention of potassium.

Similarly, *NSAIDs* (both selective and non-selective cyclooxygenase inhibitors) interfere with prostaglandin synthesis and can cause preglomerular arteriolar vasoconstriction with diminished renal flow and GFR. Patients with diminished renal perfusion due to underlying volume depletion, congestive heart failure, chronic renal failure and cirrhosis are particularly vulnerable to this effect. Renal vasodilator prostaglandins are critical in maintaining glomerular perfusion in these patients in which elevated circulating levels of renin and angiotensin II act to diminish renal blood flow and GFR. NSAIDs do not usually impair renal function in healthy persons.

Angiotensin-receptor blockers can also precipitate renal failure, most likely due to a similar mechanism as mentioned above.[1,3,4]

5. Answer: A

There is a misconception that traditional serum markers of myocardial damage (CK and troponin) are unreliable in dialysis patients presenting with chest pain. These markers are, however, not significantly elevated in ESRD patients who undergo regular dialysis and are specific markers of myocardial ischaemia in such patients.

Uraemia is a clinical syndrome and no single symptom, sign or laboratory result reflects all aspects of uraemia. Both serum urea and creatinine levels are inaccurate markers of the clinical syndrome of uraemia, although there seems to be a correlation between the symptoms of uraemia and a low GFR.

Serum and urine chemistry panels have some utility in distinguishing between prerenal and renal causes. FENa ($U_{Na}/P_{Na} \div U_{cr}/P_{cr}$) is commonly used to identify prerenal causes but has limitations that should be recognised. A FENa <1% is suggestive of prerenal causes of ARF, as is a urea to creatinine ratio >20:1.

Microscopic urine analysis is helpful in determining the underlying cause of renal failure. The urinary sediment of patients with pre- and postrenal failure is usually 'bland' and may contain hyaline casts. Intrinsic causes of ARF typically have 'active' urinary sediment with granular casts typical of tubular injury and red cell casts associated with glomerulonephritis.[1]

6. Answer: C

The risk for CIN is very closely related to the existing renal insufficiency. **An eGFR of <60 mL/min/1.73 m² represents significant renal dysfunction and is used to define the patient at high risk for developing CIN.** Similarly, the presence of other patient-related risk factors also increases the risk for CIN. These risk factors include diabetes, shock or hypotension, advanced age (>75 years), advanced congestive heart failure, sepsis and the use of nephrotoxic agents. Serum creatinine levels usually peak at 3 days after administration of the contrast medium. **Subsequently, it is generally recommended that serum creatinine levels be repeated at 48–72 hours following contrast medium in all high-risk patients.**

Recognition of the high-risk patient coupled with appropriate periprocedural management can reduce the incidence of CIN. Multiple studies have shown that **parenteral volume repletion is the cornerstone of CIN prevention**. However, data is still lacking regarding the optimal fluid regimen. One recommendation is to administer a total of at least 1 L of isotonic saline beginning at least 3 hours before and continuing at least 6–8 hours after the procedure. Initial infusion rates of 100–150 mL/hr are recommended with adjustment post procedure as clinically indicated. The appropriate caution should be taken in patients with reduced left ventricular function and congestive cardiac failure.[1,5,6]

7. Answer: C

About 20% (1 in 5 patients) of patients requiring chronic dialysis will develop pericarditis and it is usually due to either uraemia or dialysis related. Uraemic pericarditis is by far more common and is responsible for about 75% of cases. Interestingly, **the pericardial friction rub associated with uraemic pericarditis is louder than in most forms of pericarditis and is often palpable. Furthermore, the inflammatory cells in uninfected uraemic pericarditis do not penetrate into the myocardium, therefore the typical ECG changes of acute pericarditis are absent.** When the ECG has features typical of pericarditis it mandates a search for other causes including infection. The management of haemodynamically stable patients with uraemic and dialysis-related pericarditis is intensive dialysis; therefore, the dialysis team should be involved early in the diagnosis. Should the pericardial effusion persist for longer than 10–14 days with intensive dialysis, treatment is considered a failure and an anterior pericardectomy is usually performed.[1,7]

8. Answer: A

Vascular access for haemodialysis is usually obtained with the creation of an AV fistula from a native artery or vein or, if this is unsuitable, a vascular graft. Grafts are associated with a higher complication rate compared with natural AV fistulas. This is significant considering that complications of vascular access account for more inpatient hospital days than any other complication of haemodialysis. Vascular access complications include failure to provide adequate flow for dialysis, infection, bleeding, vascular access aneurysm and pseudoaneurysms, vascular insufficiency of the extremity distal to the vascular access and high-output heart failure. **Failure to provide adequate flow for dialysis and infection are by far the two most common complications.**

The inability to obtain adequate flow for haemodialysis is common. This is usually caused by thrombosis or stenosis and can clinically be determined when there is a loss of bruit and thrill over the access. This is not an emergency and can be treated within 24 hours by angiographic clot removal, angioplasty or by alteplase injection into the access. The ED clinician should rather focus on evaluating the patient for indications requiring emergency dialysis, as haemodialysis will inevitably be postponed until adequate flow is established.

The classic signs of pain, erythema and swelling of an infected vascular access are often missing. Patients more often present with signs of sepsis such as fever, hypotension or an elevated white cell count (WCC). *Staphylococcus aureus* is the most common infecting organism. Vancomycin is the drug of choice because of its effectiveness against methicillin-resistant organisms and a long half-life (5–7 days) in dialysis patients.[1,7]

9. Answer: B

The kidney is the most commonly transplanted organ and is placed in the right or left lower quadrant of the abdomen; it is easily palpable on abdominal examination. These patients require lifelong immunosuppression to prevent rejection. Current available immunosuppressant drugs are more potent than those in the past and as a result, the incidence of rejection is now lower in these patients. However, it has contributed to a greater incidence of medication-related problems.

Two common causes of ARF after kidney transplantation are acute cyclosporine or tacrolimus nephrotoxicity and acute rejection. It is difficult to distinguish between these two disorders. Traditionally, fever and allograft tenderness favoured rejection; however, these findings are now rare with current immunosuppressive regimens. Elevated

cyclosporine or tacrolimus blood levels make nephrotoxicity the more likely diagnosis. Blood levels should be obtained in all patients who present with ARF.

Fever is a common problem that brings renal transplant recipients to the ED. The causes of fever in these patients vary according to the time after transplant. Infections seen in the first post-transplant month are the usual postoperative infections seen in the general surgical population. **Opportunistic infections are uncommon in the first post-transplant month and usually occur after the first month and before the first post-transplant year.** Beyond the first year, opportunistic infections may still occur but community-acquired infections unrelated to immunosupression become more common.

The serum creatinine level is the most valuable prognostic marker of graft function at all times after transplantation.[8,9]

10. Answer: B

In severe hyperkalaemia, intravenous calcium is effective in reversing electrocardiographic changes and reducing the risk of arrhythmias. Improvement of ECG is usually visible within 1–3 minutes. Calcium administration can be repeated if no effect is seen within 5–10 minutes. The duration of action is 30–60 minutes.

It is true that CaCl 10% is about three times as potent as Calcium-gluconate (10% CaCl = 27.2 mg $[Ca^{2+}]$/mL; 10% gluconate = 9 mg $[Ca^{2+}]$/mL. **However, no specific Ca^{2+} preparation has been shown to be superior to the other and its use depends on clinician preference, patient factors and availability.** The initial and repeat doses may need to be adjusted accordingly. CaCl 10% is more likely to cause tissue necrosis if it extravasates and should preferably be given via central line.

Calcium administration should be reserved for life-threatening situations in patients on digoxin. **Calcium can potentiate cardiac toxicity to digoxin regardless of the serum Ca^{2+} levels.** If the patient's condition necessitates administration of Ca^{2+}, it is recommended to give it slowly over 20–30 minutes mixed in 100 mL of D_5W. **An alternative is to consider using magnesium instead of calcium to stabilise the myocardium.**[10-15]

11. Answer: D

Intravenous insulin is the most reliable agent for shifting potassium into cells and is regarded as the first-line treatment for hyperkalaemia. Its onset of action is rapid within 15–30 minutes.

β-receptor agonists have a similar onset of action and their effect has been shown to be additive to insulin administration. However, the effective dose is at least 4 times higher than typically used for bronchodilation. Salbutamol at doses of 10–20 mg is recommended via a nebuliser.

NaHCO$_3$ has been routinely used in the management of hyperkalaemia in the prior decades. However, latest evidence suggests that it has no effect to shift K$^+$ into cells, even after several hours. This, combined with the potential complication of increased sodium concentration and volume overload, especially relevant in patients with renal compromise, has recently caused the use of HCO$_3$ to fall out of favour. Its use is no longer routinely recommended although it may still be appropriate in patients with severe metabolic acidosis.

Cation exchange resins promote elimination of total body potassium by gastrointestinal excretion as it binds K$^+$ in the colon in exchange for sodium.[10–15]

12. Answer: C

The most common causes of rhabdomyolysis in adults are alcohol and drugs of abuse, followed by medications, muscle disease, trauma, neuroleptic malignant syndrome, seizures, immobility, infection, strenuous physical activity and heat-related illnesses. Alcohol and drugs play a role in up to 80% of adults. In many cases the aetiology is multifactorial. **The most common causes in children are trauma, viral myositis and connective tissue disease.**

Rhabdomyolysis is an extremely rare (<1%) but life-threatening complication of statin therapy. The incidence varies with the particular statin, is dose-related and increases with dual therapy.

Influenza viruses A and B are the most commonly cited infectious causes and *Legionella* is the most frequently reported bacterial cause of rhabdomyolysis. Patients will classically give a history of a viral illness 1–2 weeks prior to the onset of myalgias and myoglobinuria.

Strenuous physical activity is another common cause. High force eccentric contraction as with strength training or heavy lifting leads to a greater breakdown in muscle and higher levels of CK than concentric contractions, such as endurance-based exercise.[16,17]

13. Answer: C

The classic clinical manifestations of rhabdomyolysis include myalgia, weakness and tea-coloured urine. **Acute rhabdomyolysis may present without any of these symptoms and musculoskeletal symptoms may be present in as few as half of patients. The diagnosis of rhabdomyolysis therefore requires a high index of suspicion, particularly when patients present with an altered sensorium, and is confirmed by laboratory evaluation.**

Serum myoglobin is an insensitive marker for rhabdomyolysis. The half-life of myoglobin in plasma is 1–3 hours and can be cleared completely from plasma within 6 hours after injury. Urine myoglobin is also excreted rapidly and may also be an inaccurate measure. **Serum and urinary myoglobin may therefore be absent in patients who present late in the course of their illness.**

An elevated CK is the most sensitive and reliable indicator of muscle injury. It is present in the serum almost immediately after muscle injury, is not rapidly cleared from serum (half-life is 1.5 days) with peak levels occurring within 24–36 hours of muscle injury. Rhabdomyolysis is not defined by a specific CK level. However, in the absence of cerebral or myocardial infarction, CK levels greater than five times normal is generally thought to be diagnostic and levels above 5000 U/L indicate serious muscle injury.

The degree of CK elevation correlates with the amount of muscle injury and severity of illness but not the development of renal failure or other morbidity. Patients may have significant morbidity with only moderately elevated CK levels. There is no defined threshold value of serum CK above which the risk of acute kidney injury is markedly increased. Furthermore, only a weak correlation between peak CK levels and the incidence of acute kidney injury has been reported and it seems that the risk of acute kidney injury is low when CK levels at admission are <15,000 to 20,000 U/L. The risk of renal failure increases with comorbid conditions such as sepsis, dehydration, and acidosis and acute kidney injury may occur under these circumstances at CK levels as low as 5000 U/L.

Additionally, it seems like an initially elevated serum urea and creatinine and a large base deficit have an increased risk for developing ARF.[16-18]

14. Answer: D

HUS is primarily a disease of infancy and early childhood, especially of those aged between 6 months and 4 years and is rare after 5 years of age. It is classically characterised by the triad of microangiopathic haemolytic anaemia, thrombocytopaenia and ARF.

Two forms of HUS exist: epidemic (typical) and sporadic (atypical). The typical form is much more common and is associated with infectious diarrhoea. **The shiga toxin (also called verotoxin) producing *E. coli* serotype O157:H7 has been associated with more than 80% of infections leading to HUS.** Other infectious causes of HUS include *Shigella* organisms, *Streptococcus pneumoniae*, *Aeromonas* and *HIV*. In contrast, the sporadic form is not associated with diarrhoea but may have a genetic link. It has been associated with non-enteric infections such as invasive *S. pneumoniae* as well as non-infectious causes including drugs, malignancies, transplantation, pregnancy and other underlying medical conditions such as scleroderma and antiphospholipid syndrome. **HUS continues to be one of the most common causes of ARF in children.**

Unnecessary use of antibiotics or antimotility agents should be avoided during diarrhoeal illness as it may increase the risk of HUS. Antimotility agents slow gut motility and therefore the gut is exposed to the toxins for a longer period of time. Antibiotic-induced injury to the bacterial membrane favours the acute release of large amounts of toxins. **The use of antibiotics has been shown to increase the risk of full-blown HUS by 17-fold and, therefore, the current recommendation is to avoid its use, except in cases of sepsis.**[19-22]

15. Answer: C

HUS is primarily a clinical diagnosis coupled with consistent laboratory findings. Patients usually present with watery diarrhoea and crampy abdominal pain. Fever is only present in about 30% of cases. From 2 to 3 days after onset of symptoms, patients experience increased abdominal pain with bloody stools, the latter developing in up to 89% of patients by day 5. **Central nervous system irritability may develop in about 33% of patients and may result in seizures.** Anaemia can be profound due to haemolysis and it is not uncommon for the haemoglobin levels to be 50–90 g/L.[19-22]

16. Answer: D

Group A β-haemolytic streptococcal infections are common in children and can lead to the postinfectious complication of acute glomerulonephritis. ASPGN is characterised by the sudden onset of gross haematuria, oedema, hypertension and renal insufficiency. Peripheral oedema typically results from salt and water retention and is common; nephrotic syndrome develops in a minority (<5%) of childhood cases.

Confirmation of the diagnosis requires clear evidence of a prior streptococcal infection. Although a positive *throat culture* may support the diagnosis it may simply represent the carrier state and is not necessarily the cause of glomerulonephritis. An *ASO titer* of 250 U or higher is highly suggestive of recent streptococcal infection. However, a rise in the titer of the antibody, measured at an interval of 2–3 weeks, is more meaningful than a single measurement. Importantly, the antistreptolysin O titer is commonly elevated after a pharyngeal infection but rarely increases after streptococcal skin infections. *Anti–DNAse B* and AHase titers are more often positive following skin infections. **The *serum C3* level is significantly reduced in >90% of patients in the acute phase and returns to normal 6–8 weeks after onset. C4 is most often normal in APSGN, or only mildly depressed.**[19,21,23]

17. Answer: C

Nephrotic syndrome can be primary (involving only the kidneys) or secondary (multisystem). Primary nephrotic syndrome occurs more commonly in children younger than 5 years, whereas secondary nephrotic syndrome occurs more often in older children. Around 90% of affected children have the primary disease, with the majority having minimal change nephrotic syndrome. The diagnostic criteria for nephrotic syndrome are generalised oedema, hypoproteinemia with a disproportionately low albumin level, proteinuria (3+ or 4+ on the dipstick reading) and hyperlipidaemia. Microscopic haematuria also may be present.

Serum complements, antibodies and coagulation factors are lost as protein in the urine, making these children susceptible to severe infection and thromboembolic events. Steroid therapy further increases the infection risk. Hyperlipidaemia may lead to hyperviscosity and further increase the thrombotic risk.[19,20]

18. Answer: D

The causes of haematuria can be divided into haematologic, renal and postrenal causes. Renal causes may be further classified as glomerular or nonglomerular. Gross haematuria more often indicates a lower tract cause, whereas microscopic haematuria tends to occur with kidney disease. The presence of red cell casts and proteinuria suggest a glomerular source.

Haematuria associated with pain during urination is often due to a UTI, whereas painless haematuria is more often due to neoplastic, hyperplastic and vascular causes. **Haematuria in patients on oral anticoagulants should not be attributed to the anticoagulant alone because the incidence of underlying disease is as high as 80%.**

Patients younger than 40 years of age with a first episode of asymptomatic microscopic haematuria should have a repeat urine analysis ideally within 2 weeks. If haematuria is persistent, further urological evaluation is warranted. **Most patients older than 40 years should undergo a thorough evaluation after even a single episode of haematuria.**[24]

19. Answer: B

The most common pathogens associated with acute bacterial prostatitis are gram-negative bacilli (uropathogens), such as E. coli and Proteus spp. Additionally, ascending urethral infection with Neisseria gonorrhoeae and Chlamydia trachomatis may occur following sexual intercourse, especially in sexually active men younger than 35 years and older men who engage in high-risk sexual behaviours.

The diagnosis of acute bacterial prostatitis is usually based on symptoms alone: urinary symptoms (irritative or obstructive), pain in the suprapubic or perineal region, or in the external genitalia, as well as systemic symptoms of fever, chills or malaise. A gentle digital examination will reveal a hot, swollen, tender prostate. **Prostatic massage with sampling of prostatic fluid for culture is not recommended with acute bacterial prostatitis because it can precipitate bacteraemia.** A simple midstream urine specimen should rather be obtained for microscopy and culture. The presence of >10 WBC/hpf suggests a positive diagnosis.

Chronic prostatitis can be due to bacterial or non-bacterial causes. Chronic bacterial prostatitis usually occurs in adults who have a history of recurrent urinary tract infection. Symptoms include recurring episodes of pain or discomfort in the perineum, groin, lower back, or scrotum and voiding dysfunction. Prostatic examination is not usually helpful because findings are variable. To further classify chronic prostatitis, cultures of urine before and after a prostatic massage are necessary to rule out infection. This is obtained by collecting midstream urine followed by collecting the first 10 mL of urine after a vigorous prostate massage.[25–28]

20. Answer: D

Reinfection (within 1–6 months after treatment) is usually by different enteric organism or different serotype of same organism. Relapse of UTI is recurrence of symptoms within 1 month (caused by the same organism) and represents treatment failure.

The most common urinary tract pathogen is E. coli. In acute uncomplicated cystitis E. coli is the responsible organism in 70–90% of cases. Although E.coli are isolated in 20–50% of cases of complicated UTIs, other gram-negative bacteria (e.g. Proteus, Klebsiella), enterococci and Streptococcus agalactiae (group B streptococcus) are more common in this group.

Chlamydia trachomatis is common in dysuria-pyuria syndrome (culture negative pyuria) in which sterile or low-colony count culture results are obtained.

Pseudomonas species have a low virulence for the urinary tract and its presence suggests that normal host defenses have been altered. The most common reasons for this are incomplete emptying of the urinary tract due to obstruction, high-grade vesicoureteric reflux or voiding dysfunction.[24,25,29]

21. Answer: B

A positive u-dipstix for nitrites is caused by bacteria that convert nitrates to nitrite, usually coliform bacteria like E.coli, Enterococcus, Pseudomonas species and Acinetobacter (usually responsible for complicated UTIs) do not convert nitrates and therefore usually yield a negative nitrate test. **Although nitrate reaction by dipstix has a very high specificity (90%) and a positive result is useful in confirming diagnosis of UTI, it has a low sensitivity (about 50%) so it is not always useful as a screening exam because a negative test does not exclude the diagnosis of UTI.**

Visual inspection and assessment of the odour of urine is generally not helpful in determining infection. Cloudiness in fresh urine is usually not due to white blood cells or bacteria, but rather due to large amounts of protein or amorphous phosphate crystals. Malodour of urine may be caused by diet or medications and is not a reliable sign if infection.

The absence of pyuria and bacteriuria in a patient with clinical suspicion of UTI mandates the exclusion for an obstructed, infected kidney and an ultrasound and/or CT is therefore indicated.

In males <50 years of age, the symptoms of dysuria or urinary frequency are usually due to sexually transmitted disease-related infection of the urethra or prostate. **Withholding urination may enhance the likelihood of a positive result on urethral swab testing in a male patient with minimal discharge. Obtaining a first void specimen rather than midstream stream specimen is helpful to diagnose urethritis.**[24,25]

22. Answer: D

Asymptomatic bacteriuria is diagnosed in the presence of >10^5 CFU/mL of a single bacterial species, ideally on two successive urine cultures, in patients without symptoms. It is uncommon (5%) in healthy, non-pregnant, sexually active women aged 18–40 years but occurs in up to 30% of pregnant women and up to 40% of female nursing home residents. It is also common in patients with indwelling urinary catheters.

Screening and treatment is only indicated in pregnant women and patients before urological procedures. Complications that may result from untreated bacteriuria in pregnancy include premature labour, perinatal mortality, maternal anaemia and maternal pyelonephritis. In all other cases, antibiotic treatment does not decrease symptomatic episodes but will lead to the emergence of more resistant organisms.[24,25,29]

23. Answer: B

The presence of gross haematuria in patients with a UTI (hemorrhagic cystitis) occurs in 30–40% of female cases, most often young adults. It is unusual in males and a more serious cause must be considered. Gross haematuria is more common with lower UTI (haemorrhagic cystitis) and occurs infrequently with pyelonephritis. When present, the differential should include calculi, cancer, glomerulonephritis, tuberculosis, trauma and vasculitis.

Flank pain, costovertabral angle tenderness and renal tenderness to deep palpation may also be associated with cystitis because of referred pain. When it occurs in association with fever and chills, nausea, vomiting and prostration, the clinical diagnosis is pyelonephritis.

Internal dysuria is more associated with UTI than external dysuria. In females, external dysuria or a history of vaginal discharge or irritation is more associated with vaginitis, cervicitis or PID than with UTI.

Clinical findings cannot reliably differentiate between upper and lower tract infections. About 30–50% of women with signs and symptoms restricted to the lower urinary tract have silent (or subclinical) infection of the kidney.[24,25,30]

24. Answer: B

Children with UTI are more likely to have a family history of UTI in first-degree relatives than children without UTI. This may be explained by a genetic predisposition to risk factors such as VUR and the presence of specific blood-group antigens which, when expressed on the surface of urinary epithelium, promote adherence of bacteria.

Up to 10% of girls will have had a UTI by adulthood, with most cases occurring after the age of 2 years. Only 2–3% of boys will be diagnosed with a UTI during childhood and more than 60% of these occur before the age of 2 years. UTIs are an uncommon occurrence in boys older than 4 years of age.

VUR is present in at least 20–30% of children having their first UTI, compared with only 1–3% of the general paediatric population. A single UTI has a relatively high risk of recurrent infections, with various studies showing rates of 15%–40%. Most recurrences occur within 2 years of the initial UTI. Factors associated with recurrence include young age at first UTI, urinary tract abnormalities including VUR, and voiding dysfunction.[31,32]

25. Answer: A

Guidelines referring to the appropriate investigations that should be performed in children with a first UTI remain controversial.

It is generally recommended that *renal ultrasound* should be performed in all young children after an initial febrile UTI, mainly to detect anatomical abnormalities, ureteral and calices dilation and to exclude obstruction. This should ideally be performed within 6 weeks of diagnosis. **It is recommended that a renal ultrasound be performed at the time of UTI in the presence of**

- **a first UTI and age <6 months**
- **failure to respond to antibiotic treatment within 48 hours**
- **the child being seriously ill**
- **infection with an atypical organism**
- **severe pain or haematuria**

- **poor urinary stream**
- **an abdominal mass**
- **oliguria or renal impairment despite adequate hydration.**

MCUG (to detect VUR and posterior urethral valves) may be necessary but the decision to perform this invasive and sometimes distressing investigation needs to be individualised. The value of demonstrating vesicoureteric reflux in assisting future management is controversial. It is currently a matter of clinician preference and can be discussed with the parents at follow-up. It may be done in children under 6 months of age (especially boys), and may be necessary for older children according to circumstances. A *DMSA scan* is not routinely recommended in all patients. If performed, it should be done after 3–6 months of the UTI to detect renal scarring, as acute pyelonephritis is also associated with photopenia on DMSA scanning.

SPA is a simple and safe procedure. It can be performed in children under 2 years of age, as a full bladder in this age group normally sits above the bony pelvis.[32,33]

References

1. Sinert R, Peacock P. Acute renal failure. In: Tintinalli J, Stapczynski J, Ma O, et al, editors. Tintinalli's emergency medicine: a comprehensive study guide. 7th ed. New York: McGraw Hill Medical; 2011. p. 615–21.
2. Agrawal M, Swartz R. Acute renal failure. American Family Physician. Online. Available: http://www.aafp.org/afp/20000401/2077.html; 8 Apr 2011.
3. Hilton R. Acute renal failure. BMJ 2006;333:786–90.
4. Wolfson AB. Renal failure. In: Marx JA, Hockberger RS, Walls RM, editors. Rosen's emergency medicine: concepts and clinical practice. 7th ed. Philadelphia: Elsevier; 2009. p. 1257–81.
5. Barrett BJ, Parfrey PS. Preventing nephropathy induced by contrast medium. N Engl J Med 2006;354:379–86.
6. Schweiger MJ, Chambers CE, Davidson CJ, et al. Prevention of contrast induced nephropathy: recommendations for the high risk patient undergoing cardiovascular procedures. Catheterization and Cardiovascular Interventions 2007;69:135–40.
7. Spektor M, Sinert R. Emergencies in renal failure and dialysis patients. In: Tintinalli J, Stapczynski J, Ma O, et al, editors. Tintinalli's emergency medicine: a comprehensive study guide. 7th ed. New York: McGraw Hill Medical; 2011. p. 624–30.
8. Venkat KK, Venkat A. Care of the renal transplant recipient in the emergency department. Ann Emerg Med 2004;44:330–41.
9. Fish RM, Massa MK. The transplant patient. In: Tintinalli J, Stapczynski J, Ma O, et al, editors. Tintinalli's emergency

medicine: a comprehensive study guide. 7th ed. New York: McGraw Hill Medical; 2011. p. 1997–2012.
10. Kelen G, Hsu E. Fluids and electrolytes. In: Tintinalli J, Stapczynski J, Ma O, et al, editors. Tintinalli's emergency medicine: a comprehensive study guide. 7th ed. New York: McGraw Hill Medical; 2011. p. 117–29.
11. Gibbs MA, Tayal VS. Electrolyte disturbances. In: Marx JA, Hockberger RS, Walls RM, editos. Rosen's emergency medicine: concepts and clinical practice. 7th ed. Philadelphia: Elsevier; 2009. p. 1615–32.
12. Nyirenda MJ, Tang JI, Padfield PL, et al. Hyperkalemia. BMJ 2009;339:1019–24.
13. Weisberg LS. Management of severe hyperkalemia. Crit Care Med 2008;36(12):3246–51.
14. Hollander-Rodriguez JC, Calvert JF. Hyperkalemia. American Family Physician 2006;73(2):283–90. Online. Available: http://www.aafp.org/afp/2006/0115/p283.html; 10 Apr 2011.
15. Mahoney BA, Smith WAD, Lo D, et al. Emergency interventions for hyperkalaemia. Cochrane Database of Systematic Reviews 2005, Issue 2. Art. No: CD003235. DOI: 10.1002/14651858.CD003235.pub2.
16. Bontempo LJ, Kaji AH. Rhabdomyolysis. In: Marx JA, Hockberger RS, Walls RM, editors. Rosen's emergency medicine: concepts and clinical practice. 7th ed. Philadelphia: Elsevier; 2009. p. 1650–7.
17. Counselman F, Lo B. Rhabdomyolysis. In: Tintinalli J, Stapczynski J, Ma O, et al, editors. Tintinalli's emergency

medicine: a comprehensive study guide. 7th ed. New York: McGraw Hill Medical; 2011. p. 622–4.

18. Bosch X, Poch E, Grau JM. Review article: Rhabdomyolysis and acute kidney injury. N Engl J Med 2009;361:62–72.

19. Koerner C. Renal emergencies in infants and children. In: Tintinalli J, Stapczynski J, Ma O, et al, editors. Tintinalli's emergency medicine: a comprehensive study guide. 7th ed. New York: McGraw Hill Medical; 2011. p. 866–72.

20. Klap P, Hemphill R. Acquired hemolytic anemia. In: Tintinalli J, Stapczynski J, Ma O, et al, editors. Tintinalli's emergency medicine: a comprehensive study guide. 7th ed. New York: McGraw Hill Medical; 2011. p. 1488–93.

21. McCollough M, Sharieff GQ. Genitourinary and renal tract disorders. In: Marx JA, Hockberger RS, Walls RM, editors. Rosen's emergency medicine: concepts and clinical practice. 7th ed. Philadelphia: Elsevier; 2009. p. 2200–17.

22. Tan AJ, Silverberg MA. Hemolytic uremic syndrome in emergency medicine. Online. Available: http://emedicine.medscape.com/article/779218-overview; 10 Apr 2011.

23. Pan CG, Avner ED. Acute poststreptococcal glomerulonephritis. In: Kliegman R M, Behrman RE, Jenson HB, et al, editors. Nelson textbook of pediatrics. 19th ed. Philadelphia: Saunders Elsevier; 2011. p. 1783–6.

24. Howes D, Bogner M. Urinary tract infection and hematuria. In: Tintinalli J, Stapczynski J, Ma O, et al, editors. Tintinalli's emergency medicine: a comprehensive study guide. 7th ed. New York: McGraw Hill Medical; 2011. p. 630–40.

25. Ban KM, Easter JS. Selected urologic problems. In: Marx JA, Hockberger RS, Walls RM, editors. Rosen's emergency

medicine: concepts and clinical practice. 7th ed. Philadelphia: Elsevier; 2009. p. 1297–324.

26. Nicks B, Manthey D. Male genital problems. In: Tintinalli J, Stapczynski J, Ma O, et al, editors. Tintinalli's emergency medicine: a comprehensive study guide. 7th ed. New York: McGraw Hill Medical; 2011. p. 645–51.

27. Sharp VJ, Takacs EB, Powell CR. Prostatitis: diagnosis and treatment. American Family Physician 2010;82(4). Online. Available: http://www.aafp.org/afp.

28. Touma NJ, Nickel JC. Prostatitis and chronic pelvic pain syndrome in men. Med Clin N Am 2011;95:75–86.

29 Therapeutic Guidelines Limited. Emergency version 2008. Infectious disease emergencies. Urinary tract infections. Online. Available: www.tg.org.au; 9 Apr 2011.

30. Shoff WH, Green-McKenzie J, Edwards C, et al. Acute pyelonephritis. Online. Available: http://emedicine.medscape.com/article/245559-clinical; 12 Apr 2011.

31. Kennedy S. UTI in children – part 1. How to treat 2009. Online. Available: http://www.australiandoctor.com.au/education/how-to-treat/paediatrics/uti-in-children—part-1; 12 Apr 2011.

32. Byerley JS, Steiner MJ. Urinary tract infection in infants and children. In: Tintinalli J, Stapczynski J, Ma O, et al, editors. Tintinalli's emergency medicine: a comprehensive study guide. 7th ed. New York: McGraw Hill Medical; 2011. p. 854–60.

33. Kennedy S. UTI in children – part 2. How to treat 2009. Online. Available: http://www.australiandoctor.com.au/education/how-to-treat/paediatrics/uti-in-children—part-2:12 Apr 2011.

1. Answer: B

Fully cross-matched blood refers to blood that is: ABO and Rh typed; screened for antibodies; and compatibility tested with the donor's blood to identify the potential for a transfusion reaction. This involves mixing the donor's RBCs and serum with the recipient's red blood cells (RBCs) and serum. Testing is performed immediately after mixing, after incubation at 37°C for varying times, and with and without an antiglobulin reagent to identify surface immunoglobulin or complement. When properly cross-matched, each unit of blood product can be administered with the expectation of safety. Full cross-match takes approximately 60 minutes, which is too long in an emergency situation.

In an emergency situation, three alternatives to fully cross-matched blood, in order of preference, exist:
1. *Type-specific blood with an abbreviated cross-match* (takes approximately 30 minutes)

This includes testing for ABO and Rh compatibility. In addition, the recipient's serum is screened for unexpected antibodies, and an immediate 'spin' cross-match is performed at room temperature as opposed to 37°C.
2. *Type-specific blood* (takes approximately 2 minutes)

Testing is only done for ABO and Rh compatibility, without screen or immediate spin cross-match. Type-specific blood that is not cross-matched has been given in numerous military and civilian series without serious consequences. While the type-specific blood is being transfused, the antibody screen and the cross-match are carried out in the laboratory. It is rare that a few minutes cannot safely be expended to allow the blood bank to release type-specific blood.
3. *Group O blood* (immediately available)

Either Rh+ or Rh- blood can be given in an emergency situation because immediate transfusion reactions do not occur due to rhesus incompatibility. However, Rh- patients may become sensitised if Rh+ blood is given and they theoretically carry the risk of experiencing a transfusion reaction if exposed again to Rh-incompatible blood. However, significant, subsequent transfusion reactions with

Rh-incompatible blood sensitised to the Rh factor are very rare. Many nowadays advise the **routine use of the more widely available O Rh+ packed cells in all patients for whom the Rh factor has not been determined, except in females of childbearing age, for whom future Rh sensitisation may be an important consideration.**[1,2]

2. Answer: D

In adults, 'massive transfusion' may be defined as a transfusion of half of one blood volume in 4 hours, or more than one blood volume in 24 hours (approximately 10 units PRBC).

In trauma patients with critical bleeding, early transfusion of FFP and platelets is associated with reduced mortality and subsequent RBC requirements. **The exact ratio of PRBC to platelets to FFP that should be used during massive transfusion is controversial.** Traditionally, a ratio of PRBC to FFP of 1:4 has been used but data from both civilian and military experience reveal that patients receiving more than 10 U PRBC show decreased mortality when they simultaneously receive FFP in a ratio of PRBC to FFP of 1:1, rather than 1:4. Evidence now suggests that in trauma patients with critical bleeding requiring massive transfusion, a ratio of ≤2:1:1 of RBCs:FFP:platelets is associated with reduced mortality. Another consensus article examining the use of blood products worldwide supported the administration of platelets in a massive transfusion protocol in a 1:1:1 ratio with PRBC and FFP; however, further research is needed to recommend target ratio of RBC:FFP:platelets. **The National Blood Authority Australia recommends that institutions develop a massive transfusion protocol (MTP) that includes the dose, timing and ratio of blood component therapy for use in trauma patients with, or at risk of, critical bleeding requiring massive transfusion as the use of a protocol is associated with reduced mortality.**

There is limited data to support or refute the use of rFVIIa in trauma patients and the indications for administration of rFVIIa in cases of traumatic haemorrhage remain unclear. Much of the current use of rFVIIa is for patients with critical bleeding unresponsive to conventional measures of surgical haemostasis and adequate component therapy. This use remains controversial, particularly because of concerns about the risk of potential thrombotic complications. **Currently, the routine use of rFVIIa in trauma patients with critical bleeding requiring massive transfusion is not recommended because of its lack of effect on mortality and variable effect on morbidity**. Furthermore, rFVIIa is approved in Australia and New Zealand only for the control of bleeding and prophylaxis for surgery in patients with inhibitors to coagulation factors FVIII or FIX, congenital factor VII deficiency and Glanzmann's thrombasthenia. Any use outside of these indications is considered 'off-licence'.

In trauma patients with, or at risk of, significant haemorrhage, TXA should be considered. A recently published randomised controlled trial has demonstrated improved survival in trauma patients who received TXA. In this international, multicentre randomised controlled trial of more than 20,000 patients, TXA (loading dose 1 g over 10 minutes, followed by infusion of 1 g over 8 hours) demonstrated a significant reduction in all-cause mortality at 4 weeks after injury and risk of death from bleeding. The investigators strongly endorse the importance of early administration of TXA in bleeding trauma patients and suggest that trauma systems should be configured to facilitate this recommendation. In patients presenting late (several hours after injury) the clinician should be more cautious and make an assessment of the individual benefits and risks of this treatment, since the drug is likely to be much less effective and possibly even harmful. A recent Cochrane review demonstrated that TXA safely reduces mortality in bleeding trauma patients without increasing the risk of adverse events. **Given the above evidence, TXA should be considered as an adjunct in these patients and should be administered as part of a locally adapted MTP in the setting of overall patient management, including strict attention to the control of bleeding, physiological and metabolic parameters, coagulation status and temperature maintenance.**[2-6]

3. Answer: A

It is not uncommon for patients to develop a fever during transfusion of blood products. Although fever is usually due to a *febrile non-haemolytic reaction*, more serious *haemolytic reactions* and *bacterial contamination* can be fatal and should always be considered.

Immediate haemolytic transfusion reactions occur when the recipient's antibodies recognise and haemolyse the donor's *red blood cells*. It is most commonly due to ABO incompatibility and usually is the result of human error; incorrect cross-matching or inadvertent administration of wrong blood to the wrong patient. The clinical manifestation of acute haemolysis includes fever, chills, low back pain, flushing, dyspnoea, tachycardia, shock, haemoglobinuria and an anxious feeling of impending doom. The risk of morbidity and mortality is usually proportional to the amount of blood received before recognition of the transfusion reaction. Therefore, in non-emergent blood transfusions, the initial rate of blood transfusion is low for the first 30 minutes to allow for identification of a transfusion reaction while minimising the volume of blood transfused.

A febrile, non-haemolytic reaction is defined as an increase in temperature of 1°C or higher during or up to 6 hours after the transfusion of blood products. It is one of the more common transfusion-related complications, occurring in 1 per 300 units of PRBC infused and is not commonly due to an interaction between recipient antibodies and donor *leucocytes* with release of cytokines. The clinical manifestation includes fever, rigors, headaches, myalgias, tachycardia, dyspnoea and chest pain. Febrile reaction is usually self-limited and will respond to antipyretics.

Sepsis due to bacterial contamination is an uncommon cause of fever because both the citrate preservative and refrigeration kill most bacteria.

Initially, it may be difficult to differentiate a febrile reaction from a more serious haemolytic transfusion reaction or sepsis. Accordingly, if any patient develops a fever attributable to a transfusion, the transfusion should be stopped immediately, the blood bank should be informed and blood samples should be collected from the opposite arm to transfusion for retype and repeat cross-match, direct and indirect Coombs', full

blood count (FBC), coags, urea and electrolytes test (U&E), haptoglobin, indirect bilirubin, lactate dehydrogenase (LDH), plasma free Hb, urine for Hb and the blood returned to the bank for testing. While lab confirmation is being performed, the sequel of haemolysis is treated supportively. Transfusion reactions are due to a specific interaction between a particular unit and a particular patient, therefore if a blood transfusion is still indicated, blood can be collected for retype and cross-match and a new unit should be transfused.[1,2]

4. Answer: C

Two brands of warfarin are currently available, Coumadin and Marevan. These two brands have not been shown to be bioequivalent and are therefore not interchangeable; subsequently, it is important that a patient remains with one or other of the currently available brands.

Warfarin acts by inhibiting the synthesis of functional vitamin K-dependent coagulation factors II, VII, IX and X (extrinsic coagulation pathway). Additionally, it blocks the synthesis of antithrombin protein C and protein S, which is responsible for the transient state of increased thrombogenesis at the start of warfarin therapy. For this reason, patients with acute thromboembolic events, such as deep vein thrombosis (DVT), pulmonary embolism (PE) or embolic stroke, should be given heparin or low molecular weight heparin concurrently when starting warfarin. **The heparin or low molecular weight heparin can be ceased after a minimum period of 5 days of combined therapy with warfarin *and* after the INR has been in the therapeutic range for 48 hours. A minimum of 5 days of heparin should be given, even if the INR reaches the desired level beforehand.** Patients at less immediate risk, such as patients in stable atrial fibrillation without embolic events, may be safely started on warfarin without concurrent heparin.

The major adverse effect of warfarin is an increased bleeding tendency and many factors can increase the risk. A patient's risk of bleeding is greatest in the first 3 months of starting warfarin therapy. **Age, especially age >70 years, is one of the strongest risk factors for bleeding.** Generally, elderly people have increased sensitivity to the anticoagulant effect of warfarin and require a lower mean daily dose than younger

patients. In one study, recent antibiotic use was the second greatest risk factor (after age) for over-anticoagulation. Other risk factors include a history of past bleeding, previous stroke, history of falls, liver disease, chronic renal failure, change in interacting medications, change in, or poor, nutrition and large fluctuations of INR. **Although the bleeding risk increases as the INR increases, 50% of bleeding episodes occur while the INR is <4.0.[7,8,9]**

5. Answer: B

When managing a patient with supratherapeutic INR levels it is important to determine (1) the cause or precipitating event, (2) the presence or absence of bleeding, (3) if bleeding is absent, the risk of bleeding, and (4) the indication for warfarin therapy, as this will determine the subsequent managing strategy. The decision of which combination of reversal agents to use is based on the urgency (presence of significant bleeding or risk of bleeding), the completeness of reversal required (normalisation of INR or therapeutic INR), the level of INR and the risk of thrombosis when the anticoagulation is reversed.

In this scenario there is no evidence of clinically significant bleeding but there is also no additional information to determine this patient's risk for bleeding. **In the absence of bleeding, current consensus guidelines of the Australasian Society of Thrombosis and Haemostasis recommend the following therapy based on the *risk of bleeding* in patients with an INR >9.0:**

- Low risk of bleeding: cease warfarin therapy, give 2.5–5.0 mg vitamin K1 orally or 1.0 mg intravenously, measure INR in 6–12 hours and resume warfarin therapy at a reduced dose once INR <5.0.
- High risk of bleeding: cease warfarin therapy, give 1.0 mg vitamin K1 intravenously, consider prothrombinex-HT (25–50 IU/kg) and fresh frozen plasma (150–300 mL), measure INR in 6–12 hours and resume warfarin therapy at a reduced dose once INR <5.0. Examples of high-risk patients include the elderly, those with active gastrointestinal disorders (such as peptic ulcer or inflammatory bowel disease), those receiving concomitant antiplatelet therapy, those who underwent a major surgical procedure within the preceding 2 weeks, and those with a low platelet count.

Oral vitamin K1 is the route of choice as the *intravenous* route, although it produces a more rapid reversal, may be associated with anaphylactic reactions. There is no evidence that this rare, but serious, complication can be avoided by using low doses. In Australia and New Zealand, vitamin K1 is a mixed micelle-based formulation, and may not carry the same risk of allergies, including anaphylaxis, as earlier formulations. **The formulation of injectable vitamin K1, while not approved for oral use by government regulatory agencies in Australia and New Zealand, is preferred for the reversal of anticoagulation because of its dosing flexibility.** Additionally, intravenous administration also carries the risk of overcorrection (subtherapeutic INR). To temporarily reverse the effect of warfarin when there is a need to continue warfarin therapy, vitamin K1 should be given in a dose that will quickly lower the INR to a safe, but not subtherapeutic, range and will not cause resistance once warfarin is reinstated. For most patients, 1.0–2.0 mg of oral vitamin K1 is sufficient. If the INR is particularly high, as in this case, 5 mg orally may be required. Large doses of vitamin K1 may produce some resistance to reanticoagulation with warfarin, and this can be avoided by giving smaller doses. Larger doses are appropriate if a clinical decision has been made to discontinue further warfarin treatment.[9,10,11,12]

6. Answer: C

The onset of HIT is usually 5–10 days after initiation of heparin treatment but may occur sooner in patients who have been previously exposed to heparin. Heparin-induced thrombocytopaenia is caused by the formation of autoantibodies directed against both heparin and platelet factor IV. **This causes activation of platelets leading to both thrombocytopaenia and a tendency for thrombosis.** Thromboembolic complications can be venous, arterial,or both, and can be life or limb threatening. The platelet count usually returns to normal 4–6 days after heparin has been stopped and the risk of thrombosis is highest during this recovery phase. **HIT more commonly occurs with UFH but can also occur with LMWH, albeit approximately 10 times less frequent.** Therefore, anticoagulation with a nonheparin anticoagulant, such as fondaparinux, and not LMWH is recommended when HIT is suspected, even in the absence of thrombosis.

Bleeding is one of the major complications associated with the use of heparin. **Protamine can reverse the anticoagulant effect of UFH and is given as 1 mg per 100 U of total amount of heparin given intravenously within the past 3 hours**; although UFH half-life is dose-dependant, its anticoagulation effect can last up to 3 hours. In general, LMWH preparations cause less bleeding than UFH. Protamine will not reverse the anticoagulant effect of LMWH completely as it does not neutralise the inhibitory effect of LMWH on factor Xa. However, it still has a partial effect as it neutralises the inhibitory effect on thrombin. Enoxaparin is a LMWH commonly used in the ED. Protamine is given as 1mg intravenously for every 1mg of enoxaparin given in the previous 8 hours. If 8–12 hours since last dose of enoxaparin dose, give protamine 0.5 mg intravenously for every 1 mg of enoxaparin given.[10]

7. Answer: B

rtPA, a second-generation fibrinolytic, is the only approved treatment for acute ischaemic stroke. The total dose of rtPA is 0.9 mg/kg, with a maximum dose of 90 mg; 10% of the dose is administered as a bolus, with the remaining amount infused over 60 minutes. **No anticoagulants or antiplatelet agents should be given in the initial 24 hours following treatment;** this recommendation is mainly based on the initial NINDS protocol.

Tenecteplase, a third-generation fibrinolytic, is a modified version of rtPA that is more fibrin-specific, with potentially fewer bleeding complications, and has a longer half-life, which allows for a single-weight bolus dosing over 5–10 seconds. It has been approved for use in myocardial infarction, in which it is associated with fewer systemic bleeding complications than alteplase. **However, there are currently no randomised controlled trials of tenecteplase in acute ischaemic stroke and rtPA remains the only approved treatment.** A previous pilot dose-escalation study with intravenous tenecteplase showed promise as a potentially safer alternative. A subsequent phase IIB/III trial of tenecteplase in acute ischaemic stroke was unfortunately prematurely terminated due to slow enrolment and no convincing conclusions could be made.[10,13,14]

8. Answer: A

The mean corpuscular volume (MCV) is the most useful guide to the possible aetiology of anaemia and is used to classify the anaemic process as microcytic, normocytic and macrocytic. **The RDW measures the size variability of the RBC population and is useful in distinguishing the deficiency anaemias** (iron, vitamin B12, or folate) **from other causes**. It may be increased in early deficiency anaemia (iron, vitamin B12 or folate) even before the MCV becomes abnormal. RDW is also useful in differentiating iron deficiency (high RDW) from thalassaemia (normal RDW). Thalassaemia is a hereditary disorder caused by defective synthesis of globin chains, resulting in an inability to produce normal adult haemoglobin. The hallmark of thalassaemia is microcytic, hypochromic haemolytic anaemia.

The direct Coombs' test is used to detect antibodies on the RBCs. It is positive in autoimmune haemolytic anaemia, transfusion reactions and some drug-induced haemolytic anaemia. The indirect Coombs' test is used to detect antibodies in the serum and is routinely used in compatibility testing before transfusion.[15,16]

9. Answer: D

Severe acute pain due to a **vaso-occlusive crisis** is the most common manifestation of SCD requiring hospital admission. Acute pain frequently occurs spontaneously, but may be precipitated by hypoxia, dehydration, infections, cold weather or stress. **Initial management should be aimed at providing rapid *pain control* and *hydration*.** Opioids are usually required for severe pain but NSAIDs may have an additive role in combination with opioids for severe pain. There is currently no evidence to guide clinicians regarding the optimal choice of intravenous fluid. Dextrose (5%) can induce hyponatraemia, which may be of marginal benefit during painful crises, although significant hyponatraemia should be avoided. Once pain is controlled, the *underlying cause* should be assessed and further investigations should be undertaken for atypical pain. Although *supplemental oxygen* is commonly used routinely for painful crises, it has not been proven to be of routine benefit. Current recommendations support the use of oxygen if oxygen saturation is <95%. SCD patients are more susceptible to serious infection, especially with encapsulated organisms, and broad-spectrum *antibiotics* should be started if the patient is febrile (temperature >38°C), generally unwell, has chest symptoms or signs, or infection is suspected for some other reason. Low-grade fever is common during an acute crisis. White cell counts are routinely elevated in SCD and leucocytosis does not always equate with infection. A WCC >20,000 with an increased number of bands is not typical for sickle cell crises alone and a potential infection should be considered.

A serious complication is *aplastic crisis*. This is usually caused by infection with parvovirus B-19. This virus infects RBC progenitors in bone marrow, resulting in impaired cell division for a few days. A subsequent very rapid drop in haemoglobin occurs with few or no reticulocytes present. The leukocyte and platelet counts are usually normal. The condition is self-limited, with bone marrow recovery occurring in 7–10 days, followed by brisk reticulocytosis. Transfusion may be required in the interim.

Acute splenic sequestration is a medical emergency characterised by the onset of life-threatening anaemia with rapid enlargement of the spleen and high reticulocyte count. Treatment of the acute episode requires early recognition, volume resuscitation and aggressive transfusion support. Blood for transfusion should be leucodepleted and matched for Rh (C, D and E) and Kell antigens.[17,18]

10. Answer: A

ITP is an acquired autoimmune disease, often precipitated by intercurrent viral infections that result in the rapid destruction of platelets. **Patients usually present with petechiae and/or purpura that is flat, with the rest of the physical examination normal.** Palpable petechiae/purpura suggests vasculitis, subacute bacterial endocarditis (SBE), systemic lupus erythematosos (SLE) or rheumatoid arthritis. Occasionally, a spleen tip may be palpable, but prominent hepatosplenomegaly or lymphadenopathy should raise the suspicion of an alternative diagnosis. The laboratory hallmark of ITP is an isolated thrombocytopaenia with normal white and red blood cell counts. Review of the peripheral blood smear is important to ensure the presence of normal white blood cell morphology and differential and normal red blood cell morphology. The peripheral smear typically shows a reduced number of platelets that are large and well-granulated, suggesting a platelet destructive state. The presence of any other abnormality on peripheral smear would suggest an alternate diagnosis.[19,20]

11. Answer: D

This child most likely has idiopathic thrombocytopaenic purpura (ITP); the result of thrombocytopaenia caused by immune destruction of platelets, often precipitated by intercurrent viral infections. **Acute ITP is more common in young children and typically resolves spontaneously within 2–3 months, independent of any treatment.** Chronic ITP is more common in adults, usually lasts more than 3 months and rarely remits spontaneously or with treatment.

The treatment of childhood ITP is controversial. There is no consensus as to whether 'watchful waiting' or pharmacologic intervention is most appropriate. Both the American Society of Hematology and British Society of Haematology have published guidelines for the management of ITP in children based on expert opinions and observational studies. **The majority of children will not require treatment, as serious bleeding is rare.** The risk of bleeding in ITP is lower for any given platelet count compared with other conditions and even pronounced skin purpura and bruising do not indicate a serious bleeding risk on their own. The British Society of Haematology guidelines currently recommend that that children be classified clinically and not by platelet count as even children with severe thrombocytopaenia ($<10 \times 10^9$/L) usually have 'mild' clinical symptoms.

Treatment, if indicated, is employed to promote platelet recovery and include corticosteroids, intravenous immunoglobulins (IVIg) and anti-Rh(D) immunoglobulin. **Platelet transfusions are of no value in the management of ITP as platelets will be rapidly consumed by circulating antiplatelet antibodies.** Current treatment recommendations from the British guidelines:

- Children with acute ITP and mild clinical disease may be managed *expectantly* with supportive advice and a 24-hour contact point, irrespective of platelet count.
- If a child has mucous membrane bleeding and more extensive cutaneous symptoms, *high-dose prednisolone* 4 mg/kg/d is effective.

- *IVIg* should be reserved for emergency treatment of serious bleeding symptoms or in children undergoing procedures likely to induce blood loss.
- *Platelet transfusions* should only be given for intracerebral haemorrhage (ICH) or other life-threatening bleeding, and then in much larger doses than for marrow failure. At the same time, immunomodulatory treatment should be given with high-dose intravenous steroids or IVIg.

Regardless of whether pharmacologic therapy is used, restriction of activity should be recommended in all children with ITP. In addition, medications with antiplatelet activity, including the nonsteroidal anti-inflammatory drugs, should be avoided.[19–22]

12. Answer: C

Abnormal bleeding is usually due to platelet deficiency or dysfunction, clotting factor deficiency, or a combination. **Bleeding related to *platelets* presents with petechiae and mucosal bleeding** that manifests as easy bruising, gingival bleeding, epistaxis, haematuria, gastrointestinal bleeding or heavy menses. **Conversely, patients with spontaneous deep bruises, haemarthrosis, retroperitoneal bleeding, or intracranial bleeding are more likely to have a *coagulation deficiency* (i.e. haemophilia A and B).**

Haemophilia A is a disorder due to deficiency in factor VIII, whereas haemophilia B is due to a deficiency in factor IX. Haemophilia A and B are clinically indistinguishable from each other. In patients with haemophilia, the prothrombin time (PT), which measures the extrinsic pathway, will be normal and the aPPT, which measures the intrinsic coagulation cascade, will be abnormal.

Von Willebrand's factor (vWD) is the most common congenital bleeding disorder. Von Willebrand's factor (vWF) is a cofactor for platelet adhesion as well as the carrier protein for factor VIII. **Patients with vWD may present with features of both platelet and clotting factor dysfunction. Skin and mucosal bleeding symptoms are common.** Haemarthrosis is not typical unless severe disease is present. Common abnormalities seen in vWD include prolonged bleeding time, low or normal vWF antigen and low vWF activity. The PT should be normal and about half of patients will have mildly prolonged aPTT.[23]

13. Answer: D

Fever in cancer patients are defined as a single oral temperature ≥ 38.3°C, or an elevation of 38°C on at least 2 occasions or persisting >1 hour. All patients presenting with fever following chemotherapy should be assumed neutropenic until proven otherwise. Although rectal measurement most accurately reflects core body temperature, the theoretical risk of bacterial translocation during the procedure of inserting the thermometer into the anus is not recommended in these patients, and therefore oral or axillary measurements are preferred. **Most fevers (55–70%) occurring in cancer patients have an infectious origin.** Other causes include inflammation, transfusions, antineoplastics, antimicrobials and tumour necrosis.[24,25]

14. Answer: B

Approximately 85% of the initial pathogens are bacterial. Gram-negative bacilli, particularly *Pseudomonas aeruginosa,* used to be the most common pathogens found in the blood of febrile neutropenic patients until the 1980s. **However, the administration of prophylactic antibiotics primarily active against gram-negative pathogens during chemotherapy, the widespread use of indwelling intravascular devices and newer chemotherapy regimens have lead to an increase in gram-positive pathogens and currently gram-positive bacteria account for 60–70% of microbiologically confirmed infections in these patients.** *Staphylococcus aureus, Staphylococcus epidermidis* and *Streptococcus epidermidis* are the predominant gram-positive organisms. Once believed to be a contaminant, *S. epidermidis* has arisen as a major pathogen. *Escherichia coli, Pseudomonas aeruginosa* and *Klebsiella pneumoniae* remain the most common gram-negative pathogens. Fungal, viral and parasitic infections are also important primary and secondary complications.

Vascular access can be challenging in patients receiving chemotherapy. Therefore, indwelling vascular catheters should be retained as far as possible. Even when catheter infection is suspected, the infection can be successfully treated in most cases without removing the catheter. The collection of a blood culture from vascular catheter lumen in addition to peripheral blood cultures may further assist in the diagnosis of clinically relevant catheter-related blood stream infections (CRBSI) by allowing the time necessary for blood culture from the peripheral vein to become positive to be compared with the time until blood culture from a central venous catheter becomes positive. A differential time to positivity of ≥120 minutes has been shown to be predictive of CRBSI. This approach is particularly useful in patients in whom catheter retention is desirable. Removal of the line is indicated in the context of tunnel infections, persistent bacteraemia despite adequate treatment, atypical mycobacteria infection and candidaemia. Vancomycin should be added when infection of the line is suspected and should be administered through the line when possible.[24–28]

15. Answer: B

Tumour lysis syndrome (TLS) is a metabolic crisis that arises from massive cell death with release of cellular contents in the circulation. It is associated with either a rapid growing tumour, or after chemotherapy or radiotherapy. It most commonly occurs with haematologic malignancies because of rapid growth rates and cell turnover, bulky tumour mass and high sensitivity to antineoplastic agents. **The resultant electrolyte abnormalities include hyperkalaemia, hyperuricaemia, hyperphosphotaemia and hypocalcaemia.** Malignant cells can contain up to four times the amount of phosphorous than normal cells, and with the abrupt release into the circulation may produce a significant drop in calcium. Life-threatening complications, including arrhythmia and seizures, arise from *electrolyte abnormalities*, whereas *renal failure* is a common sequel from uric acid precipitation in the renal tubules.

Treatment is aimed at correction of electrolyte abnormalities and prevention of renal failure. Treatment of hyperkalaemia is identical to other causes of hyperkalaemia. However, administration of calcium is generally avoided unless there is evidence of cardiovascular instability (ventricular arrhythmia or widened QRS) or neuromuscular irritability (seizures), as it may cause metastatic precipitation of calcium phosphate. **Aggressive intravenous fluid hydration is the single most important intervention**. Not only does it help to correct electrolyte abnormalities by diluting extracellular fluid, but it also increases the intravascular volume with resultant improved renal flow and urine output. This counteracts precipitation of uric acid and calcium phosphate crystals in distal nephrons. The use of furosemide or mannitol for osmotic diuresis has not proven to be beneficial as first-line therapy. Instead, diuretics should be reserved for well-hydrated patients with insufficient diuresis, and furosemide alone should be considered for normovolaemic patients with hyperkalaemia or for the patients with evidence of fluid overload. Allopurinol is usually given because it inhibits the synthesis of new uric acid, but it has no effect on existing uric acid levels. Therefore, the effect is only seen after 48–72 hours. Haemodialysis should be considered if TLS is refractory to the above measures. The prognosis is good in the absence of renal failure.[24,25]

16. Answer: A

Pain **is by far the most common presenting symptom of MSCC, occurring in approximately 90% of patients.** It is typically worse at night when the patient is recumbent due to lengthening of the spine, or with Valsalva manoeuvre. Initially, the pain is localised and confined to the area of spinal metastases. As the tumour compresses or invades the nerve roots, radicular pain will be experienced. Most patients (80%) with MSCC have a prior diagnosis of cancer and it is therefore important to maintain a high clinical index of suspicion and low threshold for imaging in cancer patients presenting with back pain.

Motor deficit is the second most common symptom of MSCC (60–85%), followed by *sensory deficits* (40–80%). Weakness is most apparent in the proximal muscles. Frequently, it is rather described as clumsiness or heaviness, and can progress to complete paralysis. Sensory deficits rarely occur before motor deficits or pain, and they usually begin distally and ascend as the disease advances. *Autonomic/sphincter dysfunction* is typically a later finding (40–60%).[24,29]

17. Answer: B

There are three main mechanisms by which malignancy can cause hypercalcaemia of which the production of parathyroid hormone-related protein is responsible for 80% of cases (paraneoplastic syndrome). Other mechanisms include local bone destruction (metastases) and production of vitamin D analogues. **In general, calcium levels do not correlate with symptoms, since the acuity of the rise is more important.** Hypercalcaemia associated with cancer normally occurs rapidly and, therefore, the symptoms of hypercalcaemia are more dramatic. A slow increase in serum calcium may be relatively asymptomatic until reaching high levels.

Hypercalcaemia produces an osmotic diuresis and patients are often profoundly dehydrated; therefore, **initial treatment should begin with volume expansion with *intravenous saline.*** Volume expansion increases calcium excretion by decreasing passive reabsorption in the proximal tubule and the loop of Henle. *Furosemide* has little additive effect to the use of intravenous saline alone in the treatment of patients with normal cardiac and renal function and should be restricted to patients with heart failure and renal insufficiency to prevent fluid overload, as it may cause even greater intravascular volume depletion. The standard treatment for symptomatic hypercalcaemia is rehydration and the use of a bisphosphonate. **However, failure to rehydrate before the use of *bisphosphonates* can lead to renal failure due to deposition of calcium complexes in the kidney.** Pamidronate is a commonly used intravenous bisphosphonate. Adverse effects include transient flu-like illness attributed to an acute reaction to initial infusions, a transient exacerbation of bone pain, a fall in serum calcium concentration that is usually asymptomatic, and a transient lymphopenia. **Severe local reactions and thrombophlebitis have followed administration of pamidronate as a bolus injection, so it should be given by slow intravenous infusion (<60 mg/hour). Additionally, it should be used with caution in patients with renal impairment.** If creatinine clearance is <30 mL/min, pamidronate should be avoided unless there is life-threatening hypercalcaemia. With less severe renal impairment, the rate of infusion should be reduced to approximately 20 mg/hour. Other therapies include calcitonin and glucocorticosteroids.[24,30]

18. Answer: D

Acute leukaemia is the most common cancer in children and ALL accounts for approximately 75% of these cases. AML and ALL present in a similar manner, with symptoms and signs that are due to replacement of bone marrow by malignant cells and secondary bone marrow failure. Deep bone pain due to marrow involvement is not associated with tenderness. However, bone and periosteal leukaemic infiltration may have exquisite tenderness over the bone. Bone marrow infiltration with leukaemia 'blasts' results in anaemia, thrombocytopaenia and neutropenia, which often manifest as fever and infection, pallor, easy bleeding and petechiae. The peripheral white blood cell count may be high, low, or even normal at presentation. **In addition to *bone marrow failure*, patients with AML present with signs and symptoms that are uncommon in ALL; *extramedullary involvement* as well as signs and laboratory findings of *disseminated intravascular coagulation.* ** Manifestations of extramedullary involvement include gingival hyperplasia, subcutaneous nodules or 'blueberry muffins lesions', and discrete masses composed of AML blasts called chloromas. Gingival hyperplasia in a child is unusual and should raise alarm to the presence of a myelogenous leukaemia, even if no other signs or symptoms are present. Chloromas can occur anywhere but are common in the orbit or peri-orbital region.

The **most common complications of the acute leukaemias encountered in the ED** include:
- bleeding due to either:
  - thrombocytopenia
  - chemotherapy, or
  - disseminated intravascular coagulation (DIC)

DIC may occur in the setting of sepsis, newly diagnosed or relapsing AML, and hyperleucocytosis. Some AML blasts release a procoagulant tissue factor that can lead to life-threatening consumptive coagulopathy.
- tumour lysis
- hyperleucocytosis
- sepsis

These patients typically have functional neutropenia, even if their neutrophil count is normal, and they are at high risk for gram-positive and gram-negative bacteraemia or sepsis.[21,31,32]

19. Answer: B

Hyperleukocytosis is an extreme elevation of the blast count or white blood cell count greater than 100 × 10^9/L. The clinical presentation depends largely on the lineage and the number of circulating leukaemic blasts. Risk factors for hyperleukocytosis include age <1 year, male gender, certain subtypes of leukaemia (French-American-British (FAB) Classification M4, M5), and select cytogenetic abnormalities (11q23 rearrangements and the Philadelphia chromosome).

Complications associated with hyperleukocytosis include:
1. **Leukostasis**

Hyperleukocytosis and leukostasis should be considered a medical emergency because the mortality rate approaches 40%. It is caused by the increased viscosity and sluggish flow of circulating leukaemic blasts in tissue microvasculature resulting in microvascular obstruction with injuries to the lung (dyspnoea, hypoxaemia and respiratory failure) and central nervous system (headache, mental state changes, seizure and stroke) most commonly observed. The frequency of complications is higher in AML than in ALL because the myeloblasts are larger and more adhesive than lymphoblasts.
2. **Increased risk for TLS**
3. **Increased risk for DIC**. Disseminated intravascular coagulation occurs in 30–40% of patients with AML and in 15–25% of patients with ALL
4. **Increased risk for intracranial hemorrhage** if platelets <20 × 10^9/L

Patients with hyperleukocytosis should urgently be referred to the haematologist as rapid reduction in the number of circulating blast cells (leukocytoreduction) is essential. Prompt introduction of chemotherapy remains the mainstay of treatment with leukapheresis an important adjunct. **ED management includes aggressive intravenous hydration, prevention of TLS and avoidance of treatments that can increase blood viscosity such as pRBC and diuretics. Platelets do not increase the blood viscosity and should be administered for levels <20 × 10^9/L to decrease the risk of cerebral haemorrhage.** If coma is present and the diagnosis established, a temporising measure can be a 2 U phlebotomy with concomitant volume replacement with 2–3 L of normal saline.[21,32–34]

20. Answer: C

Brain tumours are the most common solid tumour in children, and are the second most common

childhood cancer. Medulloblastoma, a neuronal tumour of the posterior fossa, is the most common malignant brain tumour in children. A large study of 3300 newly diagnosed pediatric brain tumour patients performed by the Childhood Brain Tumor Consortium reported that nearly two-thirds of patients had chronic or frequent headaches before their first hospitalisation. However, headache is a common complaint in the pediatric population with the prevalence in elementary school children approximately 40–50% and up to 60–80% in the high school years. Additionally, **The Childhood Brain Tumor Consortium Study also showed that more than 98% of patients with newly diagnosed brain tumours presenting with headache also had objective neurologic findings.** Recommendations for further imaging in children with headache includes occipital location, association with seizures, association with recumbent position, association with vomiting, exacerbation with straining, presence of ominous signs (Cushing's triad, altered mental status), presence of objective neurologic findings (abnormal eye movements, optic disc distortion or papilledema), asymmetric examination (motor, sensory, deep tendon reflexes), coordination problems (ataxia, dysmetria) and macrocephaly in infants and toddlers.

The most common malignant abdominal tumours in children typically occur before the age of 5 years. Renal tumours and neuroblastoma are the most frequently diagnosed cancers arising in the abdomen. *Wilms' tumour* is the most common tumour of the kidney with a peak age of diagnosis at 2–3 years. The most common presentation of Wilms' tumour is the incidental discovery of a non-tender abdominal mass by parents, caregivers or primary care providers on routine examination. Most children appear well at diagnosis. *Neuroblastoma* is the most common extracranial solid tumour diagnosed in children. It is a cancer of neural crest origin and can arise in the adrenal gland or as a paraspinous mass anywhere along the sympathetic chain. As with Wilms' tumour, neuroblastoma is typically a disease of young children with 90% of cases diagnosed in children <5 years of age. Two-thirds of primary neuroblastoma tumours occur in the abdomen. Although neuroblastoma may also present as a painless abdominal mass, constitutional symptoms often occur due to a high prevalence of metastatic disease at diagnosis. Children with neuroblastoma may appear ill and are often irritable. Periorbital ecchymoses and proptosis are classic signs due to metastatic involvement of periorbital bones.[21,32,33]

References

1. Gorgas DL. Transfusion therapy: blood and blood products and reversal of warfarin-induced coagulopathy. In: Roberts JR, Hedges JR, editors. Clinical procedures in emergency medicine. 5th ed. Philadelphia: Elsevier; 2009. p. 463–80.

2. Coil CJ, Santen SA. Transfusion therapy. In: Tintinalli JE, Kelen GD, Stapczynski JS, editors. Emergency medicine: a comprehensive study guide. 7th ed. New York: McGraw-Hill; 2011. p. 1493–500.

3. The CRASH-2 collaborators. The importance of early treatment with tranexamic acid in bleeding trauma patients: an exploratory analysis of the CRASH-2 randomised controlled trial. Online. Available: http://www.thelancet.com. DOI:10.1016/S0140-6736(11)60278-X.

4. Roberts I, Shakur H, Ker K, et al. Antifibrinolytic drugs for acute traumatic injury. Cochrane Database Syst Rev 2011;1:CD004896.

5. Brunett PH, Cameron PA. Trauma in adults. In: Tintinalli JE, Kelen GD, Stapczynski JS, editors. Emergency medicine: a comprehensive study guide. 7th ed. New York: McGraw-Hill; 2011. p. 1671–6.

6. National Blood Authority Australia. Patient blood management guidelines: module 1. Critical bleeding/massive transfusion. Online. Available: http://www.nba.gov.au; 2 Aug 2011.

7. Blood product administration laboratory reference. Better Safer Transfusion (BeST) Program. December 2005. Online. Available: http://www.health.gov.au/best; 2 Aug 2011.

8. Campbell P, Roberts G, Eaton V, et al. Managing warfarin therapy in the community. Aust Prescr 2001;24:86–9. Online. Available: http://www.australianprescriber.com.

9. Baker RI, Coughlin PB, Gallus AS, et al. Warfarin reversal: consensus guidelines, on behalf of the Australasian Society of Thrombosis and Haemostasis Group. MJA 2004;181:492–7.

10. Slattery DE, Pollack CV. Anticoagulants, antiplatelet agents, and fibrinolytics. In: Tintinalli JE, Kelen GD, Stapczynski JS, editors. Emergency medicine: a comprehensive study guide. 7th ed. New York: McGraw-Hill; 2011. p. 1500–8.

11. Prasad S, Wootten MR, Kulinski N, et al. What to do when warfarin therapy goes too far. J Family Practice

2009;58(7):346–52. Online. Available: http://www. jfponline.com; 10 Aug 2011.

12. Ansell J, Hirsh J, Hylek E. Antithrombotic and thrombolytic therapy. 8th ed: ACCP guidelines. pharmacology and management of the vitamin K antagonists. Chest 2008;33(6):160S–98S.

13. Go S, Wrman D. Stroke, transient ischaemic attack and cervical artery dissection. In: Tintinalli JE, Kelen GD, Stapczynski JS, editors. Emergency medicine: a comprehensive study guide. 7th ed. New York: McGraw-Hill; 2011. p. 1122–35.

14. Haley EC, Thompson JLP, Grotta JC, et al. Phase IIB/III trial of tenecteplase in acute ischemic stroke. Results of a prematurely terminated randomized clinical trial. Stroke 2010;41:707–11.

15. Janz TG, Hamilton GC. Anemia, polycythemia, and white blood cell disorders. In: Marx JA, Hockberger RS, Walls RM, editors. Rosen's emergency medicine: concepts and clinical practice. 7th ed. Philadelphia: Elsevier; 2010. p. 1557–77.

16. Hemphill RR. Anemia. In: Tintinalli JE, Kelen GD, Stapczynski JS, editors. Emergency medicine: a comprehensive study guide. 7th ed. New York: McGraw-Hill; 2011. p. 1457–64.

17. British Committee for Standards in Haematology. Guidelines for the management of the acute painful crisis in sickle cell disease. British Journal of Haematology 2003;120:744–52.

18. Williams-Johnson J, Williams E. Sickle cell disease and other hereditary hemolytic anemias. In: Tintinalli JE, Kelen GD, Stapczynski JS, editors. Emergency medicine: a comprehensive study guide. 7th ed. New York: McGraw-Hill; 2011. p. 1480–8.

19. Dunn R. Abnormal haemostasis. In: Dunn R, Dilley S, Brookes J, editors. The emergency medicine manual. 5th ed. 2010. p. 938–50.

20. Santen SA, Hemphill RR. Acquired bleeding disorders. In: Tintinalli JE, Kelen GD, Stapczynski JS, editors. Emergency medicine: a comprehensive study guide. 7th ed. New York: McGraw-Hill; 2011. p. 1464–70.

21. Place R, Lagoc AM, Mayer TA, et al. Oncology and hematology emergencies in children. In: Tintinalli JE, Kelen GD, Stapczynski JS, editors. Emergency medicine: a comprehensive study guide. 7th ed. New York: McGraw-Hill; 2011. p. 929–47.

22. British Committee for Standards in Haematology General Haematology Task Force. Guidelines for the investigation and management of idiopathic thrombocytopenic purpura in adults, children and in pregnancy. British Journal of Haematology 2003;120(4):574–96.

23. Manson W, Hemphill RR, Kempton CL. Hemophilias and von Willebrand disease. In: Tintinalli JE, Kelen GD, Stapczynski JS, editors. Emergency medicine: a comprehensive study guide. 7th ed. New York: McGraw-Hill; 2011. p. 1475–80.

24. Blackburn P. Emergency complications of malignancy. In: Tintinalli JE, Kelen GD, Stapczynski JS, editors. Emergency medicine: a comprehensive study guide. 7th ed. New York: McGraw-Hill; 2011. p. 1508–16.

25. Ugras-Rey S, Watson M. Selected oncologic emergencies. In: Marx JA, Hockberger RS, Walls RM, editors. Rosen's emergency medicine: concepts and clinical practice. 7th ed. Philadelphia: Elsevier; 2010. p. 1590–603.

26. Therapeutic Guidelines Limited. Febrile neutropenia. Revised June 2010. (etg34, July 2011)

27. Tam CS, O'Reilly M, Andresen D, et al. Use of empiric antimicrobial therapy in neutropenic fever. Internal Medicine Journal 2011;41:90–101.

28. Marti Marti F, Cullen MH, Roila F. Management of febrile neutropenia: ESMO clinical recommendations. annals of oncology 2009;20(Suppl. 4):iv166–iv169.

29. Sun H, Nemecek AN. Optimal management of malignant epidural spinal cord compression. Emerg Med Clin N Am 2009;27:195–208.

30. Therapeutic Guidelines Limited. Hypercalcaemia of malignancy in patients receiving palliative care. Revised February 2010. eTG complete. Online. Available: www. tg.org.au; 1 Nov 2011.

31. Tubergen DG, Bleyer A, Ritchey AK. The leukemias. In: Kliegman RM, Behrman RE, Jenson HB, et al, editors. Nelson textbook of pediatrics. 19th ed. Philadelphia: Saunders Elsevier; 2011. p. 1732–9.

32. Nazemi KJ, Malempati S. Emergency department presentation of childhood cancer. Emerg Med Clin N Am 2009;27:477–95.

33. McCreight AL, Wickiser JE. Oncologic emergencies. In: Strange GR, Ahrens W R, Schafermeyer RW, editors. Pediatric emergency medicine. 3rd ed. New York: McGraw Hill; 2009. p. 835–47.

34. Adams BD, Baker R, Lopez JA, et al. Myeloproliferative disorders and the hyperviscosity syndrome. Emerg Med Clin N Am 2009;27:459–76.

1. Answer: A

The rationale for clearance antibiotics after an individual case of invasive meningococcal disease is to prevent secondary cases. Antibiotics are used to eliminate carriage in the asymptomatic carrier who was responsible for transmission of the meningococcus to the index case, therefore preventing transmission to other susceptible individuals in the carrier's close contact network. Clearance antibiotics are therefore indicated for the following contacts of the index case:

- household members and household visitors who have stayed overnight in the 7 days before the index case became unwell
- sexual and intimate kissing contacts
- family daycare attendees (i.e. where groups of children are cared for in a private home) and childcare attendees where a group stays together in a single room for a 4-hour period
- contacts sharing a hostel dormitory, military barracks or university dormitory
- travel contacts who were sitting immediately adjacent to the case for a journey/flight of over 8 hours
- the healthcare worker (HCW) who intubated the index case if a mask was not worn by the HCW (due to increased risk of disease in the HCW from respiratory droplet transmission during intubation).

The index case themselves is a poor transmitter of the meningococcus that is causing their illness. However, there is a small but definite risk of transmission of meningococci from a case to an HCW, therefore, clearance antibiotics are indicated under circumstances as mentioned above. Otherwise, saliva and low-level salivary contact is not important in the transmission of meningococcus. Therefore, contacts who have shared food, drinks, water bottles, cigarettes, bongs, lip balm, wind instruments, communion cups, referee's whistles and even dummies do **not** require antibiotics. Contacts of the case who attended classes, sporting events, parties and night clubs, childcare (unless as described above) or shared modes of travel within 7 days of the case's illness also do **not** require clearance antibiotics but

should be provided with information on invasive meningococcal disease.[1]

2. Answer: D

Neisseria meningitidis, a gram-negative intracellular diplococcus, is classified into serogroups according to their capsular polysaccharides. **Groups B and C cause the greatest disease in Australia but group C more commonly causes cases, compared with group B in most developed countries.** There is a vaccine against group C. Cases occur when organisms are transmitted to a susceptible individual from the nasopharynx of a carrier; carriers often have some immunity from invasive disease caused by the organisms they carry.

Clinical disease typically takes the form of meningitis or meningococcaemia; the two may coexist. Meningococcal disease has a wide spectrum of presentation including nausea, vomiting, myalgias, abdominal pain, leg or joint pain, pharyngitis, septic shock, pneumonia, myopercarditis and DIC. **The rash associated with meningococcal infection may be petechial or purpuric, but also may be urticarial, macular or maculopapular, particularly early in the disease. Patients with meningococcaemia without meningitis have a greater mortality than those with meningitis.**[2,3]

3. Answer: D

Blood cultures are a relatively expensive investigation with a low yield and high contamination rate that rarely changes management in the ED. **The primary determinant in detecting bacteraemia is the volume of blood taken; adult cultures should contain at least 10 mL of blood. The yield is also improved when the sample is collected at the onset of fever, and more than one set is taken over several hours.** Contamination is usually from skin organisms (coagulase negative *Staphylococci, Corynebacterium* spp., or *Propionibacterium,* or cultures where multiple bacteria are isolated).

Blood cultures are *not* recommended in immunocompetent patients with community-acquired pneumonia (CAP) who are treated as outpatients (however, they are recommended for inpatients).

Cultures are positive in 1–40% of patients with CAP but only change management in 1 in 500 patients. Anaerobic cultures are not warranted in patients with CAP, and should be reserved for patients with suspected abdominal and pelvic sources of infection. The most common organism isolated on culture in patients with CAP is *Streptococcus pneumoniae*.[4]

4. Answer: D

This patient's examination and X-ray findings are consistent with severe pneumonia as calculated by two pneumonia severity scoring systems used in CAP in Australia (CORB score >2, SMART-COP score of 5). In addition, she lives in a tropical area and is at risk of *Burkholderia pseudomallei* and *Acetinobacter baumanii* infection due to her heavy alcohol consumption. She should therefore receive broad-spectrum antibiotics which cover *B. pseudomallei* and *A. baumanii* plus *S. pneumonia*, *Legionella pneumophilia* and enteric gram-negative bacilli. **Therapeutic guidelines recommend the use of meropenem and azithromycin for patients living in tropical areas with risk factors for *B. pseudomallei* and *A. baumanii* infection;** these risk factors include diabetes, chronic lung disease, chronic renal failure and heavy alcohol consumption.

Severe CAP in patients from non-tropical regions and in patients in tropical regions who don't have risk factors for infection with *B. pseudomallei* and *A. baumanii* should again be treated with broad-spectrum antibiotics. Azithromycin should be given with ceftriaxone, cefotaxime or benzylpenicillin plus gentamicin; if the patient has an immediate/severe penicillin allergy they should receive moxifloxacin with azithromycin. (Choices A, B and C are therefore all correct choices, depending on drug allergies, for such a patient).[5,6]

5. Answer: C

Women who develop chickenpox infection within 2 weeks of likely delivery present the greatest risk to the fetus of developing neonatal varicella, which presents with a fever and vesicular rash plus potential visceral disease including pneumonia, meningoencephalitis and hepatitis. The mortality of neonatal varicella is 25% and is higher in premature babies and those whose mothers developed or were exposed to varicella zoster virus within 5 days of delivery. This patient should receive acyclovir to reduce *her* risk of complications of varicella infection such as varicella pneumonia; however, treatment does not reduce the risk of transmission of varicella to the fetus. If delivery occurs within 5 days of the patient developing a rash, the neonate should receive varicella-zoster immune globulin as PEP.

Congenital varicella syndrome usually occurs in infants whose mothers were infected between 8 and 20 weeks' gestation, but the transmission risk is low (2%) compared with the risk of other viruses.

The risk of viral transmission during delivery is not greater than at other times during pregnancy; therefore a caesarean section will not reduce the risk of neonatal varicella infection. If in a rural centre it would be prudent to discuss the case with the referral obstetrics and paediatric service prior to delivery.[7,8]

6. Answer: D

Patients may develop malaria despite appropriate chemoprophylaxis. Appropriate diagnostic testing includes full blood count, renal function and electrolytes, serum glucose, liver function tests and Coombs' tests. Results typically show a haemolytic anaemia (normochromic normocytic) with elevated unconjugated hyperbilirubinaemia, reduced serum haptoglobin, raised lactate dehydrogenase (LDH) and a positive direct Coombs' test. The serum white cell count is usually low rather than elevated, as is the platelet count. Cerebrospinal fluid analysis is undertaken to exclude other causes for a patient's altered level of consciousness, and is usually relatively normal in cerebral malaria. **Thick and thin films are examined to determine the species of parasite and the parasitic load. A negative blood film/ smear may be seen due to sequestration of the mature parasites from the peripheral blood;** in this instance antimalarial treatment should still be commenced, since delay can lead to markedly increased morbidity and mortality. Repeat films should be taken at least every 12 hours for 2–3 days to exclude malaria completely.

Falciparum malaria should be assumed to be resistant to chloroquine and treatment should be commenced with artesunate 2.4 mg/kg IV 12-hourly, or quinine IV loading followed by maintenance doses.[9,10]

7. Answer: C

Yellow fever is caused by *Flavivirus* infection transmitted by a mosquito and is endemic in parts of South America and Africa. Vaccination is mandatory prior to entering endemic areas; it is also highly effective, hence the infection is rare in travellers. Symptoms develop after an incubation period of 3–6 days and vary in severity from a flu-like illness to haemorrhagic fever with a 50% mortality rate. Typical symptoms include fever, headaches, myalgia, conjunctival infection, abdominal pain, facial flushing and relative bradycardia; some patients recover at this point while others relapse and develop high fever, vomiting, back pain, shock, multiorgan failure and coagulopathy. Treatment is supportive.

Dengue fever is caused by an *Arbovirus* prevalent in Asia, Africa and South America and including urban environments; it is transmitted by mosquitoes. The incubation period of 4–7 days is followed by sudden fever, headache, nausea, vomiting, myalgias and a fine pale morbiliform rash that spreads from the trunk to the face and limbs. If a second infection occurs, the patient may develop Dengue haemorrhagic fever, in which there is a bleeding diathesis, fatigue and a mortality of 10%; if untreated this develops into Dengue septic shock. Again, treatment is supportive.

Typhoid is caused by *Salmonella typhi* or *S. paratyphi* and is seen in travellers to Asia, Africa, Central and South America. It is spread by food contaminated with faeces or urine from infected persons or asymptomatic carriers. Vaccination is only 75% effective. Typical symptoms include high fever, chills, abdominal distension, constipation (more often than diarrhoea), and a relative bradycardia; after several days a pale red macular rash may appear on the trunk ('rose spots'). Complications include pneumonia, small bowel ulceration, DIC, anaemia, meningitis and renal failure. Diagnosis is clinical and confirmed by blood, urine, rose spot or stool culture. Treatment is traditionally with chloramphenicol, but in Australasia ceftriaxone or ciprofloxacin is commonly used.

Malaria is caused by *Plasmodia* species transmitted by infected mosquitoes. The incubation period is variable. Patients typically develop intermittent fevers with myalgia, malaise and headache, and possible chest pain, cough, abdominal pain and diarrhoea. As the illness progresses patients develop high fevers, tachycardia, orthostatic dizziness and extreme weakness; on examination these patients appear ill, and complications include splenomegaly, hepatomegaly, coagulopathy, delirium or reduced level of consciousness. Diagnosis is clinical and confirmed on blood smears (thick and thin films). Treatment will depend on the species of *Plasmodium* and possible resistance.[11]

8. Answer: D

Toxoplasmosis is the most common cause of encephalitis in patients with AIDS. Symptoms include headache, fever, seizures, altered mental status and focal neurological deficits. Diagnostic investigations include the presence of antibodies to *Toxoplasma gondii* in CSF and multiple ring-enhancing subcortical lesions on CT; these lesions may also be visible on non-contrast CT. Treatment for patients with suspected toxoplasmosis includes pyrimethamine and sulfadiazine, with folinic acid to ameliorate haematological side effects of therapy. Dexamethasone is also given to reduce oedema if necessary.

The differential diagnosis for ring-enhancing lesions in the brain of HIV-infected patients includes:

- **lymphoma** (typically a single lesion in the periventricular white matter or corpus callosum)
- **cerebral tuberculosis** (in which there is a characteristic inflammatory appearance with exudate in the basal cisterns)
- **fungal infections**

Patients with cryptococcal meningitis usually have normal neuroimaging. Patients with AIDS dementia complex usually experience a slow and subtle impairment of short-term memory and cognition, followed by more obvious changes in mental status and possible impairment of motor function and speech. Lymphoma presents with neurological deterioration over months.[12]

9. Answer: A

The risk of HIV transmission from percutaneous exposure to HIV infected blood is 0.3%. The risk is higher:

- after a deep injury
- with hollow devices
- where there is visible blood on the device

- if the procedure involved the needle being placed in an artery or vein
- if the source has a terminal illness

The prevalence of HIV among injecting drug users in Australasia is 1–2%, so the risk of HIV transmission in this case would be ~ 1:300 x 1:100 i.e. 1: 30,000. **The use of PEP should be discussed with an infectious diseases clinician**, and if prescribed, a 2 or 3 drug regime should be used (e.g. zidovudine plus lamivudine, and lopinavir/ritonavir); single-drug regimes are not indicated.

Hepatitis B immunoglobulin is indicated for PEP in patients who are not hepatitis B immune; patients who have been immunised and have evidence of hepatitis B antibodies at a level of > 10 mIU/mL do not require any HBV prophylaxis after a body fluid exposure, regardless of source status.

The risk of hepatitis C transmission after body fluid exposure is 1.8–10%. Many studies show no role for Immunoglobulin or antiviral agents (interferon, ribavirin) in PEP. Management involves early identification of infection since anti-viral treatment of acute HCV infection may increase rates of HCV clearance.[13,14]

10. Answer: C

Rabies is an invariably fatal disease transmitted by many mammals. **In Australia, no native animals carry the rabies virus but the related (and also fatal) Australian bat lyssavirus is found in several species of bats.** Disease can be transmitted by bites, scratches or mucous membrane contact.

Post-exposure prophylaxis (PEP) is required for all bite, scratch or mucous membrane exposures from bats in Australia and animals abroad, particularly dogs, monkeys and bats. It is preferably initiated within 24 hours; however, if there is a delay it should be administered regardless of the duration of the delay, as evidence exists that the incubation period of rabies can be more than a year. When followed *exactly,* PEP prevents development of rabies. The wound should be cleansed thoroughly using povidone-iodine (virucidal). Post-exposure prophylaxis should be administered as follows:

- Previously immunised patients
  - Human rabies immunoglobulin (HRIG) should not be given.

- Booster doses of rabies vaccine should be given into the deltoid (never gluteal) on days 0 and 3.
- Unimmunised patients
  - 20IU/kg HRIG; infiltrate as much volume as possible around the wound, with the remaining volume (if unable to give it all e.g. on the finger) given IM at an anatomical site distant from the vaccination site.
  - The vaccine should be given on days 0, 3, 7, 14 and 28.

HRIG is indicated only once to provide immediate antibodies before the patient responds to the vaccine by producing their own antibodies. There are no contraindications to HRIG or rabies vaccine, since the disease is fatal.[15,16]

11. Answer: D

Measles is a highly contagious endemic myxovirus infection that is now seen in sporadic cases due to widespread immunisation. An incubation period of 10 days followed by a 3-day prodrome of upper respiratory symptoms progresses to malaise, fever, conjunctivitis, cough, coryza and systemic toxicity. **The rash begins behind the ears and in the hairline and spreads to down the body and limbs; it is blanching, erythematous, maculopapular and lasts about 7 days. Koplik spots, 1 mm white spots on the buccal mucosa, are pathognomonic.**

Treatment is supportive and infection control to prevent spread of disease is vital. If the diagnosis is suspected patients should be isolated in a negative pressure room with droplet precautions (masks) taken at all times. Unimmunised contacts, including staff, should be vaccinated within 72 hours; in addition, **unimmunised exposed contacts who are at high risk of complications from the disease (infants < 1 year, pregnant women, immunosuppressed persons) should also receive immunoglobulin.**[14,17]

12. Answer: B

DGI affects up to 3% of patients with *Neisseria gonorrhoeae*. Two clinical pictures exist (although there may be overlap between them):

- a triad of a vesiculopustular rash, tenosynovitis and polyarthralgia
- purulent arthritis without skin lesions

Tenosynovitis may affect many tendons simultaneously, and is uncommon in other infectious forms of arthritis. The rash associated with DGI usually develops on the extensor surfaces of the wrists, palm and hands, as well as the dorsal aspects of the ankles and feet. Diagnosis is made on clinical findings plus skin, synovial, blood and cervical/urethral cultures, although these may be negative. Treatment involves parenteral antibiotics (ceftriaxone due to penicillin and quinolone resistance) plus azithromycin or doxycycline to cover *Chlamydia*; asymptomatic infected partners should also be treated.

Lyme disease is caused by the bacterium *Borrelia burgdorferi* and is transmitted to humans by ticks. There is little evidence that it occurs in Australia, however, it cannot be ruled out. Typical symptoms include fever, headache, fatigue, myalgia, arthralgia and a characteristic skin rash called erythema migrans (pink or red rash that starts as a small red spot and gradually spreads in a much larger circle with a characteristic bullseye appearance). The later stages involve neurological and cardiac consequences.

Reactive arthritis (formerly known as Reiter's syndrome) is characterised by an acute, asymmetric oligoarthritis occurring 2–6 weeks after an infectious illness (post venereal or post dysentery). Joint involvement typically involves the lower extremities. The classic triad of urethritis, conjunctivitis and arthritis are seldom seen. Additionally, there may be a psoriasis-like skin eruption, but petechiae, macules, papules or maculopapules do not occur.

Common manifestations of acute HIV infection (seroconversion illness) are fever, an erythmatous maculopapular rash, myalgia and arthralgia, headache and cervical lymphadenopathy. The rash is usually more generalised and joint effusions uncommon; DGI and acute HIV infection can coexist.

The differential for DGI includes:
- meningococcal arthritis
- hepatitis B (rash usually urticarial, usually polyarthritis)
- post-streptococcal arthritis (rash transient, not pustular)
- rheumatoid arthritis
- psoriatic arthritis
- reactive arthritis
- circinate balanitis (keratoderma blenorrhagicum)

- acute HIV infection (DGI and acute HIV infection can coexist)
- secondary syphilis (rash involves the palms and soles)
- Lyme disease[18–21]

13. Answer: D

Necrotising soft-tissue infections form a spectrum of disease differentiated by the depth of infection: adipositis, fasciitis and myositis (superficial to deep). They are most commonly a polymicrobial infection (caused by aerobes and anaerobes) but *Clostridium* species and group A *Streptococcus* can cause single-organism infections. *Clostridium* infections are now an uncommon cause due to improvements in hygiene and sanitation.

Clinical features of all the necrotising soft tissue infections include pain out of proportion to the clinical findings, mild erythema and oedema, brawny induration, and late in the course, possible crepitus due to gas formation. Gas formation may be due to multiple organisms, including *Clostridia*, *E. coli* and others. The patient is usually unwell but if presents early in the illness may have few systemic features. The mortality is high due to systemic toxicity, and early detection and immediate treatment are required. Management involves aggressive resuscitation and supportive care, broad-spectrum antibiotics (e.g. empiric carbapenem plus clindamycin, or benzylpenicillin plus clindamycin), surgical debridement including amputation if required, plus possible hyperbaric oxygen therapy after surgery.[22,23]

14. Answer: B

The clinical picture described is that of primary herpes gingivostomatitis, which may present in infancy or later in childhood or adulthood. Typically, vesicular lesions affect the oral cavity; these become ulcerated and then often spread to involve the lips, cheeks and chin. In young children, the presenting symptom may be oral pain or refusal to feed. The causative organism is HSV-1; HSV-2 causes neonatal herpes infections (including encephalitis) or genital lesions (seen in adults). Diagnosis can be made clinically, or confirmed with DNA swabs or viral culture of vesicle fluid. **Complications of herpes gingivostomatitis include herpetic whitlow, disseminated disease in immunosuppressed individuals, and herpes**

meningitis or encephalitis, although the latter is *not* preceded by known herpes infection in 80% of cases.

The mainstay of therapy is providing adequate analgesia and to ensure oral rehydration. Oral aciclovir may reduce the length and severity of symptoms when started early in the disease and should be considered, especially in severe cases. Topical aciclovir is ineffective.

Herpangina is an acute febrile illness usually affecting children in which there are ulcerated or vesicular lesions only over the posterior oropharynx; it is caused by enterovirus.[24,25–27]

15. Answer: C

Floods can potentially increase the transmission of:
- waterborne diseases, including
  - typhoid
  - cholera
  - hepatitis A
  - melioidosis
  - leptospirosis
- vector-borne diseases, including
  - malaria
  - dengue
  - Ross River fever
  - Barmah Forest virus
  - West Nile virus and related illnesses

It is important to consider these in any patient presenting with symptoms consistent with infection who presents during or in the few months following floods.

Symptomatology may narrow the diagnosis. *Vibrio cholera* causes watery diarrhoea and is spread by contamination of drinking water. Melioidosis due to the soil organism *Burkholderia* is seen typically in northern tropical Australia; it may present in a variety of ways including skin lesions (abscesses caused by infection of non-intact skin), pneumonia, splenic and liver abscesses. Mosquitoes transmitting dengue are predominantly seen in northern Australia. Ross River fever and Barmah Forest virus are transmitted by mosquitoes found throughout Australia; the typical presentation of illness is fever with arthralgia; there may also be a rash, deranged liver function tests (LFTs), and thrombocytopenia.[19,28–31]

16. Answer: A

Predisposing factors for cellulitis are:
- arterial or venous disease/harvest
- diabetes
- previous significant fracture
- dermatological conditions including eczema and dry skin
- trauma, bites and clenched fist injuries

The majority of cellulites are caused by gram-positive bacteria, of which the most common pathogens are β-haemolytic streptococci (*Staphylococcus pyogenes*) and *Staphylococcus aureus*, and gram-negative aerobic bacilli. Aeromonas species are associated with fresh water exposure, whereas *Vibrio* species are seen in salt water-associated infections. *Pseudomonas* is seen in infected burns, and mixed gram-negative and gram-positive aerobes and anaerobes in diabetic foot infections.

Most uncomplicated cases can be managed with outpatient antibiotics and supportive care including elevation of the affected part and addressing underlying causes; patient education is important. Certain patients should be treated aggressively including surgical debridement where needed; such patients include those with clenched fist injuries, orbital cellulitis and diabetic foot infections. Patients with diabetic foot infections will require anaerobic as well as aerobic cover. Suggested antibiotic regimes for mild–moderate diabetic foot infections include amoxicillin + clavulanic acid 875/125 mg po bd *plus* metronidazole 400 mg bd. For patients with penicillin hypersensitivity, ciprofloxacillin 500 mg bd *plus* clindamycin 600 mg tds can be given orally.

Often it is difficult to distinguish clinically between cellulitis and DVT, especially when the erythema overlaps the path of the deep veins in the leg. **Additionally, laboratory tests may not be specific enough to help differentiate between the two disease entities; there are no diagnostic lab tests for DVT and the white cell count may be normal or elevated in both conditions. An ultrasound is therefore indicated if any doubt exists regarding the diagnosis.**[23,32,33]

17. Answer: C

Primary TB occurs when mycobacterium tuberculosis (MTB) is transmitted via droplet infection to the lungs of a new host; some patients may be asymptomatic of primary TB but others manifest a pneumonitis similar to viral infection with fever, shortness of breath and possible chest pain. After a period of latent infection organisms proliferate; the lung apices are common sites of this reactivation due to their high oxygen content and blood flow.

A Mantoux test involves injection of purified protein derivative under the skin and measurement of the delayed hypersensitivity reaction generated; a positive reaction may indicate active or past infection or Bacille Calmette-Guérin (BCG) vaccination. Determining whether a patient who has a positive Mantoux test has active TB involves considering clinical features, microbiology and X-ray findings.

A positive early morning sputum smear is the best indicator of active infection; a chest X-ray may show typical features of reactivated pulmonary TB but the absence of findings is insufficient to rule out active infection that may be primary or reactivation (secondary). **Patients do not need to be isolated if they do not have a productive cough.**[34,35]

18. Answer: D

Standard precautions are used when caring for *all* patients and include handwashing, gloves, gowns, eye protection and masks, and when handling patient care equipment and linens, patient placement and environmental controls. *Airborne* precautions are used to prevent the transmission of infectious particles that may remain in the air and are dispersed widely by air currents, such as measles, varicella and TB. Patients with such illnesses should be placed in a negative pressure room with 6–12 air changes per hour from which the air is discharged to a high-efficiency filtration unit. HCW entering the patient's room should wear N95 masks and if patient movement outside their room is unavoidable the patient should also wear N95 masks during transport. *Droplet* precautions are used to prevent transmission of infectious particles that are generated by coughing, talking or sneezing such as *Neisseria meningitidis*, streptococcus, influenza and pertussis. HCW should wear masks when within 1m of the patient, and patients should be in a private room or at least 1 m from other patients or visitors. *Contact* precautions are used to prevent transmission of infections spread by direct contact with the patient or equipment in their environment

(e.g. multidrug resistant organisms, enterohaemorrhagic *E. coli*, respiratory syncytial virus (RSV), rotavirus, herpes simplex virus (HSV), impetigo scabies. Patients should be isolated in a single room and have their own dedicated multiuse equipment (e.g. BP cuffs); staff should wear gowns upon entering the room and discard these immediately before handwashing with antiseptic then leave the room.[23]

19. Answer: C

Empiric antibiotic choice is important in the care of ED patients with significant illness. Principles involve the following:

- The narrowest spectrum antibiotic should be used to cover likely pathogens.
- An antibiotic dose high enough to ensure efficacy and reduce the chance of selection resistance should be administered.
- Cultures should be taken before antibiotic administration where possible.
- Direct antigen tests etc. should be used to guide treatment before culture results are available.
- Where possible, local pathogens and their susceptibilities and drug resistance should be taken into account.
- In addition, patient factors including comorbidities (e.g. the presence of chronic kidney disease), the presence of immunosuppression, colonisation and recent infection should also guide treatment.

It is most useful to commence broad-spectrum cover and to then narrow the spectrum once pathogen and sensitivities are known. Suggested empiric antibiotic therapy for adults with sepsis of unknown source includes:

- flucloxacilin (or cephazolin or vancomycin in penicillin-sensitive patients) plus gentamicin
- in neutropenic patients: anti-pseudomonal cover with cefipime, ceftazidime or piperacillin-tazobactam
- marine infections: cephalosporin/clindamycin, fluoroquinolone plus doxycycline.

The first dose of gentamicin does not need to be reduced in the setting of renal impairment; however, subsequent doses should be reduced and the dosing interval should be increased and guided by gentamicin levels. Fluoroquinolone absorption is reduced with concurrent administration of calcium and magnesium salts, and such medications should not be given at the same time as the antibiotic.[36,37]

20. Answer: A

Food poisoning may be caused by viral (rotavirus, norovirus, astrovirus, enteric adenovirus) or bacterial pathogens. Most episodes of gastroenteritis due to food poisoning are self-limited and require only supportive care. Elderly patients, young children and the immunocompromised are more likely to have severe illness. Antibiotic therapy may be necessary in certain instances; the need is determined based on clinical symptoms and signs, disease severity, likelihood of resolution without antibiotics, and the suspected pathogen.

Botulism is caused by *Clostridium botulinum* associated with canned food, canned fish, and foods kept warm in dishes. **Patients usually present with vomiting and diarrhoea but classically develop a descending, symmetric paralysis.** The cranial nerves and bulbar muscles are first affected causing diplopia, dysarthria and dysphagia. Patients may report 'blurred vision'. Adult patients require botulinum antitoxin while infant botulism is treated with botulinum immunoglobulin.[38,39]

21. Answer: C

EBV (human herpes virus 4) is the usual cause of infectious mononucleosis (IM). After the 1–2 month incubation period a variety of illnesses can occur: typical EBV presents with fever, exudative pharyngitis, lymphadenopathy, splenomegaly and lymphocytosis. There may be elevated transaminases but jaundice and hepatomegaly are usually seen only in older adults. Splenomegaly is common, and is palpable in 50% of patients, usually during week 2 of the illness; all patients with IM should be counselled to avoid contact sports and strenuous activity for 4 weeks following the onset of symptoms to avoid the complication of splenic rupture.

Diagnosis is usually based on clinical symptoms plus rapid-result screening tests such as the monospot test, which indicates the presence of heterophile antibodies; such antibodies are induced by the EBV infection but are not specific to EBV and may be present with other infections including cytomegalovirus and toxoplasmosis.

Treatment is supportive in most cases and only in rare cases where complications such as anaemia and thrombocytopenia occur are controversial therapies such as corticosteroids used. Most patients recover fully from EBV, but resolution of symptoms including fatigue may take months; since patients may shed the virus intermittently for months or years after their infection, and the source of a case of IM is rarely known, there are no restrictions on when a patient with IM may return to school or work.[24,40]

22. Answer: D

Mycoplasma pneumonia is a cause of atypical pneumonia, seen often in older children, young adults and the elderly. Clinical features include a low-grade fever, chills, a non-productive cough, sore throat and headache; the onset is often insidious and patients may present after 2–3 weeks of symptoms. The cough can last 4–6 weeks. The chest X-ray may be relatively normal or may show patchy infiltrates, hilar adenopathy and pleural effusions but rarely shows lobar consolidation. Diagnosis is via serology and fluorescent antibody testing. Now measured less commonly than in the past, cold agglutinins are elevated in 50–70% of patients with mycoplasma pneumonia. Treatment is with macrolides or tetracyclines (in children > 10 years). The differential diagnosis includes *Chlamydia pneumoniae*, *Chlamydia psittaci* (seen with exposure to birds), viral pneumonia, or legionella pneumonia. [6, 41]

23. Answer: B

Gastrointestinal manifestations of HIV are common. *Oral thrush* affects 80% of HIV patients; it is treated with nystatin, clotrimazole or in resistant cases fluconazole or amphotericin B. However, *oesophagitis* is typically seen in patients with CD4 counts < 100 cells/uL and can be due to CMV or HSV as well as *Candida*. *Oral hairy leukoplakia* is due to opportunistic infection by EBV; adherent white patches along the lateral borders of the tongue are seen; treatment is not required and the lesions often recur after treatment with aciclovir. *Diarrhoea* is very common and may be due to drugs, bacteria, parasites (*Giardia*, *Cryptosporidium*, *Isospora*), viruses (CMV, HSV, HIV) and fungi (*Histoplasmosis capsulatum*, *Cryptococcus neoformans*). Cryptosporidium typically causes profuse watery diarrhoea and is difficult to treat, requiring both antiretroviral therapy and antiparasitic agents. *Proctitis* is also relatively common, and is usually due to

Neisseria, Chlamydia trachomatis, syphilis and HSV; it causes painful defecation, rectal discharge and tenesmus; treatment is of the causative agent.[12]

24. Answer: C

Cervicitis is commonly due to *Chlamydia trachomatis* infection; in women, infection may be asymptomatic or be a cause of infertility; other presentations include symptoms and signs of pelvic inflammatory disease, dyspareunia and vaginal discharge or lower abdominal pain if symptoms have been longstanding. Men are usually symptomatic with urethritis and a watery discharge; infection may also cause epididymitis, orchitis, proctitis and prostatitis.

Diagnosis is via PCR on an endocervical swab or 10 mL urine (men). Treatment involves either 7 days of doxycycline 100 mg po, or a single dose of azithromycin 1 g po; the latter is useful where compliance may be poor. Due to the common co-infection of patients with Chlamydial infections, treatment for *N. gonorrhoeae* should be given at the same time, with ceftriaxone 125 mg IM; sexual contacts within the last 60 days should also be treated for both infections.

Complications of chlamydial infection include pelvic inflammatory disease, infertility and ectopic pregnancy. **Chlamydia is a notifiable disease.**

Vaginal candida infections may produce cervicitis but there is a prominent white discharge present; treatment is with cotrimoxazole.[42]

25. Answer: A

Unimmunised patients are at risk for a number of now 'rare' infections including diphtheria, caused by the gram-positive rod *Corynebacterium diphtheria*, which may be toxigenic or non-toxigenic. Cutaneous diphtheria is usually due to non-toxigenic strains and produces punched out ulcers; it is treated with penicillin. Respiratory disease is usually due to toxigenic strains; a 2–5-day incubation period is followed by a sore throat with the characteristic adherent pseudomembrane coating the pharynx; patients typically develop a 'bull neck' due to soft tissue oedema; airway compromise is a major concern mandating intubation. Bacterial toxin effects are responsible for the local necrosis causing the pseudomembrane; the toxin is spread via the circulation and causes the delayed extrapharyngeal effects of myocarditis, cranial nerve palsies and skeletal muscle paralysis. Diagnosis involves isolating *C diphtheria* on culture of nasal and throat swabs (Loeffler's medium) or by fluorescent antibody testing; toxigenicity testing is also performed.

Management involves airway management, ventilation and critical care support; **specific therapy involves early intravenous administration of antitoxin 20,000–150,000 units followed by penicillin to stop further toxin production.** All patients should be nursed in isolated negative pressure rooms with staff wearing N95 masks plus gowns, gloves and eye protection. Contacts should have nose and throat swabs cultured, receive prompt erythromycin prophylaxis, and should be examined daily for 7 days for evidence of disease.[43,44]

References

1. Australian Government. Department of Health and Ageing. Management of sporadic cases of meningococcal disease. In: Guidelines for the early clinical and public health management of meningococcal disease in Australia. 2007. p. 21–4. Online. Available: http://www.health.gov.au/internet/main/publishing.nsf/Content/cda-pubs-other-mening-2007.htm; 19 Dec 2011.

2. Dilley S, Dunn R. Headache. In: Dunn R, Dilley S, Brookes J, editors. The emergency medicine manual. 5th ed. Adelaide: Venom Publishing; 2010. p. 646–71.

3. Yung A, Knott J. The approach to undifferentiated fever in adults. In: Cameron P, Jelinek G, Kelly A, editors. Textbook of adult emergency medicine. 3rd ed. Edinburgh: Elsevier; 2009. p. 402–7.

4. Dilley S, Dunn R. General infectious diseases. In: Dunn R, Dilley S, Brookes J, et al, editors. In: The emergency medicine manual. 5th ed. Adelaide: Venom Publishing; 2010. p. 723–9.

5. Therapeutic Guidelines Limited. Community acquired pneumonia in adults. In: eTG complete. Online. Available: www.tg.org.au; 18 Jul 2011.

6. Emerman CL, Anderson E, Cline DM. Community acquired pneumonia, aspiration pneumonia, and noninfectious pulmonary infiltrates. In: Tintinalli JE, Stapczynski JS, Ma OJ, editors. Emergency medicine: a comprehensive study guide. 7th ed. New York: McGraw-Hill; 2011. p. 479–91.

7. Borland M, Dunn R. Fever in children. In: Dunn R, Dilley S, Brookes J, editors. The emergency medicine manual. 5th ed. Adelaide: Venom Publishing; 2010. p. 803–14.

8. Riley LE. Varicella-zoster virus infection in pregnancy. In: UpToDate. Waltham: UpToDate Inc; 2011. Online. Available: www.uptodate.com.

9. Therapeutic Guidelines Limited. Malaria. In: eTG complete. Online. Available: https://www.tg.org.au; 2 Nov 2011.

10. Szela JJ, Tayali JJ, Band JD. Malaria. In: Tintinalli JE, Stapczynski JS, Ma OJ, editors. Emergency medicine: a comprehensive study guide. 7th ed. New York: McGraw-Hill; 2011. p. 1056–62.

11. VanRooyen MJ, Venugopal R. World travellers. In: Tintinalli JE, Stapczynski JS, Ma OJ, editors. Emergency medicine: a comprehensive study guide. 7th ed. New York: McGraw-Hill; 2011. p. 1080–93.

12. Rothman RE, Marco CA, Yang S. Human immunodeficiency virus and acquired immunodeficiency syndrome. In: Tintinalli JE, Stapczynski JS, Ma OJ, eds. Emergency medicine: A comprehensive study guide. 7th ed. New York: McGraw-Hill; 2011. p. 1031–47.

13. Arendse S, Street AC. Needlestick injuries and related blood and body fluid exposures. In: Cameron P, Jelinek G, Kelly A, editors. Textbook of adult emergency medicine. 3rd ed. Edinburgh: Elsevier; 2009. p. 456–60.

14. Cline DM. Occupational exposures, infection control and standard precautions. In: Tintinalli JE, Stapczynski JS, Ma OJ, editors. Emergency medicine: a comprehensive study guide. 7th ed. New York: McGraw-Hill; 2011. p. 1093–103.

15. Weber EJ, Ramanujam P. Rabies. In: Marx JA, Hockberger RS, Walls RM, editors. Rosen's emergency medicine: concepts and clinical practice. 7th ed. Philadelphia: Elsevier; 2009. p. 1723–31.

16. Australian Government. Australian bat lyssavirus infection and rabies. The Australian immunisation handbook. 9th ed. 2008. Online. Available: http://www.health.gov.au/internet/immunise/publishing.nsf/Content/Handbook-lyssavirus; 19 Dec 2011.

17. Moss WJ. Measles (rubeola). In: Longo DL, Fauci AS, Kasper DL, et al, editors. Harrison's principles of internal medicine. 8th ed. New York: McGraw Hill; 2011. p. 1600–4.

18. Thomas JJ, Perron AD, Brady WJ. Serious generalised skin disorders. In: Tintinalli JE, Stapczynski JS, Ma OJ, editors. Emergency medicine: a comprehensive study guide. 7th ed. New York: McGraw-Hill; 2011. p. 1614–24.

19. Meredith JT. Zoonotic infections. In: Tintinalli JE, Stapczynski JS, Ma OJ, editors. Emergency medicine: a comprehensive study guide. 7th ed. New York: McGraw-Hill; 2011. p. 1070–80.

20. NSW Department of Health. Lyme disease. Factsheet. Updated 29 June 2011. Online. Available: http://www.health.nsw.gov.au/factsheets/infectious/lyme_disease.html; 20 Dec 2011.

21. Burton JH. Acute disorders of the joints and bursae. In: Tintinalli JE, Stapczynski JS, Ma OJ, editors. Emergency medicine: a comprehensive study guide. 7th ed. New York: McGraw-Hill; 2011. p. 1926–32.

22. Therapeutic Guidelines Limited. Nectrotising skin and soft tissue infections. In: eTG complete. Online. Available: https://www.tg.org.au; 2 Nov 2011.

23. Kelly EW, Magilner D. Soft tissue infections. In: Tintinalli JE, Stapczynski JS, Ma OJ, editors. Emergency medicine: a comprehensive study guide. 7th ed. New York: McGraw-Hill; 2011. p. 1014–24.

24. Haile-Mariam T, Polis MA. Vital illnesses. In: Marx JA, Hockberger RS, Walls RM, editors. Rosen's emergency medicine: concepts and clinical practice. 7th ed. Philadelphia: Elsevier; 2009. p. 1700–22.

25. Nasser M, Fedorowicz Z, Khoshnevisan MH, et al. Cochrane review: Acyclovir for treating primary herpetic gingivostomatitis. Evidence-Based Child Health: A Cochrane Review Journal 2009;4(3):1214–40.

26. Bonfante G, Rosenau AM. Rashes in infants and children. In: Tintinalli JE, Stapczynski JS, Ma OJ, editors. Emergency medicine: a comprehensive study guide. 7th ed. New York: McGraw-Hill; 2011. p. 910–24.

27. Beaudreau RW. Oral and dental emergencies. In: Tintinalli JE, Stapczynski JS, Ma OJ, editors. Emergency medicine: a comprehensive study guide. 7th ed. New York: McGraw-Hill; 2011. p. 1572–83.

28. Barber B, Denholm JT, Spelman D. Ross River virus. Australian Family Physician 2009;38(8):586–9.

29. Russell RC, Currie BJ, Lindsay MD, et al. Dengue and climate change in Australia: predictions for the future should incorporate knowledge from the past. MJA 2009;190:265–8.

30. Queensland Government. Dengue fever. Online. Available: http://www.health.qld.gov.au/dengue/; 19 Dec 2011.

31. Queensland Government. Barmah forest virus. Online. Available: http://access.health.qld.gov.au/hid/InfectionsandParasites/ViralInfections/barmahForestVirus_fs.asp; 19 Dec 2011.

32. Therapeutic Guidelines Limited. Diabetic foot infections (revised June 2010). In eTG complete. Available: https://online-tg-org-au.cknservices.dotsec.com/ip/; 19 Dec 2011.

33. Blaivas M, Lyon M. Deep venous thrombosis: Identify the killer before it strikes. Emeregncy Medicine Practice 2005;7(11). Online. Available: http://www.empractice.net; 19 Dec 2011.

34. Sokolove PE, Derlet RW. In: Marx JA, Hockberger RS, Walls RM, editors. Rosen's emergency medicine: concepts and clinical practice. 7th ed. Philadelphia: Elsevier; 2009. p. 1793–815.

35. Phan VD, Poponick JM. Tuberculosis. In: Tintinalli JE, Stapczynski JS, Ma OJ, editors. Emergency medicine: a comprehensive study guide. 7th ed. New York: McGraw-Hill; 2011. p. 494–500.

36. Therapeutic Guidelines Limited. Skin and soft tissue infections: water-related infections. In eTG complete. Online. Available: https://www.tg.org.au; 22 Nov 2011.

37. Raasch RH. Pharmacology of antimocrobics, antifungals and antivirals. In: Tintinalli JE, Stapczynski JS, Ma OJ, editors. Emergency medicine: a comprehensive study guide. 7th ed. New York: McGraw-Hill; 2011. p. 1103–11.

38. McGauly P, Mahler S. Foodborne and waterborne diseases. In: Tintinalli JE, Stapczynski JS, Ma OJ, editors.

Emergency medicine: a comprehensive study guide. 7th ed. New York: McGraw-Hill; 2011. p. 1062–70.

39. Andrus P, Jagoda A. Acute peripheral neurologic lesions. In: Tintinalli JE, Stapczynski JS, Ma OJ, editors. Emergency medicine: a comprehensive study guide. 7th ed. New York: McGraw-Hill; 2011. p. 1159–66.

40. Takhar SS, Moran GJ. Disseminated viral infections. In: Tintinalli JE, Stapczynski JS, Ma OJ, editors. Emergency medicine: a comprehensive study guide. 7th ed. New York: McGraw-Hill; 2011. p. 1024–31.

41. Moran GJ, Talan AD. In: Marx JA, Hockberger RS, Walls RM, editors. Rosen's emergency medicine: concepts and clinical practice. 7th ed. Philadelphia: Elsevier; 2009. p. 927–38.

42. Nobay F, Promes S. Sexually transmitted diseases. In: Tintinalli JE, Stapczynski JS, Ma OJ, editors. Emergency medicine: a comprehensive study guide. 7th ed. New York: McGraw-Hill; 2011. p. 989–99.

43. Diphtheria: Queensland Health Guidelines for Public Health Units. Online. Available: http://www.health.qld.gov.au/cdcg/index/diphtheria.asp; 18 Jul 2011.

44. Dilley S, Dunn R. Weakness. In: Dunn R, Dilley S, Brookes J, editors. The emergency medicine manual. 5th ed. Adelaide. Venom Publishing; 2010. p. 685–94.

1. Answer: D

Typical target lesions can be seen in erythema multiforme (EM). In addition, erythematous macules and papules, vesiculaobullous lesions and urticaria may occur in this condition. In SJS similar lesions are seen but the target lesions can be atypical. **In TEN vesicles and bullae are the main lesions and there is associated painful and tender erythroderma and exfoliation. Furthermore, flat atypical targets may be seen in TEN.** Pyoderma gangrenosum is a dermatosis with dense dermal infiltrate of neutrophils (a neutrophilic dermatosis). It is often associated with inflammatory bowel disease, rheumatoid arthritis and leukaemia. It results in severe painful ulceration frequently in the lower limbs and it is not associated with target lesions.[1-3]

2. Answer: A

SJS and TEN are now considered two variants of the same disease process and they are different to EM. **Although very rare, these conditions are caused almost exclusively as idiosyncratic reactions to a spectrum of medications.** Mycoplasma infections may induce some cases of SJS. **The mortality in TEN can approach 40% and in SJS it is approximately 5%.** The medications that are implicated include:

- **sulphonamide antibiotics** – most commonly implicated medication
- other antibiotics – penicillins and cephalosporins
- imidazole antifungals
- nevirapine (antiviral)
- allopurinol
- nonsteroidal anti-inflammatory drugs (NSAIDs)
- anticonvulsants – carbamazepine, phenytoin, sodium valproate, lamotrigine.

As the use of medications increases with age these conditions are more frequent in older age groups than in the young.

The onset of SJS/TEN is usually within the first week from the start of antibiotic treatment but the onset may be delayed up to 2 months from the start of anticonvulsant treatment. Usually there is a prodrome resembling an 'upper respiratory tract infection' prior to the abrupt onset of a rash consisting of macules, targets and blisters. Initial misdiagnoses are common; however, a few days later the patient appears very unwell and is in severe pain. The typical features of these blisters include the following.

- They are flaccid blisters (as opposed to tense fluid-filled blisters).
- Blisters show large areas of epidermal detachment and they merge.
- The epidermis breaks, showing red and oozing dermis.
- **Positive Nikolsky's sign** – when the intact skin is rubbed gently new blisters appear due to slippage of epidermis from the dermis.

There is extensive involvement of mucosal surfaces and at least two surfaces are involved. These include eyes, lips and oral mucosa, oesophagus, trachea and bronchi, urinary tract, genital mucosa and gastrointestinal tract. Significant ophthalmic lesions occur in both conditions.

The differentiation between SJS and TEN is dependent on the maximal extent of skin detachment and the typical appearance of the rash. **In SJS, the skin detachment is <10% of the body surface area (BSA) and in TEN it is usually >30% of the BSA.** In the entity called overlap SJS/TEN the skin detachment is between 10–30% of BSA.[2,4,5]

3. Answer: D

SSSS is more commonly seen in infants and children younger than 5 years. In adults, the elderly with renal failure are more likely to get affected than others. SSSS is caused by an epidermolytic toxin produced by a strain of *Staphylococcal aureus*. It is not due to an extensive primary skin infection. Usually the focus of infection may not be significant, that is, it can be a minor skin, nasal or eye infection. Early features are fever and tender erythematous skin. The small blisters coalesce to form large flaccid blisters or bullae that usually burst giving rise to the characteristic appearance of a scalded skin. Nikolsky's sign is positive. In infants and young children the extensive exfoliation of skin is usually confined to the upper body but in neonates the whole skin surface may be affected.

Similar-looking conditions such as SJS and TEN should be considered in the differential diagnosis; skin biopsy may be required in the differentiation. The skin biopsy will show the subcorneal split in the epidermis. This means these blisters have very thin roofs and therefore break easily. **There is no mucosal involvement in SSSS as opposed to what occurs in SJS/TEN.** The mainstays of management of these children are intravenous fluid resuscitation similar to a burn patient, prompt initiation of antibiotic therapy to eliminate *Staphylococcal* focus and supportive care in a specialised burn unit or an intensive care unit.[6–8]

4. Answer: A

The term erythroderma describes an inflammatory skin disorder affecting almost the entire BSA and this can be considered as a 'skin failure'.
Erythroderma may be acute or chronic and may often proceeds to exfoliation of skin, hence called exfoliative erythroderma. The patients are often >40 years of age. The causes are varied and generally it is a cutaneous reaction to a medication, underlying systemic or cutaneous illness. The causes include:

- drug eruptions (most frequently secondary to sulphonamides, penicillins, anticonvulsants, allopurinol and antimalarials)
- dermatitis (any type)
- psoriasis (5% of cases of psoriasis)
- cutaneous T cell lymphoma
- underlying systemic malignancy
- HIV infection.

The clinical features are generalised erythema without skin tenderness, but with increased warmth, scaling or flaking, pruritus and skin tightness. Erythema starts on the face and spreads downwards to involve most or all of the body. **In the assessment, a thorough search should be conducted to identify the underlying cause. As a failure of the skin, erythroderma can cause significant complications including:**[3,9,10]

- hypovolaemia and electrolyte imbalance (due to increased transepidermal water loss)
- hypoalbuminaemia (due to exfoliation)
- high output cardiac failure (due to widespread cutaneous vasodilatation)
- sepsis (due to secondary infection)
- hypothermia (due to heat loss).

5. Answer: C

Neonates may present to the ED with pustular lesions on the skin. Some of these pustular lesions are the only manifestation of serious underlying disease processes in the neonate and therefore the correct identification of these lesions and further assessment of the neonate are important. Other pustular lesions are part of benign transient conditions.

The causes of common pustular lesions in the neonatal period include the following.

- **Erythema toxicum neonatorum: most common pustular skin lesion in the neonate.** Onset is usually 24–48 hours from birth. The lesions are present in the trunk and the upper extremities and palms and soles are usually spared. **The lesions are self-limiting and no treatment is required.**
- Infections: congenital or acquired – mainly caused by *Staphylocaccus*, group B *Streptococcus* and *Haemephilus influenzae*
- Congenital neutropenia: the appearence of pustules may be the only sign.
- Eosinophilic pustular folliculitis of scalp: these pustules are usually sterile but secondary infection may occur.

Milia are inclusion cysts and not true pustules. They appear commonly in the scalp and the face as white discrete small papules. They can be present at birth or can occur after birth. They usually resolve spontaneously after a few weeks.[7]

6. Answer: B

The diagnosis of disseminated gonococcal infection should be suspected in a sexually active patient who complains of tenosynovitis and arthralgia associated with the typical rash. **Although there are petechiae, the typical rash in disseminated gonococcal infection is more papular, vesicular or pustular skin lesions on the extensor surfaces of the wrists and hands and dorsal aspects of the ankles and feet and in the palms. The typical lesions are small papules or maculopapules with a red periphery and a petechial component.** The number of lesions in the body can be up to 20. These lesions either become vesicles filled with purulent fluid or resolve rapidly. In spite of the disseminated infection the patient is not usually systemically toxic.

Neisseria gonorrhoea can be demonstrated with gram-staining of fluid obtained from the lesions and blood cultures often become positive in the early stages of the disease. However, the cultures remain sterile from specimen obtained from mucosal surfaces (e.g. urethral, cervical, vaginal). These should be tested for gonococcal antigens.[3]

7. Answer: B

About 3% of the patients admitted to hospital have been found to have rashes due to adverse drug reactions and this number may be higher in patients presenting to the ED. Drug reactions can be due to true immunological hypersensitivity or allergy or can be due to non-immunological causes such as idiosyncratic reactions, irritant effects, toxicity and enzyme deficiencies.

One classification of drug eruptions is given below.

- Exanthematous drug reactions: the rash is most often morbilliform (symmetrical erythematous macules and papules). Other appearances of rash are scarlantiniform (tiny red spots) and confluent lesions (large erythematous patches or urticaria). These reactions are more likely in patients infected with EBV and HIV, and also in association with leukaemia and intake of allopurinol.
- DRESS (drug rash with eosinophilia and systemic symptoms) syndrome, also known as drug hypersensitivity syndrome. This is a severe reaction, most commonly caused by anticonvulsants such as phenytoin and phenobarbitone, allopurinol and sulfa medications. This syndrome is associated with exfoliative dermatitis, hepatitis, pneumonitis and renal impairment.
- Drug-induced urticaria: may be associated with angioedema and it arises up to 3 weeks from the time of first exposure or immediately after a re-challenge.
- Fixed-drug eruption: this condition consists of solitary or multiple oval plaques that may have central blisters. The lesion often occurs in mucosal surfaces as well. Lesions resolve when the culprit drug is ceased but re-occur at the same sites if it is re-introduced.
- Drug-induced photosensitivity: May be due to immunological mechanism (photoallergic, e.g.

quinine) or toxicity (phototoxic, e.g. doxycycline, chlorpromazine). It usually affects the sites of light exposure.
- Drug-induced pigmentation.

In the pathogenesis of TEN both type II (cytotoxic) and type IV (cell mediated) mechanisms are involved.[3,11]

8. Answer: A

In children, when examining a rash, the presence of blisters in the skin narrows the possible differential diagnoses. The differential diagnosis for vesicles in children include infections such as HSV, varicella zoster virus (VZV), enterovirus, scabies, impetigo and tinea, various drug eruptions, insect bites, eczema, EM, photosensitivity and the rare condition called dermatitis herpatiformis. Larger blisters may occur in SSSS, SJS, immunologically-mediated bullous eruptions and in trauma and burns.

Blisters occur as a result of accumulation of fluid within or under the epidermis. The clinical appearance of a blister may range from flaccid to tense and these blisters may remain intact or may rupture. These appearances generally depend on the level of intercellular split associated with a particular skin disorder. Three levels of epidermal split have been described:

- subcorneal: very thin roof to the blister that breaks easily (e.g. impetigo, SSSS)
- intraepidermal: thin roof, easily to rupture (e.g. varicella, HSV, acute eczema, pemphigus)
- subepidermal: tense roof and roof remains intact (e.g. bullous pemphigoid, erythema multiforme, TEN).

Some bullous disorders are autoimmune disorders and at least nine such disorders have been described. Bullous pemphigoid is the most common and it affects mainly the elderly. There are different subtypes of pemphigus and some (e.g. pemphigus vulgaris) are potentially fatal.[8]

9. Answer: B

Hand, foot and mouth disease is a common, infectious skin disorder most frequently affecting infants and young children. It can affect older children and adults occasionally. **It is usually caused by coxackievirus A16 but some cases are caused by enterovirus 71.** The condition is highly infectious and faeco-oral contamination is usually the mode of spread. The incubation period is 3–5 days and then small blisters appear on palms and soles and painful ulcers appear in the oral mucosa. The lesions may be present on buttocks of some children. **The first week appears to be the most contagious; however, infected children may shed the virus in the faeces for weeks and continue to be contagious at a lower level.** In addition the virus may be present in fluid of blisters, saliva and nasal secretions. EM, pustular psoriasis and EBV infection are some of the differentials to consider.[7,10,12]

10. Answer: D

The primary HSV infection acquired in the post-neonatal period is caused by HSV type 1 and mainly affects the face. HSV type 2 infection is often sexually transmitted and may affect older children and adults.

Type 1 infection causes herpetic gingivostomatitis and 'cold sores' in children. It also can cause infections in the fingers, particularly in thumb and index fingers and this is called herpetic whitlow. Herpetic whitlow is often misdiagnosed as bacterial infection and/or abscess formation.

Eczema herpeticum is disseminated type 1 infection in association with atopic eczema. Patients with both mild and severe atopic eczema can be affected with this infection. The most severe disease can be seen in young children and adults who are immunosuppressed. **Often the herpetic vesicles are quite atypical. The infection may appear as erosions associated with eczema and therefore misdiagnosed as exacerbation of eczema or as bacterial infection.** Patients with severe disease should be treated with parenteral antivirals.[3,7]

References

1. Oakley A. Neutrophilic dermatoses. In: DermNet NZ. The dermatology resource. New Zealand Dermatological Society Inc. Online. Available: www.dermnetnz.org.

2. Ngan V, Oakley A, Dyall-Smith D. Steven Johnson syndrome and toxic epidermal necrolysis. In: DermNet NZ. The dermatology resource. New Zealand Dermatological Society Inc. Online. Available: www.dermnetnz.org.

3. Thomas J, Perron A, Brady W. Serious generalized skin disorders. In: Tintinalli J, Stapczynski J, Ma O, et al, editors. Tintinalli's emergency medicine: a comprehensive study guide. 7th ed. New York: McGraw Hill Medical; 2011. p. 1614–24.

4. Klein P. Dermatological manifestations of Stephen Johnson syndrome and toxic epidermal necrolysis. In: Medscape reference: diseases drugs and procedures. Online. Available: http://emedicine.medscape.com/article/1124127-overview.

5. Sevketoglu E, Hatipoglu S, Akman M et al. Toxic epidermal necrolysis in a child after carbamaxepine dosage increment. Paed Emer Care 2009;25:93–5.

6. Shah M, Wiebe R. Superficial skin infections. In: Strange G, Ahrens W, Schafermeyer R, et al, editors. Pediatric emergency medicine. 3rd ed. New York: McGraw Hill Medical; 2009. p. 713–5.

7. Phillips R, Orchard D, Starr M. Dermatology. In: Cameron P, Jelinek G, Everitt I, et al, editors. Textbook of paediatric emergency medicine. Edinburgh: Churchill Livingston Elsevier; 2012. p. 281–322.

8. Oakley A. Blistering skin diseases. In: DermNet NZ. The dermatology resource. New Zealand Dermatological Society Inc. Online. Available: www.dermnetnz.org.

9. Oakley A. Erythroderma. In: DermNet NZ. The dermatology resource. New Zealand Dermatological Society Inc. Online. Available: www.dermnetnz.org.

10. Dunn R. Rashes. In: Dunn R, Dilley S, Brookes J, editors. The emergency medicine manual. 5th ed. Adelaide: Venom Publishing; 2010. p. 1061–72.

11. Oakley A. Drug Eruptions. In: DermNet NZ. The dermatology resource. New Zealand Dermatological Society Inc. Online. Available: www.dermnetnz.org.

12. Oakley A. Specific viral examthems. In: DermNet NZ. The dermatology resource. New Zealand Dermatological Society Inc. Online. Available: www.dermnetnz.org.

1. Answer: C

Pseudohyponatraemia is hyponatraemia in the setting of normal plasma osmolality (POsm 275–295). High levels of plasma proteins and lipids increase the non-aqueous and non-Na⁺ containing fraction of plasma which analysers misread as a factitious lower value of [Na⁺] than the serum truly contains. Hence, a *pseudohyponatraemia*. It is also known as *factitious hyponatraemia*. Causes of pseudo or factitious hyponatraemia include hyperlipidaemia and hyperproteinaemic states such as multiple myeloma and Waldenstrom macroglobulinaemia.[1]

Hyperglycaemia causes a hypertonic hyponatraemia (POsm > 295) by causing water to move from the ICF to the ECF. This causes a subsequent decrease in [Na⁺]. The corrected Na⁺ can be calculated by the formula:[1]

$Sodium_{corrected}$ = glucose (mmol/L)/3.5 + measured [Na⁺]

SIADH and liver cirrhosis are both causes of hypotonic hyponatraemia (POsm < 275).[1]

2. Answer: D

SIADH is generally a diagnosis of exclusion. It is a cause of **euvolaemic hypotonic hyponatraemia**, though some patients may have slightly increased ECF volume, however, are generally not clinically fluid overloaded. Total body sodium is nearly normal despite the presence of hyponatraemia. SIADH is characterised by six criteria:[1,2]

- hypotonicity
- urinary osmolality > plasma osmolality (typically > 200 mOsm/kg)
- normovolaemia
- elevated urinary [Na⁺] > 20 mmol/L
- normal adrenal, renal, cardiac, thyroid and hepatic function
- correctable with water restriction

The most common causes of SIADH can be categorised into three groups:[1]
- malignant causes
  - lung
  - ovarian
  - pancreatic
- thymoma
- haematological – lymphoma, leukaemia
- pulmonary causes
  - infective – abscess, tuberculosis (TB)
  - cystic fibrosis
  - chronic obstructive airways disease (COAD)
- neurological causes
  - trauma
  - tumour
  - infection
  - demyelinating conditions – Guillain-Barré, multiple sclerosis
  - cerebrovascular accident, subarachnoid haemorrhage

3. Answer: B

This man is likely to be seizing due to his elevated sodium concentration. Hypernatraemia is defined as a serum sodium of >150 mmol/L and can be caused by either a decrease in total body water or, less likely, from an increase in sodium load (decreased excretion or increased intake). It has a high mortality rate of around 50% due to the combination of both the effects on the body of hypernatraemia, and due to the severity of the underlying disease itself. **Nearly all hypernatraemia seen in the ED is due to volume depletion. However, overly rapid correction (unless acute hypernatraemia) can be almost as harmful, leading to cerebral oedema, further seizures and permanent neurological sequelae.**[1,3]

Diabetes insipidus is one of the causes of hypernatraemia seen in the ED. This disease can cause marked hypotonic urine excretion and consequently significant total body water loss, leading to severe dehydration partioularly in the elderly. Causes of diabetes insipidus may be central or nephrogenic. Central causes include tumours, trauma or idiopathic, and nephrogenic causes include drugs, renal disorders, haematological and familial disorders.

Lithium is a drug well known for causing nephrogenic diabetes insipidus.[1] Consequently, morphine, NSAIDs and carbamazepine are all drugs that have the potential to cause a euvolaemic hyponatraemia.[1]

4. Answer: A

The normal total serum calcium concentration is 2.15–2.55 mmol/L, and hypercalcaemia can be defined as a level higher than this. It is a relatively common condition with more than 90% of causes being attributed to hyperparathyroidism or malignancy. **Treatment should be initiated in any symptomatic patient or if the [Ca²⁺] is >3.5 mmol/L.** There are four primary treatment goals:

1. hydration

2. enhancement of renal excretion of calcium

3. inhibition of bone resorption

4. treatment of the underlying cause

Hydration replaces the ECF volume thereby diluting the calcium concentration and increasing calcium clearance. Normal saline is the fluid of choice, and Hartmann's solution or colloids are best avoided as they contain calcium.

Enhanced renal excretion, though a modest effect, is achieved by the use of *loop* diuretics such as frusemide once the patient is adequately hydrated. *Thiazide* diuretics should be *avoided* as they actually enhance calcium reabsorption in the distal convoluted tubule. While they rarely cause hypercalcaemia in isolation as the result of this enhanced reabsorption, thiazide diuretics can unmask hypercalcaemia due to other causes.

In the treatment of hypercalcaemia, corticosteroids assist only in a selected population of patients such as haematological malignancies, vitamin D toxicity and sarcoidosis. Generally, it is an ineffective treatment for hypercalcaemia due to solid tumour cancers (though breast cancer may be an exception).

Bisphosphonates inhibit osteoclast activity and therefore reduce mobilisation of calcium from bone.[1-3]

5. Answer: D

Hypercalcaemia should be immediately considered as one of the potential causes of this patient's confusion. It can cause a wide range of disturbances of the neurological, gastrointestinal, cardiovascular, renal and musculoskeletal systems. Signs and symptoms expected to be seen include all of confusion, polyuria, hyporeflexia and constipation. **The rhyme: *stones* (urinary calculi, polyuria, polydipsia), *bones* (bony pain), *groans* (abdominal pain from constipation, peptic ulcer disease, pancreatitis) and *psychic moans* (confusion, irritability, hallucinations) can be used to easily remember the key clinical features of hypercalcaemia.**

The ECG abnormalities of hypercalcaemia include depressed ST segments, widened T waves, and shortened ST segments and QTc segments. It can progress to bradyarrhythmias, bundle branch blocks and eventually complete heart block. It is hypocalcaemia that causes a prolonged QTc.[1-3]

6. Answer: B

The AG is the difference between the measured cations and the measured anions. To maintain electrical neutrality, the number anions must equal the number of cations. Hence, the difference between the two (i.e. the anion gap) is a measure of the unmeasured anions in plasma. AG = [Na⁺] −{[HCO₃⁻] + [Cl⁻]}. The normal value is < 12 mmol/L and is composed of proteins (primarily albumin), phosphate and organic anions such as lactate. Albumin is the major unmeasured anion and contributes almost the whole of the value of the AG. A normally high AG acidosis in a patient with hypoalbuminaemia may appear as a normal AG acidosis. This is particularly relevant in severely unwell and intensive care patients where lower albumin levels are common. Hypoalbuminaemic states must therefore be corrected for by *adding* 2.5 to the AG for every 10 g/L below the normal albumin level.

A reduced AG may be present in conditions of increased unmeasured cations such as calcium, magnesium and lithium. Additionally, positively charged proteins from multiple myeloma and polyclonal gammopathies can cause a reduced AG as can bromide and iodine toxicity. Elevation of the AG is most commonly associated with a metabolic acidosis, however, is not exclusive to and may be seen with many acid–base disturbances. Metabolic and respiratory alkalosis may also elevate the AG. Generally however, if the AG is >30 mmol/L, than a metabolic acidosis is present. If the AG is <30 mmol/L, then approximately one-third of these patients will not have a metabolic acidosis. Therefore, an AG should be calculated in all acid–base disturbances.[4-6]

7. Answer: D

The delta gap is a measure of the relationship between the anions in the blood and can be

TABLE 11.1 DELTA GAP MEASUREMENTS

Delta gap	Acid–base disturbance
<0.4	Hyperchloraemic normal AG metabolic acidosis
0.4–0.8	Normal *and* high AG metabolic acidosis
0.8–2.0	Pure high AG metabolic acidosis
>2.0	High AG metabolic acidosis *and* metabolic alkalosis or respiratory acidosis (suggests pre-existing elevated HCO_3 level)

Based on: Brandis K. Acid-base physiology. Online. Available: http://www.anaesthesiaMCQ.com.

calculated as the ratio of the change in AG to the change in [HCO_3^-]. It can be used in the presence of a high AG metabolic acidosis to further evaluate for a *coexistent metabolic abnormality*. In a pure high AG metabolic acidosis the rise in the AG equals the fall in bicarbonate and there is a 1 : 1 relationship between the AG and the fall in bicarbonate. If the rise in the AG is *less* than the fall of the bicarbonate then a mixed high AG and normal AG metabolic acidosis coexist. If the rise in the AG is *greater* than the fall of the bicarbonate then a mixed high AG and metabolic alkalosis coexist.[4-6]

Some general guidelines are listed in Table 11.1.

8. Answer: B

There are multiple causes for metabolic alkalosis, which can be remembered either as an increase in acid losses or increased bicarbonate retention. Causes include:[5]

- gastrointestinal acid loss – protracted vomiting, ongoing nasogastric suction
- urinary acid loss – loop and thiazide diuretics, Cushing's syndrome, Barter's syndrome, adrenogenital syndrome, primary hyperaldosteronism
- administration of bicarbonate – antacids, milk-alkali syndrome
- renal retention of bicarbonate – hypokalaemia, hypochloraemia

Adrenal insufficiency, acetazolamide and profuse diarrhoea are all causes of a normal AG metabolic acidosis.[5]

9. Answer: A

The venous blood gas shows an acidaemia with low bicarbonate, therefore indicating a metabolic acidosis.

- The expected CO_2 [1.5 x HCO_3 (8) + 8] would be 20 if a single acid–base process was occurring. The measured carbon dioxide is, however, 28, indicating a coexistent respiratory acidosis.
- The *anion gap* {[Na^+] – [HCO_3^-] – [Cl^-]} = 141–8–92 = 41 mmol/L (normal <12 mmol/L) is elevated.
- The osmolar gap (OG) = measured osmolality – calculated osmolality
- Calculated osmolality = 2 x [Na^+] + [Ur] + [glucose] + [ethanol]
- OG = 375 – 329 = 46 mmol/L (normal < 10 mmol/L) is elevated

Therefore, the venous blood gas shows a high AG metabolic acidosis, with coexistent respiratory acidosis and high osmolar gap.

All of the above drug choices cause a high AG metabolic acidosis. Ethanol and acetone are also both exogenous agents that directly cause a high OG. Cyanide poisoning causes a severe lactic acidosis and hence can cause a high OG. Paracetamol in overdose does not typically cause a lactic acidosis unless ingested in doses large enough to cause severe hepatotoxicity and fulminant hepatic failure.[4,7]

The causes of a high OG include:[7]

- exogenous agents – ethanol, methanol, ethylene glycol, acetone, mannitol, glycerol, sorbitol
- non-toxicological conditions – DKA, alcoholic ketoacidosis, severe lactic acidosis, chronic renal failure, shock, trauma, burns, hyperlipidaemia and hyperproteinaemia.

10. Answer: C

Metabolic alkalosis results from either a loss of hydrogen ions or a gain in bicarbonate. Bicarbonate and chloride ions are closely kept in homeostasis and therefore a change in concentration of one will readily alter the plasma concentration of the other. **Metabolic alkalosis can be classified as being chloride responsive or chloride unresponsive, which assists in the approach to treatment.** Conditions that produce chloride loss and fluid loss, such as vomiting, diarrhoea, diuretic therapy and cystic fibrosis reduce serum chloride concentrations and extracellular volume, leading to an increase in mineralocorticoid activity. This stimulates the kidney to reabsorb sodium and bicarbonate and secrete potassium and hydrogen ions leading to a hypochloraemic, hypokalaemic metabolic alkalosis that responds to normal saline (chloride *responsive* metabolic alkalosis). Urinary chloride is usually <10 mmol/L. Alternatively, other conditions causing mineralocorticoid excess, such as Conn's syndrome, Cushing's syndrome, adrenal hyperplasia and renal artery stenosis also produce a state of hyperaldosteronism, which also leads to a metabolic alkalosis and hypokalaemia. In these conditions, however, the extracellular volume is expanded and patients may often be hypertensive. The metabolic alkalosis in these patients is perpetuated by the hypokalaemia rather than the volume depletion and consequently is chloride *resistant*. Urinary chloride is generally >10 mmol/L.[1,6]

11. Answer: B

Hypokalaemia is defined as a [K+] of <3.5 mmol/L. It is most frequently caused by intracellular shifts and increased losses of potassium. There are multiple aetiologies for hypokalaemia one of which is metabolic alkalosis. As the pH of the extracellular fluid rises, potassium shifts into the cells in exchange for hydrogen ions thereby causing hypokalaemia. Therefore, most causes of metabolic alkalosis will also cause a hypokalaemia due to redistribution. Addisonian crisis, digoxin overdose and beta-blockers all cause hyperkalaemia.[1,2]

12. Answer: C

There are several causes of prolonged QTc:[8]
- electrolyte disturbance – hypokalaemia, hypomagnesaemia, hypocalcaemia
- metabolic/endocrine – hypothermia, hypothyroidism
- toxins/drugs – antiarrhythmics (most commonly class Ia, Ic and III), antipsychotic agents (e.g. haloperidol, quetiapine, chlorpromazine), tricyclic antidepressants (e.g. amitriptyline, dotheipin), antidepressants (e.g. venlafaxine, citalopram), antibiotics (e.g. fluorquinolones, erythromycin)
- cardiovascular disease – myocarditis, rheumatic heart disease
- cerebrovascular disease – intracranial haemorrhage, cerebrovascular accident
- hereditary – familial prolonged QTc such as Romano-Ward and Lange-Nielsen syndrome

Consequently, in alcoholics there are also multiple reasons for a prolonged QTc finding. However, hyponatraemia while common in alcoholics, does not typically cause a prolonged QTc.[8]

13. Answer: B

Clinical manifestations of hyperkalaemia result from changes in the transmembrane potential. Cardiac cells are particularly vulnerable and more sensitive in acute changes in potassium levels. ECG changes are characteristic (see Table 11.2), however, an insensitive method in evaluating the degree of hyperkalaemia. In chronic hyperkalaemia, ECG changes tend to occur at higher potassium levels.[3]

TABLE 11.2 ECG CHANGES ACCORDING TO POTASSIUM LEVELS

[K+]	ECG characteristics
6–7	Tall, peaked T waves (> 5 mm), shortened QT interval, prolonged PR interval
7–8	QRS widening, flattening of P waves
8–9	Fusion of QRS complex with T waves producing sine wave
>9	Atrioventricular (AV) dissociation, ventricular tachyarrhythmias, asystole

14. Answer: A

The role of bicarbonate therapy in the treatment of acidosis is still controversial and is currently reserved for use primarily in severe acidosis. **Bicarbonate therapy imposes a high osmotic and sodium load that may precipitate pulmonary oedema and volume overload. It also is responsible for generating large quantities of carbon dioxide that can diffuse into the CSF and into cells causing a paradoxical intracellular and CSF acidosis. The extra carbon dioxide can also cause respiratory failure. Other side effects include overshoot alkalosis, hypokalaemia and precipitation of hypocalcaemia.**

Some literature reviews have focused on the use of bicarbonate therapy in cardiac arrest, DKA and lactic acidosis. Several studies have failed to show benefit or reduced complication rates with the use of bicarbonate and other studies have found that use in patients with severe cardiac disease may have deleterious effect from the therapy. In hypoxic tissues, bicarbonate therapy can further increase the production of lactate (due to removal of glycolysis inhibition from acidotic state) and impair the removal of oxygen from haemoglobin due to increased pH (left shift of the oxygen dissociation curve), thereby causing negative effects.[2–4,6]

15. Answer: C

The treatment of metabolic acidosis should be directed at treating the primary cause and the use of intravenous bicarbonate therapy should be reserved only for a few cases. These indications include:

- poisonings – TCAs, salicylates (alkalinising the urine promotes salicylate diuresis and renal clearance), cyanide, toxic alcohols
- cardiac arrest – in young children or pregnant women
- severe hyperkalaemia with cardiac toxicity (though calcium gluconate will more rapidly protect against life-threatening toxic arrhythmias)
- severe hyperchloraemic acidaemia (normal AG metabolic acidosis) – lost bicarbonate cannot be quickly regenerated as there are no extra organic anions. Therefore, supplemental bicarbonate can assist in resolving the acidaemia more quickly. If, however, the patient is improving and is clinically stable, then its use should still be avoided.

Clinical studies have shown that bicarbonate is not indicated in DKA because it shows no beneficial effect in outcome, and may in fact slow the clearance of ketones. Additionally, as mentioned above, lactic acidosis may actually worsen if bicarbonate is administered.[2–4,6]

16. Answer: D

The venous blood gas shows an alkalaemia (pH > 7.45). A high bicarbonate level and high carbon dioxide level indicates a metabolic alkalosis. The expected carbon dioxide level as calculated from the compensation rule $(0.7 \times HCO_3 + 20)$ would be 48, which is appropriate indicating no secondary respiratory acid–base disorder. The hypochloraemia and hypokalaemia are consistent with a metabolic alkalosis. **The most common cause of a hypochloraemic hypokalaemic metabolic alkalosis that responds to saline, is protracted vomiting or diuretic use.** In this age group, vomiting due to sepsis or gastrointestinal obstruction (pyloric stenosis in this age group) needs to be excluded. Sepsis, however, will typically cause a metabolic acidosis. Surgery is performed to correct the pyloric stenosis after the acid–base and electrolyte abnormalities are corrected with normal saline replenishment.[5]

17. Answer: C

The venous blood gas shows an acidaemia (pH < 7.35). The low bicarbonate level indicates a metabolic acidosis. The expected carbon dioxide if appropriately compensated can be calculated by the formula $[CO_2 = 1.5 \times HCO_3^- + 8]$ (± 2). In this scenario, the expected carbon dioxide would be 29 (± 2) indicating a single acid–base disturbance of a metabolic acidosis. The AG is calculated to be $[Na^+] - \{[HCO_3^- + Cl^-]\} = 7$. Therefore, there is a normal AG metabolic acidosis. Renal failure can cause a high AG metabolic acidosis. However, in this case the degree of renal failure present has not been sufficient enough to elevate the AG indicating that there is not significant retention of acid anions. Furthermore, tissue perfusion is still adequate to prevent lactic acidosis.

Diarrhoea causes a normal AG metabolic acidosis due to loss of bicarbonate from the gastrointestinal system. To maintain electrical neutrality, chloride ions are retained hence the hyperchloraemia. Additionally, hypovolaemia caused by profuse diarrhoea stimulates aldosterone production, which increases sodium reabsorption and increases potassium excretion contributing to the hypokalaemia. In severe profuse diarrhoea, however, the acid–base disturbance can progress to a high AG metabolic acidosis secondary to the severe dehydration, lactic acidosis and renal failure.[4–6]

18. Answer: A

In acute asthma, there is an initial increase in respiratory rate and work of breathing, leading to an initial respiratory alkalosis. However, in severe or life-threatening asthma as patients tire and their work of breathing falls, carbon dioxide can be retained secondary to hypoventilation. Additionally, as the disease progresses and mucous plugging and V/Q mismatch occurs, gas exchange is impaired further increasing retention of carbon dioxide.

Salbutamol is the first-line pharmacological therapy used in the treatment of acute asthma. It causes a shift of potassium into cells thereby reducing the extracellular concentration of potassium. Total body potassium, however, is unchanged and is usually normal. Used in excess, it can also cause a salbutamol lactic acidosis toxicity and V/Q mismatch in the lungs.[5,9]

Keeping this in mind, working through each of the above blood gas pictures:

A. Acidaemia with a respiratory acidosis. Expected HCO_3 can be calculated to be

$HCO_3 = 24 +\{[CO_2] - 40\}/10$ i.e. ~27, therefore single acid–base disturbance.

Hypokalaemia as expected, hence answer A is correct.

B. Acidaemia with respiratory acidosis. Expected HCO_3 calculated as 27. Hyperkalaemia however, is not typically expected, hence answer B is incorrect.

C. Alkalaemia with respiratory alkalosis. Expected HCO_3 can be calculated to be

$HCO_3 = 24 - \{40 - [CO_2]\}/10$ i.e. ~ 22. However, in life-threatening asthma you would expect carbon dioxide levels to be elevated with an associated respiratory acidosis following an initial respiratory alkalosis. Additionally, hyperkalaemia is not generally expected from treatment with continuous nebulised or intravenous salbutamol.

D. Alkalaemia with respiratory alkalosis. Expected HCO_3 calculated as 22. Again, however, in life-threatening asthma you would typically expect carbon dioxide levels to be elevated with an associated respiratory acidosis following the initial respiratory alkalosis.

19. Answer: C

The A-a gradient is the difference between the alveolar (PAO_2) and arterial (PaO_2) oxygen pressures and is a measure of how well the lungs are functioning. The PaO_2 is measured from arterial blood samples and the PAO_2 can be calculated using the alveolar gas equation. The A-a gradient is essentially $[PAO_2 - PaO_2]$. A normal A-a gradient is <10 mmHg or corrected for age [10 + (age/10)]. There are multiple causes of an elevated A-a gradient including ventilation perfusion mismatch, intracardiac shunts and causes of diffusion abnormalities.[2,10]

In this scenario, using the alveolar gas equation, the PAO_2 would be:

- $PAO_2 = FIO_2 [760-47] - [PaCO_2 /0.8$ (respiratory quotient)]
- $PAO_2 = 150 - 22.5 = 127.5$
- A-a gradient = $127 - 70 = $ **57**

20. Answer: C

A 1 L bag of normal saline has equal concentrations of sodium and chloride at 154 mmol/L of each. The osmolality of the same bag is 300 mmol/L. Hartmann's solution contains 130 mmol/L of sodium and 109 mmol/L of chloride, that is, values almost equal to normal serum electrolyte concentrations.[1]

21. Answer: C

Causes of high AG metabolic acidosis can be remembered either by the mnemonic

CATMUDPILES[5]

Cyanide, carbon monoxide

Alcoholic ketoacidosis

Toluene

Methanol, metformin

Uraemia

DKA

Paracetamol, paraldehyde, propylene glycol

Iron, isoniazid

Lactic acidosis

Ethanol, ethylene glycol

Salicylates.

Or, alternatively, by dividing them into the groups defined by the cause:

- poisons (e.g. toxic alcohols, iron, paracetamol)
- metabolic (e.g. DKA, alcoholic ketoacidosis, renal failure).

Fanconi's syndrome is a disease that affects the proximal tubules of the kidney, impairing the reabsorption of glucose, amino acids, bicarbonate, phosphate and uric acid. Different forms of the disease affect different functions of the kidney. The form that affects the reabsorption of bicarbonate produces renal tubular acidosis type 2 and hence causes a *normal* AG metabolic acidosis.[11]

22. Answer: D

Complications developing from the treatment of hyponatraemia are uncommon but are more likely to occur in patients with chronic hyponatraemia. Central pontine myelinosis (CPM) (or osmotic demyelination syndrome) is a neurological condition that progressively develops over 3–5 days after the correction of sodium. It is thought to be caused by correction of sodium at a faster rate than what the brain can adapt to at the higher osmolality. Demyelination is seen in the pontine and extrapontine sites on MRI. There is an increased risk of developing CPM if the hyponatraemia has been present for >48 hours. Additionally, alcoholics, malnourished and elderly patients are more susceptible to the disease. CPM is characterised by neurological findings such as fluctuating level of consciousness, mutism, dysphagia, dysarthria, quadriparesis and seizures. Severe debilitation can ensue for several weeks and in many cases are permanent. Cardiac arrhythmias are typically not caused by a direct effect of rapid correction of hyponatraemia.[1-3]

23. Answer: C

Hypocalcaemia is defined as $[Ca^{2+}]$ of <2.0 mmol/L. The most common cause is post-thyroid or parathyroid surgery (hypoparathyroid states). It can also occur secondary to decreased calcium absorption (vitamin D deficiency, malabsorption syndromes), increased excretion (renal insufficiency, alcoholism, loop diuretics), endocrine disorders (Conn's syndrome, pseudoparathyroidism), drugs (multiple though note loop diuretics cause hypocalcaemia and thiazide diuretics cause hypercalcaemia) and conditions that sequester calcium into damaged cells (e.g. sepsis, trauma, acute pancreatitis, rhabdomyolysis).

In contrast, the most common causes of hypercalcaemia are hyperparathyroidism (primary, secondary and tertiary), malignancies (typically from the production of parathyroid hormone-related protein and bony metastases) and rarer causes (e.g. sarcoidosis, hyperthyroidism, Paget's disease, adrenal insufficiency).[1,2]

24. Answer: A

Rhabdomyolysis is a syndrome characterised by injury to the skeletal muscle and release of intracellular contents. There are numerous causes of rhabdomyolysis; however, the common terminal event appears to be disruption of the Na-K ATPase and calcium pump, leading to increased intracellular calcium and muscle cell necrosis. Additionally, the calcium activates numerous intracellular proteases and the production of free radicals further leading to cell death. Some of the causes of rhabdomyolysis includes drug and toxin abuse (e.g. cocaine, amphetamines), trauma, sepsis, heat-related injury and strenuous physical activity. Complications of rhabdomyolysis include:

- acute renal failure
- metabolic derangement
- disseminated intravascular coagulation (DIC)
- mechanical complications such as compartment syndrome.

The most common metabolic abnormality is hypocalcaemia. It usually occurs early in the disease process and is caused by the deposition of calcium salts in necrotic tissue. It is generally asymptomatic. Later in the disease process, calcium is mobilised from the damaged necrotic muscles and hypercalcaemia can ensue.

Other electrolyte abnormalities include serum phosphate levels, which are initially elevated early in the disease course. Later, however, mild hypophosphataemia may be seen but rarely requires treatment.

Hyperuricaemia occurs especially in crush injuries due to the release of muscle nucleotides, which are then converted to uric acid in the liver. These levels usually correlate well with the serum CK levels.

Hyperkalaemia occurs in 10–40% of cases due to release of potassium from injured skeletal muscle. The presence of renal failure, however, appears to be the most important determinant of the degree of elevation of the potassium. Hyperkalaemia can be a significant complication causing cardiac arrhythmias if acute renal failure occurs.[12,13]

25. Answer: D

An acidaemia exists with a low HCO_3 and high CO_2 level suggesting either a metabolic acidosis or a respiratory acidosis as the primary disorder. The calculated expected CO_2 if the primary process was a metabolic acidosis would be 31. The measure CO_2 is 50, indicating a second process of a respiratory acidosis. Conversely, if the primary process was a respiratory acidosis, then the expected HCO_3 would be 25.5. Through both calculations, you can see that there is a dual process occurring with a coexistent metabolic acidosis and respiratory acidosis. Given the scenario, it is most likely that the metabolic acidosis is the primary process with a secondary respiratory acidosis.

The AG is calculated to be 144 − [98 + 15] = 31 (i.e. elevated). The delta gap can also be calculated as 31 − 12/ 24−15 = 2.1, thereby also indicating a coexistent process to the high anion metabolic acidosis.

References

1. Kelen G, Hsu E. Fluids and electrolytes. In: Tintinalli J, Stapczynski J, Ma O, et al, editors. Tintinalli's emergency medicine: a comprehensive study guide. 7th ed. New York: McGraw Hill Medical; 2011. p. 117–29.

2. Dunn R. Investigations. In: Dunn R, Brookes J, Leach D, editors. The emergency medicine manual. 4 ed. Adelaide: Venom Publishing; 2006. p. 471–508.

3. Pasco J. Electrolyte disturbances. In: Cameron P, Jelinek G, Kelly A, editors. Textbook of adult emergency medicine. 3rd ed. Edinburgh: Elsevier; 2009. p. 497–507.

4. Nicolaou D, Kelen G. Acid–base disorders. In: Tintinalli J, Stapczynski J, Ma O, et al, editors. Tintinalli's emergency medicine: a comprehensive study guide. 7th ed. New York: McGraw Hill Medical; 2011. p. 102–12.

5. Murray L, Daly F, Little M, et al. Acid–base disorders. In: Murray L, Daly F, Little M, editors. Toxicology handbook. 2nd ed. Sydney: Churchill Livingston Elsevier; 2011. p. 109–13.

6. Brandis K. Acid–base physiology. Online. Available: http://www.anaesthesiaMCQ.com.

7. Murray L, Daly F, Little M, et al. Osmolality and osmolar gap. In: Murray L, Daly F, Little M, editors. Toxicology handbook. 2nd ed. Sydney: Churchill Livingston Elsevier; 2011. p. 107–9.

8. Murray L, Daly F, Little M, et al. The 12-lead ECG in toxicology. In: Murray L, Daly F, Little M, editors. Toxicology handbook. 2nd ed. Sydney: Churchill Livingston Elsevier; 2011. p. 113–8.

9. Brookes J, Dunn R. Respiratory. In: Dunn R, Brookes J, Leach D, editors. The emergency medicine manual. 4th ed. Adelaide: Venom Publishing; 2006. p. 765–810.

10. Slesinger T. Blood gases: pathophysiology and interpretation. In: Tintinalli J, Stapczynski J, Ma O, et al, editors. Tintinalli's emergency medicine: a comprehensive study guide. 7th ed. New York: McGraw Hill Medical; 2011. p. 112–7.

11. Fathallah-Shaykh S. Fanconi syndrome. In: Medscape reference: drugs, diseases and procedures. Online. Available: http://emedicine.medscape.com.

12. Counselman F, Lo B. Rhabdomyolysis. In: Tintinalli J, Stapczynski J, Ma O, et al, editors. Tintinalli's emergency medicine: a comprehensive study guide. 7th ed. New York: McGraw Hill Medical; 2011. p. 622–4.

13. Dunn R. Trauma: compartment syndrome. In: Dunn R, Brookes J, Leach D, editors. The emergency medicine manual. 4th ed. Adelaide: Venom Publishing; 2006. p. 1070–1.

CHAPTER 12
EMERGENCY ANAESTHESIA AND PAIN MANAGEMENT
ANSWERS

1. Answer: B

Sellick's manoeuvre, in which an assistant applies cricoid pressure during intubation to prevent aspiration, may worsen the laryngoscopic view. All of the remaining manoeuvres are associated with improved visualisation of the vocal cords but it appears that **bimanual laryngoscopy, a technique where the intubator manipulates the larynx with their right hand until visualisation, and then an assistant maintains the position, provides better visualisation.** The BURP manoeuvre is where the assistant applies backwards-upwards-rightwards pressure on the thyroid cartilage.[1–3]

2. Answer: D

For many years cricoid pressure has been advocated as the standard of care during RSI for preventing aspiration. The evidence supporting the widespread use of cricoid pressure to prevent aspiration is, however, unconvincing by current standards of evidence-based medicine. **Cricoid pressure generally impairs BVM ventilation, worsens laryngoscopic view and impairs insertion of the tube over an endotracheal introducer.** Although evidence does not support its effectiveness in RSI, many practitioners still use it. The routine use of cricoid pressure to prevent aspiration is no longer recommended. If cricoid pressure is used, the pressure should be adjusted, relaxed or released if it impedes ventilation or placement of an advanced airway.[1,4–6]

3. Answer: C

Upper airway obstruction due to laryngospasm can occur during the induction of anaesthesia or post-extubation. A variety of triggers are recognised including movement of the cervical spine, vocal cord irritation from blood, vomitus or oral secretions, pain or sudden stimulation while the patient is still in a light plane of anaesthesia. In some cases the triggers are not identified. A recent respiratory tract infection or exposure to passive cigarette smoke may predispose patients to laryngospasm on emergence.

Laryngospasm can persist long after the causative stimulus has ceased.

Laryngospasm has the potential to cause increased morbidity and mortality due to severe hypoxaemia, pulmonary aspiration and postobstructive pulmonary oedema. The proposed mechanism of pulmonary oedema is the generation of high negative pressures during respiratory effort associated with glottis closure and laryngospasm.

Although laryngospasm can occur in both adults and children, it is more common in children, being highest in infants 1–3 months of age. Bradycardia may also complicate laryngospasm and hypoxaemia, especially in young children. Bradycardia accompanied one-fifth of cases under 1 year of age in the Australian Incident Monitoring Study.[7–9]

4. Answer: C

The LMA is a useful alternative to endotracheal intubation when an advanced airway is required but it is not a definitive airway and doesn't protect the patient from aspiration. Positioning of the patient into the 'sniffing' position is not essential but it is preferable. The LMA should not be held while the cuff is being inflated to allow the LMA to seat properly. The LMA tube on average will move out of the mouth approximately 0.7% during inflation. The LMA can potentially be placed too deeply if the tube is held in place during inflation and not allowed to rise slightly.[10–12]

5. Answer: A

The optimum approach to intubation of the morbidly obese is unclear. **Positioning the patient in the 'ramp' position appears to improve the laryngoscopic view compared with the standard 'sniffing' position.** The ramp position can be achieved by elevating the head and shoulders with blankets/pillows/wedge such that the external auditory meatus and the sternal notch are horizontally aligned. Clearly this approach is not suitable in trauma patients with suspected cervical spine injuries.

Obesity alters the pharmacokinetics and pharmacodynamics of many medications. In contrast to induction agents, there is consistent evidence from the literature to guide the dosing of neuromuscular blocking agents. **Suxamethonium should be dosed according to total body weight as dosing based on ideal body weight provides inadequate paralysis and poorer laryngoscopic views.** Non-depolarising neuromuscular blocking agents such as vecuronium and rocuronium should be dosed according to ideal body weight because recovery may be prolonged when dosed according to total body weight. Ideal body weight can be estimated by various formulae. The Devine formula is the most commonly used formula and can be calculated as follows:

- male IBW = 50 kg + 2.3 kg for each inch over 5 feet
- female IBW = 45.5 kg +2.3 kg for each inch over 5 feet (1 inch = 2.5 cm, 1 foot = 30.48 cm).

Ventilation can pose another challenge. **Tidal volumes are calculated based upon the patient's ideal body weight** (obesity does not change underlying lung volumes) and then adjusted according to the clinical response, using airway pressures, oxygen saturation and blood gas results.[13,14]

6. Answer: A

Laryngoscopy and intubation stimulate reflex responses to protect the airway, such as gagging and coughing. Other reflex responses include sympathetic stimulation in adults that can cause significant increases in heart rate, blood pressure and intracranial pressure and parasympathetically mediated bronchospasm. Parasympathetic stimulation usually dominates in young children and can cause profound bradycardia. Pretreatment agents are commonly used prior to rapid sequence intubation in an attempt to attenuate these adverse physiological responses.

Lignocaine has been recommended in patients with raised intracranial pressure (ICP) and bronchospasm due to its potential ability to reduce bronchospasm and blunt increases in intracranial pressure. However, there is no high-quality evidence to demonstrate its effectiveness. Additionally, there are also no studies to demonstrate that pretreatment with lignocaine improves outcome in patients undergoing RSI.

Pretreatment with *atropine* does not consistently prevent bradycardia in children and is now only recommended for symptomatic bradycardia and not as a routine agent. Some practitioners still prefer

to use it, especially in infants, as they are more likely to develop bradycardia.

Traditionally, preadministration of a *defasciculating dose* (one tenth of a non-depolarising muscle relaxant) has been recommended to prevent fasciculations and muscle pains associated with suxamethonium. However, there is no evidence to support its use, and pretreatment with a non-depolarising agent is no longer recommended.

Fentanyl is an ultra short-acting opioid that may be used in patients with elevated ICP or cardiovascular disease that may be exacerbated by sudden elevations in blood pressure. **Adverse reaction such as chest wall rigidity and respiratory depression are minimised when fentanyl is given over 30–60 seconds.** Chest rigidity and the subsequent inability to ventilate a patient is an uncommon adverse effect of fentanyl, and is generally associated with administration of large doses and if fentanyl is given rapidly. The exact mechanism by which fentanyl induces muscle rigidity is still unknown. Suxamethonium and naloxone, an opiod recepter antagonist, might be useful in reversing chest rigidity.[1,11,15]

7. Answer: D

Propofol is presented as a white emulsion of soya bean oil and egg lecithin and should be avoided in patients with allergies to egg or soya. Saying that, most egg allergies involve a reaction to egg white (egg albumin), whereas egg lecithin is extracted from egg yolk. Hypotension is due to myocardial suppression and vasodilatation. Propofol does not cause histamine release. **Hypotension is more pronounced in the elderly and patients with hypovolaemia.** One of propofol's advantages is its antiemetic property. Propofol formulations can support the growth of bacteria, so good sterile technique must be used in preparation and handling. Administration should be completed within 6 hours of opening the ampule.[1,16]

8. Answer: C

Suxamethonium is the paralytic agent of choice for RSI in the ED due to its rapid onset (45–60 seconds) and short duration of action (3–5 minutes). It is not without any side effects and may be contraindicated in certain populations in the ED, especially those patients at risk of a life-threatening hyperkalaemic response. A clinically significant hyperkalaemic response can occur ≥5 days after a burn, denervation or crush injury due to acetylcholine receptor upregulation at the neuromuscular junction with resultant exaggerated hyperkalaemic response. Similarly, patients with pre-existing myopathies, myasthenia gravis and pre-existing hyperkalaemia are also at risk and suxamethonium should be avoided in this population.

Fasciculations and *muscle pains* **are common and the use of 1.5 mg/kg of suxamethonium is associated with less fasciculation and myalgia than occur with 1 mg/kg.** A dose of 1.5–2 mg/kg is now recommended in adults as it provides excellent intubation conditions and do not increase the risk to the patient, whereas inadequate doses can leave the patient inadequately paralysed and difficult to intubate. Neonates and infants require a slightly higher dose of suxamethonium (2 mg/kg intravenously) owing to their higher volume of distribution. Muscle fasciculation may contribute to an increase in intracranial pressure but this is not clinically significant. The benefit associated with optimal intubation conditions far exceeds this theoretical risk.

Suxamethonium can be negative chronotropic with resultant *bradycardia* following administration, especially in children. This may be due to direct cardiac muscarinic stimulation as well as stimulation of autonomic ganglia by suxamethonium. It is, however, difficult to separate the effects of suxamethonium on the heart from the effects induced by the autonomic responses to laryngoscopy and intubation. **Sinus bradycardia is treated with atropine, if necessary, but is often self-limiting. Some paediatric practitioners recommend pretreatment with atropine for children younger than 1 year old, but there is no evidence for benefit.**[1,11,15]

9. Answer: D

Lignocaine is an amide-type anaesthetic agent. When lignocaine is administered by direct infiltration, the onset of action is within seconds and lasts 20–60 minutes. When administered as a nerve block, onset occurs in 4–6 minutes and the effective duration is longer, usually 75 minutes. It may remain effective for up to 120 minutes.

The maximum safe dose of lignocaine without adrenaline is 3 to 5 mg/kg and should not exceed 300 mg at a single injection. More volume can be added safely every 30 minutes if needed. The addition of adrenaline to lignocaine causes vasoconstriction and subsequently less systemic absorption. Not only does the resulting vasoconstriction prolong the anaesthetic effect for 2–6 hours, but it also increases the safe dose to 5–7 mg/kg.

Anaesthetic solutions contain uncharged and charged forms. It is the uncharged form that crosses tissue and nerve barriers. Once the uncharged drug is through a barrier, it re-equilibrates into uncharged and charged forms in a proportion dependent on the prevailing pH. The charged form is responsible for the actual neuronal blockade. The speed of onset of any local anaesthetic agent is directly related to how quickly that agent, after injection, can diffuse through tissues to the nerve and through the nerve membrane. The concentration of the uncharged form is increased in a more alkaline environment (raised pH) and therefore a more rapid onset of action can be expected. **An alkaline environment can be achieved by adding 1 mL of sodium bicarbonate 8.4% to 10 mL of lignocaine without compromising the quality of anaesthesia.** Not only does the addition of a sodium bicarbonate solution to local anaesthetics shorten the onset of action but it also reduces the pain of injection.[17–20]

10. Answer: B

Like lignocaine, bupivacaine is an amide-type local anaesthetic agent. The onset of action is slightly slower than that of lignocaine, but the duration of anesthesia is 4–8 times longer.

The reported safe dose of bupivacaine in adults is approximately 1.5 mg/kg without adrenaline and 3 mg/kg with adrenaline. The dose can be repeated every 3 hours, not exceeding a total of more than 400 mg in a 24-hour period. Bupivacaine is not recommended in children younger than 12 years of age.

All local anaesthetics can cause rapid and profound cardiovascular depression. **Bupivacaine is a more potent cardiodepressant than lignocaine and has arrythmogenic potential as well.** The ratio of the dosage required for irreversible cardiovascular collapse (CC) and the dosage that will produce CNS toxicity (CNS), that is the CC/CNS ratio, is lower for bupivacaine than for lignocaine. Furthermore, cardiac resuscitation is more difficult after bupivacaine-induced cardiovascular collapse, and acidosis and hypoxia markedly potentiate the cardiotoxicity.[17,19,21]

11. Answer: B

Prilocaine is the drug of choice for intravenous regional anaesthesia because it is the least toxic local anaesthetic agent. It can safely be given at a dose of 2.5 mg/kg (0.5 mL/kg of a 0.5% solution). Prilocaine should be injected slowly over 90 seconds. Lignocaine is an acceptable alternative to prilocaine. The standard dose of lignocaine is 3 mg/kg injected as a 0.5% solution (without adrenaline). A high success rate has also been achieved with a minidose of 1.5 mg/kg and is preferred by some clinicians.

The minimum tourniquet inflation time should be 20–30 minutes to prevent systemic toxicity. The maximum tourniquet inflation time should not exceed 60 minutes (some suggest 90 minutes).

Anaesthesia from a fingertip-to-elbow direction occurs irrespective of the site of anaesthetic infusion. Selecting an injection site near the site of pathology will provide more rapid anaesthesia at a lower dosage. There is some evidence that indicates that the procedure is more successful when the anaesthetic is injected distally.[19,22]

12. Answer: A

Femoral nerve blocks have proven effectiveness and low complication rates. **It significantly decreases time to achieve lowest pain score as compared with intravenous narcotics, and patients have been found to require significantly lower doses of narcotics in conjunction.**

When the *blind technique* is utilised, it is common practice to elicit paraesthesia to ensure the needle tip is in close proximity to the nerve. However, when paraesthesia is elicited, it is important that the needle must be withdrawn 1–2 mm before the anaesthetic is injected to prevent intraneural injection.

Peripheral nerve stimulators are commonly used by anaesthetists in performing peripheral nerve blocks to ensure consistent delivery of the anaesthetic to the immediate vicinity of the nerve. However, this practice is not common in the ED but neither is there any evidence to discourage this practice in the ED.

Advantages of using *ultrasound* in the ED to guide femoral nerve block include the ability to achieve a more complete block with less local anaesthetic and fewer vascular punctures. Detailed knowledge of the sonographic anatomy of the femoral nerve in the inguinal region is essential to be successful with this technique.[23–27]

13. Answer: B

Opioids are frequently used in the ED for the relief of moderate to severe pain. **However, it is frequently given in inadequate doses due to the concerns for precipitation of adverse events like respiratory depression. Contrary to the belief, <1% of patients who receive opioids will develop respiratory depression.** Tolerance to this side effect develops simultaneously to tolerance to the analgesic effect. If the opioid dose is increased so that at least half the pain is relieved, the chance of respiratory depression is small. The risk of respiratory depression is increased when opioids are administered in conjunction with benzodiazepines, ethanol or other depressive drugs.

A typical adult dose of fentanyl for management of acute severe pain is 1–2 mcg/kg given intravenously. It has an onset of action within 1 minute, a peak effect at 2–5 minutes and a duration of 30–60 minutes. It does not possess any intrinsic anxiolytic or amnestic properties. *Intranasal fentanyl* has become popular for use especially in the paediatric population. Well-designed randomised controlled trials found that **intranasal administration of fentanyl provides initial pain relief comparable to intravenous opioids and may even obviate the need for intravenous access.** An initial dose of 1.5 mcg/kg is usually adequate. A second dose may be administered within 10 minutes of the first if necessary at a dose of 0.75–1.5 mcg/kg. If further analgesia is required after the second dose the patient should be reviewed and alternative or additional analgesia considered.

Traditionally, *pethidine* was preferred over morphine in the management of biliary colic as it was thought to have less of an effect on the sphincter of Oddi. However, its effect on the sphincter of Oddi is similar to morphine and there is no evidence to support the preferential use of pethidine in gall bladder or pancreatic disease. Pethidine has been removed from the Pharmaceutical Benefits Scheme and from a number of Australian hospitals because it has shown no advantage compared with other parenteral opioids, and has a number of significant disadvantages. Accumulation of the active metabolite, norpethidine can cause hyperexcitability, tremors, myoclonus and seizures, especially with repeated dosing or renal impairment. In addition, pethidine can cause serotonin syndrome when combined with other serotonergic medication and has a higher potential for abuse. It is now highly recommended that pethidine should be avoided.[28-33]

14. Answer: D

Midazolam has anxiolytic, sedative and amnestic effects but no analgesic activity. Paradoxal agitation has been reported with midazolam in 1–15% of patients and can be reversed with flumazenil. *Propofol* is frequently used for PSA in the ED. It has no analgesic activity, but it does have an excellent amnestic effect. **There is strong supportive evidence that *ketamine* does not exhibit dose-dependant adverse events within the range of clinically administered doses using standard administration techniques**. Adverse effects of ketamine include vomiting, which typically occurs well into the recovery phase when the patient is alert and can clear the airway without assistance. The peak age for vomiting is early adolescence with lesser risk in younger and older children. Vomiting seems to be more frequent with the IM route compared with IV. Hypersalivation associated with ketamine use is rare and usually not clinically significant. Anticholinergic agents are not routinely recommended but can be used if clinically important hypersalivation occurs or for patients with impaired ability to mobilise secretions.[34,35]

15. Answer: D

Depression and impairment of protective airway reflexes is a potential risk of PSA. The most significant potential risk associated with diminished airway reflexes is pulmonary aspiration. However, **the risk of aspiration is low with PSA and fasting is just one consideration.** Compared with general anaesthesia, PSA does not involve the use of volatile inhalational anaesthetics, which are particularly emetogenic, nor does it involve pharyngeal manipulation or instrumentation, again a potent stimulus for induced vomiting.

The tradition of fasting prior to a procedure is based on the intuitive recognition that vomiting and aspiration

requires something in the gut. In ED PSA, fasting is not always practical, as patients are rarely fasted at the time of presentation and they present to the ED with injuries and illnesses requiring PSA that is rarely elective in nature. **Additionally, there is insufficient evidence to support that prolonged fasting prior to sedation reduces the risk of vomiting and/or aspiration in both elective and emergency procedures.** Despite this lack of evidence, most guidelines still recommend at least 2 hours and 6 hours from the last intake of fluid and food respectively to allow for gastric emptying. Similarly, there is insufficient evidence to associate fasting time, gastric volume or gastric acidity with the probability of aspiration during procedural sedation in both children and adults. There is also no evidence to support the frequently repeated supposition that gastric emptying is delayed by acute stress or anxiety.

Despite the low risk of aspiration and lack of evidence, it is prudent to err on the side of caution. Rather than just focusing on fasting times prior to PSA, emergency clinicians should aim to:

- risk stratify the presedation aspiration risk
  – consider the potential for difficult or prolonged assisted ventilation should an airway complication occur, conditions predisposing to oesophageal reflux, extremes of age, obesity, etc.
- assess the timing and nature of recent oral intake
- determine prudent limits of targeted sedation depth and length of procedure
- assess the urgency of the procedure.[36-39]

16. Answer: B

The ASA physical class system remains the standard for assessing a child before the procedure. This risk grading system is also recommended by the paediatrics and child health division of The Royal Australasian College of Physicians in their guideline statement on the management of procedure-related pain in children and adolescents. Classes 1–2 are generally considered to be at low risk during PSA. A higher risk class is not an absolute contraindication for ED PSA, especially when performed for emergency procedures. However, emergency clinicians should strongly consider a referral for general anaesthesia or deferring the procedure.

The ASA physical classes are:

I   Normal healthy patient

II Patient with mild systemic condition

III Patient with a severe systemic condition that limits activity but is not incapacitating

IV Patient with an incapacitating systemic condition that is a constant threat to life

V Moribund patient not expected to survive for 24 hours

Children should be adequately prepared for any procedure in the ED. This entails some forethought on the part of the administrators of the ED, as a developmentally appropriate plan should be in place to deal with infants, school-aged and adolescent children. Non-pharmacological techniques in preparing the parents include coaching parents to act in a positive fashion (not a physical restrainer) during the procedure, and to address their own anxiety before participating in the procedure, as well as involving them as part of the team rather than as a passive bystander. Preparing children by allowing them to see the procedure room, explaining the procedure and practising on a doll with the equipment to be used are all good measures to alleviate stress and anxiety.

Guidelines by various anaesthetic bodies such as the American Society of Anaesthesiologists recommend that children should not consume solids for 4–8 hours or clear liquids for 2–3 hours prior to undergoing sedation for an elective procedure. Several large studies of children undergoing procedural sedation and analgesia outside of the operating theatre had no episodes of clinically evident aspiration. Therefore, although vomiting with aspiration is of great concern during procedural sedation and analgesia, the risk is low and the benefit of delaying the procedure to allow gastric emptying seems minimal. **Delaying the procedure to meet fasting guidelines may actually compromise the patient's condition in some instances.** Similarly, gastric emptying strategies for sedation procedures is not well studied in children.[39]

17. Answer: B

It is unclear whether assessing for pain before a procedure will cue the child to expect pain and therefore alter the normal pain response during a procedure. What is evident, however, from the literature is that **under-predicting pain in children has adverse consequences on any subsequent**

need for procedures, and this effect may be lifelong into adulthood. For this reason, it is better to over-predict than under-predict. Furthermore, the initial assessment of a child's pain score and his/her ability to understand and cope with a procedure is only a starting point. Re-evaluation of the progress through a given choice of procedural analgesia or sedation may need to be altered depending on the evolving pain assessment.

Measuring pain intensity is only one part of pain assessment. There are different objective and subjective methods of measuring pain: physiological monitoring of bodily processes, rating scales and observation measures (for both the child and parent/ staff).

The *FLACC* scale is commonly used for children with cognitive impairment but it has not been validated for procedures.

Self-report tools vary depending on developmental age. Commonly used self-report tools include:

- Pieces of Hurt (3–6 years)
- Faces Pain Scale (4+ years)
- visual analogue scales (6+ years)
- numerical scales (8+ years)

The Pieces of Hurt, also know as the Poker Chip Tool, were developed to allow children to rate their pain by using chips that are described as 'pieces of hurt' (one white chip representing no pain, and four red ones representing pain). The more chips the child uses, the greater their hurt.

Faces scales show a series of faces that are graded in increasing intensity from no pain to the worst pain possible. One scientifically validated and commonly used scale is Faces Pain Scale – Revised. Others include the Wong and Baker Faces scale and the Oucher scale.

Visual analogue scales require the patient to make a mark somewhere along a 100 mm line to indicate the amount of pain that they experience, with 'no pain' at one end of the scale and 'the worst pain' at the other.

Numerical scales (e.g. 0–10) use numbers to represent increasing degrees of pain. Children must understand number concepts and have sufficient abstract thinking ability to use this type of scale.[39]

18. Answer: C

The evidence is conflicted as to whether it is beneficial to have parents in attendance during painful procedures. What is important is how they behave in a given situation. Adult behaviours likely to interfere with a child's coping include:

- making reassuring comments (e.g. 'It'll be all right')
- apologising (e.g. 'I'm sorry you have to go through this')
- criticising (e.g. 'You're being a baby')
- bargaining with the child (e.g. 'I'll get you a play station if you let them do it')
- giving the child control over when to start the procedure (e.g. 'Tell me when you're ready').

Play therapists are a mainstay of non-pharmacological strategies to decrease anxiety in the periprocedural phase in paediatric oncology and EDs.[39,40]

19. Answer: A

Venepuncture is the preferred method of blood sampling when a significant volume of blood is required. It has been shown to be less painful in neonates and less likely to require resampling. Capillary sampling is often used when the volume of blood required is small. EMLA® cream, other topical anaesthetic agents and paracetamol do not relieve the pain of capillary sampling. **Administration of 15–50% sucrose is effective in neonates and may be effective up to 2 months of age.** Systematic reviews of the literature suggest doses in the order of 0.5–1.0 mL of 24% sucrose in 0.25 mL aliquots, commencing 2 minutes before the procedure. Multiple published reviews dating back to the late 1990s have clearly showed the efficacy and potency of sucrose in alleviating pain in neonates – the challenge has been converting this body of evidence into practice. Current evidence suggests that the use of EMLA® with sucrose does not result in any further analgesic efficacy than sucrose alone in neonates undergoing skin puncture.

A Cochrane review in 2006 concluded that amethocaine (Ametop®, AnGel®) is better than EMLA® for reducing pain from intravenous cannulation. A newer topical agent, LMX4® (lignocaine 4%) promises to provide more potent analgesia and longer lasting action, without requiring refrigeration. No randomised studies are available as yet to compare its use to the older formulations in children, although one published study in adults did indicate it is effective in reducing

pain from cannulation. It is the author's opinion that the best topical agent for use in children is AnGel® cream, especially for cannulation, while EMLA® is useful in settings where some vasoconstriction is desirable, for example, LP in infants and children (or adults!). LMX4® looks like a promising product for intravenous cannulation analgesia and is probably equivalent to AnGel® cream in this regard, with formal studies pending.[39,41,42]

20. Answer: D

General considerations in laceration repair in children include:

- the use of distraction techniques
- the use of skin glues rather than sutures for repair of simple lacerations
- the use of topical agents in preference to injected lignocaine if a local anaesthetic is required.

The mixture of lignocaine, adrenaline and tetracaine (ALA® or LET®) should be used in preference to cocaine-containing topical anaesthetics (such as TAC® and AC Gel®) because of equivalent efficacy and better safety profile. Laceraine® (4% lignocaine hydrochloride, 0.5% amethocaine hydrochloride, 0.1% adrenaline1.8 mg/mL) is the topical agent of choice, although specific studies are still pending.

Inhaled nitrous oxide is effective in providing analgesia and anxiolysis to facilitate *suturing* in children. Midazolam does not have analgesic properties. For more complicated lacerations, intravenous ketamine and midazolam can provide excellent conditions for laceration repair providing a high degree of motion control. Oral or intranasal midazolam may be used to facilitate laceration repair in children but the reported efficacy is significantly lower than the above-stated techniques.

The combination of ketamine and midazolam provides more effective analgesia than the fentanyl and midazolam combination for fracture manipulation, and has fewer respiratory side effects. The combination of propofol/fentanyl offers a similar level of analgesia to ketamine and midazolam but a much higher incidence of airway complications and is therefore not recommended for children at this time.

Regarding skin puncture in children, vapocoolant is more effective in relieving pain during immunisation than EMLA®. Its role in the ED during acute procedures is currently being explored and holds promise.[39,42,43]

References

1. Vissers RJ, Danzl DF. Tracheal intubation and mechanical ventilation. In: Tintinalli JE, Stapczynski JS, Ma OJ, editors. Emergency medicine: a comprehensive study guide. 7th ed. New York: McGraw-Hill; 2011. p. 198–209.

2. Henderson JJ. Direct laryngoscopy and oral intubation of the trachea. In: Hung O, Murphy MF, editors. Management of the difficult and failed airway. New York: McGraw Hill; 2007. p. 103–21.

3. Orebaugh SL. Difficult airway management in the emergency department. J Emerg Med 2002;22(1):31–48.

4. Hazinski M, Nolan JP, Billi JE, et al. 2010 International consensus on cardiopulmonary resuscitation and emergency cardiovascular care science with treatment recommendations. Circulation 2010;122(16)suppl 2:s249–s638.

5. Ellis DY, Harris T, Zideman D. Cricoid pressure in emergency department rapid sequence tracheal intubations: a risk-benefit analysis. Ann Emerg Med 2007;50:653–65.

6. Butler J, Sen A. Cricoid pressure in emergency rapid sequence induction. Emerg Med J 2005;22:815–6.

7. Padley AP. Westmead anaesthetic manual. 3rd ed. Sydney: McGraw-Hill; 2009. p. 299–300.

8. Visvanathan T, Kluger MT, Webb RK, et al. Crisis management during anaesthesia: laryngospasm. Qual Saf Health Care 2005;14:e3. Online. Available: http://www. qshc.com/cgi/content/full/14/3/e3.

9. Roman MA. Noninvasive airway management. In: Tintinalli JE, Stapczynski JS, Ma OJ, editors. Emergency medicine: a comprehensive study guide. 7th ed. New York: McGraw-Hill; 2011. p. 183–9.

10. Brown AFT. Critical care. In: Cameron P, Jelinek G, Kelly A, et al, editors. Textbook of adult emergency medicine. 3rd ed. Edinburgh: Elsevier; 2009. p. 20–6.

11. Walls RM. Airway. In: Marx JA, Hockberger RS, Walls RM, editors. Rosen's emergency medicine: concepts and clinical practice. 7th ed. Philadelphia: Elsevier; 2009. p. 3–82.

12. Agro FE, Doyle DJ, Hung OR, et al. Extraglottic devices for ventilation and oxygenation. In: Hung O, Murphy MF, editors. Management of the difficult and failed airway. New York: McGraw Hill; 2007. p. 173–90.

13. Dargin J, Medzon R. Emergency department management of the airway in obese adults. Ann Emerg Med 56(2):95–104.

14. Grant P, Newcombe M. Emergency management of the morbidly obese. EMA 2004;16:309–17.

15. Hopson LR, Schwartz RB. Pharmacologic adjuncts to intubation. In: Roberts JR, Hedges JR, editors. Clinical procedures in emergency medicine, 5th ed. Philadelphia: Elsevier; 2009. p. 99–109.

16. Padley AP. Westmead anaesthetic manual. 3rd ed. Sydney: McGraw-Hill; 2009. p. 427–30.

17. Simon B, Hern HA Jr. Wound management principles. In: Marx JA, Hockberger RS, Walls RM, editors. Rosen's emergency medicine: concepts and clinical practice. 7th ed. Philadelphia: Elsevier; 2010. p. 698–714.

18. Miner JR, Paris PM, Yealy DM. Pain management. In: Marx JA, Hockberger RS, Walls RM, editors. Rosen's emergency medicine: concepts and clinical practice. 7th ed. Philadelphia: Elsevier; 2010. p. 2410–28.

19. Dillon DC, Gibbs MA. Local and regional anaesthesia. In: Tintinalli JE, Stapczynski JS, Ma OJ, editors. Emergency medicine: a comprehensive study guide. 7th ed. New York: McGraw-Hill; 2011. p. 270–83.

20. McGee DL. Local and topical anesthesia. In: Roberts JR, Hedges JR, editors. Clinical procedures in emergency medicine, 5th ed. Philadelphia: Elsevier; 2009. p. 481–99.

21. Berde CB, Strichartz GR. Local anesthetics. In: Miller RD, Eriksson LI, Fleisher LE, et al, editors. Miller's Anesthesia. 7th ed. Elsevier; 2009. p. 913–39.

22. Roberts JR, Carney SK. Intravenous Regional Anesthesia. In: Roberts JR, Hedges JR, editors. Clinical procedures in emergency medicine, 5th ed. Philadelphia: Elsevier; 2009. p. 535–9.

23. Gray AT. Ultrasound guidance for regional anesthesia. In: Miller RD, Eriksson LI, Fleisher LE, et al, editors. Miller's anesthesia. 7th ed. Elsevier; 2009. p. 1675–704.

24. Fletcher AK, Rigby AS, Heyes FL. Three-in-one femoral nerve block as analgesia for fractured neck of femur in the emergency department: a randomized, controlled trial. Ann Emerg Med 2003;41:227–33.

25. Spektor M, Kelly JJ. Nerve blocks of the thorax and extremities. In: Roberts J R, Hedges J R, editors. Clinical procedures in emergency medicine. 5th ed. Philadelphia: Elsevier; 2009. p. 513–34.

26. Mutty CE, et al. Femoral nerve block for diaphyseal and distal femoral fractures in the emergency department. J Bone Joint Surg Am 2007;89:2599.

27. Fiechtl JF, Fitch RW. Femur and hip. In: Marx JA, Hockberger RS, Walls RM, editors. Rosen's emergency medicine: concepts and clinical practice. 7th ed. Philadelphia: Elsevier; 2010. p. 619–44.

28. The Royal Children's Hospital Melbourne. Intranasal fentanyl. The Royal Children's Hospital Melbourne clinical practice guidelines. Online. Available: http://www.rch.org.au/clinicalguide/cpg.cfm?doc_id=13553;31 May 2011.

29. Therapeutic Guidelines Limited. Pethidine. In: eTG complete. Online. Available: http://www.tg.org.au; 31 May 2011.

30. Atkinson P, Chesters A, Heinz P. Pain management and sedation for children in the emergency department. BMJ 2009;339:1074–9.

31. Ducharme J. Acute pain management in adults. In: Tintinalli JE, Stapczynski JS, Ma OJ, editors. Emergency medicine: a comprehensive study guide. 7th ed. New York: McGraw-Hill; 2011. p. 259–65

32. Fatovich DM. General pain management. In: Cameron P, Jelinek G, Kelly A, et al, editors. Textbook of adult emergency medicine. 3rd ed. Edinburgh: Elsevier; 2009. p. 692–7.

33. Green SM, Krauss B. Systemic analgesia and sedation for procedures. In: Roberts JR, Hedges JR, editors. Clinical procedures in emergency medicine. 5th ed. Philadelphia: Elsevier; 2009. p. 540–62.

34. Green SM, Roaback MG, Kennedy RM, et al. Clinical practice guideline for emergency department ketamine dissociative sedation: 2011 update. Ann Emerg Med 2011;57(5):449–61.

35. Miner J. Procedural sedation and analgesia. In: Tintinalli JE, Stapczynski JS, Ma OJ, editors. Emergency medicine: a comprehensive study guide. 7th ed. New York: McGraw-Hill; 2011. p. 283–91.

36. Bell A, Trseton G. Procedural sedation and analgesia. In: Cameron P, Jelinek G, Kelly A, et al, editors. Textbook of adult emergency medicine. 3rd ed. Edinburgh: Elsevier; 2009. p. 704–11.

37. Green SM, Roback MG, Miner JR, et al. Fasting and emergency department procedural sedation and analgesia: a consensus-based clinical practice advisory. Ann Emerg Med. 2007;49:454–61.

38. Green SM, Krauss B. Systemic Analgesia and Sedation for Procedures. In: Roberts JR, Hedges JR, editors. Clinical procedures in emergency medicine. 5th ed. Philadelphia: Elsevier; 2009. p. 540–62.

39. Guideline statement: Management of procedure-related pain in children and adolescents. Paediatrics & Child Health Division. Sydney: The Royal Australasian College of Physicians; 2005.

40. Piira T, Sugiura T, Champion GD, et al. The role of parental presence in the context of children's medical procedures: a systematic review. Child: Care, Health and Development 2005;31(2):233–43.

41. Stevens B, Taddio A, Ohlsson A, et al. The efficacy of sucrose for relieving procedural pain in neonates – a systematic review and meta-analysis. Acta Paediatrica 1997;86(8):837–42.

42. Lander JA, Weltman BJ, So SS. EMLA and amethocaine for reduction of children's pain associated with needle insertion. Cochrane Database Syst Rev 2006;3:CD004236.

43. Valdovinos NC, Reddin C, Bernard C, et al. The use of topical anesthesia during intravenous catheter insertion in adults: a comparison of pain scores using LMX-4 versus placebo. Emerg Nurs 2009;35(4):299–304.

1. Answer: D

Children are a diverse group of people and vary enormously in weight, size, shape, intellectual ability and emotional responses. The larynx is situated anteriorly and superiorly at the level of C2–C3, making intubation in children difficult. The child relies on the diaphragm for breathing with the horizontal ribs hardly contributing. The infant has a greater metabolic rate and oxygen consumption and accounts for the higher respiratory rate of infants. However, the tidal volume remains relatively constant in relation to the body weight throughout childhood. The work of breathing is also relatively unchanged at about 1% of the metabolic rate. **The child's circulating blood volume per kilogram of body weight (70–80 mL/kg) is higher than that of an adult, but the actual volume is small. This means that in severe trauma in infants and small children, relatively small absolute amounts of blood loss can be critically important.**[1]

2. Answer: B

Head trauma is the most common single organ system injury associated with death in injured children. The child's head-to-body ratio is greater, the brain is less myelinated and cranial bones are thinner, resulting in more serious head injury. However, multiple injuries are common in children because the small body size allows for a greater distribution of forces.

The chest wall of children is pliable and will take a large amount of force to fracture and their mediastinum is more mobile than in adults. Children often have significant intrathoracic injuries without signs of trauma on the thoracic wall. The presence of fractured ribs is therefore an ominous sign in children. Unlike in adults, pulmonary contusions and pneumothoraces without associated rib fractures can often occur in children.

The child's internal organs are more susceptible to injury because the abdominal wall is thin, the liver and spleen are more anteriorly placed and the diaphragm is more horizontal, causing the liver and spleen to lie lower.

In children, the bladder being mostly an intraabdominal organ, is prone to injury.[2,3]

3. Answer: B

Bruises in NAI are common to soft tissue areas rather than bony prominences. Additionally, certain fracture patterns have been found more characteristic of abuse than others. *Metaphyseal fractures* of long bones showing chip fractures at the corner of the metaphysis are due to violent torsion or traction injury and pathognomonic of NAI. *Rib fractures* are usually multiple and symmetrical and most occur posteriorly, resulting from maximal mechanical stress at the costovertebral junction as the child is grasped and shaken. *Spiral fractures of long bones* from NAI are also common, but under the age of 3 this should be differentiated from the spiral fractures of the tibia as seen in toddlers first starting to walk.[4,5]

4. Answer: A

Abusive head trauma (shaken baby syndrome or shaken impact syndrome) is a form of inflicted head trauma and is the leading cause of child abuse fatalities. It is a well-recognised clinical syndrome caused by violent shaking of infants, direct blows to the head, dropping or throwing a child, and asphyxia. **Retinal haemorrhages, subdural haematomas and diffuse axonal injury strongly suggest abusive head trauma (AHT), especially when they co-occur. Retinal haemorrhages are virtually pathognomonic of AHT.** Although retinal haemorrhages can be found in other conditions, haemorrhages that are multiple, involve more than one layer of the retina, and extend to the periphery are very suspicious for abuse. The mechanism is likely repeated acceleration-deceleration due to shaking. Retinal haemorrhages are present in 80% of children suspected of NAI, whereas 60% of acute subdural haemorrhages in children are related to NAI. Fractures are seen in approximately 35% of children with NAI.[4,6,7]

5. Answer: C

A decerebrate or extensor posture response suggests severe midbrain injury. The arms are held extended and internally rotated and the legs are extended. Decorticate or flexor response suggests severe intracranial injury above the level of midbrain. Here, the arms are held in flexion and internal rotation while the legs are in extension.[8]

6. Answer: C

One of the aims of ED resuscitation of a severe traumatic brain injury patient is to prevent any secondary insults to the brain. **Secondary insults are the clinical conditions that may worsen the outcomes of traumatic brain injury (TBI). These differ from secondary brain injury, which are changes that occur at a cellular level resulting in expansion of the primary brain injury.** Known secondary insults are increased intracranial pressure, hypotension, hypoxaemia, hypercarbia, hyperglycaemia and hyperthermia. *Hypercapnia* causes cerebral vasodilation and increased cerebral blood flow (CBF) and subsequently increases the intracranial pressure (ICP). *Hypocapnia*, secondary to hyperventilation, causes cerebral vasoconstriction. Although it potentially decreases ICP, prolonged hypocapnia through over enthusiastic hyperventilation causes cerebral ischaemia with a subsequent worse outcome. *Hyperglycaemia* in severe head injury is associated with a worse outcome, but the exact mechanism is still unknown. **Even a single event of *hypotension* or *hypoxaemia* has been described as causing significant increase in the mortality in severe TBI.** In addition to rapid correction of hypoxaemia with advanced airway management and ventilation, hypotension should be corrected with rapid fluid resuscitation and early use of vasopressors such as noradrenaline. Although not ideal, vasopressors may be commenced with peripheral intravenous access until central access is obtained. Fluid resuscitation to correct hypotension will not increase the ICP. In a trauma patient with severe TBI, early hypotension is not due to intracranial haemorrhage and therefore other sites for haemorrhage should be sought and rapidly controlled. Hypotensive resuscitation is contraindicated in these patients. **In adults, to maintain an adequate cerebral perfusion pressure (CPP), a systolic BP of at least 100 mm Hg is required with a mean arterial pressure (MAP) of 80 mm Hg.** This should overcome any modest rise in ICP due to TBI.[9,10]

7. Answer: C

Adults presenting with a Glasgow Coma Scale (GCS) of 15 and a history of head injury with loss of consciousness usually are investigated with a head CT to exclude intracranial injury. These patients are considered as having minor head injury or TBI. However, assessment of patients presenting with minor head injury but without a history of loss of consciousness can be challenging. **The absence of a history of loss of consciousness alone may not be the best predictor to rule out intracranial injury. About 2% of such patients have intracranial injury visible on CT and < 1% will require neurosurgery. These rates are similar for patients who had loss of consciousness.**

In addition to loss of consciousness, other clinical features in the history and examination, for example vomiting after head injury, posttraumatic seizure and posttraumatic amnesia, have similar odds ratios for having an intracranial lesion visible on head CT (positive head CT). Subsequently, there are a number of evidence-based decision rules developed to identify patients who have minor head injury and who need to have CT to exclude intracranial injury.[10]

8. Answer: B

Diffuse axonal injury is a severe form of traumatic brain injury secondary to severe blunt trauma such as that occurring in sudden decelerations. Additionally, it is also a well-described finding in 'shaken baby syndrome' due to NAI.

The axonal injury occurs at the grey–white matter interface in the cerebral hemispheres and in the brainstem. **In its severest form, cerebral oedema develops rapidly, increasing ICP. This acts as a secondary insult and worsens the neurological outcome. Therefore, ED interventions should be directed at preventing and reducing any increase in ICP.**

Diffuse axonal injury can be classified into four categories according to the CT appearance. In category I there are no visible abnormalities on the CT. In all other categories, lesions are present but are not of high or mixed density and always < 25 mm. In category III, significant swelling is present and in category IV this is associated with significant midline shift. However, the majority do not show any lesions or haemorrhage on CT.[10–12]

9. Answer: D

Although traumatic *subarachnoid haemorrhage* is common in TBI, this can be missed on early CT scan done within the first 6–8 hours from the time of injury. It carries a very high mortality and risk of significant permanent neurological injury. Mortality from an acute *subdural haematoma* is nearly three times higher than mortality from an *extradural haematoma* (75% vs 20–30%). This may be related to the significant neuronal injury that is often associated with acute subdural haematoma.

On non-contrast CT, an **acute subdural haematoma appears over cerebral hemispheres as a hyperdense, medially concave haematoma that crosses the suture lines**. A subacute subdural haematoma may appear isodense and a chronic subdural haematoma appears hypodense. In contrast, the **extradural haematoma appears hyperdense (white), characteristically elliptical shaped and not crossing suture lines of the skull.** Usually, it is over the temporal or temperoparietal areas and occasionally occurs in the posterior fossa. Although the history of loss of consciousness is well known to be associated with blunt trauma causing extradural haemorrhage, this feature may not be present. Even if present it is very brief in half of the patients.[10,12]

10. Answer: A

The incidence of cervical spine fractures or spinal cord injury is very uncommon in children. When suspected, the application of immobilisation to children especially to infants and young children can be a challenge. In infants, the relatively large head may cause the neck to flex when immobilising in the supine position. This can be prevented by carefully placing adequate padding under the shoulders.

The common site of cervical spine fractures in children is in the upper cervical spine where the fulcrum for the flexion-extension is situated in children. In contrast, fractures occur more commonly in the lower cervical spine in adults.

Children are more likely to have spinal cord injury without radiological abnormalities (SCIWORA). Because of increasingly easy accessibility to MRI, SCIWORA appears to be a misnomer as these injuries can be detectable on MRI. The child may initially complain of transient neurological symptoms such as paraesthesia or weakness soon after the injury and a large number of these children may not get further symptoms up to a few days.

Neither NEXUS nor the Canadian cervical spine decision rules can be safely applied to children because these studies had only small numbers of children. These rules have not been validated in children.[13–14]

11. Answer: B

During assessment of the cervical spine in trauma in awake and alert adults, both NEXUS criteria and Canadian cervical spine decision rule can be applied to identify patients who require further imaging to exclude cervical spine injury. **Both have very high sensitivities in detection of fractures (99% and 100% respectively) but their specificities are limited. The specificity of NEXUS criteria is only 12.9% and Canadian cervical spine rule is 42.5%.** Both rules can be applied together when clearing the cervical spine. However, these are only decision support tools, hence good assessment of the patient with a focused neurological examination and the checking of the range of cervical spine motion is essential before spinal clearance.

With cervical spine plain films, some of the fractures can be missed despite the adequacy of the films. Patients who have persistent symptoms in spite of having normal plain films will require CT to exclude bony injury or MRI to rule out cord and ligamentous injury. In older patients, the chance of fracture is said to be twice as high as younger patients. Odontoid fractures are common in this age group but diagnosis can be missed when plain films alone are used.[15–20]

12. Answer: C

Bilateral interfacetal dislocation occurs with disruption of all ligamentous structures secondary to hyperflexion allowing articular masses of one vertebra to dislocate superiorly and anteriorly into the intervertebral foramen of the vertebra below. On radiographs, the vertebral body is dislocated anteriorly at least 50% of its width.

Sacral injuries are relatively rare and usually occur in conjunction with pelvic fractures. Despite the rarity of sacral injuries, associated neurological injuries are not uncommon and unrecognised and inadequately treated sacral fractures may lead to painful deformity and progressive loss of neurological function. Potential neurological injuries in patients with a sacral fracture include those involving the cauda equina, the lumbosacral plexus, the sacral plexus, and the sympathetic and parasympathetic chains. Several classification systems exist to help predict the neurological deficits and establish treatment protocols. The Denis three-zone classification system is based on fracture anatomy. Zone-I fractures occur lateral to the sacral foramina and are the most common fracture pattern. Neurological injury occurs in approximately 6% of patients and typically involves the L4 and L5 nerve roots. Zone-II fractures are the second most common pattern. These injuries consist of a vertical transforaminal fracture without involvement of the sacral spinal canal. An associated neurological injury is found in 28% of patients, and it most frequently affects the L5, S1 or S2 nerve root. Any sacral fracture involving the spinal canal is classified as a zone-III injury. This fracture subtype occurs the least but is associated with the highest prevalence and severity of neurological injury, which affects approximately 57% of patients. Bowel and bladder control or sexual function is impaired in about 76% of patients with a neurological injury in this group.

A *Jefferson fracture* involves the anterior and posterior arches of C1 vertebra and occurs when the cervical spine is subjected to an axial load. The occipital condyles are forced downwards and produce a burst fracture by driving the lateral masses of C1 apart. A *Hangman fracture* involves both pedicles of C2 and occurs in extension.

Teardrop fractures to the anterioinferior part of the cervical vertebra can occur in flexion and extension and despite appearing small and insignificant on plain radiography, is associated with significant and complete disruption of the ligamentous structures at the level of the injury. These fractures are unstable.[21,22]

13. Answer: C

Cervical SCIs are associated with paralysis of intercostal and abdominal wall muscles. The phrenic nerve supplying the diaphragm originates from C3,4 and 5 nerve roots. In C5 injury diaphragmatic function is intact; however, about half of these patients still require short-term mechanical ventilation (MV). With injury at C4 level, all patients will need MV as there is a partial loss of diaphragmatic function. Injury at C3 or above, all need MV with half needing long-term ventilation. **Early hypoxaemia is very common in patients with a cervical SCI. One of the goals of ED intervention should be to prevent this hypoxaemia as it is known to cause secondary injury to the cord producing worse outcome. A patient with a cervical SCI at C5 level or above should strongly be considered for advanced airway management and MV before respiratory failure sets in.**

Unopposed vagal activity in the face of loss of sympathetic innervation may cause severe bradycardia, especially in high SCI. About 16% of patients will have asystolic cardiac arrest likely to be triggered by tracheal suctioning. Pretreatment with atropine may prevent this.

Central cord syndrome is an incomplete SCI. An incomplete SCI is where motor, sensory or both functions are partially preserved below the neurological level of injury. This functional assessment cannot be done if the patient is in the spinal shock stage and should be done when the spinal shock is resolved. Four incomplete cord syndromes have been described:

- anterior cord syndrome
- central cord syndrome
- Brown-Séquard's syndrome
- cauda equina syndrome.

Except for anterior cord syndrome, a good prognosis can be expected for patients with other incomplete syndromes if the cord injury is managed appropriately. Central cord syndrome is usually seen in elderly patients with hyperextension injuries. This results in quadriparesis where a higher degree of weakness can be elicited in the upper limbs than in the lower limbs. Some loss of pain and temperature sensation may occur with a similar pattern of distribution.[21,23]

14. Answer: C

Spinal shock **is a term used to describe the state of transient physiological, rather than anatomical, loss or depression of spinal cord sensory and motor functions (somatic functions) below the level of a complete or incomplete injury that occurs soon after the cord injury.** This may last for days to weeks. Because of the loss of functions below the level of injury during spinal shock an incomplete cord injury may appear as a complete cord injury and hence the spinal shock is not predictive of functional outcome. Flaccid paralysis below the level of the lesion including that of bladder and bowel occurs in spinal shock. Priapism is an associated feature in some patients. When spinal shock resolves, the bulbocavernous reflex usually returns first.

In contrast, the *neurogenic shock* is secondary to peripheral sympathetic denervation due to cord injury at cervical or thoracic levels. The neurogenic shock is manifested by a triad of hypotension, bradycardia and hypothermia. The sympathetic denervation causes reduced systemic arteriolar tone and systemic vascular resistance leading to hypotension. Warm and vasodilated peripheries cause heat loss leading to hypothermia. If the cord injury is above T1–T4 level sympathetic innervation to the heart is lost, but parasympathetic supply through the vagus nerve remains unopposed leading to bradycardia.[21,24]

15. Answer: D

Hypotension in a patient who had trauma and that resulted in SCI, should be considered as having ongoing blood loss (haemorrhagic shock) until proven otherwise. Other potential courses of hypotension include tension pneumothorax, cardiac tamponade, myocardial injury, intoxication with drugs and alcohol and neurogenic shock. While searching for a cause of potential haemorrhagic shock, hypotension should be promptly corrected with fluid resuscitation. Vasopressors should be used once the volume is restored. Hypotension contributes to secondary injury to the cord.

During rapid sequence intubation, suxamethonium can be used as a paralytic agent in patients with an acute spinal cord injury. **However, after the first week and up to about 6 months suxamethonium should not be used because life-threatening hyperkalaemia may occur due to denervation injury.**

There is no high-quality evidence to suggest that the use of corticosteroids is clinically beneficial. Instead, the currently available evidence suggests harmful side effects such as sepsis are associated with this therapy. The controversy remains and the current use of corticosteroids is not widespread.

Acute gastric distension and paralytic ileus develop early and abdominal distension affects ventilation. Subsequently, early insertion of a nasogastric tube should be done in the ED. Also, early urethral catheterisation prevents over distension of the bladder.[21,23]

16. Answer: A

The prominence of the zygoma (malar eminence) makes this fracture common with blunt injury but the true 'tripod' fracture is less common. The injuries in tripod fracture are:
- disruption of zygomaticofrontal suture
- disruption of zygomaticotemporal junction
- fracture of infraorbital rim.

The other associated features are:
- large lateral subconjunctival haemorrhage
- flattening of malar eminence
- inferolateral eye tilt
- trismus
- diplopia
- infraorbital anaesthesia.

Although a patient with an uncomplicated fracture of the zygomatic arch can be discharged from the ED with outpatient maxillofacial follow up, **patients with tripod fractures require admission for intravenous antibiotics and surgical repair.**[25,26]

17. Answer: C

Although rare, the danger of midfacial fractures in a multitrauma patient is the loss of mechanical support it provides to the oral cavity and the severe haemorrhage, causing obstruction to the airway. In a patient with facial trauma the early identification of this injury is important to consider interventions. Midfacial instability, and in fact the type of Le Fort fracture, can be identified by gentle rocking of the midface and hard palate during primary and secondary surveys. Types of Le Fort fractures are:
- Le Fort I: a transverse fracture separates the body of maxilla from the pterygoid plate and nasal septum
- Le Fort II: pyramidal fracture through the central maxilla and the hard palate
- Le Fort III: craniofacial dysjunction where the face is separated from the skull; fracture goes through the orbits (the only attachments between the face and the skull are optic nerves)
- Le Fort IV: the above fracture extends to the frontal bone.

In the management of unstable midfacial fractures with significant bleeding, airway control and haemorrhage control should be achieved during primary survey. Early control of posterior and anterior epistaxis with balloon devices can be attempted, with care not to place the balloon device intracranially through the fracture. For very severe oral bleeding the use of two suction devices are often needed. Two-person bag–valve–mask (BVM) ventilation is often required in the airway management. This should be done with skilled expertise and a definitive plan in hand to manage a difficult airway. Oral packing to control bleeding should be done after intubation. In an awake patient who is maintaining the airway the sitting position is more suitable to protect the airway and for better control of bleeding.[25,26]

18. Answer: C

An avulsed primary tooth should not be replaced due to possible ankylosis and failure of secondary dentition to emerge. However, a permanent tooth should be replaced as soon as possible (none will survive > 6 hours post-injury). A perforated tympanic membrane of > 50% will require tympanoplasty but smaller perforation takes 6 weeks to heal when treated conservatively. **The tongue being a muscular structure does not require repairing, but large lacerations, particularly those involving the edge of the tongue, or bleeding may do so.** Often the patient/parents need to be advised that if complications occur and the tongue is deformed, then revision will be required. Nasal septal haematoma with superadded infection can cause septal cartilage necrosis in 24 hours.[26]

19. Answer: C

In a patient presenting with a penetrating injury to the neck such as a stab wound or a gunshot wound, the presence of any hard signs should be promptly identified during the primary survey. These hard signs are well described in literature. *Hard signs* are signs of significant injury that indicate the need for immediate surgical exploration in operating theatre. In the presence of one or more hard signs the patient should be transferred to the operating theatre (OT) without further extensive diagnostic testing such as CT and the injuries should be managed in the OT. Hard signs are identified by physical examination. Hard signs detected on physical examination have a reasonably high specificity for the presence of significant injury that requires surgical intervention. Hard signs of significant injury include:

- vascular hard signs
  - severe active bleeding
  - shock – unresponsive to fluid resuscitation
  - evolving stroke
  - large or expanding haematoma
- airway hard signs
  - air bubbling through the wound
  - respiratory distress or airway compromise.

Patients with *soft signs* alone without any hard signs are suitable to have further diagnostic imaging while staying in the ED. Significant subcutaneous emphysema with a normal CXR is described as the most common soft sign. Air can originate from the airway, oesophagus, a pneumothorax or from outside through the wound.[27]

20. Answer: D

The neck is horizontally divided into three zones to aid the clinical assessment and management of penetrating neck injuries. **The surgically significant penetrating neck injuries are the injuries that penetrate platysma. Such injuries, although they may look trivial at times, should not be explored in the ED.** The neck zones are:

- zone I: between the clavicle and cricoid cartilage
- zone II: between the cricoid and angle of mandible
- zone III: between the angle of mandible and the base of skull.

In zone II, most structures are readily accessible for both physical examination as well as surgical exploration when necessary. **In zone I and III, assessment of the injuries is difficult and unreliable especially when physical examination alone is used.** This is due to the transition of zone I into the thoracic cavity and zone III into the base of skull as well as the fact that the structures in these areas are not readily visible.

External and internal jugular veins are the most commonly injured vascular structures, but injury to the carotid arteries cause most devastating effects. Occult vascular injuries are more likely to occur in zones I and III than in zone II. However, CT angiography is still reliable in detecting both vascular and aerodigestive injuries in these zones. The rate of significant cervical spine injury (cervical fracture or cord injury) is very low in stab wounds to the neck. Patients with cord injury usually present with neurological deficits.[27]

21. Answer: D

Hanging occurs when pressure is exerted on the neck and then tightened by the weight of the victim's body. *Complete hanging* refers to when the body is suspended but the feet do not touch the ground. *Incomplete hanging* refers to all other positions of the body, when the feet are in contact with the ground.

The mechanism of death usually differs depending on the method of hanging. When a victim falls from a height equal or greater than his or her height and the knot is anteriorly placed, death usually results from a fracture of the cervical spine at C2 (Hangman's fracture) and transection of the spinal cord. **If a hanging is incomplete or the victim drops a distance less than his or her height, the cervical spine is spared. In these circumstances, death is usually due cerebral anoxia from venous and arterial occlusion or bradycardic cardiac arrest from carotid stimulation.** Tracheal compression is unlikely to cause death as other immediately acting mechanisms overtake this as the cause of death.

In hanging injuries venous infarctions in the brain are common and care should be taken during resuscitation not to further compromise the venous return by interventions around the neck.[12,28]

22. Answer: B

Haemothorax is a frequent finding in patients with both blunt and penetrating thoracic trauma. **Massive haemothorax is a life-threatening injury and detection is vital during the primary survey. It is defined as >1500 mL of blood in the hemithorax or blood occupying approximately two-thirds of the available space in the hemithorax.** During the primary survey, while excluding other life-threatening chest injuries, any evidence of a massive haemothorax should be looked for. These include absent chest movement, reduced or no breath sounds and dullness to percussion on the affected side.

On a supine CXR even >1000 mL of blood in the hemithorax can be missed due to posterior layering of blood. However, bedside USS has a higher sensitivity and similar specificity compared with CXR in detecting a haemothorax in a supine patient and can show the layering of blood posteriorly.

Haemothorax is most frequently caused by bleeding from direct lung injury, with several local factors playing a role in limiting bleeding from torn lung parenchyma. This could be a possible reason for <5% of the admitted patients with chest trauma requiring tube thoracostomy. Massive haemothoraces are often caused by arterial bleeding from pulmonary, intercostal and internal mammary arteries and almost always require invasive management. Venous bleeding usually tamponades without intervention.

While massive haemothorax requires urgent tube thoracostomy, small haemothoraces may be observed in the stable patient. Drainage may still be required if the patient is symptomatic. Haemothoraces of >300–500 mL should be removed as completely and rapidly as possible because large clots can act as a local anticoagulant, preventing cessation of bleeding from small intrathoracic vessels.[29,30]

23. Answer: D

A flail chest is defined as a segment of the rib cage involving at least three adjacent ribs with fractures in two or more locations on each rib anteriorly or laterally. This segment of the chest wall moves paradoxically inward with spontaneous inspiration and outward during spontaneous expiration with associated increased work of breathing. The paradoxical chest wall movement may not be visible initially because of muscular spasms and splinting. However, as lung contusion develops and lung compliance falls, the paradoxical movement becomes more visible.

The reason for hypoxaemia in these patients is the associated underlying lung contusion. Although small flail segments without underlying lung contusion can be managed without mechanical ventilation, **all high-risk patients should be considered for early intubation and ventilation as it is associated with reduced mortality compared with delayed intubation until the onset of respiratory failure.** High-risk patients include flail segment involving eight or more ribs, patients >65 years of age and those with underlying lung disease.[29,31]

24. Answer: B

In a supine trauma patient, the USS seems to be more sensitive than a supine CXR in diagnosing a pneumothorax. A pneumothorax that is not visible on a CXR and incidentally found on a chest CT or abdomen can usually be managed conservatively without IC tube. However, if the patient is ventilated or likely to be requiring ventilation, an IC tube should be placed to prevent development of a tension pneumothorax. **Stab wounds to the chest are notorious for producing delayed onset pneumothoraces, usually 4–6 hours from the time of injury. Therefore, when the initial CXR is negative for a pneumothorax and the patient is asymptomatic, the patient should be observed and the CXR repeated in 4–6 hours.** When there is airflow obstruction as in COPD, it is more likely that more air will be pushed in to the traumatic pneumothorax form the alveoli, hence there is an increased likelihood of development of tension in such patients.[29]

25. Answer: A

One of the main concerns in managing patients with a traumatic pneumomediastinum is to exclude significant associated tracheobronchial and oesophageal injuries. **Although rare, aerodigestive tract injuries are associated with significant morbidity and mortality; therefore, assessment should be directed at detecting these important injuries.** In the majority of cases, pneumomediastinum is caused by either alveolar rupture, with dissection and coursing of free interstitial air towards the mediastinum along the connective tissues surrounding the bronchi and pulmonary vessels (Macklin effect), or by the direct extension of a pneumothorax into the mediastinum.

The features of pneumomediastinum include:

- central chest pain
- hoarseness of voice
- stridor
- subcutaneous emphysema in the neck
- a crunching sound over the heart during systole (Hamman's crunch).

Electrical alternans is a feature of a large pericardial effusion.[29,32]

26. Answer: C

Traditionally, sternal fractures have been considered a marker of serious underlying injury. **However, current evidence suggests that the incidence of associated cardiac arrhythmias requiring treatment is very low (1.5%) and mortality rate is <1%.** Subsequently, sternal fractures are no longer considered to be markers of significant blunt myocardial injury. In the given scenario the most

appropriate management is to observe the patient for 6 hours and to repeat ECG at that point. If vital signs and ECG are normal, pain control has been achieved and no other significant injuries are present, the patient can be considered for discharge.[29,31]

27. Answer: A

The pathological characteristics of myocardial contusion resembles that of acute myocardial infarction with associated myocardial haemorrhage and oedema, myocardial cell necrosis with subsequent healing with scar formation. More than 50% of patients will have small pericardial effusions but the underlying myocardial injury itself can be small. Although not accurately determined, a small proportion of patients with myocardial contusion may develop significant arrhythmias. Myocardial dysfunction including cardiogenic shock, delayed rupture of the myocardium and ventricular aneurysm formation are other rare complications.

However, definitive diagnosis of myocardial contusion in a trauma patient is difficult because there is no gold standard. Clinical features, ECG and cardiac biomarker findings in a suspected patient can be non-specific. As a result the main objective of investigating a suspected patient is to identify a low-risk patient who is less likely to develop complications, mainly life-threatening cardiac arrhythmias, therefore less likely to benefit from inpatient cardiac monitoring and further investigations. When both the 12-lead ECG and the serum troponin are normal, the negative predictive value for a myocardial contusion reaches 100% and therefore can be considered as adequate investigations for 'ruling out'.

It is important to note that a normal ECG alone, without troponin results, does not exclude the risk of developing a clinically significant cardiac event. Although the right ventricle is more prone to contusion than other chambers of the heart because of its location, the right ventricular (RV) contusions may produce relatively little ECG abnormalities. There are no gold standard ECG abnormalities that will help in the diagnosis and sinus tachycardia and supraventricular and ventricular ectopics are the most common changes. Various degrees of AV block and atrial fibrillation may be seen. Ventricular tachycardia (VT) and ventricular fibrillation (VF) are the life-threatening arrhythmias.

Myocardial cell necrosis in myocardial contusion releases troponin; however, this happens at a relatively low level when compared with acute myocardial infarction. The sensitivity of troponin as a lone test to detect blunt myocardial injury seems to be limited (12–23%). When troponin is elevated, in combination with ECG abnormalities, it indicates a high-risk patient. These patients should be cardiac monitored in an inpatient setting with further investigation with 2D echocardiography and serial ECGs and troponins until these test results return to normal levels.[30,33]

28. Answer: B

The right ventricle is at greatest risk for injury from penetrating wounds, including stab wounds, because of its anterior location and the large surface area. Gunshot wounds may produce complex injury in the heart and therefore survival from stab wound is much better than that from a gunshot wound. The injury to the pericardium and the myocardium can seal spontaneously and this is more true for stab wounds than gunshot wounds due to its small and linear defect. Additionally, ventricular wounds seal better than atrial wounds because of the thicker ventricular muscle. If the pericardial injury is sealed before the myocardial injury, the continuing blood loss into the pericardial sac can cause a cardiac tamponade. The likelihood of occurrence of cardiac tamponade is higher with stab wounds than with gunshot wounds. If both myocardial and pericardial defects remain open, exsanguinating haemorrhage can occur into the pleural cavity creating a large haemothorax.[30,33,34]

29. Answer: B

Emergency department thoracotomy (EDT) is recommended for victims of penetrating chest trauma (stab wounds or gunshot wounds) who are unstable with witnessed signs of life in the ED at least upon arrival and subsequently deteriorated and arrested. Signs of life refer to any organised electrical activity on the cardiac monitor, a palpable pulse, a recordable BP, any respiratory effort, any purposeful movement or a reactive pupil. In general, penetration with sharp objects is associated with a better outcome than penetration resulting from gunshot wounds. Two-thirds of the patients with stab wounds who are transferred to the OT may survive

neurologically intact. Patients with severe hypotension, but not in the immediate danger of cardiac arrest, will also require an emergency thoracotomy, but this is best performed immediately in OT.

The available evidence is less clear regarding the value of EDT for similar patients with blunt cardiac trauma. Patient outcome is relatively poor when EDT is done for blunt trauma – 2% survival in patients in shock and <1% survival with no vital signs. Conversely, the success of EDT approximates 35% in patients arriving in shock with a penetrating cardiac wound, and 15% for all penetrating wounds. Some undertake EDTs for patients with clear evidence of cardiac tamponade who are in similar situations to the above following blunt cardiac trauma. A FAST examination performed upon arrival may be helpful in this situation.

In the given scenarios, patient B is the most likely to benefit from an EDT. Even though he has no vital signs he still has organised cardiac activity. Patient D is most likely to benefit from emergency thoracotomy performed in theatre, rather than in the ED. Patients A and C suffered from significant blunt trauma and are unlikely to benefit from EDT.[33-37]

30. Answer: B

The primary objectives of EDT are to:

- release pericardial tamponade
- control cardiac haemorrhage
- control intrathoracic bleeding
- evacuate massive air embolism
- perform open cardiac massage
- temporarily occlude the descending thoracic aorta.

One of the main aims of EDT is to identify and stop bleeding from a cardiac wound. Once identified digital occlusion should be attempted. A Foley type catheter can be used to seal a large defect. Thereafter, the patient should be taken to theatre immediately for definitive repair. Temporary aortic cross-clamping can be done at the level of the descending thoracic aorta for either thoracic or abdominal sources of haemorrhage. This will decrease the effective circulating volume, cause a reduction in subdiaphragmatic blood loss in abdominal haemorrhage and redistribute blood volume to the myocardium and brain.[33,35,37]

31. Answer: B

Aortic injuries are usually associated with high kinetic energy injuries. The mechanism of injury is such that as much as 75% of patients have fractures of bones other than the ribs. Traumatic rupture of the aorta begins in the intima and moves outwards into the adventitia, which provides most of the tensile support. The atherosclerosis in the tunica media does not predispose the aorta to traumatic rupture. Approximately two-thirds of the tears start at the isthmus of the aorta where the descending aorta begins just distal to the left subclavian artery and the attachment of the ligamentum arteriosum.

On a supine film the sensitivity of a widened mediastinum is 90%, but its specificity is only 30% to detect traumatic rupture. The sensitivity improves to 95% for aortic injury on an erect film. A chest CT with angiography is the best screening study of choice to diagnose aortic injury. With the use of multidetector CT (MDCT) in thin-slice rapid scanning and accurate contrast bolus timing, not only aortic injury but other significant thoracic vascular injuries can be detected.[33,38]

32. Answer: C

Diaphragmatic injuries are most frequently caused by penetrating trauma to the thoracoabdominal region. A gunshot wound anywhere in the abdomen or chest may put the patient at risk for diaphragmatic injury due to the projectile's prolonged length of travel within the body. For stab wound, however, the blade has a limited length. Subsequently, **wounds below or at the nipple line and above the umbilicus are the only ones that are at risk for causing such damage**. The diaphragm normally rises to the level of the fifth rib with expiration and is frequently penetrated by wounds to the anterior chest below the nipple line.

Rupture due to blunt trauma is less frequent and occurs in <5% of patients hospitalised with chest trauma. This incidence is somewhat higher (10–15%) in patients with a fractured pelvis. In blunt trauma, diaphragmatic injuries are often associated with other abdominal and pelvic injuries. A high index of suspicion is necessary in such patients.

CXRs pick up diaphragmatic injuries in <25% cases because most of the CXR abnormalities are non-specific. However, the majority of the patients have at least one abnormality. MDCT has a relatively high sensitivity in diagnosing these injuries. When there remains a high suspicion for diaphragmatic injury, direct visualisation with either thoracoscopy or laparoscopy should be performed. Previously thought to be more common on the left, recent advances in the diagnosis suggest that the incidence of diaphragmatic rupture is similar on both sides.

Except in obvious cases such as penetrating injury to the thoracoabdominal region where diaphragmatic injury can be suspected, there is a risk of delayed diagnosis, especially in blunt abdominal trauma. In these cases, often the diagnosis is made at laparotomy. Most injuries, if undetected, will enlarge with time and delayed rupture and herniation of abdominal structures with accompanying consequences such as obstruction and infarction may occur.[29,38,39]

33. Answer: A

Localised tenderness, when present, has a relatively high sensitivity in detecting intraabdominal injury but this sign is not specific. Abdominal girth measurements or general assessment for abdominal distension have no value in identifying intraabdominal bleeding. Abdominal distension is generally due to gas and a large amount of fluid should be present in the peritoneal cavity to cause any measurable increase in abdominal girth. Neither physical examination nor FAST can identify retroperitoneal injury.

A negative FAST scan may be unreliable, especially when the following clinical findings are present:
- abrasions on the abdomen, pelvis or lower part of chest
- tenderness over the abdomen, pelvis or lower part of chest
- presence of a pelvic fracture
- fracture in the thoracic or lumbar spines

In these circumstances there could be an intraabdominal injury without producing a haemoperitoneum and an abdominal CT is usually indicated in spite of the FAST being negative.[40,41]

34. Answer: A

Splenic injury is the most common blunt intrabdominal injury in children. As with other solid organ injuries, a feature of splenic injury is slow initial bleeding. **Consequently, it may not initially produce haemodynamic instability or signs of peritonism. However, it can cause disastrous haemorrhagic** shock due to late sudden rapid bleeding if not detected early. Children tend to be more haemodynamically stable than adults for the same degree of splenic injury. Therefore, children are more likely to be managed conservatively and the vast majority of children recover fully with conservative management. A fatal haemorrhage is more likely to be associated with a liver injury than a splenic injury. Haemodynamically stable liver injuries are often managed conservatively in children.[14]

35. Answer: A

Bowel injuries as a whole are fairly uncommon, making up <5% of patients with blunt abdominal trauma. Small bowel injuries specifically are associated with other severe injuries, which accounts for the associated high mortality (~20%) in these patients. Initial symptoms and signs are often subtle and the diagnosis is often difficult, even with the use of contrast-enhanced CT. The detection may become even more difficult if patients are ventilated and sedated due to other major injuries. Small bowel injuries are often associated with some intraabdominal bleeding due to mesenteric injury. This bleeding, combined with peritonitis caused by bacterial contamination, produces features of peritonism. However, this may take 6–8 hours to develop.

On contrast-enhanced CT scan (intravenous and oral contrast) free intraperitoneal gas is present in only 40% cases and extravasation of oral contrast is present in only 5% of cases. These features, when present, are considered to be diagnostic of bowel perforation. Other markers of bowel injury may also be found with CT. Presence of free peritoneal fluid without evidence of solid-organ injury and bowel wall thickening are examples.[40,41]

36. Answer: B

Under the Young-Burgess classification for pelvic fractures, the four categories of pelvic fractures are lateral compression (50%), anteroposterior compression (25%), vertical shear (5%) and combination (mostly lateral compression and vertical shear) (15–20%). Each category is then further divided into subtypes (see Table 13.1).[42]

37. Answer: A

The ED management of pelvic fractures confirmed with a pelvic X-ray in a haemodynamically unstable trauma patient is a challenging scenario. Because of the haemodynamic instability these patients cannot be taken for CT to identify commonly associated intraabdominal, retroperitoneal and other pelvic vascular injuries, all of which can cause significant or

Table 13.1 YOUNG-BURGESS CLASSIFICATION FOR PELVIC FRACTURES

Mechanism	Subtype	Features	Stability
Lateral compression (LC)	\multicolumn{2}{}{Transverse fracture of the pubic rami (ipsilateral or contralateral to the side of the injury), *and* with one of three types of second injury:}	
	I	Sacral compression fracture on the side of the impact	Stable
	II	Crescent iliac wing fracture on the side of the impact	Unstable
	III	LC-I or LC-II injury on the side of the impact with a contralateral SI joint injury	Unstable
Anteroposterior (AP) compression	\multicolumn{2}{}{These injuries involve symphyseal diastasis and/or longitudinal rami fractures with variable SI joint disruption. There are three types:}	
	I	Slight widening (< 2.5 cm) of the symphysis pubis and/or anterior SI joint (but with intact anterior and posterior SI joints)	Stable
	II	Widen SI joint (> 2.5 cm) with disrupted ligaments, but intact posterior SI joint	Unstable
	III	Complete SI joint disruption with lateral displacement, with disrupted anterior and posterior SI joints (open book fracture)	Unstable
Vertical shear (VS)		Symphyseal diastasis or vertical displacement anteriorly with posterior diastasis and vertical displacement (usually through the SI joint, occasionally through the iliac wing/sacrum)	Unstable
Combination		A combination of the other injury pattern, LC/VS being the most common.	Unstable

exsanguinating haemorrhage. In these patients, all measures such as application of pelvic binding or C-clamp should be done to reduce the pelvic volume and increase the tamponading effect in order to slow the bleeding. The following steps are generally applicable to this scenario.[43]

- FAST scan should be the first bedside investigation.
- If FAST is grossly positive, laparotomy is indicated prior to consideration for pelvic angiography, external fixation or surgical control of pelvic bleeding.
- If FAST is negative, there is relatively low risk of significant or life-threatening intraabdominal haemorhage. Therefore, bleeding control from the pelvis is the priority.
- To control bleeding from the pelvis the following should be considered:
  - angiography and selective embolisation – this will significantly reduce mortality but requires the presence of interventional radiology
  - external fixation of pelvis – to reduce the volume of pelvis in an open book fracture and to control venous and small arterial bleeding from fracture sites
  - open surgical control – to control bleeding from large arteries such as aorta, iliacs and common femoral.

38. Answer: B

In adult patients, the degree of haematuria does not correspond to the degree of injury. For example, microscopic haematuria could correspond to significant renovascular pedicle injury. **By consensus, microscopic haematuria (defined as >5 RBC per high power field, HPF) in adults requires no further imaging studies, with the exception of where a severe deceleration mechanism is involved or hypotension is present.** Even transient hypotension should be taken as significant for further investigation. However, in children microscopic haematuria, particularly when above 50 RBC HPF, should be investigated regardless of the mechanism or the blood pressure reading.

The gold standard for diagnosing bladder rupture is a retrograde cystogram. This can be done with plain films or CT. A contrast-enhanced CT with passive bladder filling, even with a clamped catheter, is not sensitive enough to exclude bladder rupture.

Urethral injuries in the anterior urethra are seen in straddle injuries and secondary to instrumentation while posterior urethral injuries are seen with pelvic fractures.[44]

39. Answer: D

During pregnancy numerous changes take place in the anatomy and the physiology of the patient that impact on the management of trauma in the ED. *Blood volume* increases to as much as 45% during pregnancy, starting at 6–8 weeks. Recognition of traumatic bleeding is less obvious in these patients as the mother can be bleeding but not show early signs of hypotension. The uterus is not a critical organ, and its blood flow is markedly reduced when the maternal circulation must be maintained. As a result, by the time the traditional symptoms and signs of shock appear, the fetus has already been compromised. The *pressure of the gravid uterus* on the abdominal vessels increases the amount of blood in the lower limbs and causes increased bleeding from the lower limb wounds. Despite a physiological *anaemia*, the oxygen carrying capacity matches the oxygen demand of the growing uterus and the fetus by an increase in the amount of red cell mass. The *oxygen reserve* is reduced mostly by a reduction in the functional residual capacity (FRC) due to elevation of the diaphragm (20%) than by the increased oxygen demand (15%).[45]

40. Answer: C

The sensitivity of abdominal examination, blood tests and USS is questionable in the assessment of pregnant women involved in trauma. Only CTG, for a minimum of 4 hours, is predictive of fetal outcome, and therefore should be used as soon as the fetus is viable, usually after 23 weeks' gestation. The most common cause of fetal demise is placental abruption and this is best diagnosed with a CTG. Other less common causes are maternal shock and maternal death.

A posterior–anterior CXR gives <1 millirad (mrad) of radiation while anteroposterior CXR gives <5 mrad. A pelvic X-ray carries a radiation exposure of 140–2200 mrads. Less than 1% of pregnant trauma patients are exposed to >3 rads and a dose >5–10 rads is required for any radiation-induced adverse effects.[45,46]

41. Answer: B

Fetal distress on CTG, which predicts underlying occult maternal placental bleeding, is characterised by:

- an abnormal baseline heart rate (<120 or >160 bpm)
- a decreased beat-to-beat and long-term variability
- decelerations of the heart rate after uterine contractions.

The Kleihauer test needs at least 5 mL of fetomaternal haemorrhage for it to be positive. This means that the need for RhIg (or anti-D) should not be based on this test. **Any Rh negative mother with significant trauma should be given anti-D within 72 hours from the injury.** Neither anti-D immunoglobulin, nor tetanus toxoid is harmful to the fetus.

Serum HCO_3^- is low in pregnant women because of the respiratory alkalosis caused by an increase in minute volume. The increased minute volume is due to an increased tidal volume by approximately 40%, whereas the respiratory rate usually remains normal. Low HCO_3^- over and above this (<21 mmol/L) may suggest placental abruption or hypoperfusion.[45,46]

42. Answer: B

Trauma affects 7% of all pregnancies. The incidence increases with advancing gestational age. Just over half of trauma during pregnancy occurs in the third trimester. As the uterus enlarges, the diaphragm rises about an extra 4 cm. Subsequently, consideration should be given when placing an intercostal tube. It is recommended that the chest tube should be placed one or two spaces higher than the usual 5th intercostal space to allow for diaphragm elevation.

Clinical abdominal examination may be unreliable as the enlarged uterus displaces the abdominal content. The evaluation of possible injury to the abdomen is different because of the presence of the gravid uterus. In addition, stretching of the abdominal wall modifies the normal response to peritoneal irritation. Guarding and rebound can be blunted despite significant intraabdominal bleeding or organ injury, leading to an underestimation of the extent and gravity of maternal trauma.

The bladder is displaced into the abdominal cavity beyond 12 weeks' gestation and is therefore more vulnerable to injury. The bladder becomes hyperaemic, like the uterus, and injury may lead to a

marked increase in blood loss compared with a similar injury in a non-pregnant patient.

During pregnancy, the ligaments of the symphysis pubis and sacroiliac joints are loosened. A baseline diastasis of the pubic symphysis may exist and this can be mistaken for pelvic disruption on X-ray.[45-48]

43. Answer: B

Primary blast injury due to a bomb explosion is caused by the direct effects of pressure (barotrauma). The initial wave of high pressure caused by the bomb explosion is followed closely by the blast wind exposing the body organs to high and low pressure effects. If the patient is in a confined space such as a bus, the patient can be subjected to several reverberations and reflections of this pressure wave, hence a higher degree of primary blast injury is seen in such a patient.

The structures most commonly injured due to primary blast injury are air-filled structures (middle ear, lung and hollow viscera) and structures with air–fluid interfaces. Tympanic membrane rupture is most commonly seen followed by lung injury at second place. The colon is the most commonly affected visceral structure. Other important structures injured are the eyes and brain. **Detection of a tympanic membrane rupture with otoscopy or evidence of middle or inner ear injury (deafness, tinnitus, vertigo) when the tympanic membrane is not visible is a sensitive marker of potential primary blast injury to other critical structures such as the lung.** If there is no evidence of tympanic membrane rupture, primary blast injury to other organs is less likely. However, in a small number of patients primary blast injury to the lung and other organs can occur without tympanic membrane rupture. Primary blast injuries to the lung include alveolar disruption, pulmonary contusion, pneumothorax, pneumomediastinum, haemothorax, pulmonary oedema, parenchymal haemorrhage and systemic air embolism. These are the most common critical injuries in patients who were close to the blast centre. Abdominal solid organ injuries are usually due to secondary or tertiary injury.[49]

44. Answer: D

Injuries occurring in a blast or a bomb explosion can be categorised into four categories according the mechanism of injury:

- *primary blast injury* – injuries due to direct barotrauma to organs by over pressurisation or under pressurisation
- *secondary blast injury* – due to penetrating trauma by fragments of the bomb as well as those that result from the explosion
- *tertiary blast injury* – due to structural collapse and blunt trauma due to patient being thrown by the blast wind
- *quaternary blast injury* – due to burns, asphyxia and exposure to toxic inhalants.[49]

45. Answer: A

The total body surface area (TBSA) of burns can be estimated in a variety of ways. **The 'rule of nines' is useful in adults and children >10 years of age. It should not be used for younger children because their head is larger and their extremities are smaller in proportion compared with adults.** This rule divides the body into segments that are approximately 9% or multiples of nine and puts the percentages allocated for the head at 9%, the front of the trunk at 18%, the back of the trunk at 18%, the upper limbs at 9% and the lower limb at 18%, with the perineum forming the remaining 1%. The *Lund-Browder chart* is useful for estimating the extent of burns in children. These charts are age adjusted and allows for changes in children at different ages. For instance, an infant's head is approximately 18% of the TBSA, compared with 9% in an adult. Another way of working out the extent of the burn is to use the *palm with the adducted fingers* to calculate the extent of the burn as this will be approximately equivalent to 1% TBSA.[50–53]

46. Answer: C

The Parkland formula is the most commonly used resuscitation fluid prediction formula in both adults and children with moderate-severe burns. It calculates the 24-hour fluid requirement, of which half should be infused in the first 8 hours (counted from the time of the burn injury) and the other half over the following 16 hours. This 24-hour fluid requirement is:

4 ml/kg body weight × total burn surface area (TBSA)

In children, maintenance fluid requirement should also be added.

In this child, the initial IV fluid requirement is (without maintenance fluids) 165 mL/h for the first 8 hours.

Organ perfusion should be monitored and fluid requirement should be adjusted accordingly.[50]

47. Answer: D

The SAFE Study compared the use of albumin and normal saline in resuscitation of ICU patients and showed that there is no significant difference in mortality, ICU length of stay (LOS) or duration of mechanical ventilation.

Class I haemorrhagic shock (<15% or 750 mL of blood loss) where there is no or minimal tachycardia and no change in BP, is typically not associated with orthostatic changes to the BP, provided the patient was not initially dehydrated. Class II haemorrhagic shock (15–30% or 750–1500 mL blood loss) is associated with tachycardia, narrowed pulse pressure, mild–moderate hypotension with peripheral vasoconstriction and potential changes in mentation.

The basis of hypotensive resuscitation in trauma is to prevent increased arterial blood loss from uncontrolled bleeding sites due to overly aggressive fluid resuscitation until surgical control of bleeding is achieved. **In hypotensive resuscitation, the systolic BP is maintained at 80 mm Hg unless there is evidence of end-organ hypoperfusion**. End-organ damage may be seen as myocardial ischaemia, renal failure or cerebral ischaemia and in these situations adequate end-organ perfusion should be maintained with fluid resuscitation and emergent surgical control of bleeding. Hypotensive resuscitation is contraindicated in a head-injured patient where maintenance of cerebral perfusion pressure is dependent on the blood pressure.

The standard haemodynamic measurements do not measure the physiologic derangements of a patient in haemorrhagic shock. **The initial lactate level and base deficit seem to be useful in quantifying the degree of ongoing fluid resuscitation requirements and one of the targets of resuscitation is to normalise this during the first 24 hours.**
Additionally, the time taken to normalise the same is considered as circulatory predictors of survival of a trauma patient.[54–56]

48. Answer: B

The DCR is indicated in patients with severe class IV haemorrhage who require massive transfusion and immediate damage control surgery (DCS). The clinical scenario could be traumatic or non-traumatic in nature. **The aim of DCR is to avoid the 'lethal triad' of hypothermia, coagulopathy and metabolic acidosis, which is made worse with the injudicious use of crystalloid.**

The components of DCR include:
- haemostatic resuscitation with a use of a massive transfusion protocol (e.g. early transfusion of PRBCs, FFP and platelets in the ratio of 1:1:1)
- restriction of crystalloids
- systolic blood pressure is ideally maintained between 80–100 mm Hg until bleeding is surgically controlled
- restoration and maintenance of normothermia
- use of cryoprecipitate to keep fibrinogen >1.0 g/L
- administration of calcium to maintain calcium >1.0 mEq/L
- early use of recombinant factor VIIa
- immediate damage control surgery, which includes control of haemorrhage, prevention of contamination and protection from further injury.

Once the coagulopathy, hypothermia and metabolic acidosis are subsequently corrected in a critical care facility, the definitive surgical procedure can be carried out as necessary.[60,61]

49. Answer: C

Massive transfusion is defined, in adults, as replacing >50% of the patient's blood volume in 4 hours or 100% over 24 hours. The adult blood volume is approximately 70 mL/kg. **In children, it is defined as transfusion of >40% of blood volume.** The blood volume in a child over 1 month of age is approximately 80 mL/kg.

The aetiology of high mortality associated with massive transfusion is usually multifactorial. The factors that could contribute to high mortality include hypotension, acidosis, coagulopathy, shock and the underlying pathologies in the patient. **The triad associated with highest mortality are acidosis, hypothermia and coagulopathy.**

A massive transfusion may be required in the clinical situation of severe trauma, surgery, ruptured aortic aneurysm, gastrointestinal haemorrhage and during obstetric complications. It is recommended that individual institutions should develop a massive transfusion protocol to be used in patients who potentially require massive transfusions. It has been shown that there is a survival advantage when a massive transfusion is associated with a decreased ratio of RBCs to FFP, platelets or cryoprecipitate/fibrinogen concentrate. In trauma patients, a ratio of ≤2:1:1 seems to be associated with improved survival. In non-trauma patients currently there is insufficient evidence to support or refute the use of a defined ration of blood components.

During massive transfusion, the monitoring of the following is recommended every 30–60 minutes:
- full blood count
- coagulation screen
- ionised calcium
- arterial blood gas.

The following should be aimed during massive transfusion:[57–59]
- temperature: >35°C
- acid–base status: pH >7.2, base excess <–6, lactate <4 mmol/L
- ionised calcium: >1.1 mmol/L
- haemoglobin: Interpret in the context with haemodynamic status, organ and tissue perfusion (do not use alone as a transfusion trigger)
- platelet: ≥50 × 10^9/L
- PT/APTT and INR: ≤1.5 × of normal
- fibrinogen: ≥1.0 g/L.

50. Answer: A

The essential characteristics of level 1 trauma centres are:
- 24-hour availability of surgeons in all subspecialities (including cardiac surgery/bypass capabilities)
- 24-hour availability of neuroradiology and haemodialysis
- a program that establishes and monitors the effects of injury prevention and education efforts
- an organised trauma research program.

Death from trauma shows a trimodal distribution with the first peak in the prehospital stage where deaths are from devastating head and vascular injuries, then the first hour in the ED where deaths occur from major head injury, chest and abdominal injuries. The third peak occurs in the ICU where the cause of death is from the SIRS response, severe sepsis and multiorgan failure.

Trauma calls are initiated on the basis of anatomical, physiological or dangerous mechanism criteria – any one or a combination of these.[15]

References

1. Mackway-Jones K, Molyneux E, Phillips B, editors. Advanced paediatric life support: the practical approach. 4th ed. Why treat children differently? Oxford: Blackwell Publishing; 2005. p. 7–14.

2. Mackway-Jones K, Molyneux E, Phillips B, editors. Advanced paediatric life support: the practical approach. 4th ed. The structured approach to the seriously injured child. Oxford: Blackwell Publishing Ltd; 2005. p. 151–66.

3. Alterman D. Considerations in pediatric trauma. Medscape reference: drugs diseases and procedures. Online. Available: http://emedicine.medscape.com.

4. Borland M, Dunn R. Paediatrics. In: Dunn R, Dilley S, Brookes J, editors. The emergency medicine manual. 5th ed. Adelaide: Venom Publishing. 2010. p. 791–802.

5. Shilt J, Green N, Cramer K. Nonaccidental trauma. In: Kliegman RM, Behrman RE, Jenson HB, et al, editors. Nelson textbook of pediatrics. 19th ed. Philadelphia: Saunders Elsevier; 2011. p. 585–607.

6. Dubowitz H, Lane W. Abused and neglected children. In: Kliegman RM, Behrman RE, Jenson HB, et al, editors. Nelson textbook of pediatrics. 19th ed. Philadelphia: Saunders Elsevier; 2011. p. 135–47.

7. Kellogg N. Evaluation of suspected child physical abuse. Pediatrics 2007;119(6):1232–41.

8. Talley N, O'Connor S. Clinical examination: a systemic guide to physical diagnosis. 6th ed. The nervous system. Sydney: Churchill Livingstone Elsevier; 2010. p. 323–407.

9. Wallis L, Cameron P. Neurotrauma. In: Cameron P, Jelinek G, Kelly A, et al, editors. Textbook of adult emergency medicine. 3rd ed. Edinburgh: Elsevier; 2009. p. 75–80.

10. Wright D, Merck L. Head trauma in adults and children. In: Tintinalli J, Stapczynski J, Ma O, et al, editors. Tintinalli's emergency medicine: a comprehensive study guide. 7th ed. New York: McGraw Hill Medical; 2011. p. 1692–709.

11. Myburgh J. Severe head injury. In: Berston AD, Soni N, editors. Oh's intensive care manual. 6th ed. Philadelphia: Elsevier; 2009. p. 765–82.

12. Dunn R. Head trauma. In: Dunn R, Dilley S, Brookes J, editors. The emergency medicine manual. 5th ed. Adelaide: Venom Publishing; 2010. p. 1137–47.

13. Mackway-Jones K, Molyneux E, Phillips B, editors. Advanced paediatric life support: the practical approach. The child with injuries to the extremities or the spine. 4th ed. Oxford: Blackwell Publishing Ltd; 2005. p. 189–97.

14. Hauda WE. Trauma in children. In: Tintinalli J, Stapczynski J, Ma O, et al, editors. Tintinalli's emergency medicine: a comprehensive study guide. 7th ed. New York: McGraw Hill Medical; 2011. p. 1676–83.

15. Burnett P, Cameron P. Trauma in adults. In: Tintinalli JE, Kelen GD, Stapczynski JS, editors. Emergency medicine: a comprehensive study guide. 7th ed. New York: McGraw-Hill; 2011. p. 1671–6.

16. Ma OJ, Edwards JH, Meldon SW. Geriatric trauma. In: Tintinalli JE, Kelen GD, Stapczynski JS, editors. Emergency medicine: a comprehensive study guide. 7th ed. New York: McGraw-Hill; 2011. p. 1683–7.

17. Dunn R. Spinal trauma. In: Dunn R, Dilley S, Brookes J, editors. The emergency medicine manual. 5th ed. Adelaide: Venom Publishing; 2010. p. 1148–63.

18. Hoffman JR, Mower WR, Wolfson AB, et al. Validation of a set of clinical criteria to rule out injury to the cervical spine in patients with blunt trauma. N Engl J Med 2000;343:94–9.

19. Steill IG, Wells GA, Vandemheen KL, et al. The Canadian c-spine rule for radiography in alert and stable trauma patients. JAMA 2001;286:1841–8.

20. Widder S, Doig C, Burrowes P, et al. Prospective evaluation of computed tomographic scanning for the spinal clearance of obtunded trauma patients: preliminary results. J Trauma 2004;56:1179–84.

21. Baron BJ, McSherry KJ, Larson JL, et al. Spine and spinal cord trauma. In: Tintinalli J, Stapczynski J, Ma O, et al, editors. Tintinalli's emergency medicine: a comprehensive study guide. 7th ed. New York: McGraw Hill Medical; 2011. p. 1709–30.

22. Vaccaro AR, Kim DH, Brodke DS, et al. Diagnosis and management of sacral spine fractures. JBJS-Am 2004;86(1):166–75.

23. Gutteridge G. Spinal injuries. In: Berston AD, Soni N, editors. Oh's intensive care manual. 6th ed. Philadelphia: Elsevier; 2009. p. 803–13.

24. Garret P. Shock overview. In: Cameron P, Jelinek G, Kelly A, et al, editors. Textbook of adult emergency medicine. 3rd ed. Edinburgh: Elsevier; 2009. p. 45–56.

25. Bailitz J. Trauma to the face. In: Tintinalli J, Stapczynski J, Ma O, et al, editors. Tintinalli's emergency medicine: a comprehensive study guide. 7th ed. New York: McGraw Hill Medical; 2011. p. 1730–8.

26. Dunn R. Facial trauma. In: Dunn R, Dilley S, Brookes J, editors. The emergency medicine manual. 5th ed. Adelaide: Venom Publishing; 2010. p. 1173–81.

27. Casey S, de Alwis W. Emergency department assessment and management of stab wounds to the neck. Emerg Med Austral 2010;22:201–10.

28. Baron BJ. Trauma to the neck. In: Tintinalli J, Stapczynski J, Ma O, et al, editors. Tintinalli's emergency medicine: a comprehensive study guide. 7th ed. New York: McGraw Hill Medical; 2011. p. 1738–44.

29. Brunett P, Yarris L, Cevik A. Pulmonary trauma. In: Tintinalli J, Stapczynski J, Ma O, et al, editors. Tintinalli's emergency medicine: a comprehensive study guide. 7th ed. New York: McGraw Hill Medical; 2011. p. 1744–58.

30. Eckstein M, Henderson S. Thoracic trauma. In: Marx J, Hockberger R, Walls R, editors. Rosen's emergency medicine: concepts and clinical practice. 7th ed. Philadelphia: Elsevier; 2010. p. 387–413.

31. Fitzgerald M, Gocentas R. Chest trauma. In: Cameron P, Jelinek G, Kelly A, et al, editors. Textbook of adult emergency medicine. 3rd ed. Edinburgh: Elsevier; 2009. p. 104–9.

32. Rezende-Neto JB, Hoffmann J, Al Mahroos M, et al. Occult pneumomediastinum in blunt chest trauma: Clinical significance. Injury 2010;41(1):40–3.

33. Ross C, Schwab TM. Cardiac trauma. In: Tintinalli J, Stapczynski J, Ma O, et al, editors. Tintinalli's emergency

medicine: a comprehensive study guide. 7th ed. New York: McGraw Hill Medical; 2011. p. 1758–65.

34. Embrey R. Cardiac trauma. Thorac Surg Clin 2007;17:87–93.

35. Dunn R. Penetrating trauma. In: Dunn R, Dilley S, Brookes J, editors. The emergency medicine manual. 5th ed. Adelaide: Venom Publishing; 2010. p. 1197–210.

36. Demetriades D, Velmahos GC. Penetrating injuries of the chest: indications for operation. Scandinavian Journal of Surgery 2002;91:41–5.

37. Cothren CC, Moore EE. Emergency department thoracotomy for the critically injured patient: Objectives, indications, and outcomes. World Journal of Emergency Surgery 2006;1:4. Online. Available: http://www.wjes.org/content/1/1/4.

38. Dunn R. Thoracic trauma. In: Dunn R, Dilley S, Brookes J, editors. The emergency medicine manual. 5th ed. Adelaide: Venom Publishing; 2010. p. 1164–72.

39. Scharff JR, Naunheim K. Traumatic diaphragmatic injuries. Thorac Surg Clin 2007;17:81–5.

40. Dunn R. Abdominal and pelvic trauma. In: Dunn R, Dilley S, Brookes J, editors. The emergency medicine manual. 5th ed. Adelaide: Venom Publishing; 2010. p. 1182–96.

41. Scalea TM, Boswell SA, Baron BJ, et al. Abdominal trauma. In: Tintinalli J, Stapczynski J, Ma O, et al, editors. Tintinalli's emergency medicine: a comprehensive study guide. 7th ed. New York: McGraw Hill Medical; 2011. p. 1765–71.

42. Heetveld MJ, Harris I, Schlaphoff G, et al. Guidelines for the management of haemodynamically unstable pelvic fracture patients. ANZ J Surg 2004;74:520–8.

43. McArthur C. Abdominal and pelvic injuries. In: Berston AD, Soni N, editors. Oh's intensive care manual. 6th ed. Philadelphia: Elsevier; 2009. p. 815–21.

44. McManus J, Gratton MC, Cuenca PJ. Genitiurinary trauma. In: Tintinalli J, Stapczynski J, Ma O, et al, editors. Tintinalli's emergency medicine: a comprehensive study guide. 7th ed. New York: McGraw Hill Medical; 2011. p. 1773–8.

45. Bhatia K, Cranmer O. Trauma in pregnancy. In: Marx JA, Hockberger RS, Walls RM, editors. Rosen's emergency medicine: concepts and clinical practice. 7th ed. Philadelphia: Elsevier; 2010. p. 252–61.

46. Delorio NM. Trauma in pregnancy. In: Tintinalli J, Stapczynski J, Ma O, et al, editors. Tintinalli's emergency medicine: a comprehensive study guide. 7th ed. New York: McGraw Hill Medical; 2011. p. 1687–92.

47. Barraco RD, Chiu WC, Clancy TV, et al. Trauma in Pregnancy. J Trauma 2010;69(1):211–14.

48. Desjardins G. Management of the injured pregnant patient. Online. Available: http://www.trauma.org/archive/resus/pregnancytrauma.html; 29 June 2012.

49. DePalma R, Burris DG, Champion HR, et al. Blast injuries. N Engl J Med 2005;352(13):1335–42.

50. Mackway-Jones K, Molyneux E, Phillips B. Advanced paediatric life support: the practical approach. 4th ed. The burned or scalded child. Oxford: Blackwell Publishing Ltd; 2005. p. 199–P204.

51. Schwartz LR, Balakrishnan C. Thermal burns. In: Tintinalli J, Stapczynski J, Ma O, et al, editors. Tintinalli's emergency medicine: a comprehensive study guide. 7th ed. New York: McGraw Hill Medical; 2011. p. 1374–80.

52. Dunn R. Burns. In: Dunn R, Dilley S, Brookes J, editors. The emergency medicine manual. 5th ed. Adelaide: Venom Publishing; 2010. p. 1222–9.

53. Singer AJ, Taira BR, Lee CC, et al. Thermal burns. In: Marx JA, Hockberger RS, Walls RM, editors. Rosen's emergency medicine: concepts and clinical practice. 7th ed. Philadelphia: Elsevier; 2010. p. 758–66.

54. Dunn R. Principles of trauma. In: Dunn R, Dilley S, Brookes J, editors. The emergency medicine manual. 5th ed. Adelaide: Venom Publishing; 2010. p. 1127–36.

55. Finfer S, Rinaldo B, Neil B, et al. A comparison of albumin and saline for fluid resuscitation in the intensive care unit. N Engl J Med 2004;350:2247–56.

56. Cabanas J, Manning J, Cairns C. Fluid and blood resuscitation. In: Tintinalli J, Stapczynski J, Ma O, et al, editors. Tintinalli's emergency medicine: a comprehensive study guide. 7th ed. New York: McGraw Hill Medical; 2011. p. 172–7.

57. Dunn R, Leach D. Circulatory support. In: The emergency medicine manual. 5th ed. Adelaide: Venom Publishing; 2010. p. 96–138.

58. National Blood Authority. Patient blood management guidelines: module 1. Critical bleeding. Online. Available: www.nba.gov.au; 10 Jan 2012.

59. Australian Red Cross Blood Service. Massive transfusion. Online. Available: www.transfusion.com.au; 10 Jan 2012

60. Zalstein S, Pearce A, Scott DM, et al. Damage control resuscitation: a paradigm shift in the management of hemorrhagic shock. EMA 2008;20:291–3.

61. Brohi K. Damage control surgery. Online. Available: http://www.trauma.org/archive/resus/DCSoverview.html.

1. Answer: C

In Salter-Harris type I injuries the fracture goes through the growth plate, completely separating the epiphysis from the metaphysis. However, the epiphysis is not always displaced, hence there may not be any abnormalities visible on X-ray. The epiphysis is displaced when the periosteum is damaged or torn. Usually the displaced epiphysis is easily reduced as the two surfaces are covered with cartilage.

In Salter-Harris type V injury, the growth plate is crushed, all or in part. Other mechanisms have been described for type V injury. It may be associated with a long bone fracture away from the growth plate injury such as a midshaft femur fracture. Consequently, growth arrest at the growth plate may occur, resulting in limb length discrepancy or angular deformity at the joint (e.g. angular deformity at the wrist due to normal growth of the ulna and growth arrest of the radius).

Type I and V injuries are difficult to differentiate clinically and there may not be any X-ray changes. The history might give a clue where a type I injury is due to shearing or avulsion forces and a type V injury is due to axial compression.[1,2]

2. Answer: B

The most common site of a Salter-Harris type III fracture is the distal end of tibia (Tillaux fracture). As type III fractures occur in partially closed growth plates, the distal tibia is affected towards the end of growth when the medial half of the growth plate is closed. Type III fractures are intra-articular, therefore, requires accurate reduction – often open reduction. As the growth plate is already closing growth arrest is not a major concern.

Type IV injuries (fracture line passes from the joint surface across the epiphysis, growth plate and into the metaphysis) **most commonly affect the lateral condyle of the humerus**. Accurate reduction, usually open with internal fixation, is required for this fracture because any failure will produce growth arrest, nonunion, causing joint deformity and stiffness.

The growth plate is injured in approximately one-third of all bony injuries in children. When fracture separation occurs, some epiphyses such as head of femur and head of radius are prone to avascular necrosis. However, most epiphyses (e.g. distal radius, distal tibia and distal femur) survive because their circulations are maintained.[1,2]

3. Answer: D

The assessment for a potential nerve injury is essential in every child who presents to the ED with a supracondylar fracture. In displaced supracondylar fractures the rate of nerve injury is reported to be 15%. **The most commonly affected nerve is the anterior interosseous branch of the median nerve, but median, radial and ulnar nerve injuries may occur.**

The following screening tests can be used in a young child to check the motor function of the individual nerves.

- **Okay sign**: touch the tips of index and thumb together. If the anterior interosseous nerve is intact the child is able to do this with *visible flexion* at the distal interphallangeal joint of the index finger and at the interphalangeal joint of the thumb. These actions are due to flexor digitorum profundus to the index finger and flexor pollicis longus to the thumb. If these joints are not flexed but remain extended the anterior interosseous nerve is damaged.
- **Benediction sign**: ask the child to make a fist. When the anterior interosseoous nerve is injured, the fist is made without flexion of the index finger and the thumb.
- **Thumbs up sign**: ability to fully extend the thumb. This tests extensor pollicis longus (EPL) supplied by the radial nerve.
- **Retropulsion of thumb**: with the palm facing down resting on a surface such as a pillow and extend the thumb. Tests EPL supplied by the radial nerve.
- **Starfish sign**: ability to fully abduct all fingers, making a starfish. Tests finger abductors supplied by the ulnar nerve.
- **Cross fingers one over other**: tests palmar and dorsal interossei supplied by the ulnar nerve.

When assessing these movements it is important to provide the child with adequate analgesia first, but any deficit should not be attributed to the presence of pain.[3]

4. Answer: C

Gartland classification of extension type (98%) supracondylar fractures:

- Gartland type I: undisplaced – fracture line may or may not be visible on AP and lateral views; an effusion can usually be recognised on X-ray
- Gartland type IIa: posterior angulation with intact posterior cortex; <20 degrees angulation
- Garland type IIb: posterior angulation with intact posterior cortex; in addition, the distal fragment can be rotated or have a varus/valgus angulation
- Gartland type III: grossly displaced or rotated fracture.

Gartland type I fractures (undisplaced fractures) can be managed with elbow immobilisation using a simple plaster slab or collar and cuff because they are stable. Gartland type IIa fractures may be managed conservatively with orthopaedic input at the time of presentation. Under sufficient analgesia the elbow should ideally be flexed to at least 90 degrees and the forearm should be kept at a neutral position. However, increasing flexion may cause vascular compromise because of the associated swelling of the elbow. If the radial pulse is lost during hyperflexion of the elbow, the elbow should be extended until the radial pulse is palpable again and a further relaxation of 10 degrees is advised before splinting is applied. Once the pulse is palpable and vascular supply is established, a plaster slab can be applied. The child can usually be discharged home with appropriate advice and a definitive arrangement to follow up within the next 24 hours.

Children with Gartland type IIb and III fractures should be referred for admission under orthopaedics for manipulation under anaesthetic (MUA) in the OT, internal fixation or open reduction and management of any associated complications.

Splinting the elbow in a relative extension is an acceptable method for a grossly swollen elbow to prevent compartment syndrome while waiting for MUA.[2–4]

5. Answer: A

Vascular compromise due to supracondylar fracture is most likely to be associated with Gartland type III fractures where there is complete displacement of the distal fragment with no intact cortical contact. Brachial artery injuries include arterial entrapment, laceration, intimal tear and compression due to compartment syndrome developing in the forearm. The brachial artery injury may occur in up to 15% of this type of fracture.

The child may present with a pulseless hand. The hand should be closely assessed to determine whether it is *warm and pink* or *cool and pale*. **When the hand is cool and pale, the fracture needs emergent reduction and stabilisation with K wires in the OT. This will usually establish the arterial supply to the forearm and hand.** This should be achieved in the OT with the use of an image intensifier; however, only in circumstances where this is practically impossible to achieve, the reduction should be attempted in the ED to reestablish the vascular supply. On repeated attempts it is likely that the artery can be injured further; therefore, failure to establish blood supply requires emergent transfer to the OT. Vascular surgeons should be alerted in such cases.

If the hand is pulseless but warm and pink, there is a little more time for the emergency clinician to arrange definitive management on an urgent basis. The arm should be splinted to prevent further vascular compromise. In these children the collateral branches of the brachial artery maintain an adequate blood supply to the forearm and hand despite the injury to the brachial artery.[3,4]

6. Answer: B

Lateral condylar fractures account for 15–20% of all elbow fractures in children (most common between 6 and 10 years) and should be sought in elbow injuries in children. The ossification centre for the lateral condyle appears between 18 months and 2 years of age and the ossification centre for the lateral epicondyle appears between 11–13 years. These fractures are unstable even with cast immobilisation due to the pull from the forearm extensors. The diagnosis can be difficult because the fracture line may not be visible on AP view or the fracture line appears 7–10 days later. When there is significant displacement there is marked swelling over the lateral elbow both clinically and on X-ray. The lateral view may show the fracture line more clearly, but oblique views are considered the best to determine the degree of displacement and rotation. Multiple oblique views may be needed to accurately differentiate a non-displaced fracture from a displaced one.

A truly non-displaced fracture or fracture that is truly <2 mm displaced (minimal lateral elbow swelling) can be treated with cast immobilisation with the elbow at 90 degrees and the forearm in pronation. Early orthopaedic follow-up should be arranged. A fracture that is >2 mm displaced requires open reduction and internal fixation.

Medial condylar fractures are rare (<1%), in contrast medial epicondylar fractures/avulsions occur in 5–10% of children. The ossification centre for the medial epicondyle appears around 5–6 years of age; it fuses with the humerus at 18–20 years of age. Therefore, it does not occur in children <5 years of age. In children older than this, the presence of the medial epicondyle ossification centre should be confirmed when reviewing X-rays in elbow injuries. A medial epicondylar fracture that is <5 mm displaced can generally be treated with cast immobilisation. Surgical management is indicated for fractures that are >5 mm displaced.[4–8]

Compared with supracondylar fractures vascular compromise is uncommon with condylar fractures.

7. Answer: C

Galeazzi's fracture is one of the most likely fractures to be missed in the ED. This is a fracture of the distal one-third of the radius with dislocation or subluxation of the distal radioulnar joint. Sometimes overdiagnosis may happen due to the inability to obtain a true AP view. In a slightly oblique view of the radius and ulna, unlike in a true AP view, the distal radio ulnar joint may appear subluxed when in fact it is not. The way to circumvent this problem is to look at the ulna styloid and the direction it points to. **The ulnar styloid should be pointing to the triquetrum at all times irrespective of an AP or oblique view. If it doesn't, it is likely that there is a dislocation or subluxation of the distal radio ulnar joint.**

In Monteggia's fracture dislocation, there is fracture of the proximal one-third of the ulna with dislocation of the radial head.[9]

8. Answer: C

Femoral shaft fractures in children are relatively common and may be secondary to a variety of mechanisms.

- In children <1 year of age, the majority of the fractures are secondary to NAI.
- In toddlers the fractures are mainly secondary to mechanisms other than non-accidental injury and spiral fractures are common in them.
- In young children, minimal trauma and twisting injuries during ordinary play may cause fractures.
- In older children and teenagers major mechanisms including multitrauma may be responsible.

Shock is very unlikely to be resulting from an isolated femur fracture in a child. If shock is present, other traumatic causes for the shock such as splenic, liver or pelvic injury should be considered.[2,10]

9. Answer: A

Toddler's fracture is an occult tibial fracture that occurs in children younger than 2 years of age. This usually occurs after a fall; however, often the mechanism is not witnessed by the caregiver. The rotational stress on the distal tibia during the fall causes an oblique distal tibial fracture. The child usually presents refusing to walk or with a painful limp. It is essential to rule out fractures in other sites and issues with the hips through a carefully obtained history, examination and laboratory tests, especially when the fall is not witnessed. **The diagnosis of toddler's fracture is challenging because the fracture is not usually visible on the X-ray during the first week after the injury.** When suspected, the fracture should be treated with a long leg cast and the child should be referred for orthopaedic follow-up. Repeat X-ray done in 3 weeks often shows the evidence of the fracture as periosteal new bone formation.[5,11]

10. Answer: C

In children both acute septic arthritis and osteomyelitis occur most commonly secondary to haematogenous spread. In a smaller number of children this can be due to direct inoculation from an overlying wound. Osteomyelitis in the metaphysis can spread to the joint, causing septic arthritis in the joint. Direct inoculation to the hip joint may occur during less careful femoral venous access in children. Osteomyelitis in children occur characteristically in the metaphysis of long bones, especially in femur, tibia and humerus. Brodie abscess is a form of subacute pyogenic osteomyelitis usually affecting the metaphysis of long bones or metaphyseal equivalent bones (tarsal and carpal bones, pelvis and vertebrae) mainly in children.

In acute septic arthritis, plain X-ray is frequently normal. Due to a joint effusion, a widening of the joint space may been seen; however, this is a late sign. Ultrasound, CT and MRI should show evidence of septic arthritis including the presence of a joint effusion. Although the spectrum of infecting organisms is dependent on a child's age, *Staphylococcus aureus* is the most commonly isolated organism in both acute septic arthritis and osteomyelitis in children across all age groups. There seems to be an increasing incidence of infections due to community-acquired MRSA.[5]

11. Answer: A

Diagnosing transient synovitis of the hip in a limping or non-weight-bearing but otherwise well young child can be a challenge. This is a diagnosis that should be arrived at by exclusion of significant causes affecting the hip in this age group (3–6 years). History, examination, radiological and laboratory findings generally overlap between transient synovitis and other conditions.

Differential diagnosis of conditions affecting the hip include:
- septic arthritis
- osteomyelitis
- Legg-Calvé-Perthes disease
- malignancy
- rheumatoid arthritis
- acute slipped upper femoral epiphysis
- osteoid osteoma.

Predictors of septic arthritis of the hip have been described. **The presence of all four of fever, inability to weight bear, WCC of >12 × 10⁶/L and ESR > 40 mm gives a 93–99% likelihood of having septic arthritis. If none of these predictors are present the likelihood of septic arthritis seems to be very low.**

Two-thirds of the cases of transient synovitis is associated with a joint effusion. In transient synovitis,

medial joint space widening, lateral displacement of the femoral epiphysis with flattening of the surface (Waldenstrom's sign) secondary to joint effusion can be seen. However, these findings are not specific to transient synovitis and the finding of an effusion on ultrasound cannot be used to confirm the diagnosis of transient synovitis. In some patients, joint aspiration under ultrasound guidance, MRI and nuclear scanning may need to be used to exclude other potential conditions.

A child with transient synovitis is more likely to appear well and have a hip that is pain free on passive movements carried out by the examiner. Internal rotation and abduction can be slightly restricted.[4]

12. Answer: D

In children younger than 8 years of age, upper cervical spine injuries (above C 3–4) level are more common than lower cervical spine injuries. These injuries are often fatal but survivors may only have subtle radiological abnormalities. Children over 8 years of age typically sustain lower cervical spine injuries. Compounding the difficulties in assessing a young child's cervical spine and neurology, interpretation of radiology is challenging because many features may mimic fractures in the growing cervical spine. Some of these features include:[12,13]
- absence of lordosis
- anterior arch of C1 is not visible until approximately 2 years of age – consequently, predental space cannot be measured on the lateral view in this age group
- wedging of the anterior parts of vertebral bodies
- notching of anterior and posterior vertebral bodies by vascular channels in infants – this may mimic vertebral body fracture
- pseudosubluxation of C2–3 – this should be ≤4 mm
- anterior atlantodental (predental) space is <5 mm in children <8 years of age and <3 mm in children ≥8 years
- synchondrosis at base of odontoid process – this fuses at 3–7 years of age and may mimic a fracture or a fracture can be mistaken for synchondrosis
- apical odontoid epiphysis, which appears at 7 years and fuses at 12 years and may mimic a fracture.

13. Answer: B

The sternoclavicular joint is the most frequently mobile non-axial joint of the body. It is one of the most stable joints because it is strengthened by the surrounding strong ligaments. Consequently, dislocations are rare unless a high degree of forces are involved. Similarly, fractures involving the medial (proximal) clavicle account only for 5% of all clavicular fractures. **Routine clavicular X-ray may not precisely show the fracture and dislocations in this area.** Comparison with the normal side and special views of the medial clavicle may be helpful. Contrast CT scan is indicated where uncertainty of the fracture or dislocation exist or when there is high suspicion for injuries to the superior mediastinal vessels and other structures secondary to posterior dislocation or displacement of the fracture.

In these injuries pneumothorax should be excluded by both clinical examination and CXR. Evidence for impingement on superior mediastinal structures should be sought during physical examination. Injuries and compresssion to the great vessles, trachea and oesophagus can occur. Posterior strenoclavicular dislocations will require closed or open reduction under anaesthetic to prevent significant functional impairment.[14]

14. Answer: D

Acute rotator cuff tears occur as a result of significant traumatic mechanisms such as hyperabduction and hyperextension, as occurs when falling on an outstretched arm or lifting a very heavy object. Individuals with chronic impingement syndrome due to repetitive overhead use of an arm (as in heavy labour and in sports) may progress to an advanced stage of injury (stage 3 inpingement syndrome) to a rotator cuff injury that involves acute tears. They are more prone to tears during acute injury as well.

Rotator cuff tears can be partial or complete. The most commonly affected component is the supraspinatus tendon and muscle.

In the acute stage the diagnosis is based on clinical features. Tears cause pain and weakness typically on abduction of the shoulder at 60–120 degrees and also on external rotation. A positive *drop arm test* is due to the inability to hold and lower an abducted arm at 90 degrees without dropping it. Other tests of shoulder impingement may become positive. **Most rotator cuff tears can be adequately assessed using ultrasound, although this test is operator-dependent. USS has a relatively high sensitivity in identifying and assessing both partial and full thickness tears.**[15,16]

15. Answer: B

Only 2% of the shoulder dislocations are posterior and can be classified according to the final resting postion of the humeral head – subacromial (most common), subglenoid, subspinous (both are rare). The mechanism of injury in posterior shoulder dislocations is often forced internal rotation and adduction. This may occur in falls and sudden muscular contractions as in convulsions and due to accidental electric shock. A direct anterior force to the shoulder can dislocate it posteriorly as well.

Posterior dislocations are notoriously difficult to diagnose on standard X-rays of the shoulder. The AP view may appear normal unless careful attention is directed to identify subtle indications of posterior dislocation. These include:

- 'loss of half moon overlap' sign: on AP view, the normal overlap between the humeral head and the glenoid fossa is lost
- rim sign: the distance between the articular surface of the humeral head and the anterior glenoid rim is increased
- lightbulb or drumstick sign: the internally rotated humeral head appears this way
- trough line sign: posterior dislocation is associated with a fracture of the anteromedial humeral head causing this sign. This lesion is called *reverse* Hill-Sachs deformity. (Hill Sachs deformity is associated with anterior dislocations. It is a compression fracture of the humeral head).

The transcapular ('Y') view confirms the posterior location of the humeral head. Other specific views such as axillary and posterior oblique can be obtained. These views can identify any associated humeral head and posterior glenoid rim fractures.[15,17]

16. Answer: C

When fractures of the distal radius are manipulated in the ED, all important abnormalities should be identified in the pre-reduction X-rays, corrected during manipulation and checked for adequacy of reduction in post-reduction X-rays. The following abnormalities should be properly corrected.[18]

- **Dorsal tilt** (on lateral view): should be reduced if the tilt is >neutral. Some allow up to 10 degrees of dorsal tilt.
- **Radial shortening** (on PA view): loss of 2 mm or more should be corrected (normally radial styloid extends 9–12 mm beyond articular surface of distal ulna).
- **Radial shift** (on PA view): any shift should be corrected.
- **Radial inclination** (on PA view): <15 degrees should be corrected (the slant of radial styloid to transverse plane is normally 15–25 degrees).
- **Volar tilt** (on lateral view): >20 degrees should be corrected (normal volar tilt is 10–25 degrees).
- **Intra articular step off** (on PA view): >1 mm should be corrected.
- **Dorsal displacement.**

17. Answer: C

Scapholunate dislocation is an easily missed ligamentous injury unless careful attention is directed when reviewing the injured wrist and the X-ray. This injury may occur due to a simple mechanism such as falling on an outstretched hand where the dominant force is extreme dorsiflexion of the wrist. A missed injury could cause osteoarthritis of the wrist with resultant functional impairment, as well as ischaemic necrosis of the lunate (Kienbock disease).

For the radiological identification of the injury, on a PA view of the wrist a widened gap is visible between the two carpal bones. This gap is normally <3 mm in adults and if it is wider it is due to scapholunate dislocation ('Terry-Thomas sign'). On routine X-ray this increased gap may not be obvious and a clenched fist AP view may be required. This injury may also be associated with rotary subluxation of the scaphoid. This gives a 'signet ring sign' over the scaphoid.

Arthroscopy is the gold standard in diagnosing and grading of scapholunate injuries. Sensitivity of MRI is relatively low (63%) and its specificity is 86%.

This injury is treated with closed reduction or open reduction with internal fixation in the OT.[18,19]

18. Answer: B

Perilunate dislocation belongs to a continuum of ligamentous injuries in the wrist, which include scapholunate dissociation, perilunate dislocation and lunate dislocation. These injuries typically occur with falling on an outstretched hand where wrist hyperextension is the dominant mechanism. Scapholunate dissociation is generally associated with less severe force, whereas perilunate dislocation and lunate dislocation with their associated carpal bone fractures are due to progressively more severe forces.

The four stages of ligamentous injuries in the wrist are:

- stage I: scapholunate dissociation
- stage II: perilunate dislocation
- stage III: perilunate dislocation with associated dislocation/fracture of triquetrum
- stage IV: lunate dislocation.

Perilunate dislocation is best seen on the lateral view. In this injury the lunate remains in position relative to the distal radius but the capitate is dorsally dislocated. On a normal lateral view four C-shaped curved articular surfaces can be identified. They are distal radius, the proximal and distal articular surfaces of the lunate and the proximal articular surface of the capitate. This arrangement is disrupted because of the dorsal displacement of the capitate.

On PA view there is overlap of proximal and distal carpal rows.

This injury can be associated with fractures of multiple carpal bones. Most often a scaphoid fracture/subluxation or capitate fracture is seen.

On examination, wrist swelling and tenderness are present but gross deformity is surprisingly absent in perilunate dislocation. The patient should be referred to the orthopaedics department for arthroscopy guided or open reduction and stabilisation.[18,20,21]

19. Answer: A

When a patient presents to the ED with complete amputation of a digit or multiple digits with the amputated parts, the injury should be carefully assessed and the patient should be urgently referred to the relevant surgical specialty involved in replantation. Amputated parts that were subjected to severe crush, severe avulsion, severely comminuted bones and prolonged ischaemia due to improper preservation techniques are generally not suitable for replantation. If a digit is cooled without freezing it may survive for a prolonged period. An amputated finger proximal to the insertion of flexor digitorum superficialis tendon insertion is not suitable for replantation. All other conditions mentioned are definitive indications for referral for replantation. If the digit is partially amputated and still attached to the proximal stump, surgical re-attachment is called revascularisation.[22,23]

20. Answer: B

Compartment syndrome may occur due to a variety of causes but is most commonly due to fractures of the tibia (40% of the cases) and forearm. Other conditions such as haemorrhage, oedema secondary to ischaemic reperfusion injury, constrictive casts, intraarterial drug injection, extravasation of intravenous contrast and crush injury, all of which can increase intracompartmental pressure, may cause compartment syndrome.

Compartment syndrome is treated with urgent surgical fasciotomy, which is done at the time of clinical diagnosis and/or confirmation of compartmental pressure. At the time of diagnosis any restrictive casts and dressings should be removed.

'Delta pressure', which is the pressure difference between diastolic BP and the intracompartment pressure, has been found to better correlate with potentially irreversible muscle injury. Normal intracompartmental pressure is <10 mm Hg and pressure >30–50 mm Hg is detrimental if left untreated for several hours. Delta pressure equal or <30 mm Hg is commonly used as the critical pressure causing compartment syndrome. It is easy to reach this critical delta pressure in hypotensive trauma patients and therefore they are more prone to irreversible damage due to compartment syndrome. In these patients supporting BP is essential to limit this damage. Elevation of the limb above the level of the heart reduces the perfusion pressure of the limb by reducing the arteriovenous pressure gradient, and this can be detrimental to the limb. Elevation should not be done in compartment syndrome.[24]

21. Answer: A

The initial symptom of compartment syndrome in an awake patient is pain and this becomes excessive and out of proportion to the extent of the injury. Pain has an usual onset within a few hours from the injury. However, the onset can be delayed up to 48 hours. Both active and passive stretching of the affected muscles cause excessive pain. Accompanied with pain are the symptoms secondary to dysfunction of the nerves in the compartment, especially paraesthesia in the nerve distribution occurs. Motor dysfunction can occur but this is usually late. Permanent nerve damage can occur within approximately 8 hours. Limb ischaemia is a late feature, therefore the limb may be warm to touch and there could be an easily palpable pulse in the early stage.

In compartment syndrome irreversible damage to the nerves and muscles occur 8 hours after the onset. Functional impairment can be prevented by prompt diagnosis and treatment within 6 hours.[24]

22. Answer: C

A fractured neck of femur in the elderly is associated with high mortality and morbidity. The aims of ED management in these patients are: early diagnosis; detailed medical evaluation to identify and stabilise concurrent medical issues such as associated acute myocardial infarction, cardiac arrhythmia, stroke, sepsis and dehydration; provision of adequate analgesia; and prevention of complications such as pressure sores, hypoxia and deep venous thrombosis or pulmonary embolism. Delay to surgery beyond 48 hours has been identified as a compounding factor affecting survival in these patients and is associated with an increased major complication rate. As early surgery is recommended in most patients, detailed medical assessment should be done to identify and stabilise associated medical conditions. In the ED a three-in-one femoral nerve block is recommended as an effective method of providing analgesia (NHMRC grade A recommendation). In this method, in addition to the femoral nerve, the obturator nerve and the lateral cutaneous nerve of the thigh are blocked because these nerves substantially supply the hip joint.

Preoperative skin or skeletal traction is not useful because there is no evidence to support its use (Grade A recommendation). There is some evidence to support the use of oxygen therapy in these patients (Grade B). A regular pulse oxymetry check should be performed and oxygen should be provided as required in the ED. In addition, the patient should be placed on a pressure-relieving mattress and appropriate measures should be taken to prevent pressure sores (Grade A). The patient should be wearing pressure-gradient stockings (Grade A).[25,26]

23. Answer: A

This is a relatively frequent scenario where an elderly patient presenting to the ED with hip pain and inability to fully weight-bear but has normal-appearing pelvic and hip radiography. In this scenario, a thorough examination is necessary to exclude other possible injuries such as a missed femoral shaft fracture. Hip radiographs should be examined for subtle signs of a nondisplaced neck of femur fracture. These subtle signs of a nondisplaced fracture include a:

- cortical break in the continuity, especially visible along the superior surface of the neck
- angulation at the superior or inferior cortical surface
- distorted trabecular pattern in the neck
- band of increased bone density across the neck where fracture is impacted
- band of reduced density across the neck where fracture is separated
- shortened femoral neck
- distorted angle between femoral head and neck.

To prevent delay in the diagnosis of an occult fracture and complications such as avascular necrosis, and late displacement associated with it, the best approach would be to proceed to either CT or MRI. **MRI is more sensitive than CT in detecting occult fractures.** When subtle signs of occult fractures are present on plain radiography, CT is useful to confirm the fracture. However, in a patient with clinical findings that are suggestive of a fracture, if the CT is normal, a further MRI may be necessary to exclude a fracture. MRI is able to identify an alternative injury such as a pelvic fracture, intertrochanteric fracture or soft tissue injury. Diagnosis of a hip sprain or contusion in an elderly patient should be made only after a careful exclusion of an occult fracture. Bone scans are not frequently used as an imaging modality to exclude occult neck of femur fractures. Although a bone scan could detect fracture (sensitivity 90–95%), it takes 3–5 days for new bone formation at the fracture site and hence a bone scan will be negative until that time. Bone scans are relatively non-specific because other conditions may cause abnormal uptake.[27,28]

24. Answer: B

About 90% of hip dislocations are posterior and 10% are anterior. Anterior dislocations can be anterior superior or anterior inferior. Acetabular and femoral head fractures are frequently associated with hip dislocations. These fractures may not be easily identifiable on initial X-rays and therefore should be evaluated using a post-reduction X-ray, especially Judet views or CT scans.

Any delay in reduction of a dislocated hip increases the rate of avascular necrosis of the femoral head, therefore all hip dislocations should be reduced within 6 hours either in the ED or in the OT. Interposition of the capsule or tendons in the joint may interfere with easy reduction in the ED. Numerous repeated attempts at reducing the hip in the ED should be avoided and emergent closed reduction should be arranged in the OT under general anaesthetic.[28]

25. Answer: B

Injuries to the medial collateral ligaments are more common than lateral ligaments as in most instances the forces such as abduction, flexion and internal rotation of the femur on the tibia are applied to the medial side. There could be a sprain, partial tear or complete tear involving the collateral ligaments. During examination laxity should be elicited with valgus and varus strain, first at a 30-degree knee flexion and then with the knee fully extended. Examination findings should be compared with the normal knee. When the knee is flexed at 30 degrees, and there is no laxity but pain is produced, the injury can be considered a sprain. **If the laxity is <1 cm and it stops with a firm end point the injury is likely to be a partial tear. If the laxity is >1 cm and there is no end point it is a complete tear. If the laxity is present in full extension of the knee it indicates a more severe injury to the knee, with involvement of the capsule and cruciate ligaments.**[29]

26. Answer: A

The clinical diagnosis of ACL injury has the following characteristics:[29,30]

- At the time of injury it is associated with a characteristic 'pop' sensation in the knee.
- **The Lachman test is more sensitive than the commonly performed anterior drawer test (sensitivity 84% and 62% respectively).** The lateral pivot shift test has a sensitivity of 38%.
- Although most ligamentous injuries can cause haemarthrosis in the knee, **75% of all**

haemarthroses are due to ACL injuries.
Haemarthrosis can also be caused by peripheral meniscal tears and intraarticular fractures.

- A cruciate ligament injury may present without haemarthrosis and even without much pain. This usually occurs when there is disruption to the capsule, causing a leakage of blood into the surrounding soft tissues.
- A Segond fracture (an avulsion fracture on the lateral tibial condyle at the site of attachment of the lateral capsular ligament) indicates an ACL tear.
- It is associated with medial meniscal injuries.

PCL tears less frequently present as isolated injuries than anterior cruciate tears.

27. Answer: A

Although presentations with meniscal injuries are relatively frequent, studies describing the accuracy of physical examination findings are limited. A combination of examination findings gathered from various examinations of the knee has a reasonably high sensitivity and specificity in the diagnosis of meniscal, ACL and PCL injuries. This is described as 'composite examination of the knee' in the literature without elaborating what specific examinations were included. **No single examination or test has high sensitivity and specificity, although some of these tests are performed routinely. Therefore, findings from a number of examinations will be more useful in the ED diagnosis.**

Mean sensitivity for composite examination is 77% and specificity is 91%. In contrast, joint line tenderness has a mean sensitivity of 79% but its specificity is very low at 15%. With a 95% confidence interval it has a positive likelihood ration (LR) of 0.9 and negative LR of 1.1. The mean sensitivity of the commonly performed McMurray test is 53% and specificity is 59%, with a positive LR of 1.3 and negative LR of 0.8. Other tests and examination findings (knee effusion, Apley compression test, medial-lateral grind test) have not been formally evaluated in more than one study.[31,32]

28. Answer: D

Sprains to the lateral ankle are more common than that to the medial ankle and occur secondary to significant inversion and plantar flexion. Isolated sprains to the anterior talofibular ligament occur in two-thirds of cases. Medial ankle sprains, especially deltoid ligament sprains, are less likely to occur in isolation. With medial collateral ligamental sprains a fracture of the proximal (Maisonneuve fracture) or midshaft fibula should be sought. **If there is no associated fibular injury, injury to the talofibular syndesmotic complex at the distal lower leg may be present. This can be identified with a crossed-leg test, which can elicit pain at the syndesmotic complex site indicating syndesmotic sprain.** Peroneal tendon subluxation or dislocation from its site at the posterior aspect of the lateral malleolus may occur with sudden hyperdorsiflexion of the foot with eversion. This results in tenderness and bruising over the posterolateral aspect of the lateral malleolus, which may mimic lateral ankle sprain.[33,34]

29. Answer: C

In a patient with a clinical diagnosis of an acute ankle sprain, X-rays should be obtained following application of the Ottawa ankle rule. X-rays help to exclude fractures and to detect joint instability. Three standard views of the ankle (antero-posterior, lateral and mortise) should be obtained.

The presence of avulsion fractures usually indicate the location of ligamentous injuries and they may be present at malleoli, posterior malleolus, the lateral process of the talus, the lateral aspect of the calcaneus and the base of the fifth metatarsal.

In the presence of a joint effusion, the distended joint capsule can be seen anterior and posterior to the lower end of the tibia as a 'tear drop' on the lateral view. The presence of a joint effusion may suggest a subtle intra-articular fracture such as a fracture of the talar dome. In the mortise view, articular surfaces between the dome of the talus and the mortise should be parallel. The medial part of the joint space should not exceed 4 mm.

Anteroposterior view is important to assess the distal tibiofibular syndesmosis. In this view, usually there is an overlap between the distal tibia and fibula. Measurements outside the following suggest distal tibiofibular diastasis:

- The distance between the medial fibular cortex and posterior edge of lateral tibial groove should be ≤5 mm.

- Bone overlap between the distal tibia and fibula should be at least 10 mm.[34]

30. Answer: B

In the diagnosis of Achilles tendon rupture the following may be helpful:
- Thompson test: On a prone patient with feet extending over the edge of the examination bed, squeezing the calf muscles should cause plantar flexion when the tendon is intact.
- Hyperdorsiflexion sign: On a prone patient with their knees kept at 90 degrees, the examiner passively and maximally dorsiflexes the ankles. The passive dorsiflexion of two sides are compared. This is easy to do on the injured side.
- Palpation for the location and size of the defect on the tendon. A larger defect will have a worse prognosis than a smaller defect with non-operative management.
- Lateral ankle X-ray may show Kager's triangle (fatty tissue filled space anterior to the Achilles tendon) opacification with irregularity of the tendon.
- If doubt exists USS or MRI can confirm the diagnosis.

Weak active plantar flexion is still possible with a complete rupture as tibialis posterior, peroneal and long flexor muscles contribute to this movement. Weak plantar flexion should not be attributed to a partial tear. This is frequently a reason for misdiagnosis of a complete rupture.

In selected patients, especially older patients with smaller defects, non-operative management with a below-knee cast with the foot in gravity or maximal equinus position is indicated. Operative repair is mainly indicated in younger patients with large defects.[34,35]

31. Answer: A

Although **talar dome fractures** are relatively uncommon, they can easily be missed as the clinical findings are non-specific. **They can mimic and accompany ankle sprains.** The mechanism generally is an inversion injury at the ankle. The talar dome fracture is an osteochondral fracture, meaning a fracture involving both the cartilage and subchondral bone. The fractures can be located medially or laterally on the talar dome with equal frequency.

This fracture should be considered in any ankle sprain with gross oedema and also when a patient represents to the ED after the initial presentation with an ankle sprain. In lateral talar dome fractures, the tenderness is usually located anterior to the lateral malleolus. In medial talar dome fractures, the tenderness is located posterior to the medial malleolus.

Careful review of standard AP, lateral and mortise views of the ankle may identify these fractures. The lateral X-ray may show a joint effusion. Lateral lesions are best seen on a mortise view as thin, wafer-shaped lesions. Medial lesions are best seen on an AP view as deep cup-shaped lesions. In suspected cases with negative radiographs CT and MRI can identify the lesions.

Potential sequelae of inadequately managed talar dome fractures are chronic ankle pain, osteoarthritis and osteochondritis dissecans (with stiffness, crepitance and recurrent swelling with activity). Definitive management involves cast immobilisation or surgical excision of the fracture.[34,36]

32. Answer: A

Pilon fracture is an often comminuted fracture of the distal tibial metaphysis secondary to a massive primary axial force driving the talus into the tibial plafond in major traumatic mechanism such as falling from a height. Some of these fractures are open. **Frequently, these fractures are associated with other injuries such as fractures of the calcaneus, tibial plateau, neck of femur, acetabulum and lumbar spine, caused by axial mechanism.** The majority of medial malleolar fractures do not occur in isolation. They are usually associated with fractures at the lateral malleolus or posterior malleolus. These bimalleolar fractures are unstable. A potential proximal fibular fracture should be considered in the presence of an apparent isolated medial malleolar fracture.

A lateral malleolar fracture above the ankle joint line (Danis-Weber type C) is more likely to be associated with distal tibiofibular syndesmosis disruption than a fracture below that level (Danis-Weber types B and A).[34]

33. Answer: C

Lisfranc's injury occurs in the midfoot with significant mechanisms such as plantar flexion of the foot with an axial load. The injury spectrum consists of sprains to the Lisfranc's ligament to complete disruption to the midfoot with displacement and fractures. The very high strength Lisfranc's ligament runs between medial cuneiform and the base of the second metatarsal, and the disruption of this ligament is inevitable in significant injuries. **Consequently, bony diastasis between the first and second metatarsal bases occurs and if this diastasis is ≥1 mm it should be considered an unstable injury**. Due to the significance of mechanisms causing this injury, associated metatarsal and tarsal fractures and loss of foot arch height are relatively common. The soft tissue swelling could cause compartment syndrome in the foot.

Injuries to the foot due to significant traumatic mechanisms should be assessed for Lisfranc's injury. If suspected, CT scan is the investigation of choice because it can reveal otherwise occult injuries that cannot be identified with plain films.[19,33]

34. Answer: D

Unilateral and bilateral facet joint dislocations are important cervical spine injuries that cause recognisable signs on cervical spine X-ray. The mechanisms involved are:

- distractive flexion with rotation in unilateral injury
- severe distractive flexion in bilateral facet dislocation.

In facet joint dislocation, the inferior facet of the vertebra above dislocates anteriorly over the superior facet of the vertebra below. Therefore, on the lateral view, vertebral body above is anteriorly displaced. **In unilateral facet dislocation this displacement is <50% of the vertebral body width and in bilateral dislocation it is 50% or more. Unilateral dislocation is usually associated with nerve root injury and bilateral injury causes complete cord injury.** When there are no associated fractures the unilateral injury is considered to be mechanically stable but bilateral injury is always unstable. However, as a matter of caution, as with any spinal injury with radiographic abnormality or neurological deficit, this injury may be considered as unstable for practical purposes in the ED.

A lesser degree of distractive flexion can cause bilateral perched facets as compared with complete facet dislocation and the facet may not have a

significant neurological deficit. This injury is considered unstable as well.[37,38]

35. Answer: A

Ligaments such as the anterior longitudinal ligament, posterior longitudinal ligament and posterior ligamental complex provide stability to the cervical spine. During significant mechanisms of injury isolated ligamental injuries can occur without associated fracture or dislocations. However, these injuries are rare, even with high-risk mechanisms. **Once bony injury has been excluded with plain radiography and CT, these patients generally continue to have *excessive pain* and *limited range of motion*.** If missed these injuries may cause delayed mechanical and neurological instability.

Three types of isolated ligamentous injuries have been described:

- Hyperflexion sprain: distractive flexion tears posterior cervical ligaments to various degrees. There may be subtle separation (fanning) of the spinous processes, loss of parallel appearence of the facet joints or focal kyphosis at the level of injury on X-ray.
- Hyperextension sprain: distractive extension tears the anterior longitudinal ligament. On plain film there may be subtle widening of the anterior part of the intervertebral disc space
- Transverse ligament tear (in the atlas): on lateral view the predental space is >3 mm wide in adults and on CT >2 mm wide.

The presence of equivocal or subtle findings on the plain films have been found to increase the chance of having ligamentous injury in patients with excessive pain and limited motion. These findings include:

- vertebral body malalignment <2 mm
- intervertebral disc space narrowing
- slight facet joint malalignment
- slight widening of the distance between spinous processes
- isolated prevertebral soft tissue swelling.

As CT cannot exclude ligamentous injury, MRI is the investigation of choice in their diagnosis. Flexion and extension views are only rarely used in the ED.[37,39]

36. Answer: C

Acute lumbosacral pain (acute low back pain) is normally referred to as low back pain that is confined to the lumbosacral region and is not associated with radicular pain (sciatica). Most patients have no identifiable abnormailites, even with radiological imaging. Therefore imaging of these patients is unlikely to be helpful unless red flag features are present. The causes include:

- muscular and ligamentous sprain due to trauma to the lumbar spine
- facet joint sprain
- internal disruption of the annulus fibrosus of the disk (without herniation of nucleus pulposus or disk prolapse).

About 60–70% of these patients, even with radicular symptoms, recover within 6 weeks and 80–90% recover by 12 weeks. If the symptoms persist for more than 12 weeks, the recovery will be unpredictable and slow.

The advice to stay active rather than to have bed rest has been found to improve the pain at 3–4 weeks as well as functional status.[40]

37. Answer: D

In sciatica the pain is mainly localised to the leg and is due to stimulation of the nerve roots or dorsal root ganglion. Therefore it is a radicular pain. This radicular pain can be associated with a radiculopathy, that is, symptoms of numbness, weakness and loss of deep tendon reflexes corresponding to a specific nerve root. Causes of acute radicular pain include:

- HNP (also called disc prolapse)
- hypertrophy of facet joints and calcification of ligamentous structures causing narrowing of one or more intervertebral foramina (this is common in the elderly and patients with severe lumbar spondylosis)
- scarring around the nerve root causing spinal nerve compression (this usually happens in a patient who has had surgery and may cause chronic radicular leg pain; it may be reversible).

In most patients without progressive neurological deficits such as worsening weakness and numbness, bladder or bowel dysfunction, the initial treatment should be symptomatic. 'Red flag' features should be excluded in the history and physical examination. CT and/or MRI imaging are not indicated for acute sciatica if the above features are not present.

Symptoms usually resolve in 90% of patients without specific treatment. Most patients with HNP do not require surgical intervention to control pain.

When persistent radicular pain is present, it is important to look for reversible causes. Staying active versus bed rest has not been shown to make any difference to the pain or functional outcome in sciatica.

Sciatica is essentially a neuropathic pain. **Tricyclic antidepressents and selective noradrenaline reuptake inhibitors (e.g. venlafaxine) and antiepileptics (e.g. gabapentin) have been shown to be effective in the management of other common forms of neuropathic pain. These medications can be tried in patients with persistent symptoms of sciatica.**[40]

38. Answer: C

Lumbar spinal canal stenosis is a relatively common condition causing low back pain secondary to compression on lumbar spinal nerve roots. The elderly often present to the ED with disabling low back pain due to this condition. The most common symptom complex caused by lumbar spinal canal stenosis is called neurogenic claudication. The symptoms are mechanical low back pain radiating to the buttocks and thighs, or often to the entire leg. The pain typically gets worse on walking and standing and subsides or resolves with sitting, flexion of the lumbar spine or lying. Unlike in vascular claudication due to peripheral vascular disease, the pain does not resolve when the patient stops walking. Symptoms are bilateral and often asymmetrical in the majority of cases. Lower limb weakness occurs in less than half of these patients. Associated cauda equina syndrome and lumbosacral radiculopathy are uncommon in this condition.

In lumbar spinal canal stenosis the narrowing may occur either in the central canal, the area under the facet joints or at the neural foramina. The causes of spinal canal stenosis in the elderly are mainly degenerative and they include:

- disc degeneration, facet osteoarthritis and hypertrophy of the ligamentum flavum causing central canal stenosis
- lateral recess stenosis – this produces sciatica-like symptoms
- spondylolisthesis – this produces mainly low back pain.

Other causes include post-laminectomy and post-fusion surgeries.

ED management includes analgesia and orthopaediac referral for outpatient follow-up or admission for patients with disabling symptoms.[41,42]

39. Answer: D

Although septic arthritis of interphalangeal joints cannot be excluded in this patient, it is more likely that this patient has flexor tendon sheath infection (infectious flexor tenosynovitis) secondary to direct inoculation of the organisms during the injury. The most common organism involved is *Staphylococcus aureus* followed by *Streptococcus* species; both are native skin flora.

The presence of four *Kanavel signs* clinically confirms infectious flexor tenosynovitis:

- finger held in slight flexion
- fusiform swelling of the finger/phalanx
- tenderness along the flexor tendon sheath
- worsening pain on passive extension of the finger.

Flexor tendon sheaths of the thumb and the little finger extend into the carpal tunnel and the infection in these sheaths can easily spread to the carpal tunnel and forearm. The proximal ends of the flexor tendon sheaths of the index, middle and ring fingers overlie the midpalmar space and therefore the infection can extend to the midpalmar space.

If the patient presents within the first 24 hours from infection onset, and especially if the extent of the infection is mild, conservative treatment with in-hospital intravenous antibiotics can be tried. However, if there is no significant improvement with this treatment in 24 hours surgical drainage is indicated without further delay. If the injury is more than 48 hours old, conservative management is likely to fail and urgent surgical drainage is advised to achieve the best functional outcome. Complications associated with delayed diagnosis and treatment are flexor tendon necrosis and digital contracture.[43]

40. Answer: D

In adults, acute osteomyelitis arises from direct inoculation of the organisms following injury or surgery or due to spread from the contiguous structure such as a joint. In children haematogenous spread is more common. In adults the site most commonly involved is the spine, whereas in children long bones are most commonly involved. Overall, *Staphylococcus aureus*, both methicillin-sensitive (MSSA) and methicillin-resistant (MRSA – both non-multiresistant and multiresistant) is the most commonly implicated organism. In the elderly the most common organism causing osteomyelitis is *Staphylococcus aureus*; however, enteric gram-negative organisms are commonly involved in oeteomyelitis affecting the spine.[44,45]

References

1. Rang M, Wenger D. The physis and skeletal injury. In: Rang M, Wenger D, Pring M, editors. Rang's children's fractures. 3rd ed. Philadelphia: Lippincott Williams & Wilkins; 2005. p. 11–25.

2. Brady R, Walsh J. Fractures and dislocations. In: Cameron P, Jelinek G, Kelly A, et al, editors. Textbook of paediatric emergency medicine. 2nd ed. Edinburgh: Churchill Livingston Elsevier; 2012. p. 532–43.

3. Allen S, Hang J, Hau R. Review article: Paediatric supracondylar humeral fractures: Emergency assessment and management. Emerg Med Austral 2010;22:418–26.

4. McQuillen K. Musculoskeletal disorders. In: Marx J, Hockberger R, Walls R, et al, editors. Rosen's emergency medicine: concepts and clinical practice. 7th ed. Mosby Elsevier; 2009. p. 2245–67.

5. Hopkins-Man C, Ogunnaike-Joseph D, Moro-Sutherland D. Musculoskeletal disorders in children. In: Tintinalli J, Stapczynski J, Ma O, et al, editors. Tintinalli's emergency medicine: a comprehensive study guide. 7th ed. New York: McGraw Hill Medical; 2011. p. 892–910.

6. Ryan L. Evaluation and management of condylar elbow fractures in children. Online. Available: www.uptodate.com; 8 Aug 2011.

7. Wheeless CR. Frx of lateral condyle in children. In: Wheeless CR, editors. Wheeless' textbook of orthopedics. Online. Available: http://www.wheelessonline.com/frx_of_the_lateral_condyle_in_children; 8 Aug 2011.

8. Wheeless CR. Medial epicondyle frx of the humerus. In: Wheeless CR, editors. Wheeless' textbook of orthopedics. Online. Available: http://www.wheelessonline.com/medial_epicondyle_frx_of_the_humerus; 8 Aug 2011.

9. Rang M, Stearns P, Chambers H. Radius and ulna. In: Rang M, Wenger D, Pring M, editors. Rang's children's fractures. 3rd ed. Philadelphia: Lippincott Williams & Wilkins; 2005. p. 135–50.

10. Pring M, Newton P, Rang M. Femoral shaft. In: Rang M, Wenger D, Pring M, editors. Rang's children's fractures. 3rd ed. Philadelphia: Lippincott Williams & Wilkins; 2005. p. 181–200.

11. Lalonde F, Wenger D. Tibia. In: Rang M, Wenger D, Pring M, editors. Rang's children's fractures. 3rd ed. Philadelphia: Lippincott Williams & Wilkins; 2005. p. 215–26.

12. Cordle R, Canter R. Pediatric trauma. In: Marx J, Hockberger R, Walls R, et al, editors. Rosen's emergency medicine: concepts and clinical practice. 7th ed. Mosby Elsevier; 2009. p. 262–80.

13. Gillingham B, Cassidy J, Wenger D. Spine. In: Rang M, Wenger D, Pring M, editors. Rang's children's fractures. 3rd ed. Philadelphia: Lippincott Williams & Wilkins; 2005. p. 253–70.

14. Rudzinski J, Pittman L, Uehara D. Shoulder and humerus injuries. In: Tintinalli J, Stapczynski J, Ma O, et al, editors. Tintinalli's emergency medicine: a comprehensive study guide. 7th ed. New York: McGraw Hill Medical; 2011. p. 1830–41.

15. Della-Giustina D, Harrison B. Shoulder pain. In: Tintinalli J, Stapczynski J, Ma O, et al, editors. Tintinalli's emergency medicine: a comprehensive study guide. 7th ed. New York: McGraw Hill Medical; 2001. p. 1893–900.

16. Malanga G, Visco C, Andrus S, et al. Rotator cuff injury. Online. Available: http://emedicine.medscape.com/article/92814-overview.

17. Daya M, Nakamura Y. Shoulder. In: Marx J, Hockberger R, Walls R, et al, editors. Rosen's emergency medicine: concepts and clinical practice. 7th ed. Mosby Elsevier 2009. p. 567–90.

18. Woolfrey K, Woolfrey M, Eisenhauer M. Wrist and forearm. In: Marx J, Hockberger R, Walls R, et al, editors. Rosen's emergency medicine: concepts and clinical practice. 7th ed. Mosby Elsevier 2009. p. 525–44.

19. Mandavia D, Newton E, Demetriades D. Musculoskeletal injury. In: Mandavia D, Newton E, Demetriades D, editors. Color atlas of emergency medicine. Cambridge: Cambridge University Press. 2003. p. 167–218.

20. Mital R, Beeson M. The wrist and forearm. In: Schwartz D, Reisdorff E, editors. Emergency radiology. New York: McGraw-Hill; 2000. p. 47–75.

21. Escarza R, Loeffel III M, Uehara D. Wrist injuries. In: Tintinalli J, Stapczynski J, Ma O, et al, editors. Tintinalli's emergency medicine: a comprehensive study guide. 7th ed. New York: McGraw Hill Medical; 2011. p. 1807–21.

22. Koman A. Replantation. Online. Available: http://emedicine.medscape.com/article/1240554-overview#showall.

23. de Alwis W. Fingertip injuries. Emerg Med Austral 2006;18(3):229–7.

24. Haller P. Compartment syndrome. In: Tintinalli J, Stapczynski J, Ma O, et al, editors. Tintinalli's emergency medicine: a comprehensive study guide. 7th ed. New York: McGraw Hill Medical; 2011. p. 1880–4.

25. Fletcher A, Rigby A, Heyes F. Three-in-one femoral nerve block as analgesia for fractured neck of femur in the emergency department: a randomised controlled trial. Ann Emerg Med 2003;41:227–33.

26. Mak J, Cameron I, March L. Evidence based guidelines for the management of hip fractures in older persons: an update. Med JAustral 2010;192:37–41.

27. Schwartz D. Chapter IV-4: Lower extremity: Patient 4. In: Schwartz D, editor. Emergency radiology: case studies. New York: McGraw-Hill; 2008. p. 317–32.

28. Steele M, Stubbs A. Hip and femur injuries. In: Tintinalli J, Stapczynski J, Ma O, et al, editors. Tintinalli's emergency medicine: a comprehensive study guide. 7th ed. New York: McGraw Hill Medical; 2011. p. 1848–56.

29. Glaspy J, Steele M. Knee Injuries. In: Tintinalli J, Stapczynski J, Ma O, et al, editors. Tintinalli's emergency medicine: a comprehensive study guide. 7th ed. New York: McGraw Hill Medical; 2011. p. 1856–64.

30. Spindler K, Wright R. Anterior cruciate ligament tear. N Engl J Med 2008;359:2135–42.

31. Solomon D, Simel D, Bates D, et al. Does this patient have a torn meniscus or ligament of the knee: value of the physical examination. JAMA 2001;286:1610–20.

32. Strayer R, Lang E. Does this patient have a torn meniscus or ligament of the knee? Ann Emer Med 2006;47: 499–501.

33. Gaines S, Handel D, Ramsey P. Foot injuries. In: Tintinalli J, Stapczynski J, Ma O, et al, editors. Tintinalli's emergency medicine: a comprehensive study guide. 7th ed. New York: McGraw Hill Medical; 2011. p. 1875–80.

34. Abu-Laban R, Ho K. Ankle and Foot. In: Marx J, Hockberger R, Walls R, et al, editor. Rosen's emergency medicine: concepts and clinical practice. 7th ed. Mosby Elsevier 2009. p. 670–97.

35. Wheeless C. Achilles tendon rupture. Online. Available: www.wheelessonline.com/achilles_tendon_rupture.

36. Judd D, Kim D. Foot fractures frequently misdiagnosed as ankle sprains. Am Fam Physician 2002;66:785–94.

37. Baron B, McSherry K, Larson J, et al. Spine and spinal cord trauma. In: Tintinalli J, Stapczynski J, Ma O, et al, editors. Tintinalli's emergency medicine: a comprehensive study guide. 7th ed. New York: McGraw Hill Medical; 2011. p. 1709–30.

38. Schwartz T. Cervical Spine Radiology. In: Schwartz D, editor. Emergency radiology: case studies. New York: McGraw-Hill; 2008. p. 359–72.

39. Schwartz T, Chapter V-6: Cervical Spine: Patient 6. In: Schwartz D, editor. Emergency radiology: case studies. New York: McGraw-Hill; 2008. p. 413–43.

40. Rathmell J. A 50-year-old man with chronic low back pain. JAMA 2008;299(17):2066–77.

41. Katz J, Harris M. Lumbar spinal stenosis. N Engl J Med 2008;358:818–25.

42. Levin K. Lumbar spinal stenosis. Online. Available: www.uptodate.com.

43. Likes R, Gellman H. Infectious and inflammatory flexor tenosynovitis. Online. Available: http://emedicine.medscape.com/article/1239040-overview.

44. O'Keefe K, Sanson T. Hip and knee pain. In: Tintinalli J, Stapczynski J, Ma O, et al, editors. Tintinalli's emergency medicine: a comprehensive study guide. 7th ed. New York: McGraw Hill Medical; 2011. p. 1900–11.

45. Therapeutic Guidelines Limited. Osteomyelitis. In: eTG complete. Online. Available: www.etg.org.au.

1. Answer: A

In retrocaecal appendicitis the pain may be localised to the flank. Pregnant women with appendicitis may present with right flank or right upper quadrant pain as the gravid uterus may displace the appendix. In males acute appendicitis can present with testicular pain if the appendix lies in a retroileal position. Appendicitis can also cause suprapubic pain and the sensation of the need to defaecate if the appendix lies in the pelvis.

- Rovsing sign: pain in the right iliac fossa with palpation of the left lower quadrant
- Obturator sign: pain in the right iliac fossa with internal rotation of the hip (with the hip is flexed)
- Psoas sign: pain in the right iliac fossa with hyperextension of the right hip

Table 15.1 illustrates the MANTRELS scoring system (Alvarado score) for acute appendicitis. Patients with a score of 7 points or higher should be referred to surgery as the probability of acute appendicitis is 50%. If the score is < 7, the probability is 5%.

TABLE 15.1 MANTRELS SCORE

Criteria	Points
Migration of the pain	1
Anorexia	1
Nausea and vomiting	1
Tenderness in the right iliac fossa	2
Rebound tenderness	1
Elevated temperature > 37.3°C	1
Leucocytosis – WCC > 10, 000	2
Left shift or >75% neutrophils	1

The maximum score is 10 (score of 9–10 equals very probably appendicitis). Score of >7 patient should be referred for surgery as the patient most likely has appendicitis.

The perforation rate is high in children under the age of 5 because appendicitis is commonly misdiagnosed. Signs of peritonitis in a young child can be vague and the child may present with lethargy or hypothermia. In elderly patients most cases of appendicitis are perforated at the time of surgery. This is attributed to delayed presentation, atypical presentation and age-related anatomical changes of the appendix.[1–4]

2. Answer: D

Diverticulitis is the most common clinical presentation of diverticular disease. It is more common in the older age group. It presents with left lower quadrant abdominal pain and tenderness, low-grade fever and a history of altered bowel habit. Occasionally pain can be right-sided. Diverticulae accounts for 40% of all lower gastrointestinal bleeds.

Pyelonephritis is more likely to present with urinary symptoms such as frequency, dysuria and urgency, fever and rigors. Pain is usually in the flank rather than the lower quadrant.

The diagnosis of irritable bowel syndrome is based on clinical presentation – both history and examination – because there are no diagnostic investigations able to provide the diagnosis. It is characterised by abdominal pain that is usually eased by defaecation, changes in bowel habit, changes in stool consistency and other features such as bloating. It is not usually associated with a fever. Romes II criteria assists with the diagnosis of irritable bowel syndrome and consists of symptoms for 12 weeks or more plus two or more of;

- rolief with defaecation
- change in frequency of stool
- change in consistency of stool
- other symptoms such as tenesmus, bloating, mucus, dyspepsia and headaches

Sigmoid volvulus more frequently occurs in patients who have chronic constipation. The presentation is that of abdominal distension and generalised abdominal tenderness.[3,5–8]

3. Answer: C

Acute mesenteric ischaemia can present in a variety of ways. Nausea and vomiting occurs in about 75% of patients, and diarrhoea in about 50%. The patient can have a low-grade fever and poorly localised abdominal pain that radiates to the back. **Classically, the pain**

is out of keeping with the physical findings on examination and often refractory to analgesia. The WCC may be normal initially; however, it usually rises to >15,000 cells/mm³. Elevated lactate is a late sign and if it remains within normal limits then another diagnosis should be sought. Metabolic acidosis is a non-specific late sign. Often the abdominal X-ray is normal; however, the following features if present suggest the diagnosis of acute mesenteric ischaemia:

- thumb printing (thickened bowel wall due to oedema from necrosis)
- pneumatosis intestinalis (gas within the bowel wall from necrosis)
- portal venous gas (rare)

Approximately 50% of cases of acute mesenteric ischaemia are due to arterial embolism, 20% arterial thrombosis, 20% non-occlusive mesenteric ischaemia and 10% venous thrombosis.

Patient A is more likely to have bowel obstruction. Classic features of bowel obstruction are nausea, vomiting, abdominal distention and obstipation.

Patient B is more likely to have a perforated appendicitis. Pain initially in the right lower quadrant, now generalised with fever, nausea and vomiting, suggests perforated appendicitis.

Patient D has acute pancreatitis. Lipase may be elevated in acute mesenteric ischaemia, however, at much lower levels than in acute pancreatitis. The presence of umbilical bruising can be seen in pancreatitis and is known as Cullen's sign.[3,9,10]

4. Answer: D

This patient has a perforated peptic ulcer.

The peak age for perforated peptic ulcer is between 40–60 years and the incidence of duodenal perforation is 7–10 per 100,000 people per year. The perforation site typically involves the anterior wall of the duodenum (60%). Less commonly the perforation may occur in the antral region of the stomach (20%) or the lesser curvature of the stomach (20%). Duodenal ulcers are more commonly found in the Western population and gastric ulcers more predominantly in the Asian community. Gastric ulcers are associated with higher morbidity and mortality.

The patient in the question has two risk factors identified from the stem – aspirin and smoking. Risk factors for peptic ulcers include:

- smoking
- alcohol
- nonsteroidal anti-inflammatory medications
- steroids
- stress
- shock
- *Helicobacter pylori* infection

The pain from a perforated duodenal ulcer is of sudden onset and the sharp pain is first noticed in the epigastric region; however, it can rapidly become generalised. The pain can radiate to the back or to the shoulders (due to sub-phrenic air). About 50% of patients with a perforated peptic ulcer will experience vomiting. A mild tachycardia is common; hypotension and fever are usually late signs. **Free air under the diaphragm is visible on erect CXR in 80–85% of cases.**

Other complications of peptic ulcers include:

- upper gastrointestinal bleeding (from rupturing into an artery)
- penetration – similar to perforation only the ulcer ruptures into another organ (gastric ulcer may rupture into the liver, a duodenal ulcer may erode into the pancreas)
- gastric outlet obstruction occurs in approximately 2% and is a result of oedema and scarring at the gastroduodenal junction.

Management of this patient in the ED should concentrate on fluid resuscitation and maintaining an adequate blood pressure. The patient should be kept nil by mouth and a nasogastric tube should be inserted. Intravenous broad-spectrum antibiotics and a proton pump inhibitor should be administered. An urgent surgical opinion should be sought.[11–13]

5. Answer: B

Postoperative adhesions are responsible for small bowel obstruction (SBO) in more than 50% of cases in the developed world. It has been found that adhesions have a higher incidence following intestinal and gynaecological surgeries.

Hernias and neoplasms are each responsible for 15% of cases of SBO.

Gallstone ileus is more common in older patients and accounts for 25% of cases of non-strangulated SBO in those over 65 years of age.

Although intussusception is frequently associated with young infants and children, it can occur in the adult population and contributes to 5% of SBO in adults. The aetiology is more likely to be mechanical

(90% cases). Tumours, malignant or benign are responsible for 65% of adult intussusceptions.

Obturator hernia is an uncommon cause of SBO in adults. It is frequently diagnosed when it causes SBO.[14,15]

6. Answer: B

Hernias or adhesions rarely cause large bowel obstructions. The most common reason for large bowel obstruction is colorectal cancer. Following neoplasms, diverticulitis and sigmoid volvulus are the next most common causes. Diverticulitis can cause mesenteric oedema and scarring from chronic inflammation, which results in strictures. Adhesions are the most common cause of SBO but account for only 1–8% of large bowel obstructions.[3,16]

7. Answer: C

This patient has sigmoid volvulus. Sigmoid volvulus is more prevalent in the elderly population and in those who are institutionalised and debilitated. It presents with features similar to large bowel obstruction with abdominal distension, abdominal pain, nausea and obstipation. Vomiting is uncommon in sigmoid volvulus.

A distended loop of large bowel, lacking haustra markings, that extends from the pelvis towards the right upper quadrant and can extend as high as the diaphragm is consistent with the diagnosis of sigmoid volvulus. It is often described as a 'bent inner tube'. Often multiple air fluid levels are visualised in the small bowel. It can be seen as often on the right side of the abdomen as it is on the left.

Patients with caecal volvulus have a presentation similar to that of SBO (nausea, vomiting, distension, abdominal pain and obstipation). It more frequently occurs in younger patients and those patients who have increased caecal mobility, which may be congenital. Other risk factors include previous abdominal surgery and adhesions, pregnancy or a history of Hirschsprung's disease.

Caecal volvulus looks more like a coffee bean or kidney shape on abdominal X-ray. The air-filled caecum can be found in the mid-abdomen and extends towards the left upper quadrant. Interestingly abdominal X-ray is not helpful in about 50% of cases.

If the diagnosis of sigmoid volvulus is unclear a contrast enema can be helpful in establishing the diagnosis. The classic appearance is described as a 'bird beak' due to tapering of the colon at the torsion. The investigation is not therapeutic but is diagnostic.

Management is directed at preventing the bowel becoming gangrenous.

Sigmoid volvulus should be initially treated with decompression via sigmoidoscopy and insertion of a rectal tube. If this fails then surgical intervention is required.

Mortality rate for sigmoid volvulus is 20%, but rises to 50% if the bowel becomes gangrenous. There is a very high recurrence rate for sigmoid volvulus so it is suggested that patients who are fit for surgery undergo a corrective procedure.[3,5,16–18]

8. Answer: A

It has been demonstrated from several studies that limited ED ultrasound for aortic aneurysm performed by emergency clinicians has a high sensitivity. Furthermore, the skill required to perform this can be acquired with minimal training.

A low-frequency curvilinear probe (or small phased array probe) with a frequency of 3.5–5 mHz should be used for abdominal aortic ultrasound. The lower frequency penetrates tissue better than higher frequency probes that have better resolution.

The diameter of the aorta should be measured from outer wall to outer wall. A false negative result may occur from measuring inner wall to inner wall because of intraluminal clot or plaque. The aorta should be measured in both transverse and longitudinal planes to ensure consistency of the measurements in providing an estimate of the true aortic diameter. Measurements should be taken of the proximal aorta and the distal aorta just proximal to the bifurcation. The study should include documentation of the maximum aortic diameter. Measurements >3 cm are suspicious of abdominal aortic aneurysm.

The use of bedside ultrasound in the ED is a rule-in test not a rule-out. Ultrasound is subject to operator factors and patient factors that can confound or assist the investigation. If there is high suspicion of a ruptured AAA but the bedside ultrasound is negative the patient should proceed to have further investigations, as it cannot be reliably ruled out.

It should be performed by trained emergency clinicians to answer specific clinical questions.[19–22]

9. Answer: C

An aortoenteric fistula is formed when an aortic aneurysm erodes into the gastrointestinal tract. When this occurs between the aorta and the duodenum, gastrointestinal haemorrhage can occur. It can present with back pain or signs of intraperitoneal infection. If a patient over the age of 50 with a history of AAA presents with gastrointestinal bleeding, then aortoenteric fistula should be considered as a cause.

The size of the aortic diameter is the strongest risk factor for rupture. This risk increases when the diameter is >5 cm (1% risk of rupture if <5 cm, 17% if >5 cm). Rupture risk is also higher in women, smokers and patients with hypertension.

Most cases of ruptured abdominal aortic aneurysms present with pain, which may be present in the abdomen, chest, flank, back or groin. A pulsatile mass may not be present if the patient is hypotensive and it can be difficult to palpate if the patient is obese or has abdominal guarding or distension. Hypotension is not present in every patient with rupture because patients present at various stages. It is often a late sign and can occur unexpectedly. Nausea and vomiting are often present and can confuse the presenting complaint. On examination the abdomen may be tender, however, a non-tender abdomen isn't always indicative that the aorta is intact. Cullen's sign (periumbilical ecchymosis) and Grey Turner's sign (flank ecchymosis) may be seen if there is retroperitoneal haematoma present. Other less common features include scrotal haematoma, inguinal mass and femoral nerve neuropathy secondary to compression.[23-25]

10. Answer: A

Given the history of recent radiotherapy the patient most likely has acute radiation proctocolitis.

Pelvic radiotherapy can result in proctitis in up to 50–70% of those receiving radiation therapy. It can be acute or chronic. The patient in question has acute radiation proctocolitis.

Acute radiation proctocolitis occurs during or shortly after (up to 6 months) the course of therapy. It presents with abdominal pain, tenesmus and rectal bleeding. An unfortunate effect may be urgency and faecal incontinence.

Some patients with severe acute radiation proctocolitis may progress to chronic proctocolitis, though most cases of acute proctocolitis are self-limiting. Chronic radiation proctocolitis can develop up to 2 years and rarely up to 30 years following cessation of radiotherapy. It occurs in 5–10% of patients who have undergone pelvic radiation therapy. Presentation can be similar to that of acute radiation proctocolitis. However, it can also present with symptoms and signs of obstruction, perforation, ulcerative disease or fistulas between the rectum and neighboring organs. Rectovaginal fistula is the most common.

Endoscopy may be helpful in the diagnosis. Chronic radiation proctocolitis can be difficult to differentiate between infectious colitis, inflammatory bowel disease or ischaemic colitis.

Treatment of acute radiation proctocolitis is supportive. Steroid enemas may be helpful in reducing inflammation. Reducing the radiation dose or ceasing therapy may improve symptoms.

Management of chronic proctocolitis is also supportive. Stool softeners and anti-inflammatory agents such as sulfasalazine are frequently prescribed. Complications should be addressed and referred on to the appropriate specialty. Fistulas and strictures generally require surgical intervention. Recurrence of the disease should also be excluded.[5,26]

11. Answer: D

Although appendicitis in pregnant patients is the most common abdominal surgical emergency it occurs with equal frequency as it does in the non-pregnant population. Appendiceal rupture, however, occurs more frequently in gravid patients (up to 60% risk in the gravid patient versus up to 20% in the non-pregnant patient) and the risk of perforation is higher in the second and third trimesters. This is most likely due to the enlarging uterus impairing the process of omentum walling off the infection.

The presenting features of appendicitis in a pregnant patient are similar to those of the non-pregnant population with fever, anorexia, nausea, vomiting and right lower quadrant pain. Because nausea and vomiting and leukocytosis can occur with normal pregnancy, diagnosis of appendicitis is frequently delayed.

By a gestation of 20 weeks the appendix starts to become displaced by the expanding uterus. While pain may become less localised, the patient still generally experiences pain in the right lower quadrant. If the patient presents with right flank pain then a retrocaecal appendix, pyelonephritis or renal colic should be suspected.

Laboratory investigations are not helpful in making the diagnosis of appendicitis in a pregnant patient because leukocytosis is frequently seen in normal pregnancies. Radiological imaging can assist in the diagnosis. Ultrasound seems to be as sensitive and specific in the pregnant population and is the investigation of choice. It has 67–100% sensitivity and 83–96% specificity compared with 86% and 96% respectfully in the non-pregnant group. There is no contraindication for MRI; however, it is time consuming and not always readily available.

Pregnancy-specific complications of appendicitis include uterine contractions, miscarriage, premature labour and fetal death. Fetal loss occurs in 1–5% of uncomplicated and up to 30% of complicated cases of appendicitis.[3,27,28]

12. Answer: D

Gallstones is a common disorder affecting up to 20% of the population. There are two main types of stones: cholesterol stones and pigmented stones.

Cholesterol stones are associated with:
- female gender
- fertility, pregnancy (progesterone reduces gallbladder contractility, oestrogens increase the risk of cholesterol stones)
- oral contraceptive pill
- obesity and metabolic syndrome
- family history
- increasing age
- rapid weight loss
- biliary stasis

Pigmented stones are associated with:
- chronic haemolytic disorders, such as sickle cell disease, β-thalassaemia or hereditary spherocytosis
- biliary infection such as Escherichia coli, ascaris lumbricoides/liver fluke, opisthorchissinensis
- some gastrointestinal disorders such as Crohn's disease, ileal resection and pancreatic insufficiency from cystic fibrosis

In haemolytic disorders, such as sickle cell anaemia, β-thalassaemia or hereditary spherocytosis, there is increased unconjugated bilirubin due to the increased

breakdown of the red cells. This leads to the formation of calcium biliruninate which can crystallise and form stones. These stones with time develop a black colour and have earned the nickname of black pigment stones.

Biliary infection from any of the organisms mentioned above leads to increased generation of unconjugated bilirubin. This contributes to the formation of the calcium bilirubin salts and stone formation.[3,29–31]

13. Answer: D

- Patient A has cholangitis.
- Patient B has biliary colic.
- Patient C has features of an SBO from gallstone ileus.
- Patient D has and inferior myocardial infarct until proven otherwise.

Cholangitis results from extrahepatic bile duct obstruction and bacterial infection. **Right upper quadrant pain, fever and jaundice is the classical triad of findings for cholangitis as described by Charcot's. These features can also be seen in cholecystitis and hepatitis. When signs of hypotension and altered mental state are present it is referred to as Reynold's pentad.** As occurs in cholecystitis, polymorphonuclear leukocytosis is present in patients with cholangitis. However, elevated bilirubin, alkaline phosphatase and transaminases occur more often. A patient with cholangitis generally has a higher fever and appears more unwell than a patient with acute cholecystitis. The presence of jaundice can be used to differentiate between the two as elevated bilirubin is an uncommon feature of acute cholecystits. Ultrasound findings also differ with the presence of dilated common and intrahepatic ducts supporting the diagnosis of cholangitis. The patient should be fluid resuscitated, commenced on broad-spectrum antibiotics and requires prompt surgical consultation.

Patient C has features of SBO secondary to gallstone ileus. This is an uncommon complication and is seen in the elderly population. The gallstone erodes through the gallbladder wall and becomes lodged at the terminal ileum causing obstruction. It is associated with a 15–18% mortality rate.

Patient D has an inferior myocardial infarction until proven otherwise. A patient with an inferior myocardial infarction tends to present with vagal symptoms such as nausea, vomiting, abdominal pain, diaphoresis and bradycardia.[32–34]

14. Answer: B

Acalculous cholecystitis occurs in approximately 10% of cases. Acalculous cholecystitis is thought to be due to ischaemia. Predisposing factors include:

- postoperatively following major surgical procedures
- major trauma
- severe burns
- sepsis with hypotension and multi-organ failure
- intensive care patients, particularly those on TPN (total parental nutrition)
- immunosuppression
- diabetes
- elderly
- CMV (cytomegalovirus) infection in AIDS

Acalculous cholecystitis has a more acute course than calculous cholecystitis and has a higher mortality rate.

Ultrasound is the imaging modality of choice. It is highly sensitive, and has a very high negative predictive value for cholecysitits. The positive predictive value for cholecysitis is high when the gallbladder wall is thickened (>3 mm thick) and pericholecystic fluid is seen with the presence of stones in the gallbladder.

CT has 92% sensitivity and 99% specificity so is useful but not as sensitive as ultrasonography for detecting gallbladder stones. It is more useful than ultrasound in detecting stones in the common bile duct.

Laboratory investigations in biliary colic or uncomplicated cholelithiasis are commonly normal; however, in acute cholecystits, polymorphonuclear leukocytosis is seen in two-thirds of patients. Mild elevation of liver transaminases can be seen and occasionally bilirubin and alkaline phosphatase can also be elevated.

Only 10% of stones are visible on plain X-ray.[30–32]

15. Answer: D

Hypocalcaemia rather than hypercalcaemia is associated with acute pancreatitis. It is one of the Ranson criteria for assessing severity of acute pancreatitis. Hypocalcaemia can result from sequestration of calcium in areas of fat necrosis and also hypoalbuminaemia and hypomagnesaemia which can occur in pancreatitis.

Up to 30% of patients will develop some degree of respiratory complication. ARDS is an uncommon complication of acute pancreatitis but carries a high mortality rate. It is caused by diffuse alveolar damage from inflammatory mediators and results in leaky capillaries. There may also be a reduction in surfactant in patients with pancreatitis. Pleural effusion can occur and is more frequent on the left side.

Other complications of pancreatitis include pseudocyst formation, systemic inflammatory response syndrome (SIRS), shock, coagulopathy, pancreatic oedema or haemorrhage and metabolic complications such as hyperglycaemia, hypocalcaemia and acute tubular necrosis.

Late complications include abscess formation, fistula formation, pseudocyst formation, diabetes and chronic pancreatitis.[3,33,35]

16. Answer: B

Ranson criteria is a clinical prediction tool frequently used for predicting the severity of acute pancreatitis (see Table 15.2a).

At 48 hours combine the total number of criteria present (see Table 15.2b).

TABLE 15.2a RANSON CRITERIA FOR ACUTE PANCREATITIS AT PRESENTATION

At presentation	Within 48 hours
Age < 55	Base excess > 4 meq/L
WCC > 16,000/mm³	Drop in haematocrit by >10%
Glucose > 10 mmol/L	Rise in urea > 5mg/dL
LDH > 350 IU/L	PaO_2 < 60 mmHg
AST > 250 IU/L	Calcium < 2 mmol/L
	Estimated fluid sequestration > 6 L

TABLE 15.2b RANSON CRITERIA FOR ACUTE PANCREATITIS AT 48 HOURS

Number of criteria present	Associated mortality rate
0–2	1%
3–4	15%
5–6	40%
>7	100%

TABLE 15.3 RANSON CRITERIA FOR
GALLSTONE-RELATED PANCREATITIS

At presentation	Within 48 hours
Age > 70	Base excess > 5 meq/L
WCC > 18,000/mm3	Drop in haematocrit by >10%
Glucose > 12.2 mmol/L	Rise in urea > 2 mg/dL
LDH > 400 IU/L	PaO2 < 60 mmHg
AST > 250 IU/L	Calcium < 2 mmol/L
	Estimated fluid sequestration > 4 L

TABLE 15.4 GLASGOW CRITERIA FOR PREDICTING
THE SEVERITY OF PANCREATITIS

At presentation	Within 48 hours
Age > 55 yrs	Serum calcium < 2 mmol/L
WCC > 15, 000/mm3	Serum albumin < 34 g/L
Blood glucose > 10 mmol/L	LDH > 600 IU/L
Urea > 16mmol/L with no response to IV fluids	AST > 200 IU/L
PaO2 < 76 mmHg	

The criteria for gallstone-related pancreatitis varies slightly (see Table 15.3).

Another system that can be used for predicting the severity of pancreatitis is the Glasgow and Modified Glasgow criteria. These have been validated for gallstone and alcoholic associated pancreatitis (see Table 15.4).

The *Modified Glasgow criteria* can be remembered by the following pneumonic.

PANCREAS

PaO$_2$ < 60 mmHg

Age > 55 years

Neutrophils, WCC > 15

Calcium < 2 mmol/L

Renal function, urea > 16 mmol/L

Enzymes, LDH > 600 IU/L, AST > 200 IU/L

Albumin < 32 g/L

Sugar, glucose > 10 mmol/L

If ≥ three of these are present within 48 hours of onset then the patient most likely has severe pancreatitis.[3,36-38]

17. Answer: D

Jaundice may be detected clinically when the serum bilirubin levels are >40mmol/L. It is seen in tissues with a high albumin concentration such as the skin and sclera.

Bacteria acting on bilirubin in the gastrointestinal tract produce urobilinogen. It is water soluble and is excreted in the urine. A non-obstructed biliary system is required for its presence in the urine as the bilirubin has to reach the gastrointestinal tract.

Testicular atrophy and caput medusa are signs of chronic liver disease and not pancreatic cancer.

Mirizzi syndrome manifests in a presentation of gallstones lodged in either the cystic duct or Hartmann's pouch of the gallbladder causing obstructive jaundice. The mechanism is presumed to be from external compression of the common hepatic duct.[39-42]

18. Answer: B

Umbilical hernias in children are congenital and rarely become incarcerated. They usually resolve spontaneously in children. In adults, however, it is an acquired defect where risk factors include obesity, pregnancy and ascites. They usually increase in size, are at higher risk of complications (e.g. incarceration) and frequently require operative repair.

Incisional hernias are recognised as a complication of abdominal surgery. Risk factors include extensive or complicated surgery, postoperative wound infection and obesity. They occur in 10–20% of laparotomies. The origin is usually wide and therefore complications are uncommon. Surgical repair may be required; however, the recurrence rates are high.

Direct inguinal hernias pass medial to the inferior epigastric artery, while indirect hernias pass lateral to the inferior epigastric artery. Direct inguinal hernias are due to a weakness in the transversalis fascia and the anterior abdominal wall through which they protrude. They do not pass through the inguinal canal and do not extend into the scrotum. They are less symptomatic and have fewer complications (incarceration or strangulation) than indirect inguinal hernias. They are more likely to recur following surgery than indirect inguinal hernias.

Indirect inguinal hernias are due to a patent processus vaginalis. They are more common in males secondary to the embryological decent of the testis and occur more frequently on the right side due to the later decent of the right testis. The hernia passes through the inguinal canal and into the scrotum as it enlarges. Complications are frequent particularly in females and infants. Around 5% of term and 30% of preterm infants will have an inguinal hernia. Surgery is recommended, if they are symptomatic or complications arise.[3,43,44]

19. Answer: D

Indications for attempting to reduce a hernia are the presence of a hernia and the absence of strangulation. Strangulated hernias, bowel obstruction secondary to the hernia, or hernia contents containing ovaries or testes are contraindications to hernia reduction in the ED. A surgical opinion should be sought in such instances. Repetitive attempts at reducing the hernia should be avoided as this will only lead to increased swelling. Analgesia and sedation may be required if an attempt at reduction is to be performed in the ED. For an inguinal hernia, placing the patient in a Trendelenburg position can help facilitate reduction.

Femoral hernias occur more commonly in women than men. They have a high incidence of strangulation and should therefore always be repaired electively when the diagnosis has been made.[44,45]

20. Answer: A

Patient A has a urinary tract infection. She has mild symptoms and no signs of peritonism. She has no signs or symptoms of pyelonephritis. She will most likely be suitable for discharge on oral antibiotics.

Patient B potentially has a large bowel obstruction and should not be discharged.

Bowel obstruction is the most common cause of abdominal pain in the elderly population. Patients with large bowel obstruction can present with abdominal distention, colicky abdominal pain and obstipation. Vomiting may or may not be present.

Patient C could have an abdominal aortic aneurysm (AAA) and requires urgent management.

Risk factors for abdominal aortic aneurysms include hypertension, atherosclerosis and a positive family history. AAA can present with sudden onset of abdominal, back or flank pain. Hypotension associated with a ruptured AAA can be transient. The most common misdiagnosis of AAA in the elderly is

renal colic. It is estimated that this misdiagnosis occurs approximately 16–30% of the time. The mortality of AAA rupture is high 50–70%.

Patient D could have anything from gastroenteritis to acute myocardial infarction. He requires further investigation and management.[3,15,46]

21. Answer: C

Femoral artery pseudoaneurysm or false aneurysm is a recognised complication of femoral artery catheterisation occurring in approximately 7.5% of femoral artery catheterisations. It is due to oozing of the arterial blood into the surrounding tissues through the puncture site, which has failed to seal. The haematoma is confined by the surrounding fascia and eventually becomes encapsulated by fibrous tissue. It does not contain all three layers (intima, media and adventitia) of the femoral artery wall so it is a pseudoaneurysm and not a true aneurysm. The presentation is typically with an expanding pulsatile mass, pain or tenderness. They may also present with paraesthesia or limb weakness from compression of surrounding structures. Complications of pseudoaneurysms include rupture, distal embolisation, thrombosis leading to ischaemia, local skin ischaemia, neuropathy and pain. An ultrasound is diagnostic and the patient should be referred to the vascular team for ongoing management (thrombolysis or embolectomy).

It is difficult to differentiate between periarterial haematoma and femoral artery pseudoaneurysm in the immediate postprocedural period; however, this patient is several weeks after the procedure so false aneurysm is the more likely diagnosis.

Femoral hernias originate below the inguinal ligament. They are less common than inguinal hernias but are more likely to become incarcerated or strangulated. They are generally asymptomatic; however, they can cause groin discomfort that is worse on standing and can present with nausea, vomiting and abdominal pain. Given the history of this patient the diagnosis of femoral hernia is unlikely.

In incarcerated inguinal hernia, the patient will present with pain, nausea, vomiting, low-grade fever and a hernia that is no longer reducible. Complications include strangulation, bowel obstruction and bowel perforation. If the hernia becomes strangulated then the patient appears more toxic and can be in septic shock.[43,47–49]

22. Answer: A

Boerhaave's syndrome is a transmural oesophageal rupture that results from sudden raised intraluminal pressure caused by uncoordinated vomiting with the pylorus and cricopharyngeus closed. In the majority of cases it occurs secondary to this forceful emesis. Less commonly Boerhaave's syndrome can occur as a result of coughing, straining, seizures or during labour. The most common location for the rupture to occur is the left lower posteriolateral wall of the oesophagus. The highest incidence occurs in middle aged males (age 40–60 years).

CXR can be normal in up to 30% of patients. The most common CXR finding in a patient with Boerhaave's syndrome is a left-sided pleural effusion. Other findings include pneumothorax, hydropneumothorax, pneumomediastinum and subcutaneous emphysema.

Mackler's triad, which consists of vomiting, chest pain and subcutaneous emphysema, is the classic presentation of Boerhaave's syndrome. Other clinical features that may be present include hoarse voice, tracheal shift and cervical vein distention. If left untreated these patients are at a high risk of developing sepsis, multiorgan failure and death as a result of chemical and bacterial mediastinitis. The mortality rate varies depending on the length of delay to treatment and can range from 20 to 90%.

Swallowing can exacerbate the pain and precipitate coughing due to the communication between the pleural cavity and the oesophagus. Haematemesis is not typically seen and if present can help differentiate a Mallory-Weiss tear from Boerhaave's syndrome.[50-52]

23. Answer: A

The patient most likely has an acute embolic arterial occlusion secondary to his recent diagnosis of atrial fibrillation. Atrial fibrillation is associated with peripheral emboli in at least 60% of cases.

Acute arterial occlusion of a limb is most commonly a result of embolism (90% of cases). Emboli usually lodge at arterial bifurcation points with the most common site being the femoral artery bifurcation (up to 50% of cases). Atheroemboli originate in the large proximal arteries. They tend to be smaller and therefore lodge in the smaller arteries such as the digital arteries resulting in ischaemic toes.

The typical presentation of an acute ischaemic limb involves one or more of the six Ps:
- pale
- pulseless
- painful
- paresthesia
- paralysis
- perishing with cold.

Interestingly, acute ischaemia may be masked in patients with peripheral vascular disease because they often have good collateral circulation.

The aim of management is to resuscitate the patient and restore blood flow to preserve the limb. If acute limb ischaemia is suspected the patient should promptly be given intravenous unfractionated heparin.

This patient has acute limb ischaemia from arterial embolism so should have intravenous unfractionated heparin and referral to the vascular surgeon for consideration of an embolectomy. Fibrinolysis is not suitable for this patient because it is a limb-threatening event that is time critical. Clot lysis can take up to 72 hours to be effective and is therefore not a suitable treatment. Thrombolysis should be considered for non-limb-threatening ischaemia.[49,53,54]

24. Answer: B

Please see the explanation under answer 25.

25. Answer: D

This patient has inadvertently injected a drug (such as benzodiazepine) intraarterially and is starting to develop compartment syndrome secondary to the consequential oedema and limb swelling.

When a drug has been injected into an artery the patient experiences immediate burning pain (sometimes known as a 'flash' or a 'hand trip' – intense burning pain from the site of injection to the digits, fingers or toes depending on site of injection). Within a few hours, constant severe pain and mottling of the limb appears, the hand may be cool with decreased capillary refill. As time progresses the limb becomes swollen but distal pulses are often still palpable. Signs and symptoms of compartment syndrome develop if treatment has not been sought and occasionally intraarterial drug injection can present as an acute ischaemic limb.

The presence of compartment syndrome in this case is demonstrated by pain on active and passive movement of the wrist. Time taken to develop compartment syndrome is variable.

Tissue loss, rhabdomyolysis and renal failure are also recognised complications of inadvertent intraarterial injection.

The presentation is not consistent with deep vein thrombosis (DVT). DVT would be more likely to present with a red warm swollen arm and tenderness to palpation along the deep veins.

There are similarities to an acute ischaemic limb; however, this diagnosis is excluded as peripheral pulses are present.

The mechanism of injury from the intraarterial artery drug delivery is not well understood but there are several thoughts on how it occurs:

- vasospasm – depending on the drug injected
- endothelial injury – increased tissue factor, which can trigger thrombosis, increased permeability and oedema leading to the increased compartment pressure
- precipitation of the poorly soluble or poorly diluted substance causing obstruction or embolisation
- irritation of the vessels – depending on substance injected (can cause local inflammation, vasculitis and local thrombosis)

There is no agreed ideal management of such patients. However, this patient should be given analgesia, limb elevation, commenced on a heparin infusion, compartmental pressures should be measured and a Doppler ultrasound, plus or minus angiography (arteriography) should be done to evaluate the extent of the vascular damage. The patient should have urgent consultation with a vascular surgeon as signs of compartment syndrome are present and fasciotomy may be indicated.

Other management options that have been mentioned in the literature include:

- local thrombolysis – recombinant tissue type plasminogen activator (rtPA)
- vasodilation – for example, with intraarterial or intravenous glyceryltrinitrate

A combination of the above can produce good results.[55–58]

26. Answer: D

The biggest risk factor for aortic dissection is hypertension. Other risk factors include Marfan's syndrome, other connective tissue disorders such as Ehlers-Danlos, aortic valve disease, Turner's syndrome and coarctation of the aorta. Atherosclerosis has no clear role in aortic dissection and is rarely found at the site where dissection occurs.

Presentation varies depending on the patient, the location and the extent of the dissection. The most common feature is pain, often described more as sharp than tearing or ripping pain. Nausea, vomiting, lightheadedness, diaphoresis and apprehension are also commonly present. The location of the pain suggests where the lesion could be, for example, anterior chest pain – ascending aorta, neck and jaw – aortic arch, interscapular – descending and lumbar/abdominal pain – below the diaphragm. Neurological symptoms such as focal neurological deficits, cerebralvascular accident (CVA), altered mental state or coma, occur in <20% cases. Syncope may occur as a result of extension into the pericardium causing tamponade or as a result of interruption of cerebral vascular blood flow.

CXR is a useful test; however, it is not very specific and is abnormal in about 80–90% patients. The abnormalities can be quite subtle. **Some of the CXR features suggestive of aortic dissection include widening of the mediastinum, left pleural effusion, apical capping, loss of aorto-pulmonary window and deviation of the trachea and oesophagus to the right. It is an inadequate test to rule out an aortic dissection.** Angiography is still thought of as the gold standard as it provides anatomical information regarding the path of the dissection; however, the risks of intravenous contrast and time delay doesn't make it a favourable investigation.

MRI is the ideal investigation as there is no radiation, it is 100% sensitive and specific and it demonstrates the anatomical features and extent of aortic dissection well. However, availability can be an issue, it is time consuming and is not suitable for unstable patients. CT is the imaging modality of choice for most, despite the exposure risk of radiation and contrast and it not providing the best anatomical information or assessment of the aortic valve and the aortic branching vessels. It has the advantage of accessibility and it is a more rapid test than MRI or angiography. Its sensitivity is up to 90%, specificity 90–100%.

Transoesophageal echocardiogram is also an investigation that can be considered. It can be as good as angiography if the operator is experienced. However, though accessibility is on the increase it can still be limited. As this investigation is invasive and sedation is necessary, it can be unsuitable in unintubated unstable patients.

DeBakey I (ascending, aortic arch and descending aorta) and II (ascending aorta) or Stanford type A (DeBakey I and II, proximal aorta and varying length of descending aorta) proximal dissections require surgical intervention.

Patients with distal dissections – DeBakey III (descending aorta only) or Stanford type B (distal aorta) – are considered high surgical risk therefore tend to be managed medically in the first instance. Surgical intervention is considered if these patients have ongoing pain, major vessel involvement, poorly controlled hypertension or aortic rupture but they have a higher mortality rate. Medical therapy is aimed at reducing the shearing forces and reducing the blood pressure to around systolic BP 100–120 mmHg with a HR of 60 bpm.[51,59,60]

27. Answer: B

Bright red rectal bleeding with defaecation is the most common presenting compliant in patients with haemorrhoids. Other presenting features include a swelling that may be painful if thrombosed, pruritis ani or mucoid discharge. Internal haemorrhoids can prolapse and need surgical referral if they do not spontaneously reduce or cannot be manually reduced.

Portal hypertension is not a cause of haemorrhoids. Rectal varices can cause rectal bleeding in a patient with portal hypertension.

About one-third of pregnant women develop haemorrhoids, predominantly in the later stages of pregnancy. This is a result of direct pressure on the haemorrhoidal vein reducing venous drainage. Traumatic delivery increases the incidence of thrombosed haemorrhoids.

Internal haemorrhoids lie above the dentate line, have visceral innervation, are submucosal and appear beefy red when they prolapse. External haemorrhoids originate below the dentate line, have somatic innervation, are subcutaneous, and are covered by squamous epithelium so appear skin coloured when they prolapse. External haemorrhoids have a blue/purple appearance when they are thrombosed.

Thrombosed external haemorrhoids should not be incised because this can lead to incomplete

evacuation of the clot, rebleeding, swelling and is associated with formation of perianal skin tags. They should be excised and this can be done in the ED. Most benefit is achieved if this procedure is done within the first 48 hours of symptoms, as this is when the thrombosed haemorrhoid is most tense and most painful. After 48 hours it starts to become softer and the pain is more tolerable.[61-63]

28. Answer: B

Pilonidal sinus is most frequently seen in patients under the age of 40. Recurrence rates are 20–40%. It is uncommon in those over 40 years even if they experienced an episode when they were younger.

Although there is still much controversy over the exact pathophysiology of pilonidal sinus, it is thought by most that it is caused by an infected hair follicle. When it ruptures the infection spreads into the subcutaneous tissue causing a foreign body reaction and abscess formation. The contents of the abscess then track to the skin through a sinus tract. The sinus usually contains hair and debris.

Pilonidal sinus is more common in males than females and more common in patients who are overweight and hirsute. Patients with a family history of the same, those with a sitting occupation or have repetitive trauma to the region may have an increased incidence of the disease.

Definitive management is surgery. It should not be done in the ED. The patient can be treated with antibiotics such as augmentin plus metronidazole if there is evidence of cellulitis or abscess formation.[61,63]

29. Answer: D

Oral antibiotics, analgesia and encouraging milk flow either by continued breastfeeding or expression via manual methods or the use of a breast pump is the mainstay of treatment. This strategy reduces the rate of abscess formation.

Staphylococcus aureus is the most common pathogen, including MRSA. Other causative organisms include *Streptococci* and *Staphylococcus epidermidis*. In non-lactating women, breast infections can also be caused by the aforementioned organisms, as well as enterococci and anaerobes such as bacteroides.

Therapeutic guidelines suggest:
- flucloxacillin 500 mg orally, 6-hourly for at least 5 days

- cephalexin 500 mg orally, 6-hourly for 5 days can be used if the patient has a penicillin allergy
- clindamycin 450 mg orally, 8-hourly for at least 5 days can be used if the patient has severe penicillin hypersensitivity.

If the patient has severe infection, cellulitis or signs of sepsis then intravenous antibiotics should be administered.

Co-amoxiclav or a macrolide can also be used to treat lactating infection. Tetracyclines, ciprofloxacin and chloramphenicol should be avoided as they are expressed in the breast milk and are harmful to the baby.

Regarding analgesia, there has been a small trial that compared the use of cold or room temperature cabbage leaves with ice packs in relieving the breast pain associated with infection. The results demonstrated they have similar efficacy.

In Australia about 20% of lactating women develop mastitis, the incidence is most common before the baby is three months of age. Approximately 10% of those who have mastitis develop a breast abscess. Breast abscess requires surgical management with either percutaneous aspiration or open drainage.

Risk factors for mastitis in lactating women include:
- maternal age > 30 years old
- gestational age > 41 weeks
- past history of mastitis
- poor attachment to the breast by the baby
- abnormalities of the baby's mouth such as cleft lip and palate and short frenulum
- sore or cracked nipples

Risk factors for developing a breast infection in non-lactating women include smoking and diabetes. In this group recurrent episodes are common.

An important diagnosis to consider if the patient's condition is not improving with adequate treatment or if presentation is atypical, is inflammatory breast cancer.[64–67]

30. Answer: B

Animal or human bite wound(s) to the hand should not be closed primarily. The wound in question should be cleaned, irrigated and debrided then packed with sterile saline-soaked gauze and dressed. Wound review should occur daily.

By day 4 or 5 the wound may be closed if there is no evidence of infection. When wound closure is performed at this stage in the healing process, the proliferative phase, there is no interruption of the process and therefore no delay in final healing. The results are similar to that of primary healing.

The treating clinician should assess each wound for risk of infection. If the wound is contaminated or remains so despite cleaning, irrigating and debridement then wound closure options include delayed primary closure or letting the wound heal by secondary intention. If the wound is deemed to be clean or has low risk of infection then it may be closed primarily.

An example of wounds that should be considered for delayed primary closure include:
- wounds contaminated by organic matter or contaminated soil
- wounds that are displaying signs of infection
- gunshot wounds, explosion injuries and other wounds that cause extensive tissue damage and wounds where the viability of underlying tissue are a concern
- complex crush injuries
- most wounds caused by bites (animal or human)
- puncture wounds

Laceration from glass can be treated by primary closure if there is no underlying tendon injury that requires surgical exploration and repair.

The laceration from the surfboard is not a contaminated wound and is easily cleaned with irrigation. This wound may be closed primarily. High pressure irrigation is the most effective method of cleaning wounds. In the ED using an 18-gauge needle or cannula attached to a 50 or 60 mL syringe may suffice (this generates approximately 5–8 PSI of pressure, which is the recommended irrigation pressure). Irrigation reduces the risk of infection and assists in the removal of foreign bodies.

Tap water or 0.9% normal saline can be used for irrigation. Evidence has demonstrated that there is no significant difference between the two.

Pretibial skin flaps in elderly patients should not be sutured and are better left to heal by secondary intention. The skin is usually thin and friable, there is little subcutaneous fat and it can be tricky to get good wound apposition. If sutured these wounds are prone to necrosis.

Management of pretibial lacerations involves a variety of factors. As well as taking into account the time since the injury and the extent of the injury, it is important also to consider the patient's mobility, medications, level of independence and comorbidities, as these effect wound healing.

It is advisable not to suture pretibial lacerations. Where possible skin edges should be gently apposed and Steri-strips applied with a non-adherent dressing. It is essential that the wound is not placed under any tension as this increases the chance of necrosis and delayed wound healing. If the wound is larger, the skin flap should be spread, a non-adherent silicon-based dressing applied followed by a double layer of tubular bandage. A flap that is deeper (e.g. involving 50% of the dermal layer) can be treated in a similar way using a hydrogel sheet dressing. The hydrogel sheet dressing is also useful if there is some degree of necrosis and haematoma. Wounds that involve the entire dermis require surgical intervention; debridement and skin grafting is likely.[68–72]

31. Answer: A

Wound dehiscence usually presents 7–10 days after surgery. Both patient factors and surgical factors contribute to the occurrence of wound dehiscence. Some predisposing factors include: emergency surgery, malnutrition, diabetes, immune-compromised host, intraabdominal infection, raised intraabdominal pressure, obesity and poor wound closure technique.

Dehiscence of abdominal wounds if left untreated can progress to evisceration. Generally surgical exploration is necessary to establish the extent of the dehiscence.[73–75]

32. Answer: C

Arteriovenous malformations are usually the cause in younger patients who present with SAH. In older patients SAH is usually secondary to a berry aneurysm.

Risk factors for SAH include: previous history of SAH, family history of SAH, hypertension, smoking, excessive alcohol intake, connective tissue disorders such as autosomal dominant polycystic kidneys, Marfan's syndrome, Ehler-Danlos syndrome and α_1-antitrypsin deficiency. Increasing age is also a risk factor. The average age at presentation is between 40 and 60 years.

The most common presenting feature is headache classically described as a sudden onset, severe

thunderclap headache. The headache can last up to 2 weeks. Other presenting symptoms include sudden death, transient loss or prolonged loss of consciousness, nausea, vomiting, neck stiffness, photophobia, seizures, focal neurological deficit including III or VI cranial nerve palsy. Intraocular haemorrhages occur in one in seven patients with ruptured aneurysms and are more likely to be observed in patients with a reduced level of consciousness. They are as a result of obstruction of the central retinal vein from sustained elevation in cerebrospinal fluid pressure.

ECG changes can occur that can mimic those of acute myocardial infarction. Other ECG changes that can occur in SAH include deep T wave inversion and QT prolongation.[76–81]

33. Answer: D

Rebleeding is a recognised complication and usually occurs in the 3–5 days following the initial bleed. Vasospasm occurs in approximately one-third of patients and is detected between days 4 and 14. Other complications of SAH are fever, hypertension, hypotension, hyperglycaemia, hyper or hyponatraemia, hypomagnesaemia, cardiac failure, arrhythmias, pulmonary oedema and pneumonia. Diabetes insipidus, syndrome of inappropriate antidiuretic hormone hypersecretion (SIADH) and cerebral salt wasting can develop in patients with SAH. Hydrocephalus is also a recognised complication that occurs in one-third of patients; it develops over days to weeks. Seizures occur in <25% cases.

A non-contrast head CT is an ideal investigation if it is performed soon after the onset of headache. As time passes the blood in the subarachnoid space degrades therefore increasing the likelihood of a normal-appearing CT. A non-contrast head CT is more reliable at 12 hours than it is at 48 hours. At 12 hours only 2–3% of SAHs are not detected, the pick-up rate at 48 hours is 80–85%, at 1 week it is only 50%. By day 10 almost all of the subarachnoid blood has been reabsorbed.

Lumbar puncture should be carried out 12 hours after the event occurred. By 12 hours blood in the subarachnoid space will have started to break down and bilirubin will have been formed as a result – xanthochromia. Xanthochromia is not present in a traumatic lumbar puncture because this blood has not been exposed to and broken down by the CSF enzymes.

Nimodipine 60 mg 4-hourly should be administered orally for 7 days. It has been shown to decrease the incidence of vasospasm, prevent secondary ischaemia and reduce the mortality associated with SAH.[76–80]

34. Answer: D

This patient most likely has malrotation with volvulus. It is a life-threatening condition. In this case there is a strong suspicion that the patient is in shock as she is lethargic and mottled. She requires immediate resuscitation and surgical attention.

Malrotation occurs in one in 500 births. The majority of presentations are in the first year of life. Three-quarters present within the first month. It has a mortality rate of 3–15%.

During embryological development the gastrointestinal tract rotates around the superior mesenteric artery (SMA) and the duodenum and caecum lie a good distance apart but loosely connected by mesentery. Bands of tissue called Ladd's bands fix them in position. When malrotation occurs, the distal duodenum and the caecum do not completely rotate and end up in close proximity to each other. This results in a short pedicle of mesentery that can rotate easily on itself causing obstruction of the bowel and compression of the SMA. This can lead to ischaemia and eventually necrosis of the bowel. Ladd's bands are also in the incorrect position and can cross over causing various degrees of duodenal obstruction when twisting of the pedicle occurs.

A patient with malrotation will look unwell and often presents with features of shock. Bilious vomiting is a characteristic feature of malrotation with volvulus.

Differentials to consider include:
- pyloric stenosis – projectile vomiting, dehydrated but hungry infant
- necrotising enterocolitis, which is more common in the premature neonate
- gastro-oesphageal reflux – vomiting is not bilious
- gastroenteritis

In this case the patient has bilious vomiting, is lethargic and mottled, suggesting she is extremely unwell and likely shocked. Answers A and B are suitable for mild and moderate dehydration/

gastroenteritis and is inappropriate for the management of this patient. Answer C is appropriate management for a patient with pyloric stenosis not malrotation of the bowel with volvulus.[82–84]

35. Answer: A

Pyloric stenosis is caused by progressive thickening of the pyloric muscles and results in gastric outlet narrowing and obstruction. It most commonly presents in the first 6 weeks of life (between 3–6 weeks of age) and is uncommon after the age of 6 months.

There is a higher incidence in:
- males (4 : 1)
- first borns
- infants with a family history of pyloric stenosis
- Caucasians

An infant with pyloric stenosis typically has non-bilious projectile vomiting after feeds; occasionally it can be bloodstained. The infant is usually hungry afterwards; however, if the condition goes unrecognised the patient may become dehydrated and either lose weight or fail to gain weight. There is a decrease in bowel movements. About 1% of infants with pyloric stenosis have jaundice secondary to unconjugated (indirect) hyperbilirubinaemia.

On examination the infant may be dehydrated and gastric peristalsis may be visible, particularly following a feed and on palpation a small mass may be felt in epigastrum to the right of midline about the size of an olive or cherry.

A blood gas may demonstrate hypokalaemic and hypochloraemic metabolic alkalosis. Abdominal ultrasound is the investigation of choice.

The infant should be fluid resuscitated and electrolyte imbalances corrected, kept nil by mouth and a nasogastric tube inserted if vomiting persists. The patient should be referred to the a paediatric surgeon for further management.[85–87]

36. Answer: B

Congenital adrenal hyperplasia is a broad term for deficiencies in enzymes responsible for the production of aldosterone and or cortisol. Each is an autosomal recessive disorder.

The most common form of congenital adrenal hyperplasia is 21–hydroxylase deficiency, accounting for approximately 95% of cases. Features of this enzyme deficiency are related to androgen excess.

It presents as masculinisation of females and can range from ambiguous genitalia and pseudohermaphroditism in infants to oligomenorrhoea, hirsutism and acne in postpubertal females. In males it can cause enlarged external genitalia and precocious puberty.

Severe enzyme deficiency can be life threatening, presenting with vomiting, severe dehydration, electrolyte abnormalities (severe hyponatraemia from salt wasting and hyperkalaemia), metabolic acidosis and occasionally hypoglycaemia. The patient should be resuscitated and treated with hydrocortisone. The patient will require treatment with long-term steroids.

All of the other conditions mentioned are a cause of abdominal pain.[88–92]

37. Answer: C

Intussusception is the most common cause of intestinal obstruction in young children. The peak incidence occurs between 5–12 months of age and more common in males (3:2). In children under the age of 5 years the aetology is either idiopathic or secondary to an enlarged Peyer's patch from viral infection. Over the age of 5 an underlying lesion is more likely to be the cause. These include Meckel's diverticulum, haematoma from Henoch-Schönlein purpura or other bleeding diathesis, coeliac disease, cystic fibrosis, postsurgical scars, lymphoma and polyps.

The majority of intussusceptions are ileocolic (80–90%); however, colocolic and, rarely, ileoileal intussusceptions can occur.

Intermittent crampy abdominal pain, a palpable abdominal mass and bloody 'currant-jelly' stool is the classical triad of signs and symptoms. At presentation all three are only found in 30% of patients while 75% of patients have two of these present. The child will experience episodes of severe abdominal pain that occurs at frequent intervals. It may last for 10–15 minutes each time, during which the child will be inconsolable and draw the legs up towards the chest. **Lethargy is a significant finding and is out of proportion to the degree of dehydration. As the intussusception progresses the child will become more lethargic and weak.**

Stools will be normal in the first few hours but will decrease as time progresses. Bloody stool may be passed within the first 12 hours but sometimes will not be present for 1–2 days. This, 'currant-jelly' stool (which is sloughed mucosa, mucus and blood) is present in up to 50% of cases.

Vomiting can occur and is initially non-bilious; however, as the duration of obstruction continues the vomiting may become bilious.

On examination the child is well in between episodes early in the illness. As the illness progresses the child may become very lethargic with a low-grade temperature. On palpation of the abdomen a sausage-shaped mass can be felt in the right upper quadrant in 30% of cases. The long axis of the mass lies cephalocaudal. This mass represents the intussusceptus. Along with the mass there is a hollowness in the right lower quadrant because the caecum has moved from its usual position. The abdomen may be distended and on auscultation there is a paucity of bowel sounds in the right lower quadrant (Dance's sign). If perforation has occurred, peritonitis may be evident.

X-ray is not sensitive or specific and is frequently normal. Absence of bowel gas in the right upper and lower quadrants may be detected or there can be the impression of a soft tissue mass in the right upper quadrant. Abdominal ultrasound is highly sensitive (98–100%) and specific (88%) – a doughnut sign is visualised and is due to several concentric rings of bowel loops. Contrast enemas can be both diagnostic and therapeutic; however, air enema is preferred because it is associated with few complications and lower radiation exposure.[83,93–95]

38. Answer: A

Meckel's diverticulum is the most common congenital anomaly of the gastrointestinal tract and occurs in 2% of the population. Symptoms can occur at any age but the majority present around the age of 2 years. It is a 2–6 cm out-pouching of the ileum approximately 2ft proximal to the ileocaecal valve. Only 2% of affected patients become symptomatic (rule of twos for Meckel's diverticulum). It is a remnant of the embryonic omphalomesenteric duct, contains bowel wall and 60% contain ectopic mucosa, most commonly gastric mucosa.

Symptoms include crampy abdominal pain and painless rectal bleeding, from bright red to melena, depending on the site and how rapid the bleeding is. The highly acidic gastric tissue in the diverticulum causes ulcerations that bleed. If the diverticulum contains pancreatic tissue, ulcerations and bleeding can result from the alkaline envirnment. Bleeding is usually self-limiting because the splanchnic vessels constrict secondary to hypovolaemia. Anaemia is usually transient. Meckel's diverticulum can be a lead point for intussusception and can present as bowel obstruction or perforation.

Diagnosis is aided by a technetium 99m scan. If bleeding is present the sensitivity and specificity of this test is 75–85% and 95% respectfully.

Abdominal X-rays are of no assistance and barium studies rarely fill the diverticulum. Treatment of Meckel's diverticulum involves fluid resuscitation and blood transfusion if required. If the patient is unstable then urgent surgical intervention is necessary. Definitive treatment is surgical excision.

Gastrointestinal bleeding is a less common presentation of haemophilia. It is more likely to manifest with easy bruising or haemarthrosis in mobile patients. Intracranial haemorrhage in neonates or following head trauma is another common presentation. The coagulation profile will be abnormal with a prolonged APTT (activated partial thromboplastin time) and a normal PT (prothrombin time).

An anal fissure is a tear or laceration of the anal margin, at the anal mucocutaneous junction. It is diagnosed on examination. In the paediatric population it is more frequent in age <1 year. It presents with bright red rectal bleeding, pain on defaecation and constipation.[83,92,96,97]

39. Answer: C

A button battery that is stuck in the oesophagus requires urgent removal. An impaction time of as little as 2–2.5 hours can result in significant injury. Batteries >15 mm size are more likely to become lodged and cause significant complications. Complications from button batteries arise from one of four mechanisms:
- release of toxic substances (e.g. lithium or mercury)
- local electrical burn
- caustic injury from electrolyte leakage
- pressure necrosis

If the object has made it to the stomach it will likely continue to pass without complication. Most will pass within 48–72 hours. If they are still in the stomach after this time then removal is usually recommended.

Button batteries look very similar to coins on X-ray; however, the battery displays a double ring shadow on X-ray (junction between the anode and the cathode). As the oesophagus is wider in the coronal plane, coins that get lodged are seen to lie in the coronal plane on plain AP X-ray. They tend to lie in the sagittal plane if they are in the trachea.

Complications of oesophogeal foreign bodies are similar to that of any object that has prolonged impaction time and include:
- oesophageal necrosis
- oesophageal perforation
- oesophageal stricture
- mediastinitis
- tracheal compression leading to airway compromise
- tracheaoesophageal fistula
- aortic-oesophageal fistula
- extra-luminal migration
- pneumothorax
- pneumomediastinum
- aspiration pneumonia
- mucosal abrasion
- vocal cord paralysis

Foreign body ingestion occurs most frequently in the paediatric age group. It is most commonly seen between the ages of 3 months to 12 years old. It is important to note from a history-taking and risk assessment point of view that the grasping and pinching motion are seen at 6 and 7 months respectively. Other populations that may have foreign bodies in the alimentary canal include, intellectually impaired patients, psychiatric patients, prisoners, body packers, patients who have a history of oesophageal anatomical abnormalities such as strictures, webs or malignancy or those with a muscular dysfunction such as achalasia or scleroderma.

There are three main areas where the oesophagus narrows, it is around one of these regions that objects are most likely to become lodged. They are:
- The region of the cricopharyngeal muscle
- At the level where the left main stem bronchus and aortic arch cross over the oesophagous
- At the lower oesophageal sphincter

Children are more likely to have a foreign body stuck at the level of the cricopharyngeus muscle, adults more frequently at the level of the lower oesophageal sphincter.[98–101]

40. Answer: D

Cervical lymphadenitis is the most likely diagnosis in this child. However, other differentials that should be considered include:

- Reactive lymph node secondary to a viral infection – this is unlikely in this case as reactive lymph nodes are generally small, firm and non-tender.
- Kawasaki disease is an important differential to consider; however, she does not fulfill the criteria for this.
- Other differentials to consider include: infectious mononucleosis, mycobacterium avium complex, mycobacterium tuberculosis, cat scratch disease, toxoplasmosis, HIV, lymphoma, leukaemia, juvenile chronic arthritis or systemic lupus erythematosus (SLE).

This patient should have analgesia and blood work to assist with exclusion of some of the abovementioned differential diagnosis including serology or cultures to identify any causative organism and sensitivities. The patient will require IV antibiotics and admission. An ultrasound scan would be helpful to confirm the presence of an abscess prior to incision and drainage.

The estimated weight of a 6-year-old is 20 kg. Therefore, the correct dose of paracetamol is (15 mg/kg) 300 mg. PR paracetamol comes in 125 mg, 250 mg and 500 mg. So answer A is incorrect.

The correct dose for ibuprofen is 200 mg (10 mg/kg) not 400 mg (20 mg/kg), so answer C is incorrect.

Blood work helps to exclude differential diagnoses such as lymphoma and leukaemia. Cultures should be taken to identify any bacterial causative organism and its antibitotic sensitivities.

Unilateral cervical lymphadenitis is usually due to either *Staphylococcus aureus* or *Streptococcus pyogenes*. Anaerobes should be considered if there is evidence of periodontal disease. In this case the IV antibiotics of choice include flucloxacillin (12.5–50 mg/kg) 6-hourly or cephazolin (10–50 mg/kg) 6-hourly, not 12-hourly. So, answer D is correct and answer B is incorrect. Clindamycin or lincomycin can be used if there is a penicillin allergy. Metronidazole should be added if anaerobic infection is suspected.[102–104]

References

1. Wolfe JM, Henneman PL. Acute appendicitis. In: Marx JA, Hockberger RS, Walls RM, et al, editors. Rosen's emergency medicine, 7th ed. Philadelphia: Mosby Elsevier; 2010. p. 1193–9.
2. DeKoning EP. Acute appendicitis. In: Tintinalli JE, Stapczynski JS, Ma OJ, et al, editors. Emergency medicine: a comprehensive study guide. 7th ed. New York: McGraw-Hill; 2011. p. 574–8.
3. Dunn R, Maclean A. Abdominal pain. In: Dunn R, et al, editors. The emergency medicine manual. 5th ed. Adeleide: Venom Publishing; 2010. p. 555–83.
4. Alvarado A. A practical score for the early diagnosis of acute appendicitis. Ann Emerg Med 1986;15:557–64.
5. Peterson MA. Disorders of the large intestine. In: Marx JA, Hockberger RM, Walls RM, et al, editors. Rosen's emergency medicine, 7th ed. Philadelphia: Mosby Elsevier; 2010. p. 1228–42.
6. Ban KM, Easter JS. Selected urological problems. In: Marx JA, Hockberger RS, Walls RM, et al, editors. Rosen's emergency medicine, 7th ed. Philadelphia: Mosby Elsevier; 2010. p. 1297–325.
7. Jacobs DO. Diverticulitis. N Engl J Med 2007;357(20): 2057–66.
8. Thompson DG. Irritable bowel syndrome and functional bowel disorders. In: Warrell DA, editor. Oxford textbook of medicine. 5th ed. Oxford; 2010. Online. Available: http://online.statref.com/Notes/ResolveNote.aspx?NoteID=44223&grpalias=QH.
9. Nishijima D. Mesenteric ischaemia in emergency medicine. Medscape reference: drugs, diseases and procedures. Online. Available: http://emedicine.medscape.com/article/756735-overview.
10. Dang CV. Acute mesenteric ischaemia. Medscape reference: drugs, diseases and procedures. Online. Available: http://emedicine.medscape.com/article/189146-overview.
11. Lowell MJ. Esophagus, stomach and duodenum. In: Marx JA, Hockberger RS, Walls RM, et al, editors. Rosen's emergency medicine, 7th ed. Philadelphia: Mosby Elsevier; 2010. p. 1137–52.
12. Bertleff MJ, Lange JF. Perforated peptic ulcer disease: a review of history and treatment. Digestive Surgery 2010;27(3):161–9.
13. Morris A, Midwinter MJ. Perforated peptic ulcer. In: Brooks A, Cotton BA, Tai N, et al, editors. Emergency surgery. Oxford: BMJ Books; 2010. p. 43–5.
14. Torrey SP, Henneman PL. Disorders of the small intestine. In: Marx JA, Hockberger RS, Walls RM, et al, editors. Rosen's emergency medicine, 7th ed. Philadelphia: Mosby Elsevier; 2010. p. 1184–92.
15. Velez LI, Benitez FL, Villanueva SE. Acute abdominal pain in special populations. Part II: elderly,

immunocompromised and pregnant patients. Emergency Medicine Report 2004;25(23). Online. Available: www. EMRonline.com.

16. Vicario SJ, Price TG. Bowel obstruction and volvulus. In: Tintinalli JE, Stapczynski JS, Ma OJ, eds. Emergency medicine a comprehensive study guide. 7th ed. New York: McGraw-Hill; 2011. p. 581–3

17. Hodin RA. Cecal volvulus. UpToDate. Last updated March 5 2009.Online. Available: www.uptodate.com.

18. Hodin RA. Sigmoid volvulus. UpToDate. Last updated May 20 2010. Online. Available: www.uptodate.com.

19. Dent B, Kendall RJ, Boyle AA, et al. Emergency ultrasound of the abdominal aorta by UK emergency physicians: A prospective cohort study. Emerg Med J 2007;24(8):547–9.

20. Australasian College of Emergency Medicine (ACEM). Policy document P21 – Policy on the use of bedside ultrasound by emergency physicians. Online. Available: www.acem.org.au.

21. Wu S, Blackstock U, Lewiss R, et al. Focus on: bedside ultrasound of the abdominal aortal. ACEP clinical and practice management. ACEP news May 2010. Online. Available: http://www.acep.org/content.aspx?id=48651.

22. Kuhn M, Bonnin RLLL, Davey MJ, et al. Ultrasound for abdominalaorticaneurysm. Annals of emergency medicine 2000;36(3):219–23.

23. Streat SJ. Abdominal surgical catastrophes. In: Bersten AD, Soni N, editors. Oh's intensive care manual. 6th ed. Philadelphia: Elsevier; 2003. p. 499–505.

24. Prince LA, Johnson GA. Aortic dissection and aneurysms. In: Tintinalli JE, Stapczynski JS, Ma OJ, eds. Emergency medicine: a comprehensive study guide, 7th ed. NewYork: McGraw-Hill; 2011. p. 453–8

25. Bessen HA. Abdominal aortic aneurysm. In: Marx JA, Hockberger RS, Walls RM, et al, editors. Rosen's emergency medicine, 7th ed. Philadelphia: Mosby Elsevier; 2010. p. 1093–102.

26. Irizarry L, Yarde I. Proctitis in emergency medicine. Updated Jun 2 2010. Medscape reference: drugs, diseases and procedures. Online. Available: http://emedicine. medscape.com/article/775952-overview#a0199.

27. Wolfe JM, Henneman PL. Acute appendicitis. In: Marx JA, Hockberger RS, Walls RM, et al, editors. Rosen's emergency medicine, 7th ed. Philadelphia: Mosby Elsevier; 2010. p. 1193–9.

28. Gilo NB, Amini D, Landy HJ. Appendicitis and cholecystitis in pregnancy. Clinical Obstetrics and Gynecology 2009;52(4):586–96.

29. Walby A, Bryant M. Bilary tract disease. In: Cameron P, Jelinek G, Kelly A, et al, editors. Textbook of adult emergency medicine. 3rd ed. Edinburgh: Churchill Livingstone; 2009. p. 344–7.

30. Crawford JM, Liu C. Liver and biliary tract. In: Kumar V, Abbas AK, Fausto N, et al, editors. Robbins and Cotran pathologic basis of disease. 8th ed. Philadelphia: Saunders Elsevier; 2009. p. 833–90.

31. Heuman DM. Cholelithiasis. Available online at Medscape reference: drugs, diseases and procedures. Online. Available: http://emedicine.medscape.com/article/175667-overview.

32. Guss DA, Oyama LC. Disorders of the liver and bilary tract. In: Marx JA, Hockberger RS, Walls RM, et al, editors. Rosen's emergency medicine. 7th ed. Philadelphia: Mosby Elsevier; 2010. p. 1153–71.

33. Hemphill RR, Santen SA. Disorders of the pancreas. In: Marx JA, Hockberger RS, Walls RM, et al, editors. Rosen's emergency medicine, 7th ed. Philadelphia: Mosby Elsevier; 2010. p. 1172–83.

34. Atilla R, Oktay C. Pancreatitis and cholecystitis. In: Tintinalli JE, Stapczynski JS, Ma OJ, eds. Emergency medicine: a comprehensive study guide. 7th ed. New York: McGraw-Hill; 2011. p. 558–66.

35. Zhou MT, Chen CS, Chen BC, et al. Acute lung injury and ARDS in acute pancreatitis: mechanisms and potential intervention. World Journal of Gastroenterology 2010;16(17):2094–9.

36. Ranson JH, Rifkind KM, Roses DF, et al. Prognostic signs and the role of operative management in acute pancreatitis. Surgery, Gynecology & Obstetrics 1974; 139(1): 69–81.

37. Corfield AP, Cooper MJ, Williamson RC, et al. Prediction of severity in acute pancreatitis: prospective comparison of three prognostic indices. Lancet 1985;2(8452):403–7.

38. Heng K, Seow E. Pancreatitis. In: Cameron P, Jelinek G, Kelly A, et al, editors. Textbook of adult emergency medicine. 3rd ed. Edinburgh: Churchill Livingstone; 2009. p. 347–50.

39. Wheatley MA, Heilpern KL. Jaundice. In: Marx JA, Hockberger RS, Walls RM, et al, editors. Rosen's emergency medicine, 7th ed. Philadelphia: Mosby Elsevier; 2010. p. 187–92.

40. Dunn R, Maclean A. General gastroenterology. In: Dunn R, et al, editors. The emergency medicine manual, 5th ed. Adelaide: Venom Publishing; 2010. Chapter 36. p. 547–54.

41. Dunn R, Maclean A. Liver disease. In: Dunn R, Dilley SJ, Brookes JG, et al, editors. The emergency medicine manual. 5th ed. Adelaide: Venom Publishing; 2010. p. 588–97.

42. Mirizzi PL. Syndrome del conductohepatico. J Int de Chir 1948;8:731–77.

43. Byars D. Hernia in adults. In: Tintinalli JE, Stapczynski JS, Ma OJ, eds. Emergency medicine: a comprehensive study guide. 7th ed. NewYork: McGraw-Hill; 2011. p. 583–7.

44. Fitch MT, Manthey DE. Abdominal hernia reduction. In: Roberts JR, Hedges JR, editors. Clinical procedures in emergency medicine, 5th ed. Philadelphia: Saunders Elsevier; 2009. p. 790–7.

45. Malangoni MA, Rosen MJ. Townsend: Sabiston textbook of surgery, 18th ed. Saunders Elsevier; 2007. p. 1156–7.

46. Dunn R, Maclean A. Urinary disorders. In: Dunn R, et al, editors. The emergency medicine manual. 5th ed. Adelaide: Venom Publishing; 2010. p. 895–904.

47. Lenartova M, Tak T. Iatrogenic pseudoaneurysm of femoral artery: case report and literature review. Clinical Medicine and Research 2003;1(3):243–7.

48. Newton EJ, Arora S. Peripheral vascular injury. In: Marx JA, Hockberger RS, Walls RM, et al, editors. Rosen's

emergency medicine. 7th ed. Philadelphia: Mosby Elsevier; 2010. p. 456–66.

49. Dilley S, Dunn R. Vascular emergencies. In: Dunn R, Dilley SJ, Brookes JG, et al, editors. The emergency medicine manual. 5th ed. Adelaide: Venom Publishing; 2010. p. 479–86.

50. Khan AZ, Strauss D, Mason RC. Boerhaave's syndrome: diagnosis and surgical management. Surgeon 2010; 5(1):39–44.

51. Dunn R, Dilley S, Brookes J. Non ACS Chest pain. In: Dunn R, Dilley SJ, Brookes JG, et al, editors. The emergency medicine manual. 5th ed. Adelaide: Venom Publishing; 2010. p. 387–406.

52. Mendelson MH. Esophageal emergencies, gastroesophageal reflux disease and swallowed foreign bodies. In: Tintinalli JE, Stapczynski JS, Ma OJ, eds. Emergency medicine: a comprehensive study guide. 7th ed. New York: McGraw-Hill; 2011. p. 548–54.

53. Chopra A, Carr D. Occlusive arterial disease. In: Tintinalli JE, Stapczynski JS, Ma OJ, eds. Emergency medicine: a comprehensive study guide. 7th ed. New York: McGraw-Hill; 2011. p. 458–63.

54. Aufderheide TP. Peripheral arteriovascular disease. In: Marx JA, Hockberger RS, Walls RM, et al, editors. Rosen's emergency medicine, 7th ed. Philadelphia: Mosby Elsevier; 2010. p. 1103–23.

55. Eddey DP, Westcott MJ. The needle and the damage done: Intraarterial temazepam. Emergency Medicine 2000;12:248–52.

56. Righini M, Angellillo-Scherrer A, Gueddi S, et al. Management of severe ischemia of the hand following intraarterial injection. Thrombosis and Haemostasis 2005;94(1):219–21.

57. Sen S, Chini EN, Brown MJ. Complications after unintentional inra-arterial injection of drugs: risks outcomes and management strategies. Mayo Clinic Proceedings 2005;80(6):783–95.

58. Mullan MJ, Magowan H, Weir C. Femoral artery necrosis due to parenteral intravascular drug misuse: a case report and literature review. Ulster Medical Journal 2008; 77(3):203–4.

59. Ankel F. Aortic dissection. In: Marx JA, Hockberger RS, Walls RM, et al, editors. Rosen's emergency medicine. 7th ed. Philadelphia: Mosby Elsevier; 2010. p. 1088–92.

60. Prince LA, Johnson GA. Aortic dissection and aneurysms. In: Tintinalli JE, Kelen GD, Stapczynski JS, et al, editors. Emergency medicine: a comprehensive study guide. 7th ed. New York: McGraw-Hill; 2010. p. 450–3.

61. Coates WC. Disorders of the anorectum. In: Marx JA, Hockberger RS, Walls RM, et al, editors. Rosen's emergency medicine, 7th ed. Philadelphia: Mosby Elsevier; 2010. p. 1243–56.

62. Coates WC. Anorectal procedures. In: Roberts JR, Hedges JR, editors. Clinical procedures in emergency medicine. 5th ed. Philadelphia: Saunders Elsevier; 2009. p. 798–809.

63. Burges BE, Bouzoukis JK. Anorectal disorders. In: Tintinalli JE, Stapczynski JS, Ma OJ, editors. Emergency medicine: a comprehensive study guide. 7th ed. New York: McGraw-Hill; 2011. p. 587–601.

64. Dixon MJ, Khan LR. Treatment of breast infection. BMJ 2011;342:484–9.

65. Charles R. Skin and soft-tissue infections. In: Cameron P, Jelinek G, Kelly A, et al, editors. Textbook of adult emergency medicine. 3rd ed. Edinburgh: Churchill Livingstone; 2009. p. 426–33.

66. Therapeutic Guidelines Limited. Mastitis. In: eTG complete. Online: Available: https://online-tg-org-au. cknservices.dotsec.com/ip/.

67. Spencer JP. Management of mastitis in breastfeeding women. American Gamily Physician 2008;78(6):727–31.

68. Lammers RL. Principles of wound management. In: Roberts JR, Hedges JR, editors. Clinical procedures in emergency medicine, 5th ed. Philadelphia: Saunders Elsevier; 2009. p. 563–91.

69. Simon B, Hern HG Jr. Wound management principles. In: Marx JA, Hockberger RS, Walls RM, et al, editors. Rosen's emergency medicine. 7th ed. Philadelphia: Mosby Elsevier; 2010. p. 698–714.

70. Moscati RM, Mayrose J, Reardon RF, et al. Irrigation of simple lacerations with tap water or sterile saline in the emergency department did not differ for wound infections. Evid Based Med 2007;12(6):181.

71. Ahmad M, Martin B. Closure of pretibial lacerations. J Accid Emerg Med 2000;17(4):287–8.

72. Beldon P. Classifying and managing pretibial lacerations in older people. British Journal of Nursing 2008;17(11):S4–S16.

73. Hooker EA. Complications of general surgical procedures. In: Tintinalli JE, Kelen GD, Stapczynski JS, et al, editors. Emergency medicine: a comprehensive study guide. 6th ed. New York: McGraw-Hill; 2004. p. 577–82.

74. Kulaylat MN, Dayton MT. Surgical complications. In: Townsend CM Jr, Beauchamp RD, Ever BM, et al. Sabiston textbook of surgery. 18th ed. Philadelphia: Saunders Elsevier; 2008. p. 328–70.

75. Eke N, Jebbin NJ. Abdominal wound dehiscence: a review. Int Surg 2006;91(5):276–87.

76. Van Gijn J, Kerr RS, Rinkel GJE. Subarachnoid haemorrhage. Lancet 2007;369:306–18.

77. Al-Shahi R, White PM, Davenport RJ, et al. Subarachnoid haemorrhage. BMJ 2006;33:235–40.

78. Dilley S, Dunn R. Headache. In: Dunn R, Dilley SJ, Brookes JG, editors. The emergency medicine manual. 5th ed. Adelaide: Venom Publishing; 2010. p. 646–71.

79. Kwiatkowski T, Alagappan K. Headache. In: Marx JA, Hockberger RS, Walls RM, et al, editors. Rosen's emergency medicine, 7th ed. Philadelphia: Mosby Elsevier; 2010. p. 1356–66.

80. Gomersall C, Calcroft R. Subarachnoid haemorrhage. ICU web. Online. Available: http://www.aic.cuhk.edu.hk/web8/subarachnoid_haemorrhage.htm.

81. Mattu A, Brady W. ECGs for the emergency physician. London: BMJ Books, Blackwell Publishing; 2003. p. 140, 151.

82. Holland AJA. Bilious vomiting. In: Cameron P, Jelinek G, Kelly A, et al, editors. Textbook of paediatric emergency medicine. Edinburgh: Churchill Livingstone, Elsevier; 2006. p. 180–2.

83. Hostetler MA. Gastrointestinal disorders. In: Marx JA, Hockberger RS, Walls RM, et al, editors. Rosen's emergency medicine, 7th ed. Philadelphia: Mosby Elsevier; 2010. p. 2168–87.

84. Kennedy M, Liacouras CA. Malrotation. In: Kliegman RM, Stanton BF, Schor NF, editors. Nelson textbook of pediatrics. 19th ed, Philadelphia: Saunders Elsevier; 2011. p. 1280–1.

85. The Royal Children's Hospital Melbourne. Pyloric stenosis. Clinical practice guidelines, Available online at: http://www.rch.org.au/clinicalguide/cpg.cfm?doc_id=8402.

86. Ong KL. Hypertrophic pyloric stenosis. In: Cameron P, Jelinek G, Kelly A, et al, editors. Textbook of paediatric emergency medicine. 1st ed. Edinburgh: Churchill Livingstone; 2006. p. 178–9.

87. Collins JL. Pyloric stenosis. In: Schwartz MW, Bell LW, Bingham PM, et al, editors. The 5-minute pediatric consult. 5th ed. Philadelphia: Lippincott Williams & Wilkins; 2008. p. 169–76.

88. White PC. Congenital adrenal hyperplasia and related disorders. In: Kliegman RM, Stanton BF, Schor NF, editors. Nelson textbook of pediatrics. 19th ed. Philadelphia: Saunders Elsevier; 2011. p. 1930–7.

89. The Royal Children's Hospital. Neonatal handbook. Congential adrenal hyperplasia. Online. Available: http://www.rch.org.au/nets/handbook/index.cfm?doc_id=818.

90. Merke DP, Bornstein SR, Avila NA, et al. Future directions in the study and management of congenital adrenal hyperplasia due to 21–hydroxylase deficiency. Ann Intern Med 2002;136(4):320–34.

91. Wilson TA. Congenital adrenal hyperplasia. Updated Sep 17 2010. Medscape reference: drugs, diseases and procedures. Online. Available: http://emedicine.medscape.com/article/919218-overview.

92. Hort J. Abdominal pain. In: Cameron P, Jelinek G, Kelly A, et al, editors. Textbook of paediatric emergency medicine. 1st ed. Edinburgh: Churchill Livingstone; 2006. p. 165–70.

93. Grossman AB. Intussusception. In: Schwartz MW, Bell LM, Bingham PM, et al, editors. The 5-minute pediatric consult. 5th ed. Philadelphia: Lippincott Williams & Wilkins; 2008. p. 132–5.

94. Kennedy M, Liacouras CA. Intussusception. In: Kliegman RM, Stanton BF, Schor NF, editors. Nelson textbook of pediatrics. 19th ed. Philadelphia: Saunders Elsevier; 2011. p. 1287–9.

95. Ong KL. Intussusception. In: Cameron P, Jelinek G, Kelly A, et al, editors. Textbook of paediatric emergency medicine. 1st ed. Edinburgh: Churchill Livingstone; 2006. p. 207–8.

96. Kennedy M, Liacouras CA. Meckel diverticulum and other remnants of the omphalomesenteric duct. In: Kliegman RM, Stanton BF, Schor NF, editors. Nelson textbook of pediatrics. 19th ed. Philadelphia: Saunders Elsevier; 2011. p. 1281–2.

97. Reilly F. Disorders of coagulation. In: Cameron P, Jelinek G, Kelly A, et al, editors. Textbook of paediatric emergency medicine. Edinburgh: Churchill Livingstone, Elsevier; 2006. p. 311–3.

98. Munter DW. Esophageal foreign bodies. In: Marx JA, Hockberger RS, Walls RM, et al, editors. Rosen's emergency medicine, 7th ed. Philadelphia: Mosby Elsevier; 2010. p. 715–33.

99. Jarugula R, Dorofaeff T. Oesophageal button battery injuries: think again. Emergency Medicine Australasia 2011;23:220–3.

100. Rempe B, Iskyan K, Aloi M. An evidence-based review of pediatric retained foreign bodies. Pediatric Emergency Medicine Practice 2009;6(12):1–19. Online. Available: www.ebmedicine.net.

101. Kumar S. Management of foreign bodies in the ear, nose and throat. Emergency Medicine Australasia 2004;16:17–20.

102. The Royal Children's Hospital Melbourne. Cervical lymphadenopathy. Clinical practice guidelines. Online. Available: http://www.rch.org.au/clinicalguide/cpg.cfm?doc_id=5166.

103. Therapeutic Guidelines Limited. Cellulitis and cervical lymphadenitis. In: eTG complete Online. Available: https://online-tg-org-au.cknservices.dotsec.com/ip/.

104. Shann F. Drug doses. 15th ed. Melbourne: Collective P/L; 2010.

1. Answer: C

Testing for an afferent pupillary defect is important and should be performed consistently during examination of the eye in the ED. This is done with the *swinging flashlight test*. **A positive RAPD means there is a disturbance in the anterior afferent visual pathway that carries the light perception to the central nervous system.** The disturbance or the defect may be present at any level along the pathway including:

- a dense or diffuse anterior chamber or vitreous due to haemorrhage
- retinal pathology such as macular oedema, central or branch retinal artery or vein occlusion, and retinal detachment
- optic neuritis, optic nerve or chiasm compression and optic tract lesions.

RAPD should not be assumed to be caused by a cataract because light can still penetrate the lens with a cataract.

It should be noted that prior to testing with the swinging flashlight test, the pupillary defect will not be apparent and the pupil of the affected side will be the same size as on the normal side. This is because of the normal consensual light response on the affected side. During the swinging flashlight test when the light is moved from the normal side to the affected side, that pupil will dilate paradoxically, therefore producing a positive RAPD.[1,2]

2. Answer: A

Bacterial conjunctivitis is more common in children than viral conjunctivitis although viral syndromes affect children more commonly. Streptococcus *pneumoniae*, *Staphylococcus aureus* and non-typeable *Haemophilus influenzae* are the most commonly implicated bacterial organisms, whereas adenovirus conjunctivitis is the most common viral conjunctivitis. The patient may present with a conjunctivitis as part of a viral syndrome or it can be an isolated conjunctivitis. **The presence of preauricular lymphadenopathy in viral conjunctivitis is one of the differentiating factors**. A more severe and highly contagious form of adenovirus infection is epidemic keratoconjunctivitis. Slit lamp examination shows a diffuse superficial keratitis without corneal ulceration.

Slit lamp examination is important during examination of the eye; the cornea should be viewed with fluoresceine staining to exclude dendritic ulcers caused by herpes simplex virus (HSV). However, this is a challenging but necessary examination in children. **The diagnoses of conjunctivitis is clinical and appropriate swabs for bacterial culture and viral studies should only be performed in severe cases and in patients who have not responded adequately to initial therapy.**[2]

3. Answer: D

These infections are more common in children, and differentiating between the two conditions is important because disposition, treatment and sequelae associated with the conditions vary. Orbital (postseptal) and periorbital (preseptal) cellulitis are described in relation to the location of the soft tissue infection relative to the orbital septum. The orbital septum extends from the periosteum into the upper and lower eyelids. Subsequently, it is unlikely that the infection will spread from one area to the other. However, because of the location of the paranasal sinuses in relation to the orbit, infection in these sinuses can cause osteitis, periosteal abscesses, orbital abscesses and orbital cellulitis. This infection does not spread to the periorbital area. In this area, the main source of infection is the skin secondary to conditions such as insect bites, impetigo, hordeolum, chalazion and dacrocystitis.

Differentiating the two entities clinically may be difficult at times; however, a contrast CT scan is able to differentiate between the two conditions. MRI is useful as well.

- Both conditions present with periorbital erythema, swelling and tenderness.
- Extraocular eye movements are normal and painless in periorbital cellulitis but greatly limited and painful in orbital cellulitis.
- **Limited swelling of the upper eyelid is the differentiating factor in orbital cellulitis. As the orbital septum is attached to the superior**

orbital rim it prevents the swelling to spread to the upper eyebrow and eyelid in orbital cellulitis.

- In orbital cellulitis reduced visual acuity, proptosis, chemosis and abnormal pupillary response are present, whereas in periorbital cellulitis the visual acuity and pupillary reactions are preserved.
- Patients are more likely to be systemically unwell in orbital cellulitis.

The organisms involved in orbital cellulitis are respiratory pathogens (*S. pneumoniae, H. influenzae* in non-immunised patients), *S. aureus* and anaerobes spreading from the paranasal sinuses. Periorbital cellulitis is more commonly caused by gram-positive skin flora, mainly *S. aureus, Staphylococcus epidermidis and Streptococcal* species. It can also be associated with upper respiratory tract infections, especially paranasal sinusitis. Other causes include insect bites, periorbital trauma and spread from eyelid infections (e.g. hordeolum and chalazion).[2]

4. Answer: C

Anterior uveitis is the inflammation of the anterior portion of the uveal tract, especially the iris and ciliary body, hence it is referred to as iridocyclitis. The causes could be due to systemic diseases (e.g. juvenile rheumatoid arthritis or ulcerative colitis), infections, malignancies and trauma. This is not a true ocular emergency but needs discussion and follow-up with ophthalmology. The symptoms and examination findings include:

- sudden onset unilateral, red and painful eye – symptoms may affect both eyes and the pain is due to ciliary muscle spasm and irritation of ciliary nerves
- the pain becoming worse with ocular movements and accommodation
- photophobia both direct and consensual (photophobia is due to ciliary muscle spasm; consensual photophobia is not seen in other causes of photophobia and is highly suggestive of anterior uveitis)
- tearing without purulent discharge
- **perilimbal or circumcorneal injection (this is a differentiating feature from conjunctivitis)**
- a constricted, often irregular and sluggish pupil
- reduced visual acuity if the condition is severe

- flare and cells in the anterior chamber on slit lamp examination (flare is due to proteinaceous transudate from the ciliary vessels; cells are the white cells in the anterior chamber)
- in severe inflammation, white cells settling in the anterior chamber to produce a hypopyon (this may visible to the naked eye)
- keratitic precipitates on the corneal endothelium – these are deposits of white cells seen with slit lamp and this is a hallmark of anterior uveitis.[2,3]

5. Answer: B

In AACG there is a blockage of the outflow of aqueous humor caused by a number of mechanisms. There is usually an abrupt onset of symptoms and severe pain and redness in the eye are prominent features. Headache on the affected side, as well as nausea and vomiting, tearing, blurred vision and 'halos around lights', are usually present. **The eye examination shows:**

- a mid-dilated non-reactive pupil
- corneal oedema (steamy or hazy cornea)
- keratitic precipitates
- shallow anterior chamber with cells and flare
- optic nerve cupping on funduscopy.

The eyeball may feel hard on palpation.

If the pupil reacts, the AACG diagnosis is generally incorrect and an alternative diagnosis should be considered.

Normal intraocular pressure (IOP) is 10–20 mmHg. In AACG the IOP is above this level and in severe disease may be as high as 60–80 mmHg. If the IOP is >30 mmHg emergent treatment is indicated to prevent visual loss.

In contrast, primary open angle glaucoma (POAG) is a chronic and progressive condition causing visual field loss. In POAG, pain is not a prominent feature. There is a familial predilection in first-degree relatives. In one in three, IOP may be normal (normal tension glaucoma) and examination of the optic disc is much more important in the diagnosis. These patients generally present to their general practitioners rather than to the ED.[2-4]

6. Answer: B

In optic neuritis, the eye pain is associated with unilateral visual loss or reduction in over 90% of patients. It is an acute demyelinating condition affecting the optic nerve and a large proportion of these patients develop multiple sclerosis subsequently. Other causes include viral infections (measles, mumps, varicella, Epstein-Barr virus), bacterial infections (tuberculosis, cryptococcus, syphilis), sarcoidosis, post vaccination in children, and idiopathic. **Eye pain with eye movements and afferent pupillary defect are typical features in optic neuritis.** Visual acuity in the affected eye could be greatly decreased and colour vision may be affected. Although the classic visual field defect is central scotoma, other focal visual field defects may be found. Features of optic disc swelling (anterior optic neuritis) can be seen in approximately one-third of patients. In others the optic disc will appear normal (retrobulbar neuritis). The symptoms will improve over the course of several weeks even without treatment. Use of intravenous steroids is controversial.

All the other conditions cause painless acute visual loss.[2,5,6]

7. Answer: C

In both CRAO and CRVO the unilateral visual loss is abrupt and painless. In CRVO the visual loss may be present when the patient wakes up in the morning. It can range from blurred vision to complete loss. Optic disc and diffuse retinal haemorrhages can occur in CRVO (in contrast to optic neuritis) due to venous stasis oedema, hence the term 'blood and thunder' has been given to this appearance on funduscopy. Unlike in papilloedema, the unaffected fundus appears normal. Immediate referral to the ophthalmology is indicated in CRAO but there is no specific treatment available for CRVO, and a patient with CRVO can be seen by ophthalmology within a few days. The medical therapies, which are described, can be used in the ED for CRAO; however, they have not been shown to be highly beneficial.[2,5,6]

8. Answer: A

CRAO is an ischaemic stroke involving the retina due to emboli. Carotid artery atherosclerosis is present in approximately half of the patients and a cardiac source for embolism is found in up to 20% of cases. The features include:
- sudden severe painless loss of vision in one eye developing over seconds
- marked afferent pupillary defect

- funduscopy showing a pale grey-white and oedematous retina with a cherry red spot.

CRAO is devastating to the vision. Less than one-third of patients recover to gain a reasonable visual acuity in spite of adequate emergent care. The recommended emergent care is aimed at increasing perfusion to the retina and dislodging the clot. They include:
- digital globe massage to dislodge the clot
- reduce IOP to improve retinal perfusion using topical timolol, acetazolamide IV or PO, IV mannitol
- retinal artery vasodilation: increase $PaCO_2$ by rebreathing into a paper bag for 10 minutes
- anterior chamber paracentesis done by ophthalmology to lower the IOP.

None of the above therapies have been investigated for their effectiveness.

Both intravenous and intraarterial thrombolysis have been attempted but currently there is not enough evidence to support or refute their use.[2,5,6]

9. Answer: C

Horner's syndrome causes constriction of the pupil on the affected side. It occurs due to damage to the sympathetic fibres on the affected side. Therefore, the affected pupil is constricted and the normal pupil on the opposite side may appear 'dilated'.

Isolated third nerve palsy presenting as an isolated dilated pupil (without ophthalmoplegia and/or ptosis) is a rare event. More common emergency presentations of an isolated dilated pupil include:
- local exposure to a drug that can cause mydriasis
- trauma to the iris or ciliary ganglion
- glaucoma
- Adie's tonic pupil.

Up to 20% of the population have minor (up to 1 mm difference) anisocoria.

Adie's tonic pupillary defect affects more females (70%) than males. In this condition parasympathetic fibres are affected after leaving the ciliary ganglion. Adie's tonic pupil presents as an isolated dilated pupil on the affected side. It affects the accommodation of the eye, therefore the patient may have blurred near vision with relative sparing of the distant vision. Half of these patients usually will recover within 2 years.

Orbital blunt trauma can cause mydriasis. Acute angle closure glaucoma is another cause of isolated dilated pupil.

Isolated third nerve palsy can be classified based on 'the rule of the pupil':

- A pupil involving third nerve palsy is usually secondary to a compressive lesion such as posterior communicating artery aneurysm or basilar tip aneurysm. The anatomic basis for the pupillary involvement is the arrangement of the pupillary constrictor fibres superficially on the dorsomedial aspect of the nerve when it runs through the subarachnoid space. These fibres can be compressed with an expanding aneurysm.
- A pupil-sparing third nerve palsy is secondary to intrinsic pathological changes in the nerve in patients with vascular risk factors such as hypertension and diabetes.

Patients presenting with pupil-involving isolated third nerve palsy should be urgently imaged using MRI/MRA or CT angiography to diagnose posterior circulation aneurysms and also to identify an alternative cause when an aneurysmal cause is not present. Posterior circulation aneurysms have the highest rates of rupture (2.5–50% per year) among all the cerebral aneurysms.[7]

10. Answer: A

Unless strong acids and alkali are involved, initial examination and visual acuity are often normal. Even with strong acids rapid complete loss of epithelium of the cornea may occur and this may mask the severity of the injury. **Most ophthalmologists advise continuous irrigation with normal saline until normal pH is restored. The pH should be checked every 30 minutes while irrigation is done and 30 minutes after the restoration of normal pH.** This is especially important in an alkali injury because further injury may occur from alkali deposited in the inaccessible areas of the conjunctival sac. (There is a wide variation in normal tear pH – approximately 6.5–7.5 – and this is partly dependent on the measurement technique as well. Except very minor exposures all patients should be referred for ophthalmology follow-up as initial assessment may not reveal the full extent of the injury.[2,8]

11. Answer: B

Orbital blowout fracture occurs with blunt injury to the orbit (e.g. punch over the orbit). **It is an isolated orbital floor or medial wall fracture. The fracture line does not extend to the orbital rim.** The fracture opens up the ethmoid sinus through the medial wall, or maxillary sinus through the orbital floor. If it involves the ethmoid sinus, subcutaneous emphysema can develop, especially with sneezing. Herniation of the contents of the lower part of the orbital cavity may occur through the fracture into the maxillary sinus. The inferior rectus muscle can get physically entrapped in the fracture. Therefore the following clinical and radiological features may be present:

- enophthalmos
- **restricted upward gaze and diplopia due to inferior rectus muscle entrapment (this is the most common feature)**
- difference in the horizontal level of the pupils
- paraesthesia, anaesthesia or hyperaesthesia in the infraorbital region due to damage to the infraorbital nerve.

This fracture cannot be diagnosed using the facial X-ray views. However, the 'tear drop' sign on a facial X-ray, produced by the herniation of orbital contents into the maxillary sinus, and opacification or an air-fluid level in the maxillary sinus may indicate the presence of this fracture. CT is highly sensitive in the diagnosis.[2,9]

12. Answer: C

Urgent surgical repair is not indicated for an isolated orbital blowout fracture, even when it is associated with entrapment. **Generally surgical repair is done electively when the swelling has subsided, usually around 7–10 days. However, during this time oral antibiotic treatment is indicated because of the communication with the paranasal sinuses.**

Significant injury to the eye can occur with orbital blowout fractures. A complete examination of the eye with full dilatation of the pupil should be done at least as an outpatient to exclude: retinal tears and detachments; lens dislocations and subluxations; hyphaema; and corneal injuries. Retrobulbar haematoma and compressive orbital emphysema are important complications and should be recognised. These patients may represent with worsening severe eye pain, reduced vision and proptosis.[2,9]

13. Answer: C

Patients might occasionally present to the ED with signs of retrobulbar haemorrhage following a severe degree of blunt trauma to the orbit. Patients on anticoagulant therapy may present in a similar way. The orbit can be an uncompromising soft tissue space due to the presence of the globe in the front and the firm attachments of the eyelids to the orbital rim with the lateral and medial canthal ligaments. As a result, undisplaced orbital fractures are more commonly associated with complications due to retrobulbar haemorrhage than displaced fractures. Increased intraocular pressure due to the tamponading effect in the orbital space can cause severe compression of the central retinal artery and optic nerve, and its blood supply. The resultant ischaemia of the retina and optic nerve causes visual loss. The symptoms are:

- worsening pain
- proptosis
- relative afferent pupillary defect
- restricted eye movements
- increased IOP in patients with extensive periorbital ecchymoses suggesting severe blunt trauma.

If there is no visual loss and there are signs of increased IOP, medical therapy (topical beta-blockers and IV mannitol or acetazolamide) can be attempted to reduce the increased intraocular pressure until the patient is tranferred for definitive ophthalmology care. In the presence of visual loss in a suspected case of retrobulbar haematoma lateral canthotomy is indicated emergently without waiting for a confirmatory CT scan. Although most clinicians do not have prior experience in this procedure in the correct setting, this is the only procedure that can save permanent loss of sight due to ischaemia. However, there should be enough clinical evidence to suggest there is vision-compromising retrobulbar haematoma. Complications and scarring caused by lateral canthotomy are limited and acceptable in such a patient.[9,10]

14. Answer: C

The usual source for posterior nasal bleeds is the sphenopalatine artery, which is supplied by the external carotid arterial system. It cannot be seen through examining the anterior nose and requires nasoendoscopy or surgical exposure to visualise.

Posterior epistaxis is usually diagnosed late in the ED, often after failed attempts at controlling bleeding with direct pressure, use of vasoconstrictors and anterior nasal packing with balloon devices or nasal tampons. In addition, significant bleeding in the elderly and continuous bleeding into the nasopaharynx may indicate posterior bleeding. **Thrombogenic foams and gels such as Gelfoam, Surgicel and Floseal can be convenient and effective in controlling anterior bleeds but cannot be used to control posterior bleeds.**

Transpalatal injection of a local anaesthetic or vasoconstrictor solution (2 mL of 1% lignocaine with adrenaline) close to the sphenopalatine artery may help to reduce significant posterior bleeds. This can be achieved by inserting a 25-gauge needle, bent at 2.5 cm from the tip, through the descending palatine foramen just medial to the upper second molar tooth.

Posterior nasal packs stop posterior epistaxis in approximately 70% of patients. Endoscopic surgical ligation or embolisation is used to control bleeding once posterior nasal packing has failed. The success rate for surgical ligation of the sphenopalatine artery is reported to be equal or better than the success rate for embolisation, which is 80–90%.[11,12]

15. Answer: D

About 90% of epistaxis are anterior and 10% are posterior. Posterior epistaxis is most common in elderly patients. Although hypertension is often seen in patients who present to the ED with epistaxis, the association has not been proven. Often anxiety may elevate BP and therefore rapid reduction of elevated blood pressure (BP) is not recommended. Gentle reduction in BP may be helpful to allow clot formation.

Once clots have been removed, and local vasoconstrictor solution and direct pressure have been applied, chemical cautery with silver nitrate sticks can be attempted to control a visualised anterior bleed. **Chemical cautery should only be attempted on one side of the nasal septum and even a second attempt on the same side should be avoided for 4–6 weeks to prevent perforation of the septum.**

When the balloon of a Foley catheter is used to control a posterior bleed, the balloon should be inflated with saline up to a volume of about 15 mL (not 30 mL) to prevent pressure necrosis. The balloon device should then be retracted anteriorly to provide the tamponade in the choanae and sphenopalatine foramen areas.[11,12]

16. Answer: C

A peritonsillar abscess is formed secondary to an infection in the mucous salivary glands located superior to the tonsils in the soft palate. With infection, peritonsillar cellulitis develops in the soft palate and later pus formation occurs with the development of an abscess. It is a polymicrobial infection; however, group A streptococcus is found most frequently. Oral anaerobes are involved as well. The diagnosis of peritonsillar abscess is mainly clinical. If the diagnosis is in doubt, then needle aspiration of pus, contrast CT scan, MRI or transcutaneous ultrasound can confirm the diagnosis. Transcutaneous ultrasound has a moderate sensitivity and specificity.

Regarding treatment, both needle aspiration and incision and drainage of a peritonsillar abscess produce similar outcomes if performed by trained medical staff.[13,14]

17. Answer: A

The diagnosis of adult epiglottitis (supraglottitis) in a patient presenting to the ED is based mainly on the history and examination findings. This can be supported by lateral soft tissue X-ray of the neck, which is generally easy and safe to obtain. The features on history and clinical examination that supports the diagnosis include:

- an unwell patient with a 24–48-hour history (some patients give a little longer history)
- severe sore throat
- fever and tachycardia
- odynophagia and dysphagia
- hoarse voice
- tenderness caused by gentle palpation of the larynx
- soft, low-pitched inspiratory stridor (most patients present with mild stridor).

These subtle features are often not recognised early. Such patients may rapidly develop features of severe airway obstruction including drooling, severe stridor, and the inability to lie flat. Bilateral submandibular swelling is a feature of Ludwig's angina and does not usually occur with adult epiglottitis.

Lateral soft tissue X-rays of the neck are easy to obtain in the ED, with the most frequently searched for sign being the enlarged thumb-shaped epiglottis. Examination of the larynx with nasoendoscopy can confirm the diagnosis, but this should be done with extreme caution by otolaryngologists as this may worsen the airway obstruction.[13,14]

18. Answer: B

Most nasal foreign bodies in children can be removed using appropriate techniques without sedation. If sedation is required, the preservation of gag-and-cough reflexes is important to prevent aspiration of the foreign body should it slip backwards. Positive pressure techniques are recommended as first-line methods for foreign bodies that are not highly impacted because they are easy to apply to a non-sedated child. The positive pressure techniques include:

- repeated nose blowing (at least 15 times) by the child with adult coaching
- 'big kiss' (a parent or carer blows air mouth to mouth with closure of the unaffected nostril) and 'modified big kiss' (the same method but with the use of a drinking straw or an endotracheal tube to blow air into the child's mouth) techniques
- Bag–valve–mask insufflation
- the Beamsley blaster technique (blowing wall oxygen or air into the unaffected nostril to dislodge the foreign body from the other side).

There is a risk of barotrauma with all these methods but that happens very infrequently with the big kiss or modified big kiss methods. The Beamsley blaster technique has a higher risk of causing barotrauma.

The success rates when using balloon catheters is high for anteriorly located foreign bodies. The most widely available is the 5–8 F Foley catheter.[15,16]

19. Answer: A

Nasal fractures in children are significant injuries because potential greenstick fractures, injuries to the cartilage, growth plate injuries and septal injuries may occur. Because of relatively small nasal passages in children the fracture may cause an obstruction that may be worsened later by formation of synechiae. The risk for poor cosmetic outcome is higher for children with nasal fractures than for adults with similar fractures. **Plain X-ray does not help in the** management of nasal fractures and CT scans are unnecessary.

Nasal fractures are often reduced under general anaesthetic and that should be done very early (within 4 days) to overcome the faster fracture healing time in children.[12]

20. Answer: D

Malignant otitis externa is a less common but potentially life-threatening form of otitis externa. The presence of diabetes and immunosuppression increases the risk of having this condition. **In >90% of patients the causative organism is *Pseudomonas aeruginosa* and therefore if suspected initiation of parenteral IV antibiotic therapy to cover this organism is essential.** In addition, surgical debridement may be necessary. The clinical features that are helpful in the diagnosis are:

- worsening otitis externa despite appropriate treatment for more than 2–3 weeks
- otalgia out of proportion with that expected from the condition
- evidence of spread of infection: infection in the soft tissue and cartilage of the pinna (also called necrotising otitis externa), infection in the parotid and mastoid, infection in the skull base (also called skull base osteomyelitis)
- trismus due to masseter and temporomandibular joint (TMJ) involvement.

In severe disease the following may occur:

- cranial nerves VII, IX, X and XI involvement
- lateral and sigmoid sinus thrombosis
- meningitis.[17]

21. Answer: D

All lacerations involving the pinna of the ear should be repaired after achieving meticulous control of bleeding to prevent haematoma formation. **All cartilage should be covered with skin to prevent infection of the cartilage. If the cartilage cannot be covered due to avulsed skin the patient should be referred to plastic surgery.** Significant debridement at the skin edges should not be done as there will not be adequate skin to cover the cartilage. In a through-and-through laceration, approximation of the skin ideally with the perichondrium is sufficient to promote healing of the cartilage and to preserve the shape of the pinna. There is a risk of haematoma formation a

few days after the repair and if unattended this may lead to deformity of the pinna ('cauliflower ear') due to the pressure it exerts on the cartilage. With a haematoma, the patient may present with swelling and increasing pain. Sutures should be removed to completely drain the haematoma and haemostasis should be achieved; the laceration should be repaired again. **To prevent haematoma formation, after repair of any significant laceration it should be covered with a properly placed pressure dressing.** The skin sutures should be removed in 4–5 days.[18]

22. Answer: C

Ludwig's angina is a rapidly spreading infection in the submandibular space, and has a dental origin in majority of cases. It is potentially lethal as the rapidly increasing infection in the submandibular space causes elevation of the floor of the mouth and swelling of the tongue, tightly closing the airway. It may cause trismus, further compromising the ability to secure the airway. It is essential to evaluate the airway immediately upon the patient's presentation to the ED. Some of the features of a compromised or threatened airway are:

- tachypnoea
- inability to talk in full sentences
- trismus
- patient distress
- confusion
- stridor
- elevated floor of the mouth
- swollen tongue.

Appropriate other specialties such as anaesthetics and ENT should be involved early in the assessment and management of the airway as this is a potentially hazardous exercise.

Any actual or potential airway compromise requires consideration for urgent tracheal intubation. In one Australian study, eight out of 29 patients that presented with Ludwig's angina required emergent securing of the airway. Fibre optic nasal intubation was attempted in all of these patients and seven were successful. The patient with failed fibre optic nasal intubation required emergent tracheostomy.[20] **Attempts at securing the airway should be done in the operating theatre.**

The anterior wall of the submandibular space is formed by the taut investing layer of deep cervical fascia running between the under surface of the mandible and hyoid bone. The mucous membrane of the floor of the mouth forms the roof of the submandibular space. The non-distensible nature of the investing layer of deep cervical fascia causes any swelling in the submandibular space to upwardly displace the floor of the mouth and tongue, compromising the airway.

Any attempt at obtaining a CT without thoroughly evaluating and securing the airway where necessary is a potential hazard to the patient and is not useful in immediate patient management. However, in patients with Ludwig's angina who present with hard induration of the suprahyoid region, it may be difficult to clinically differentiate an abscess with liquefaction requiring drainage from induration and phlegmon. In these patients, once the airway is evaluated and/or secured, CT may be helpful.[19]

23. Answer: C

An avulsed tooth is a true dental emergency if it involves a permanent tooth. In the majority of cases presenting to the ED, the tooth will not survive for a number of reasons. One of the main reasons is the lack of placement of the tooth in a suitable transport media and the amount of time that has elapsed outside the oral cavity. The survival once implanted depends on the viability of the periodontal ligament of the tooth. Periodontal ligament necrosis occurs within 60 minutes if the tooth is not placed in a suitable transport medium. **By placing the tooth in milk, it can preserve the periodontal ligament for 4–8 hours. Saliva is another acceptable transport medium.** (Commercially available transport media will preserve it for 12–24 hours). In a prehospital situation where a suitable transport media is not generally available, the most appropriate step is to rinse the root, taking care to touch the crown of the tooth only, and replacing it into the socket. However, primary teeth and fractured teeth should not be replaced. Also, when there is associated significant maxillary/mandibular trauma (e.g. alveolar ridge fracture) the avulsed tooth should not be replaced. An avulsed primary tooth if replaced can fuse to the alveolar line and can distort the eruption of permanent tooth. Additionally, it also increases the risk of infection. Between ages 6–12, children have both primary and permanent teeth, therefore identification of the type of the avulsed tooth is important.[20,21]

24. Answer: D

Patients often present to the ED with persistent bleeding from the socket post extraction. Displacement of the clot from the socket is generally the cause. The tooth socket should be carefully examined and any remaining clot in the socket kept intact. The clotted blood from the surrounding area should be removed with suction and the area can be rinsed with saline. Direct pressure should be applied to the bleeding socket with firmly clenched teeth using gauze carefully packed into the socket; this direct pressure should be maintained for at least 15 minutes. Gauze impregnated with a vasoconstrictor such as adrenaline may help to stop the bleeding. Local infiltration of lignocaine with adrenaline into the surrounding gingiva can cause vasoconstriction as well as anaesthesia for adequate application of direct pressure. If the bleeding doesn't stop, suitable coagulation sponge material can be applied to the tooth socket and these can be kept in place by loosely suturing the gingiva over the socket. Tight suturing of the gingiva is not recommended because it may cause necrosis of the gingiva.[20,21]

25. Answer: C

In adults most repairs of tongue lacerations can be done in the ED under local anaesthetic infiltration or with a lingual block. To achieve both anaesthesia and haemostasis, lignocaine with adrenaline can be used on the tongue. In a large gaping laceration, the edges should be approximated when the laceration is repaired. If such a laceration is not repaired properly, the subsequent epithelial coverage over the gap may result in a grooved or a bifid tongue. Other lacerations that need primary repair are flap-shaped lacerations and lacerations at the edge of the tongue, as well as deep lacerations that involve the muscle and that are causing significant bleeding. When the laceration penetrates both the mucosa and the muscle, it can be sutured using non-absorbable stitches that penetrate both into the mucosa and the muscle. Absorbable sutures can be used as well.[20]

References

1. Duong D, Leo M, Mitchell E. Neuro-ophthalmology. Emerg Med Clin N Am 2008;26:137–80.
2. Walker R, Adhikari S. Eye emergencies. In: Tintinalli JE, Stapczynski JS, Ma OJ, editors. Emergency medicine: a comprehensive study guide. 7th ed. New York: McGraw-Hill; 2011. p. 1517–49.
3. Prentiss K, Dorfman D. Pediatric ophthalmology in the emergency department. Emerg Med Clin N Am 2008;26:181–98.
4. Mahmood A, Narang A. Diagnosis and management of the acute red eye. Emerg Med Clin N Am 2008;26:35–55.
5. Zegers R, Reinders E, de Smet M. Primary open angle glaucoma: the importance of family history and role of intraocular pressure. MJA 2008;188(5):312–3.
6. Vortmann M, Schneider J. Acute monocular visual loss. Emerg Med Clin N Am 2008;26:73–96.
7. Sharma R, Brunette D. Ophthalmology. In: Marx JA, Hockberger RS, Walls RM, editors. Rosen's emergency medicine: concepts and clinical practice. 7th ed. Philadelphia: Elsevier; 2009:859–76.
8. Woodruff M, Edlow J. Evaluation of third nerve palsy in emergency department. J Emerg Med 2008;35(3):239–46.
9. Spector J, Fernandez W. Chemical, thermal, biological ocular exposure. Emerg Med Clin N Am 2008;26:125–36.
10. Bord S, Linden J. Trauma to the glove and orbit. Emerg Med Clin N Am 2008;26:97–123.
11. Knoop K, Dennis W, Hedges J. Ophthalmologic procedures. In: Roberts JR, Hedges JR, editors. Clinical procedures in emergency medicine, 5th ed. Philadelphia: Elsevier; 2009. p. 1141–77.
12. Schlosser R. Epistaxis. N Engl J Med 2009;360:784–9.
13. Summers S, Bey T. Epistaxis, nasal fractures and rhinosinusitis. In: Tintinalli JE, Stapczynski JS, Ma OJ, editors. Emergency medicine: a comprehensive study guide. 7th ed. New York: McGraw-Hill; 2011. p. 1564–72.
14. Shah R, Cannon T, Shores C. Infections and disorders of the neck and upper airway. In: Tintinalli JE, Stapczynski JS, Ma OJ, editors. Emergency medicine: a comprehensive study guide. 7th ed. New York: McGraw-Hill; 2011. p. 1583–91.
15. Dunn R. Other ENT disorders. In: Dunn R, Dilley S. Brookes J. The emergency medicine manual. 5th ed. Adelaide: Venom Publishing; 2010. p. 1083–95.
16. Brown J, Osincup D. Pediatric procedures: nasal and otic foreign bodies. In: Tintinalli JE, Stapczynski JS, Ma OJ, editors. Emergency medicine: a comprehensive study guide. 7th ed. New York: McGraw-Hill; 2011. p. 976–82.
17. Kiger J, Brenkert T, Losek J. Nasal foreign body removal in children. Paed Emerg Care 2008;24:785–9.
18. Siverberg M, Lucchesi M. Common disorders of the external, middle and inner ear. In: Tintinalli JE, Stapczynski JS, Ma OJ, editors. Emergency medicine: a comprehensive study guide. 7th ed. New York: McGraw-Hill; 2011. p. 1550–7.
19. Coates W. Laceration to the face and scalp. In: Tintinalli JE, Stapczynski JS, Ma OJ, editors. Emergency medicine: a comprehensive study guide. 7th ed. New York: McGraw-Hill; 2011. p. 315–22.
20. Greenberg SLL, Huang J, Chang RSK, et al. Surgical management of Ludwig's angina. ANZ J Surg 2007;77:540–3.
21. Benko K. Emergency dental procedures. In: Roberts JR, Hedges JR, editors. Clinical procedures in emergency medicine, 5th ed. Philadelphia: Elsevier; 2009. p. 1217–34
22. Beaudreau R. Oral and dental emergencies. In: Tintinalli JE, Stapczynski JS, Ma OJ, editors. Emergency medicine: a comprehensive study guide. 7th ed. New York: McGraw-Hill; 2011. p. 1572–83.

CHAPTER 17
UROLOGICAL EMERGENCIES

ANSWERS

1. Answer: C

Although no minimal bladder volume has been determined, a poorly defined bladder is a contraindication for SPC insertion. **A history of lower abdominal surgery, intraperitoneal surgery or irradiation places the patient at increased risk of complications such as bowel injury because they may result in adherence of the bowel to the bladder wall.** Other contraindications to percutaneous insertion include coagulopathies and pelvic trauma; however, SPC via open surgical insertion is commonly used in pelvic trauma with urethral injury.

Complications of insertion include:
- bowel perforation
- intraperitoneal extravasation (without a prior history of surgery)
- extraperitoneal extravasation
- infection of space of Retzius
- obstruction of the catheter by blood, mucus or kinking
- haematuria
- infection (intraabdominal, urinary tract, cellulitis)
- haematoma formation
- vesical calculi formation
- bypassing around the catheter site

Indications for SPC insertion include:
- when urethral catheter insertion is indicated but unsuccessful
- when urethral catheterisation is contraindicated in cases such as
  - urethral trauma/disruption
  - urethral stricture
  - urinary retention secondary to phimosis
  - gynaecological malignancies
  - when it is associated with a urethral false passage

SPC is associated with less bacteriuria as the periurethral area has a higher concentration of bacteria and the length of the tract is shorter in SPC.[1–3]

2. Answer: A

Around 90% of stones are radio-opaque.

Magnetic resonance imaging (MRI) can show anatomical changes of ureteric obstruction such as hydronephrosis, hydroureter and nephromegaly but is typically unable to identify ureteric stones.

Up to 20% of patients who have proven renal calculi do not have haematuria. There is no relationship between the degree of obstruction and the presence or absence of haematuria.

UTIs from urea-splitting organisms such as *Proteus*, *Klebsiella*, *Pseudomonas* and *Staphylococcus* can cause the formation of struvite stones. A urinary pH of >7.5 is suggestive of a urine infection from these urea-splitting organisms.

A pH <5 is associated with uric acid calculi.[4–6]

3. Answer: B

Patient B has heavy gross haematuria and is at high risk of developing clot retention and bladder outlet obstruction. He requires a three-way catheter insertion and bladder irrigation with normal saline. If this is unsuccessful he requires further investigation such as a cystoscopy. The patient should not be discharged with a triple lumen catheter in situ.

Criteria for admission for patients with renal colic include:
- one functioning kidney with a moderate to high degree of obstruction
- infected obstructed kidney
- ongoing pain (>4 hours) despite adequate analgesia
- a proximal stone >5 mm in size

The larger and more proximal the stone the less likely it is to pass.

A 4mm stone has 90% chance of passing, whereas an 8 mm stone has only 5% chance. Therefore, the patient A may be discharged with outpatient follow up.

Young otherwise healthy patients with uncomplicated acute pyelonephritis (patient C) can be managed as outpatients. Admission would need to be considered if the patient were immunocompromised,

pregnant or had a chronic illness and a unilateral functioning kidney.

Torsion of the testicular appendage is a common cause of testicular pain in the 7–14-year age group. Onset is gradual, usually over 1–2 days, and the patient is still able to ambulate as normal. On examination the affected testicle itself is non-tender, of normal size and normal lie, and there is maximal tenderness at the upper pole of the testis. A small, hard, tender nodule may be palpated at the upper pole of the affected testicle. In 10% of patients the torted appendage may appear as a blue dot. Management of this is reassurance and supportive therapy such as scrotal support, ice and simple analgesia. It usually settles down in 7–10 days.[4,5,7–9]

4. Answer: D

In a patient with acute pyelonephritis, mild infections (with low-grade fever, no nausea or vomiting) can be treated with amoxicillin 875 mg + clavulanate 125 mg 12-hourly for 10 days or with cephalexin 500 mg 6-hourly for 10 days or trimethoprim 300 mg once daily for 10 days.

For severe infection, IV gentamicin 4–6 mg/kg (7 mg/kg if severe sepsis) plus 2 g IV ampicillin or amoxicillin 6-hourly is required. Gentamicin 4–6 mg/kg as the sole antibiotic agent is suitable if the patient has a penicillin allergy. Ceftriaxzone 1 g IV daily or cefotaxime 1 g IV 8-hourly can be used if gentamicin is contraindicated.

The total duration of antibiotic therapy is usually for 10–14 days.[10]

5. Answer: C

Priapism is a prolonged painful erection and can be divided into two types:
- low-flow
- high-flow

Low-flow is the far more frequent type and a true urological emergency, requiring rapid (within 4 hours) treatment to prevent long-term complications such as impotence. It is due to reduced venous outflow.

High-flow priapism is due to increased arterial blood flow. It is frequently painless and often doesn't cause ischaemia and once resolved erectile function is usually retained. It is a very rare presentation caused typically by an arteriovenous fistula following trauma.

The erection in high flow priapism is usually not fully rigid.

Some causes of low-flow priapism include:
- intracavernosal injection of drugs such as papaverine, phentolamine and prostaglandin E1 (PGE1)
- sickle cell disease (23% of adult cases and 63% of paediatric priapism presentations)
- other haemaglobinopathies
- chronic granulocytic leukaemia (priapism occurs in ~50% of patients with this disease)
- hypercoaguable states
- Fabry's disease
- immunosuppressive disorders
- other medications such as SSRIs, phenothiazines and antihypertenives (e.g. prazocin and hydralazine)
- recreational drugs such as cocaine, alcohol and marijuana
- trauma (direct penile and perineal trauma, traumatic needle insertion with intracavernosal injections)[11–13]

6. Answer: B

If a patient has low-flow priapism due to thombosis from sickle cell crisis then he should be treated with intravenous rehydration, oxygen, analgesia, and exchange transfusion as required.

Otherwise, low-flow priapism is typically managed with aspiration of blood from the corpus cavernosum +/− injection of diluted phentolamine or adrenaline into the corpus cavernosum. If the patient is in urinary retention a urethral catheter should be inserted. A urologist should always be consulted. Treatment should be commenced rapidly, preferably within 4 hours of onset to reduce the incidence of long-term sequelae.

High-flow priapism is a very rare presentation. It is not a urological emergency and patients typically have an erection that is not fully rigid; however, the fully flaccid state is not reached either. The diagnosis can be confirmed by penile Doppler ultrasound. Angiography is typically required as arteriovenous fistula formation is the usual aetiology.[7,12,13]

7. Answer: A

About 80% of ureteral injuries are iatrogenic, mostly related to intraabdominal or pelvic surgery. The ureter

Table 17.1 GRADING OF RENAL TRAUMA

Grade	Description	Treatment
I	Contusion, microscopic or gross haematuria, urological investigations normal Subcapsular non-expanding haematoma without laceration	Observation Spontaneous resolution
II	Parenchymal laceration < 1 cm depth of renal cortex No extravasation of collecting system injury Non-expanding haematoma, confined to retroperitoneum	Observation Spontaneous resolution
III	Parenchymal laceration > 1 cm depth of renal cortex with no urinary extravasation or injury to the collecting system	Surgery Occasionally observation
IV	Laceration that extends through the renal cortex, medulla and collecting system Vascular pedical injury (main renal vein or artery injury) with haemorrhage contained	Surgery
V	Shattered kidney Devascularised kidney – avulsed renal hilum	Surgery

is well protected during its course to the bladder so ureteral trauma is rare accounting for ~1% of genitourinary injuries. **Injury to the ureter is more likely to be due to penetrating trauma (usually from gunshot injuries) than blunt trauma because a significant amount of force is required to injure the ureter.**

The majority of cases of urogenital injury including ureteral injury secondary to blunt trauma have other major organ involvement, about one-third of which can be life threatening. Ureteral injury from blunt trauma occurs as a result of rapid deceleration. Significant deceleration forces can cause avulsion of the ureter from its fixed points, namely the pelvoureteric junction (PUJ) or less frequently the vesicoureteric junction (VUJ).

Approximately 10% of trauma involves the genitourinary tract, with the kidney being the most frequently injured genitourinary organ.

In blunt trauma, the degree of haematuria and the severity of the genitourinary injury do not always correlate well.

Gross haematuria can occur as a result of minor injury such as minor renal contusions; microscopic haematuria (or no haematuria) may be seen in renovascular injuries. However, gross haematuria should be investigated. **Microscopic haematuria (≤50 RBCs/hpf) doesn't require further investigation unless there are signs of unexplained haemodynamic compromise.**[14–19]

Table 17.1 shows the American Association for the Surgery of Trauma (AAST) grading system for renal

trauma. A grade III renal injury does not have urinary extravasation or rupture of the collecting system.

8. Answer: D

In the majority of cases, testicular torsion is a result of medial rotation of the spermatic cord. Lateral rotation occurs in about one-third of cases.

The peak age of occurrence is puberty – ages 12–16 years old. A typical presentation of an abrupt onset of pain in the affected testis, groin or lower abdomen may follow sudden movement, sporting or strenuous physical activity or trauma. Many occur spontaneously, particularly at night (where contraction of the cremasteric muscle results in torsion). Other common associated features of presentation include nausea, vomiting and fever (20% of cases).

The examination findings include swelling and tenderness in the affected side of the scrotum; the affected testis may have a high riding position and a horizontal lie. The cremasteric reflex may be absent. The more delayed the presentation the more swollen the scrotum is likely to be and assessment of the cremasteric reflex and scrotal structures may be difficult.

Scrotal ultrasound scan (USS) is useful when investigating testicular torsion. It also can identify testicular and extratesticular masses, epididymitis, orchitis, hydroceles, hernias and varicoceles. **However, the time delay to get a USS can be detrimental to the patient because testicular torsion is a time-critical diagnosis.** The testis can usually be salvaged up to 12 hours after onset; the chances of testis survival at 24 hours is near zero. **Ideally, the patient should undergo surgery within 6 hours of symptom onset.**

Doppler USS can produce both false positives and negatives. Even the torted testis can demonstrate intra-testicular blood flow on Doppler USS, which can be misleading and lead to an incorrect diagnosis. It has only 80% sensitivity for diagnosis of testicular torsion.[7,9,12,20]

9. Answer: D

Abdominal aortic aneurysm and renal colic can cause referred pain to the scrotum.

Viral infections such as mumps can cause orchitis. Orchitis develops in approximately 20% of prepubertal boys with mumps but in almost no postpubertal males with mumps. It tends to arise several days after the onset of parotitis. Owing to the testes' relatively high threshold of resistance to infection, bacterial orchitis more commonly results from local bacterial spread from epididymis. **The most frequent bacterial pathogens are *Neisseria gonorrhoeae*, *Chlamydia trachomatis*, *Escherichia coli*, *Klebsiella*, and *Pseudomonas aeruginosa*.** These organisms tend to infect postpubertal males and men older than 50 years of age with benign prostatic hypertrophy (BPH).[5,7]

10. Answer: C

Urinary retention is the inability to void; however, the patient may pass small volumes of urine frequently. This suggests retention with overflow.

Most cases of urinary retention presenting to the ED are due to an obstructive cause such as:
- BPH
- prostate cancer
- urethral stricture secondary to
  - urethral instrumentation such as cystoscopy or previous indwelling catheter
  - infection
  - radiation therapy
- occasionally phimosis or paraphimosis.

Approximately 25% of men who present to the ED with acute urinary retention have a diagnosis of prostate cancer (the majority of which was not diagnosed previously).

Medications that can cause urinary retention include anticholinergics (e.g. antispasmodics and tricyclic antidepressants), analgesics such as opiates and NSAIDs, antihistamines and beta-blockers.

Most presentations of acute urinary retention can be classified as 'low-pressure' retention. In these cases the detrusor pressure remains low while storing urine and there is no associated hydronephrosis or renal impairment. Less commonly, men present with 'high-pressure' urinary retention that is associated with high bladder storage pressures, bilateral hydronephrosis and renal impairment. Men with high-pressure retention frequently describe nocturnal enuresis.[4,5]

11. Answer: A

The presence of nitrites on a urinary dipstick is highly specific (up to 95% specific) and not sensitive (45%) for diagnosis of a UTI. It detects bacteria that convert urinary nitrates to nitrites such as *E. coli*. Other bacteria such as *Enterococcus*, *Pseudomonas* and *Acinetobacter* are not detected by the nitrite test.

The accurate diagnosis of a UTI in a paediatric patient is important because a child with a UTI requires further investigations to exclude urinary tract abnormalities. A UTI can also lead to renal scarring that may cause significant morbidity later in life such as hypertension and renal impairment.

Many studies have lead to the conclusion that the bag urine sample is not suitable for detecting a UTI in a child. However, it may have some use in a child who is at a low to moderate risk for a UTI. If the bag specimen dipstick (+/– microscopy) is negative, then a UTI can be ruled out in such children. If it is positive then either a midstream clean catch or suprapubic aspiration or in-out catheter specimen should be taken. The bag specimen is also acceptable to use if only a chemical evaluation is required (glucose, ketones etc.).

Even when stored as per the manufacturer's instructions a urine dipstick can lose its accuracy. There are many reasons why the test can be inaccurate and leaving the top off the container is one example. Many of the 10 tests on the stick are subject to interference by a variety of conditions or medications the patient is taking. Some of the examples are:
- protein: false negative can occur with dilute urine or low urinary pH; false positive can occur if urinary pH >7 and use of chlorhexadine

- nitrites: false negative if high specific gravity (SG), low pH, specimen standing a long time prior to testing; false positive if the testing stick is exposed to air, with pyridium
- ketones: false positive with levodopa, valproate, N-acetyl cysteine, high-protein diet, high SG of urine.[4,21]

12. Answer: B

As little as 1 mL of blood in 1L of urine can cause gross haematuria. **Both microscopic and gross haematuria are caused by similar disorders. The amount of blood in the urine does not always correlate to the severity or seriousness of the condition.**

Causes of haematuria include:
- **prostate**: BPH, prostatitis
- **renal tract**: infection, calculi, iatrogenic, trauma, tumour
- **bladder**: urothelial carcinoma, vascular malformations, radiation cystitis
- **urethra**: stricture, diverticulosis, foreign body
- **renal**: glomerular nephritis, IgA nephropathy, toxaemia of pregnancy, serum sickness, erythema multiforme, interstitial nephritis, polycystic kidneys, medullary sponge kidneys, tuberculosis
- **other**: coagulopathy, sickle cell disease, malignant hypertension, exercise-induced haematuria, AAA
- **ureteric**: stricture dilation

While urothelial carcinoma is an important cause of macroscopic haematuria (especially in smokers), the most common cause of haematuria in males is BPH.

Approximately 5–15% of patients with urolithiasis do not have haematuria.

The presence of blood clots in the urine suggests a nonglomerular cause. Large clots suggest a bladder origin for the bleeding while stringy clots are more suggestive of a ureteric bleeding source. Brown muddy urine suggests a renal source of the bleeding.[5,8,13,22]

13. Answer: C

Fournier's gangrene is a polymicrobial, necrotising infection of the perineum that predominately occurs in males. The infection originates from the skin, urethra or rectum. Risk factors include diabetes, immunosuppression, perianal trauma, perianal disease and UTIs. On examination, the patient may be extremely unwell with florid sepsis. There may be crepitus on palpation and areas of demarcated gangrene.

Fournier's gangrene can progress extremely rapidly and can extend to involve the abdomen, back, thighs, genitalia and retroperitoenum.

The treatment involves fluid resuscitation, broad-spectrum intravenous (IV) antibiotics and prompt surgical debridement. Hyperbaric oxygen therapy can be considered as an adjunct to surgical debridement. Antibiotics should target anaerobic and gram-negative aerobic bacteria. An example of an empirical therapy regime is meropenem 1g IV 8-hourly and either lincomycin 600 mg IV 8-hourly or clindamycin 600 mg IV 8-hourly. This should continue until culture results are obtained.[20,23,24]

14. Answer: A

Patient A most likely has gonococcal urethritis and should be treated with 500 mg IM ceftriazone but should also be covered with azithromycin 1g as a single oral dose to cover co-infection with *Chlamydia*.

The presence of clue cells on a wet mount preparation of vaginal discharge is diagnostic of bacterial vaginosis caused by organisms such as *Gardnerella vaginalis*. *Bacterial vaginosis* causes grey/white creamy discharge.

Trichomonas is a protozoa and is the most common non-viral sexually transmitted disease; trichomonads can be visualised on a wet mount. It causes vulvo-vaginitis, dysuria, itch and a yellow-green thin offensive-smelling discharge. It is usually asymptomatic in males and is responsible for ~ 20% of cases of non-specific (non-gonococcal) urethritis. *Trichomonas* infection can be treated with metronidazole. Painful vesiculopustular lesions on an erythematous base on the perineum, which after several days ulcerate, is classical of herpes simplex infection. A first presentation of herpes can be treated with an antiviral such as acyclovir, valacyclovir or famcyclovir.

Patient D has prostatitis. At his age this may be sexually acquired or as a complication of bacterial lower UTI. The fluoroquinolone antibiotics have excellent prostatic penetration so ciprofloxacin or norfloxacin are the drugs of choice. Bactrim or trimethoprim are alternatives for bacterial prostatitis depending on culture results. Nitrofurantoin is not a good choice for prostatitis because it does not penetrate the prostate and it is bacteriostatic not bacteriocidal.[25]

15. Answer: D

Ureteric stents are well tolerated by most patients; however, patients with stents often present to the ED with complications. The most common complications of these devices seen in the ED include:

- stent irritation: flank and suprapubic pain, dysuria, haematuria
- encrustation
- UTI
- stent migration
- stent fragmentation

Ureteric stents cause a mild degree of hydronephrosis (not obstruction). Stents cause the ureter to dilate.

The upper urinary tract may remain obstructed despite insertion of a ureteric stent. This is particularly common with cases of extrinsic compression of the ureter where despite ureteric stenting the obstruction persists or returns. Ureteric stents do not cause low-grade fever.[3,26]

References

1. Silverman M, Schneider R. Urologic procedures. In: Roberts J, Hedges J, editors. Clinical procedures in emergency medicine. 5th ed. Philadelphia: Saunders Elsevier 2009. p. 1001–41.

2. Patel N, Kaji AH. Suprapubic catheterization. In: Shah K, Mason C. Essential emergency procedures. Philadelphia: Lippincott Williams & Wilkins 2008. p. 123–7.

3. Josephson E, McCarty M. Complications of urologic procedures and devices. In: Tintinalli J, Stapczynski J, Ma O, et al, editors. Tintinalli's emergency medicine: a comprehensive study guide. 7th ed. New York: McGraw-Hill. 2011. p. 657–64.

4. Dunn R, Maclean A. Urinary disorders. In: Dunn, R, Dilley S, Brookes J, et al. The emergency medicine manual. 5th ed. Adelaide: Venom Publishing; 2010. p. 895–904.

5. Ban K, Easter J. Selected urologic problems. In: Marx J, Hockberger R, Walls R, et al, editors. Rosen's emergency medicine: concepts and clinical practice. 7th ed. Mosby Elsevier 2009. p. 1297–325.

6. Pais Jr, VM, Strandhoy JW, Assimos DG. Pathophysiology of Urinary Tract Obstruction. In: Wein AJ, Kavoussi LR, Novick AC, et al. Campbell-Walsh urology. 9th ed. Philadelphia: Saunders Elsevier. 2007. p. 1017–121.

7. Dunn R, Maclean A. Genitourinary disorders. In: Dunn, R, Dilley S, Brookes J, et al. The emergency medicine manual. 5th ed. Adelaide: Venom Publishing; 2010. p. 905–10.

8. Howes D, Bogner M. Urinary tract infections and hematuria. In: Tintinalli J, Stapczynski J, Ma O, et al, editors. Tintinalli's emergency medicine: a comprehensive study guide. 7th ed. New York: McGraw-Hill. 2011. p. 630–40.

9. Kikiros CS. Acute scrotum. In: Cameron P, Jelinek G, Kelly A, et al, editors. Textbook of paediatric emergency medicine. Edinburgh: Churchill Livingston Elsevier 2006. p. 655–6.

10. Therapeutic Guidelines Limited. Acute pyelonephritis in adults. In: eTG complete. Online. Available: www.etg.org.au.

11. Kikiros CS. Acute problems of the penis and foreskin. In: Cameron P, Jelinek G, Kelly A, et al, editors. Textbook of paediatric emergency medicine. Edinburgh: Churchill Livingston Elsevier 2006. p. 657–8.

12. Liu D. Urologic and gynaecologic problems and procedures in children. In: Tintinalli J, Stapczynski J, Ma O, et al, editors. Tintinalli's emergency medicine: a comprehensive study guide. 7th ed. New York: McGraw-Hill. 2011. p. 860–6.

13. McCollough M, Sharieff GQ. Renal and genitoruinary tract disorders. In: Marx J, Hockberger R, Walls R, et al, editors. Rosen's emergency medicine: concepts and clinical practice. 7th ed. Mosby Elsevier; 2009. p. 2200–17.

14. McManus J, Gratton M, Cuenca P. Genitourinary trauma. In: Tintinalli J, Stapczynski J, Ma O, et al, editors. Tintinalli's emergency medicine: a comprehensive study guide. 7th ed. New York: McGraw-Hill. 2011. p. 1773–8.

15. Dunn R. Abdominal and pelvic trauma. In: Dunn R, Dilley SJ, Brookes JG, et al. The emergency medicine manual. 5th ed. Adelaide: Venom Publishing; 2010. p. 1182–96.

16. McAninch JW, Santucci RA. Renal and ureteral trauma. In: Wein AJ, Kavoussi LR, Novick AC, et al. Campbell-Walsh Urology 9th ed. Philadelphia: Saunders Elsevier; 2007. p. 1169–89.

17. Husmann D. Paediatric genitourinary trauma. In: Wein AJ, Kavoussi LR, Novick AC, et al. Campbell-Walsh urology. 9th ed. Philadelphia: Saunders Elsevier; 2007. p. 3731–53.

18. Runyon MS. Genitourinary system. In: Marx J, Hockberger R, Walls R, et al, editors. Rosen's emergency medicine: concepts and clinical practice. 7th ed. Mosby Elsevier 2009. p. 435–56.

19. Abdominal and pelvic injuries. Bersten AD, Soni N. Oh's intensive care manual. 5th ed. Edinburgh: Butterworth Heinemann; 2003. p. 744.

20. Nicks B, Manthey D. Male genital problems. In: Tintinalli J, Stapczynski J, Ma O, et al, editors. Tintinalli's emergency medicine: a comprehensive study guide. 7th ed. New York: McGraw-Hill. 2011. p. 645–51.

21. Dean A, Lee D. Bedside laboratory and microbiologic procedures. In: Roberts JR, Hedges JR: Clinical procedures in emergency medicine. 5th ed. Philadelphia: Saunders Elsevier 2009. p. 1283–306.

22. Wolfson AB. Renal failure. In: Marx J, Hockberger R, Walls R, et al, editors. Rosen's emergency medicine: concepts and clinical practice. 7th ed. Mosby Elsevier 2009. p. 1257–82.

23. Charles R. Skin and soft tissue infections. In: Cameron P, Jelinek G, Kelly A, et al, editors. Textbook of adult emergency medicine. 3rd ed. Edinburgh: Churchill Livingston Elsevier; 2009. p. 426–33.

24. Therapeutic Guidelines Limited. Necrotising skin and soft tissue infections. In: eTG complete. Online. Available: www.tg.org.au.

25. Therapeutic Guidelines Limited. Genitial and sexually transmitted infections. In: eTG complete. Online. Available: www.tg.org.au.

26. Yang PK, Agarwal D, Corcoran N. A disastrous sequela of a missed ureteric stent. Med J Aus 2009;191(10):567–8.

1. Answer: B

Various definitions for hyperemesis gravidarum (HG) exist but the important features are unexplained intractable vomiting associated with weight loss of more than 5% of pre-pregnancy weight, dehydration, electrolyte imbalances (especially hyponatraemia and hypokalaemia), ketosis and vitamin deficiencies. **By far the most important serious complication of HG is Wernicke's encephalopathy as a result of thiamine (vitamin B1) deficiency**. In some cases, Wernicke's encephalopathy has been precipitated by infusion of dextrose-containing solutions before administration of thiamine. In order to prevent this serious complication, **it is recommended that when a patient's vomiting is sufficient to require intravenous hydration, thiamine (100 mg) should be administered parenterally on the assumption there is thiamine deficiency.**

Rehydration with 0.9% normal saline or Hartmann's solution is the first-line initial treatment. Although it is often thought that infusions of dextrose-containing fluids (5% dextrose, 10% dextrose or dextrose saline) are useful to provide the patient with energy, this assumption is erroneous as Wernicke's encephalopathy may be precipitated by intravenous dextrose, especially in cases of severe or prolonged vomiting. Fluid and electrolyte balance must be reassessed frequently and management adjusted according to clinical assessment and fluid balance.

In cases of ongoing vomiting, *antiemetics* should be prescribed. Combinations of several parenteral antiemetics may be needed. There is no evidence that any one antiemetic is superior to another and most antiemetics are safe in pregnancy. The TGA risk categorisation of commonly used antiemetics is metoclopromide (A), ondansteron (B1) and promethazine (C).

Vitamin supplementation is essential. **Thiamine supplements should be given routinely to all women admitted to hospital for prolonged vomiting.** Pyridoxine (vitamin B6) (10–25 mg, three times daily) has been shown to reduce nausea and vomiting of pregnancy, although the effect on vomiting is not clear. In many countries, including Australia, pyridoxine is used first line in combination with an antiemetic. *Ginger* (in doses equivalent to 1 to 2 g of powdered ginger daily) may also be helpful. If vomiting continues, it is appropriate to consult an obstetrician and consider treatment with *corticosteroids* and/or hospital admission for rehydration/nutrition.[1-3]

2. Answer: C

The first sonographic sign of early pregnancy is the *intradecidual sign* – a small sac seen at 4–5 weeks, only a few millimeters in diameter, which is completely embedded within the endometrium on one side of the uterine midline, not deforming the midline stripe. The *gestational sac* is seen shortly thereafter, at about 5 weeks. It is characterised by a sonolucent centre, surrounded by a thick symmetric echogenic ring. If a clear *double decidual sign* is seen with the gestational sac, an IUP is likely. The double decidual sign consists of two concentric echogenic rings surrounding a gestational sac. **A gestational sac with a vague or an absent double decidual sign is not diagnostic of an IUP and may be a pseudogestational sac associated with an ectopic pregnancy.** For this reason, many authors consider the *yolk sac* as the first definitive evidence of an IUP, rather than the gestational sac.

The yolk sac is the first structure visualised inside the gestational sac and is seen by transvaginal (TV) sonography at about 5–6 weeks. When a high-resolution transvaginal probe (≥6.5 MHz) is used, a yolk sac is usually seen within the gestational sac when the mean sac diameter (MSD) ≥10 mm. However, in the ED, transabdomial scanning or TV scanning with a lower frequency probe is usually performed, where a yolk sac may not be seen until the MSD ≥20mm. **Therefore, for the ED purpose, an empty gestational sac ≥20 mm is a good predictor of fetal demise and is referred to as a blighted ovum.**

An indeterminate ultrasound examination in early pregnancy demonstrates no signs of intrauterine *or* ectopic pregnancy and could still indicate an early pregnancy, embryonic demise or ectopic pregnancy. Serial βHCG and ultrasounds are useful in such cases but for ED purposes, **all patients without a confirmed IUP (gestational sac plus yolk sac) should be regarded as an ectopic pregnancy until proven otherwise and the obstetricians should urgently be informed.**[4]

3. Answer: C

Major risk factors for ectopic pregnancy include PID, history of tubal surgery, use of an intrauterine device (IUD), assisted reproduction techniques and a previous ectopic pregnancy. **However, more than 50% of cases of ectopic pregnancy occur in patients without recognised risk factors.**

Abdominal discomfort or pain is the most common presenting symptom of ectopic pregnancy and occurs in 90% of patients. Pain is due to tubal distention or rupture. Vaginal bleeding occurs in 50–80% of cases and is often scant. However, heavy bleeding does not exclude ectopic pregnancy. **Although heavy bleeding and the passage of clots are more common with failed IUP, the history of passage of products of conception should not be used as the basis for diagnosis as blood clots or a decidual cast in an ectopic pregnancy may be misinterpreted as products of conception.** The menstrual history is often, but not always, abnormal. No missed menses are reported in 15% of ectopic pregnancies.

Ectopic pregnancy cannot reliably be diagnosed or excluded on physical examination. The cervix may have a blue discoloration, as in normal pregnancy. Furthermore, the uterine size for estimated gestational age is most often normal. The adnexae may be enlarged, particularly unilaterally, due to a cystic corpus luteum or ectopic pregnancy. Interestingly, when an adnexal mass is palpated, one-third of patients will have a contralateral ectopic pregnancy.[5–8]

4. Answer: A

Vaginal bleeding is the most common presentation of a threatened miscarriage. However, the severity of bleeding does not correlate with the risk of the patient proceeding to a complete miscarriage. About 50% of pregnant patients with vaginal bleeding will proceed to have a viable pregnancy. **However, the presence of cardiac activity on ultrasound significantly reduces this risk, as at least 90% will continue with a normal pregnancy.** At the same time, embryonic bradycardia predicts a poor prognosis. A heart rate

<100 bpm prior to 6 weeks and <120 bpm between 7 and 8 weeks is associated with a poor outcome.

Advice such as bed rest is commonly given to patients to 'prevent' miscarriage. This advice is not useful because there is no evidence that any therapy influences outcome. Furthermore, most fetuses can be shown to be nonviable 1 to 2 weeks before actual symptoms occur. In the vast majority of cases, spontaneous miscarriage is the body's natural method of expelling an abnormal or undeveloped (blighted) pregnancy. Patients should be advised that modern daily activities would not affect pregnancy. Tampons, intercourse and other activities that might induce uterine infection should be avoided as long as the patient is bleeding.[4,7,9]

5. Answer: A

A common misconception is that a very low βHCG rules out an ectopic pregnancy. However, **studies show that about 40% of ectopic pregnancies present with a βHCG <1000 mIU/mL and about 20% with a βHCG <500 mIU/mL.**[62,63] Furthermore, the risk of tubal rupture has been found to be similar across a wide range of βHCG levels and a low level does not predict a benign course. Approximately 30–40% of ectopic pregnancies with a βHCG level <1000 mIU/mL will be ruptured at the time of diagnosis. In another review study, a very low level <100 mIU/mL, 30% were found to be ruptured on laparoscopy.[64]

The discriminatory zone is the lowest concentration of βHCG at which a viable pregnancy should be visible on an ultrasound scan. An intrauterine gestation is usually visible on a transvaginal scan at a βHCG concentration of ≥1500 mIU/mL, and on transabdominal ultrasound if ≥6500 mIU/mL. Diagnostic accuracy is subsequently better if the transvaginal route is used for ultrasound examination but ultrasound is still inconclusive regarding the exact location of a pregnancy in 8–31% of women. In such cases, measurement of *serial βHCG* concentrations is used to guide management and is best used in conjunction with ultrasound findings. Serial measures of βHCG are used to either heighten or lower the suspicion of ectopic pregnancy, but are not diagnostic.

The pattern of rise or fall in βHCG after 48 hours is useful in distinguishing between pregnancy of

unknown locations (PUL) that will develop into failing PUL from intrauterine and ectopic pregnancy, particularly whenever the βHCG levels are lower than the discriminatory zone or when an ultrasound diagnosis cannot be made despite the βHCG being above the discriminatory zone. A doubling of βHCG concentrations over 48 hours is often used to predict viability but an increase of at least 66% is generally regarded as suggestive of a viable pregnancy. However, a large study published in 2004 suggests that the slowest increase associated with viability is 53% after 2 days and many authors now use a minimum rise of >50% as suggestive of viable pregnancy.[65] However, an increase in of βHCG >50% does not rule out an ectopic pregnancy. If βHCG levels fall by at least 15%, the most likely outcome is a failing PUL. When the rise or fall in βHCG is suboptimal, the most likely outcome is ectopic pregnancy. However, failing PUL may and 15% of normal pregnancies will have an abnormal doubling time.[4–8,10,11]

6. Answer: B

Rh D immunoglobulin (RhIG) is usually given to Rh D negative women with no preformed anti-D antibodies during pregnancy if they experience a 'sensitising' event in which there is a risk of fetal blood crossing into the maternal circulation. **The administration of RhIG has been shown to decrease maternal sensitisation and fetal complications during late pregnancy; however, it is unclear whether first trimester events lead to sensitisation as there is a paucity of well-designed studies addressing this issue.**

A 2003 National Health and Medical Research Council (NHMRC) report[16] recommends the administration of RhIG to every Rh D negative women in the first trimester (up to and including 12 weeks' gestation) with no preformed anti-D to ensure adequate protection against immunisation after the following sensitising events (level IV evidence):

- miscarriage
- termination of pregnancy (TOP)
- ectopic pregnancy
- chorionic villus sampling

The report further elaborates on the use of RhIG in miscarriage stating that there is insufficient evidence to support the use of RhIG in bleeding prior to

12 weeks' gestation in an ongoing pregnancy (threatened miscarriage), but if the pregnancy then requires curettage, or if the bleeding is particularly heavy or associated with a visible subchorionic haemorrhage, these patients should be considered at higher risk of sensitisation and RhIG given. The Royal Australian and New Zealand College of Obstetricians and Gynaecologists (RANZCOG) guidelines for the use of RhIG in obstetrics are based on this report. The *Australian Therapeutic Guidelines* support the above four indications for RhIG in first trimester bleeding; however, it refers to 'miscarriage' only and does not extrapolate on threatened miscarriage. Regardless, the tradition of giving Rh prophylaxis to all Rh negative patients with first trimester bleeding, including threatened miscarriage, is well established among practitioners albeit not evidence based. Additionally, most expert opinion is in favour of RhIG administration during the first trimester due to the extremely low incidence of complications from RhIG administration and the potential grave risks of maternal sensitisation that have been extrapolated from experience with late pregnancy bleeding and subsequent sensitisation.

Because the volume of fetal cells potentially involved in the fetomaternal haemorrhage (FMH) is small, the recommended does of RhIG is 250 IU. For successful prophylaxis, Rh(D) immunoglobulin should be given as soon as possible after the sensitising event but always within 72 hours (level I evidence). **If RhIG has not been offered within 72 hours, a dose offered within up to 10 days may provide protection.** Blood should be taken prior to administration to exclude the presence of antibodies. In cases of ongoing bleeding, it is recommended that RhIG be given every 6 weeks.[12–18]

7. Answer: D

Current national recommendations for the administration of RhIG after sensitising events beyond the first trimester include:

- chorionic villus sampling, amniocentesis, cordocentesis and fetoscopy
- abdominal trauma considered sufficient to cause FMH
- each occasion of revealed or concealed APH (where the patient suffers unexplained uterine pain the possibility of concealed APH should be considered, with a view to immunoprophylaxis)

- external cephalic version
- miscarriage or termination of pregnancy

Studies have shown that Rh(D) immunoglobulin 100 IU is sufficient to protect against a FMH of 1.0 mL of fetal red cells (2.0 mL whole blood). The majority of fetal bleeds are <5 mL of red blood cells, therefore **a dose of RhIG 625 IU is sufficient to protect against most cases of FMH but not all, and it is recommended that the magnitude of the FMH following a sensitising event be quantified to ensure an adequate dose of Rh(D) immunoglobulin is offered, as more than one dose may be required.** The Kleihauer-Betke acid elution test is one such test that is commonly used to establish the extent of FMH and requires the collection of 7 mL of maternal venous blood in an EDTA® tube.

The occurrence and degree of FMH after trauma is difficult to establish at the bedside. **Since sensitisation can occur in pregnant patients exposed to a transplacental haemorrhage of <0.1 mL, it seems sensible to administer RhIG to all pregnant patients following abdominal trauma.** The recommended standard dose in Australian is 625 IU. The Kleihauer-Betke acid elution test can be performed in addition to assess if further doses of RhIG are required.

The Australian Rh immunoglobin product can only safely be given intramuscularly. In some circumstances such as severe thrombocytopenia or a coagulation disorder, access to an intravenous Rh(D) preparation may be warranted. A quantity of intravenous Rh(D) immunoglobulin has been reserved for this purpose and is available from the Australian Red Cross Blood Service.[13,14,16,17,19]

8. Answer: B

Preeclampsia is a multisystem disorder usually diagnosed in the presence of hypertension associated with proteinuria after the 20th week of gestation in women known to be normotensive beforehand. **Oedema is no longer included in the definition of preeclampsia because it is commonly found in many women with normal pregnancies.** The International Society for the Study of Hypertension in pregnancy defines hypertension as 'a diastolic BP of 90 mmHg or higher on 2 consecutive occasions at least 4 hours apart or a single diastolic BP greater than 110 mmHg'.[65] Blood pressure during pregnancy should be measured with the patient in the sitting position or lying at a 45° angle with the arm at the level of the heart. Alternatively, the left lateral recumbent position can be used. An appropriate size cuff (length 1.5 times upper circumference or a cuff with a bladder that encircles 80% or more of the arm) should be used. A mercury sphygmanometer is preferred as it is more accurate than electronic devices. Phase V Korotkoff sound (sound disappearance) should be used to measure diastolic BP. **Although the use of antihypertensive drugs in women with preeclampsia and severe rises in BP have been shown to prevent cerebrovascular problems, such treatment does not prevent or alter the natural course of the disease in women with mild-moderate elevations of BP. Antihypertensive therapy have been remarkably unsuccessful in improving fetal outcome or prolonging pregnancy.**

Proteinuria is defined as the presence of ≥300 mg of protein in a 24-hour urine collection. This usually correlates with 1+ protein on a random urine dipstick. However, proteinuria may be variable at any given time and may not be detectable in a random urine specimen. Furthermore, it is important to be aware that preeclampsia may occur without proteinuria. Diagnosis in such cases rests on confirming hypertension and evidence of multisystem involvement.[20–25]

9. Answer: D

This patient satisfies the criteria for severe preeclampsia and has signs of imminent eclampsia. **Symptoms and signs suggestive of imminent eclampsia include headache, visual disturbances, epigastric/RUQ pain and hyperreflexia.** However, about one-quarter of cases of eclampsia occur without preceding signs or symptoms suggestive of imminent eclampsia. The definition of severe preeclampsia is not standardised but most regard it as the presence of any one of the following in the setting of preeclampsia: (1) BP ≥160/110 mmHg, (2) severe proteinuria >5 g/24 h, or (3) end-organ involvement including visual disturbances, persistent headache, epigastric or right upper quadrant pain, pulmonary edema, oliguria, renal impairment, haematologic disturbances, intrauterine growth restriction and oligohydramnios.

Severe preeclampsia is managed in the same way as eclampsia. The focus of treatment of severe preeclampsia is on the prevention of seizures (eclampsia) and treatment of hypertension to prevent permanent damage to maternal organs.

(1) *Prevention of seizures*: Magnesium sulfate is given as prophylaxis against the development of eclampsia in severe preeclampsia. **There is now robust evidence that, for women with severe preeclampsia, magnesium sulphate more than halves the risk of eclampsia and also reduces the risk of maternal death.** The MagPie trial (magnesium in the prevention of eclampsia), the largest prospective multi-centre placebo controlled study to date, found a significant reduction in the rate of eclampsia in women treated with magnesium sulphate. Similarly, a Cochrane review of magnesium sulfate use for preventing eclampsia has also shown that magnesium sulfate provided a 50% risk reduction of developing eclampsia and a reduced the risk of maternal death.[28] However, no overall difference has been found in the risk of stillbirth or neonatal death.

(2) *Treatment of hypertension*: The risk of end-organ compromise is proportional to the degree of BP elevation. The objective of treatment is to minimise the risk of end-organ damage without compromising cerebral and uteroplacental blood flow. **It is generally recommended that systolic and diastolic BP should be maintained below 160 and 105 mmHg respectively to reduce the risk of cerebral bleeds and end-organ damage.** Intravenous hydralazine is most commonly used in Australia at repeated doses of 2.5 – 5 mg every 20 minutes to keep the diastolic BP below 105 mmHg.[20,22–26]

10. Answer: A

Eclampsia should be suspected and treated in any pregnant patient who is >20 weeks of gestation or <4 weeks postpartum who develops seizures. The diagnosis of eclampsia is secure in the presence of generalised oedema, hypertension, proteinuria and convulsions. While hypertension is considered the hallmark for the diagnosis of eclampsia, it may not always be present. The hypertension can be severe (≥160/110 mmHg) in 20–54% of cases or mild (140–160/ 90–110 mmHg) in 30–60% of cases. **However, in 16% of cases, hypertension may be absent, hence, although control of BP is important, it will not necessarily prevent or treat**

eclampsia. Similarly, the diagnosis of eclampsia is usually associated with proteinuria (at least 1 + on dipstick) but it may be absent in 14% of cases.

The standard of care for women with eclampsia is to use an anticonvulsant drug to control the immediate fit, and to continue maintenance treatment to prevent further seizures. **Magnesium sulphate is the first-line treatment in termination of acute seizures as well as prevention of further seizures.** It has been shown to be more effective than diazepam or phenytoin in the treatment and prophylaxis of eclamptic seizures. The use of phenytoin should be confined only to patients who have persistent seizures despite magnesium. Various regimes exist but a loading dose of magnesium 4–6 g is usually given over 10–20 minutes followed by a maintenance infusion of 2g/hour by intravenous infusion. Approximately 10% of eclamptic women will have a second convulsion after receiving magnesium sulfate. In these women, another bolus of 2 g magnesium sulfate can be given intravenously over 3–5 minutes.

The hypertension associated with eclampsia is often controlled adequately by terminating the seizures. **Rapid lowering of BP can result in uterine hypoperfusion, so specific antihypertensive treatment is usually initiated only if the diastolic BP remains above 105 mmHg after control of seizures.** Additionally, many patients do not require specific antihypertensive treatment after treatment with magnesium sulfate. Intravenous hydralazine is most commonly used in Australia at repeated doses of 2.5–10 mg every 20 minutes to keep the diastolic BP below 105 mmHg. Labetalol has also been reported to be safe and effective; however, the intravenous preparate is not available in Australia.[23,27–31]

11. Answer: D

$MgSO_4$ is indicated in pregnant patients with severe preeclampsia to prevent seizures and in eclamptic patients for the treatment and prophylaxis of seizures. **Routine monitoring of serum levels is not useful, as there is no 'therapeutic range' established for its use in eclampsia.** Adverse effects include flushing, nausea, drowsiness and weakness with respiratory depression and respiratory and cardiac arrest the most serious complications. However, the adverse effects follow a dose response; deep tendon reflexes are lost at a serum magnesium level of

10 mEq/L, respiratory depression occur at 15 mEq/L and cardiac arrest at more than 15 mEq/L. **This dose response relationship means that clinical monitoring should ensure that toxicity and adverse effects are avoided.** For this reason, deep tendon reflexes and respiratory rate should routine be monitored and can be used as an early indicator of toxicity.

Magnesium is excreted in the urine and raised serum levels will quickly occur in patients with impaired renal function and be at risk of significant adverse effects if the dose is not reduced. Decreased urine output may therefore lead to earlier toxicity and measuring hourly urine output should be included in the clinical monitoring. **Magnesium levels should be checked if there is loss of deep tendon reflexes or in the presence of renal dysfunction.** Nevertheless, some clinicians still prefer to routinely measure magnesium levels to detect toxicity. If toxicity does develop, calcium gluconate is an effective antidote.[23,30]

12. Answer: A

Paracetamol is the analgesic of choice in pregnancy and lactation but is often inadequate for severe migraine attacks. Metoclopramide is safe to use in pregnancy, and may be added to paracetamol to increase its effectiveness. Dihydroergotamine and the triptans should be avoided throughout pregnancy. **NSAIDs can be continued into the second trimester (up to 32 weeks) as there are no data suggesting increased fetal malformations.** However, NSAIDs should not be used in late pregnancy because they can cause premature closure of the fetal ductus arteriosus, delay labour and birth, or cause oligohydramnios via an effect on fetal renal function. NSAIDs are classified as compatible with breastfeeding. Diclofenac or ibuprofen are the preferred drugs. Oxycodone is another medication that is commonly prescribed postpartum that is compatible with breastfeeding if given as occasional doses.

Trichomoniasis in pregnancy is associated with adverse pregnancy outcomes (premature rupture of membranes, preterm delivery and low birth weight) and a single dose of metronidazole 2 g orally is generally recommended. However, metronidazole treatment does not necessarily result in a reduction in perinatal morbidity and some trials suggest the possibility of increased prematurity, particularly if treatment is given during the midtrimester. Gentamicin has a TGA pregnancy classification D and should be avoided where possible. It is often used in severe sepsis in pregnancy where the benefits outweigh the risks. A cephalosporin would be a more appropriate antibiotic in the setting of pyelonephritis. Gentamicin is compatible with breastfeeding but may cause diarrhoea in the infant.[17,32–35]

13. Answer: C

The clinical presentation of abruption varies widely from totally asymptomatic cases to those where there is fetal death with severe maternal morbidity. The classic description of placental abruption is painful vaginal bleeding, severe uterine pain or tenderness, uterine hypertonicity and hypotension. It is important to realise, however, that **severe abruption may occur with neither or just of one of these signs.** Additionally, symptoms can be subtle with minimal or no bleeding and only minimal abdominal cramping. The amount of vaginal bleeding correlates poorly with the degree of abruption. Back pain may be the only symptom, especially when the placenta is posteriorly located. **The severity of symptoms depends on the location of the abruption, whether it is revealed or concealed, and the degree of abruption.** There are often features of fetal distress, with fetal death occurring in most cases in which there is >50% placental separation.

Placental abruption is often associated with the development of disseminated intravascular coagulation (DIC). **The risk of DIC is highest when there is such a large placental detachment as to cause fetal death**. Haemorrhage associated with DIC leads to further consumption of coagulation factors, setting off a vicious cycle. Bleeding may occur into the uterine myometrium, leading to a beefy boggy uterus called a Couvelaire uterus. The normal fibrinogen level in pregnancy is 4–4.5 g/L; values below <3 g/L indicates significant consumption of coagulation factors.

Ultrasonography has a limited sensitivity in detecting abruptio placenta, with a reported negative predictive value of 63–88%. The ultrasonographic appearance of abruption depends to a large extent on the size and location of the bleed as well as the duration between the abruption and the time the ultrasonographic examination was performed, as the echogenicity of fresh blood is so similar to that of the placenta. Placental abruption is primarily a clinical diagnosis. Ultrasound is purely an adjunct in the diagnosis and helps exclude other causes of vaginal bleeding such as placenta praevia.[20,22,23,36,37]

14. Answer: A

In contrast to abruption, the classic presentation of placenta praevia is painless, bright red vaginal bleeding occurring at the end of the second trimester. Bleeding is usually painless because the blood is expelled and does not cause uterine distension. **Fortunately, this 'sentinel bleed' is rarely massive and usually stops spontaneously, though it often recurs and may become profuse during labour.** The degree of bleeding is often proportional to the degree of haemodynamic compromise. Some degree of uterine irritability is present in about 20% of the cases, which may make it difficult to distinguish from abruptio.

Digital vaginal examination should be avoided in all patients presenting with antepartum haemorrhage in the second half of the pregnancy until the diagnosis of placenta praevia is excluded as the possibility of tearing or dislodging a placenta praevia may result in profuse and potentially fatal haemorrhage. Ultrasound is the diagnostic procedure of choice for diagnosing placenta praevia in any patient who presents with vaginal bleeding during the latter half of pregnancy. Transabdominal ultrasound has a sensitivity of 95%. Multiple studies have shown that transvaginal ultrasound is safe and more accurate than transabdominal ultrasound. Once an ultrasound has excluded placenta praevia, a careful speculum examination may be performed to look for other causes of bleeding. **In the rare case where an ultrasound cannot exclude placenta praevia or is not available, a digital and speculum examination should be performed in the operating theatre with the patient prepared and draped for an urgent caesarean section.**

Vasa praevia refers to the velamentous insertion of the cord below the presenting part of the fetus. Normally, the vessels run from the middle of the placenta via the umbilical cord to the fetus. Velamentous insertion means that the vessels, unprotected by Wharton's jelly, traverse the membranes before they come together into the

umbilical cord. These unprotected vessels may rupture at any time during pregnancy but usually in association with rupture of the amniotic membranes. When this occurs, bleeding is from the fetus, which may quickly lead to fetal exsanguination and death. Perinatal mortality with vessel rupture ranges from 75 to 100%.[17,20,22,23,38,39]

15. Answer: D

Shoulder dystocia refers to impaction of the fetal shoulders at the pelvic outlet occurring after delivery of the head. Typically, the anterior shoulder is trapped behind the symphysis pubis, which leads to delay of delivery of the rest of the infant. In addition, the fetal shoulders are in the vertical position rather than the normal oblique position. Impaction of the fetal shoulders and thorax in the maternal pelvis prohibits adequate respiration, and compression of the umbilical cord frequently compromises fetal circulation. Fetal hypoxia results from impaired respirations due to impaction of the fetal shoulders and thorax in the maternal pelvis. Fetal circulation is compromised due to compression of the umbilical cord as well as compression of the neck and central venous congestion. The aim is to deliver the fetus under 5 minutes to prevent asphyxia.

Various manoeuvres exist and can be employed in an attempt to dislodge the anterior shoulder. With the McRoberts' manoeuvre the mother is placed in the extreme lithotomy position, with legs sharply flexed up to the abdomen. **The McRoberts' manoeuvre does not change the actual dimension of the maternal pelvis. Rather, the manoeuvre straightens the sacrum relative to the lumbar spine, allowing cephalic rotation of the symphysis pubis sliding over the fetal shoulder.** Commonly, suprapubic pressure is applied by an assistant, directing the anterior shoulder downward and laterally in an attempt to rotate the shoulder and infant under the symphysis pubis. **Fundal pressure should never be applied, as this will further impact the shoulder on the pelvic rim.**

Shoulder dystocia is typically a 'bony' obstruction and not a result of obstructing soft tissue. Management by episiotomy has been associated with an increase in the rate of perineal trauma without benefit of reducing the occurrence of neonatal depression or brachial plexus palsy. The decision to cut a generous episiotomy must be based upon clinical circumstances, such as a narrow vaginal fourchette in a primigravid patient or the need to perform fetal manipulation. Draining the bladder with a Foley catheter may give more room anteriorly. Other manoeuvres include Wood's corkscrew manoeuvre, Rubin's manoeuvre and delivery of the posterior arm.[17,37,40–42]

16. Answer: C

Rupture of membranes that occur prior to the onset of labour, regardless of gestation, is called premature rupture of membranes. If rupture occurs before 37 weeks' gestation, it is termed preterm premature rupture of membranes. **The majority of patients with premature rupture of membranes will go into labour within 24 hours; however, a small proportion will have prolonged rupture of membranes with the increased risk of chorioamnionitis.** Ultrasound examination may show reduced liquor volume but volume can appear normal with a small leak. A sterile speculum examination is therefore indicated to confirm the presence of amniotic fluid by visualisation of fluid draining through the cervical os, change of nitrazine paper to blue or presence of ferning on microscopy. At the same time cord prolapse can be excluded. Assessment of the fetal heart with a cardiotocography (CTG) is essential to determine fetal wellbeing; however, patients should not be discharged until obstetric consultation has been sought to determine the presence or absence of ruptured membranes and to facilitate subsequent management.[17,42]

17. Answer: A

PPH can be defined as bleeding from the birth canal >500 mL in the first 24 hours after vaginal delivery and >1000 mL post caesarean section. Primary PPH refers to bleeding within the first 24 hours after delivery and secondary PPH to bleeding after 24 hours. **The most important aspect of the management of PPH is probably its prediction and prevention**. Risk factors for PPH include antepartum haemorrhage, prior postpartum haemorrhage, over distention of the uterus from polyhydramnios, multiple pregnancy or macrosomia, prolonged labour, instrumental delivery and abnormal placentation. Active management of the third stage has been shown to reduce the risk of PPH. **The most common cause of immediate PPH is uterine atony, contributing to approximately 80% of cases.** If the uterus is contracted, the leading causes of primary PPH are genital tract trauma and pathologic placentation. Secondary PPH is most frequently caused by retained products, subinvolution of the uterus, and uterine infection.

Strategies to treat primary PPH first must ensure uterine contraction and then identify and repair any genital tract injuries. **Uterine atony is initially managed with firm manual massage of the uterine fundus through the abdominal wall in conjunction with the administration of oxytocic agents.** Medical treatment of PPH is aimed at achieving uterine contractions. These include oxytocin, ergot alkaloids and prostaglandins. Oxytocin is the most common medication used to achieve uterine contraction and therefore is the first-line agent for prevention and treatment of PPH. Oxytocin is commonly administered by an intravenous infusion, which can be prepared by adding 20–40 units of oxytocin to 1 L of crystalloid and infusing it at a rate of 200–500 mL/hr. Titrate to sustain uterine contractions and control uterine haemorrhage. Slowing of haemorrhage should be observed within minutes of administration. If an intravenous line is unavailable, administer 10 units of oxytocin intramuscularly. **Administration of oxytocinin as an intravenous bolus should preferably be avoided as it may cause profound hypotension and arrhythmias**.[17,37,41,43]

18. Answer: B

The most common infectious causes of vaginitis in symptomatic women include bacterial vaginosis (22–50%), candidiasis (17–39%) and trichomonas (4–35%). Alkaline secretions from the cervix before and after menstruation, as well as semen (alkaline), reduce acidity and predispose to infection.

Bacterial vaginosis (BV) is a polymicrobial clinical syndrome caused by a change in the balance of microorganisms found in a healthy vagina. The resultant reduction of the normal hydrogen peroxide–producing *Lactobacillus* species in the vagina leads to overgrowth with high concentrations of anaerobic (e.g. *Mobiluncus* species) and other fastidious bacteria (including *Gardnerella vaginalis* and *Atopobium vaginae*), and *Mycoplasma* *hominis*. The most common symptom of bacterial vaginosis is an increase in a greyish white vaginal discharge. The discharge often has a fishy smell. The diagnosis of BV can be confirmed by examination of the discharge, including vaginal swab wet preparation and gram-stained smear. Typical features on examination of the discharge include:

- pH >4.5 (normal vaginal pH varies between 3.8 and 4.5)
- the presence of 'clue cells' (epithelial cells covered with small curved coccobacilli) on wet mount
- a positive 'whiff test'; several drops of a potassium hydroxide (KOH) solution are added to a sample of vaginal discharge (release of amine with alkalinisation of vaginal fluid, producing a fishy odour)
- a gram stain showing few or absent pus cells and lactobacilli morphotypes and, in addition to 'clue cells', abundant curved gram-variable coccobacilli and mixed anaerobes

Culture adds little to microscopy. Additionally, gardnerella organisms are part of the normal vaginal flora and therefore positive culture alone does not indicate infection.[44–46]

19. Answer: B

PID refers to a clinical syndromes resulting from infection or inflammation of the usually sterile upper genital tract. **PID is usually polymicrobial and due to sexually acquired organisms.** Other risk factors for PID include procedures or conditions that involve disruption of the normal cervical barrier (pregnancy termination, delivery, surgery or following insertion of an intrauterine contraceptive device). Additionally, there is an increased risk of PID early in the menstrual cycle or at the end of menses, which is attributed to low progesterone levels and coincident thinning of the cervical mucosal barrier.

Diagnosis of PID is usually based on clinical criteria with or without laboratory evidence. **Adnexal tenderness alone is the single most sensitive examination finding (95%) but has a specificity of 3.8%.** Other findings with high sensitivity of over 90% include lower abdominal tenderness, uterine tenderness and cervical motion tenderness. However, as isolated findings, they again lack sensitivity. The presence of white blood cells (WBCs) in the vaginal discharge is a sensitive marker for PID. The diagnosis

of PID is therefore unlikely if the cervical discharge appears normal and there are no WBCs on the wet slide preparation.[47–49]

20. Answer: C

Sexually transmitted PID is usually caused by *Chlamydiae* or *Neisseria gonorrhoeae* and antibiotic regimens traditionally were directed primarily against these organisms. However, it is now recognised that these agents are instrumental in the initial infection of the upper genital tract, causing epithelium damage that allows further entry of opportunistic infections including anaerobes, *Mycoplasma genitalium* and other bacteria. **Polymicrobial infection is therefore common and antibiotic treatment should include antibiotics with activity against the major sexually transmitted pathogens and anaerobic bacteria.** Current guidelines suggest that empiric treatment should be initiated in those women at risk who exhibit lower abdominal pain, adnexal tenderness, and cervical motion tenderness. **Early empirical treatment of sexually acquired PID is important and recommended because it may reduce the risk of tubal damage, which predisposes to infertility or ectopic pregnancy.** Furthermore, whereas a positive microscopy, culture or PCR result on endocervical swab retrospectively supports the diagnoses of PID, defines antibiotic sensitivities and identifies the need to treat sexual partners, the absence of microbiological evidence of infection does not exclude PID. Current Australian antibiotic recommendations for mild to moderate infection are:

ceftriaxone 500 mg IM or IV, as a single dose (for gonorrhoea)
plus

metronidazole 400 mg orally, 12-hourly for 14 days
plus

azithromycin 1 g orally, as a single dose
and

azithromycin 1 g orally, as a single dose 1 week later, *or* doxycycline 100 mg orally, 12-hourly for 14 days.

Azithromycin, 1 g orally as a single dose, is effective in treating *Chlamydia* of the lower genital tract; however, single-dose therapy is inadequate to treat a chlamydial infection of the upper female genital tract.[47–51]

21. Answer: A

There are two options for **postcoital (emergency) contraception** that should be given within 72 hours of unprotected sexual intercourse:

1. *Progestin-only method* (prevents 85% of the pregnancies that would be expected from unprotected mid-cycle sexual intercourse):

   - single dose of levonorgestrel 1.5 mg, or
   - levonorgestrel 750 µg with the same dose repeated 12 hours later

2. *Yuzpe method* (prevents 75% of pregnancies resulting from unprotected mid-cycle sexual intercourse):

   Consists of four tablets of ethinyloestradiol 30 µg + levonorgestrel 150 µg with the same dose repeated 12 hours later. Approximately 60% of women will experience nausea with this regimen, so an antiemetic should be prescribed at the same time.

Australian guidelines currently recommend the following regimen of **single-dose antibiotic prophylaxis**:

- ceftriaxone 250 mg IV or IM, as a single dose, *plus*
- azithromycin 1 g orally, as a single dose, *plus either*
- metronidazole 2 g orally, as a single dose, *or*
- tinidazole 2 g orally, as a single dose

Administration of post-exposure prophylaxis against HIV is not routinely recommended but should be considered if high-risk features for transmission are present after assessment of the risk of HIV transmission. The risk of HIV transmission should be assessed and is determined by: the method of exposure with its estimated risk/exposure; the risk that the source is HIV positive; and cofactors associated with the source and exposed individuals. Initiation of prophylaxis should be the responsibility of, or with advice from, an infectious diseases clinician.

Hepatitis B virus (HBV) prophylaxis should be considered if the victim is not immune. Administer a dose of hepatitis B immunoglobulin (HBIG), as soon as possible after exposure (preferably within 24 hours). In addition, a course of immunisation should be commenced as soon as possible (preferably within 24 hours).[52–54]

22. Answer: D

Ovarian cysts may become symptomatic due to rupture, torsion, bleeding into the cyst or local pressure effects. Rupture or bleeding into the cyst is mostly managed expectantly, whereas torsion is a surgical emergency. **Although adnexal torsion can occur in normal ovaries, it is almost always associated with ovarian enlargement.** Risk factors for developing ovarian torsion are pregnancy (enlarged corpus luteum cyst), presence of large ovarian cysts or tumours, and chemical induction of labour. Ultrasound with Doppler sonography remains the primary imaging modality for suspected torsion. **However, the sensitivity of Doppler flow study is not considered adequate to confirm the diagnosis in all cases, and the clinician must maintain a high level of clinical suspicion to determine which patients need immediate surgical intervention.**

Ultrasound is commonly used in the work-up of patients with suspected endometriosis and it may reveal endometriomata, or focal endometriotic lesions. However, transvaginal ultrasound is not useful in diagnosing the majority of cases of endometriosis because the peritoneal implants and adhesions involved are not detectable. A negative ultrasound does not confirm the absence of endometriosis. Laparoscopy is the gold standard investigation for diagnosing endometriosis and now provides the main tool of treatment.[55–58]

23. Answer: C

Fitz-Hugh–Curtis syndrome is an uncommon cause of abdominal or pelvic pain in females and is due to a perihepatitis secondary to PID. Usually it is an incidental finding in patients with PID, but occasionally it is the presenting symptom and there may be no clinical findings of PID on examination. *Chlamydia* **is isolated from most patients, regardless whether they have symptoms of PID or not.** Liver function studies are normal. Other than excluding other causes of abdominal pain, ultrasound is not helpful in making the diagnosis. Diagnosis is typically made with CT demonstrating perihepatic inflammation.[47,55]

24. Answer: C

A diagnosis of anovulatory bleeding is classically made from the history of irregular menses with periods of amenorrhoea followed by heavy bleeding, in the absence of features suggesting a structural or histological uterine abnormality. The underlying pathology is a relative lack of progesterone (which is released by the corpus luteum after ovulation) to oppose the oestrogenic stimulation of the endometrium and so treatment should include progestin therapy to stabilise the endometrium.

The initial treatment for most cases of abnormal uterine bleeding should be commenced in the ED. But it is important that the patient be referred for ongoing management and further evaluation. **Short-term hormonal manipulation allows the endometrium to stabilise with subsequent slowing or stopping of the bleeding. Various treatment regimes exist and the use of cyclical progestins is one of the treatment options. These are usually given for at least 10 days.** Current guidelines recommend the use of medroxyprogesterone acetate 10 mg orally, 1–3 times daily for 12 days or norethisterone 5 mg orally, 2–3 times daily for 12 days for the first month. After treatment stops, the woman should experience a withdrawal bleed within 3–10 days and this should be explained to the patient. In subsequent cycles, progestins (medroxyprogesterone acetate 10 mg orally once daily or norethisterone 5 mg orally once daily) should be administered on days 12–25 of each cycle or every other month and will usually control anovulatory bleeding. Follow up management with the GP should be arranged to continue management.

Medical therapy is usually successful in managing dysfunctional uterine bleeding and dilation and curettage are seldom used for treatment of menorrhagia.[59–61]

25. Answer: D

Ovulatory bleeding is usually occurs in regular cycles. However, a menstrual cycle of <21 days or >35 days, even if regular, is usually anovulatory.

Thyroid function testing should not routinely be performed in women with abnormal uterine bleeding. Indications for testing are women with menorrhagia and anovulatory bleeding, with evidence of thyroid endocrinopathy.

The menstrual blood in women with abnormal ovulatory bleeding has been shown to have increased fibrinolytic activity and/or increased prostaglandins. Subsequently, **NSAIDs and tranexamic acid are two drugs commonly used to control ovulatory bleeding**. NSAIDs inhibit the local action of prostaglandins in the endometrium and reduce menstrual blood loss. The usual dose of mefenamic acid is 500 mg three times a day or ibuprofen 400 mg three times a day. Tranexamic acid is a plasminogen activator inhibitor that promotes local haemostasis. Tranexamic acid 1 g orally 6- to 8-hourly are typically given for the first 3–4 days of menstruation as over 90% of menstrual loss occurs in the first three days of menstruation. Despite concerns for the development of thromboembolism, large-scale studies have not shown any increased risk of venous thromboembolism. The main adverse effects are nausea and gastrointestinal upset. **In addition to its use in ovulatory bleeding, both tranexamic acid and NSAIDs can be added to hormonal therapy for heavy anovulatory bleeding.**[59–61]

References

1. Therapeutic Guidelines Limited. (Nausea and vomiting during pregnancy. Revised February 2011. etg34. Online. Available: www.etg.org.au.
2. Jarvis S, Nelson-Piercy C. Clinical review. Management of nausea and vomiting in pregnancy. BMJ 2011;342:d3606. Online. Available: www.bmj.com; 29 Aug 2011.
3. Goodwin TM. Hyperemesis gravidarum. Obstet Gynecol Clin N Am 2008;35:401–17.
4. Reardon RF, Joing SA. First trimester pregnancy. In: Ma OJ, Mateer, JR, Blaivas M, editors. Emergency ultrasound. 2nd ed. New York: McGraw-Hill; 2008. p. 279–318.
5. Krause RS, Janicke DM, Cydulka RK. Ectopic pregnancy and emergencies in the first 20 weeks of pregnancy. In: Tintinalli J, Stapczynski J, Ma O, et al, editors. Tintinalli's emergency medicine: a comprehensive study guide. 7th ed. New York: McGraw Hill Medical; 2011. p. 676–84.
6. Bryan S. Ectopic pregnancy and bleeding in early pregnancy. In: Cameron P, Jelinek G, Kelly A, et al, editors. Textbook of adult emergency medicine. 3rd ed. Edinburgh: Elsevier; 2009. p. 592–5.
7. Houry D, Keadey M. Complications in early pregnancy. Part 1: Early pregnancy. Emergency Medicine Practice 2007;9(6):1–26. Online. Available: http://www.ebmedicine.net; 21 Aug 2011.
8. Jurkovic D, Wilkinson H. Clinical review. Diagnosis and management of ectopic pregnancy. BMJ 2011;342:d3397. Online. Available: www.bmj.com; 21 Aug 2011.

9. Griebel CP, Halvorsen J, Golemon TB, et al. Management of spontaneous abortion. American Family Physician 2005;72(7):1243–50.

10. Dunn R, Leach D. Pelvic pain. In: Dunn R, Dilley S, Brookes J, editors. The emergency medicine manual. 5th ed. Adelaide: Venom Publishing; 2010. p. 857–63.

11. Sagili H, Mohamed K. Review. Pregnancy of unknown location: an evidence-based approach to management. Obstet Gynecol 2008;10:224–30.

12. ACEP clinical policies committee and the clinical policies subcommittee on early pregnancy. Clinical policy. Critical issues in the initial evaluation and management of patients presenting to the emergency department in early pregnancy. Ann Emerg Med 2003;41:123–33.

13. Therapeutic Guidelines Limited. Bleeding in pregnancy: Rh (D) immunoglobulin use. Revised February 2008. Amended July 2008, October 2010. etg34. Online. Available: www.etg.org.au.

14. Royal Australian and New Zealand College of Obstetricians and Gynaecologists (RANZCOG). Guidelines for the use of Rh(D) immunoglobuin (anti-D) in obstetrics in Australia. Online. Available: http://www.ranzcog.edu.au/publications/statements/C-obs6.pdf; 24 Aug 2011.

15. Royal Australian and New Zealand College of Obstetricians and Gynaecologists (RANZCOG). Frequently asked clinical questions about the use of Rh (D) immunoglobulin. Online. Available: http://www.transfusion.com.au/FILES/RhD/ranzcogclinical.pdf; 24 Aug 2011.

16. National Health and Medical Research Council. Guidelines on the prophylactic use of Rh(D) immunoglobulin (anti-D) in obstetrics. Commonwealth of Australia, 2003. Online. Available: http://www.nba.gov.au/PDF/glines_anti_d.pdf; 24 Aug 2011.

17. Leach D, Dunn R. Obstetrics. In: Dunn R, Dilley S, Brookes J, editors. The emergency medicine manual. 5th ed, Adelaide: Venom Publishing; 2010. p. 875–94.

18. Hannafin B, Lovecchio F, Blackburn P. Do Rh-negative women with first trimester spontaneous abortions need Rh immune globulin? American Journal of Emergency Medicine 2006;24:487–9.

19. Weinberg L, Steele RG, Pugh R, et al. The pregnant trauma patient. Anaesthesia and Intensive Care 2005;33(2):167–80.

20. Keadey M, Houry D. Complications in pregnancy Part II: Hypertensive disorders of pregnancy and vaginal bleeding. Emergency medicine practice 2009;11(5):1–22. Online. Available: http://www.EBmedicine.net; 27 Aug 2011.

21. Sibai B, Dekker G, Kupferminc M. Pre-eclampsia. Lancet 2005;365:785–99.

22. Echevarria MA, Kuhn GJ. Emergencies after 20 weeks of pregnancy and the postpartum period. In: Tintinalli J, Stapczynski J, Ma O, et al, editors. Tintinalli's emergency medicine: a comprehensive study guide. 7th ed. New York: McGraw Hill Medical; 2011. p. 695–703.

23. Houry DE, Salhi BA. Acute complications of pregnancy. In: Marx JA, Hockberger RS, Walls RM, editors. Rosen's emergency medicine: concepts and clinical practice. 7th ed. Philadelphia: Elsevier; 2010. p. 2279–97.

24. ACOG Committee on practice bulletins. Diagnosis and management of preeclampsia and eclampsia. ACOG Practice Bulletin 2002; Number 33. Online. Available: http://www.acog.org; 27 Aug 2011.

25. Duley L, Meher S, Abalos E. Management of preeclampsia. BMJ 2006;332:463–8.

26. Lew M, Klonis E. Emergency management of eclampsia and severe pre-eclampsia. Emergency Medicine 2003;15:361–8.

27. Therapeutic Guidelines Ltd. Management of eclampsia. Revised June 2008. etg34. Online. Available: www.etg.org.au.

28. Duley L, Henderson-Smart DJ, Walker GJA, et al. Magnesium sulphate versus diazepam for eclampsia. Cochrane Database of Systematic Reviews 2010, Issue 12. Art. No: CD000127. DOI: 10.1002/14651858.CD000127.pub2. Online. Available: www.cochrane.org.

29. Duley L, Henderson-Smart DJ, Chou D. Magnesium sulphate versus phenytoin for eclampsia. Cochrane Database of Systematic Reviews 2010, Issue 10. Art. No: CD000128. DOI: 10.1002/14651858.CD000128.pub2. Online. Available: http://www.cochrane.org.

30. Sibai BM. Diagnosis, prevention, and management of eclampsia. Obstet Gynecol 2005;105(2):402–10.

31. Lee M. Pre-eclampsia and eclampsia. In: Cameron P, Jelinek G, Kelly A, et al, editors. Textbook of adult emergency medicine. 3rd ed. Edinburgh: Elsevier; 2009. p. 608–12.

32. Therapeutic Guidelines Limited. General information on drug use in pregnancy: analgesic drugs. Amended February 2007. Amended September 2008. etg34. Online. Available: www.etg.org.au.

33. Therapeutic Guidelines Limited. General information on drug use in pregnancy. etg34. Online. Available: www.etg.org.au.

34. Therapeutic Guidelines Limited. Trichomoniasis (Trichomonas vaginalis). Revised June 2010. etg34. Online. Available: www.etg.org.au.

35. Therapeutic Guidelines Limited. Migraine in women. Revised June 2011. etg34. Online. Available: www.etg.org.au.

36. Oyelese Y, Ananth CV. Placental abruption. Obstet Gynecol. 2006;108:1005–16.

37. Probst BD. Emergency childbirth. In: Roberts JR, Hedges JR, editors. Clinical Procedures in Emergency Medicine. 5th ed. Philadelphia: Elsevier; 2009. p. 1042–62.

38. Abbrescia K, Sheridan B. Complications of second and third trimester pregnancies. Emerg Med Clin N Am 2003;21:695–710.

39. Bhide B, Thilaganathan B. Recent advances in the management of placenta previa. Curr Opin Obstet Gynecol 2004;16:447–51.

40. Gottlieb AG, Galan HL. Shoulder dystocia: an update. Obstet Gynecol Clin N Am 2007;34:501–31.

41. Priestly S. Emergency delivery. In: Cameron P, Jelinek G, Kelly A, et al, editors. Textbook of adult emergency medicine. 3rd ed. Edinburgh: Elsevier; 2009. p. 585–92.

42. VanRooyen MJ, Scott JA. Emergency delivery. In: Tintinalli J, Stapczynski J, Ma O, et al, editors. Tintinalli's emergency medicine: a comprehensive study guide. 7th ed. New York: McGraw Hill Medical; 2011. p. 703–11.

43. Oyelese Y, Scorza WE, Mastrolia R, et al. Postpartum hemorrhage. Obstet Gynecol Clin N Am 2007;34:421–41.

44. Zeger W, Holt K. Gynecologic infections. Emerg Med Clin N Am 2003;21:631–48.

45. Kuhn GJ, Wahl RP. Vulvovaginitis. In: Tintinalli J, Stapczynski J, Ma O, et al, editors. Tintinalli's emergency medicine: a comprehensive study guide. 7th ed. New York: McGraw Hill Medical; 2011. p. 711–6.

46. Therapeutic Guidelines Limited. Bacterial vaginosis. Revised June 2010. etg34. Online. Available: www.etg.org.au.

47. Bryan S. Pelvic inflammatory disease. In: Cameron P, Jelinek G, Kelly A, et al, editors. Textbook of adult emergency medicine. 3rd ed. Edinburgh: Elsevier; 2009. p. 601–3.

48. Shepherd SM, Shoff WH, Behrman AJ. Pelvic inflammatory disease. In: Tintinalli J, Stapczynski J, Ma O, et al, editors. Tintinalli's emergency medicine: a comprehensive study guide. 7th ed. New York: McGraw Hill Medical; 2011. p. 716–20.

49. Therapeutic Guidelines Limited. Pelvic inflammatory disease. Revised June 2010. etg34. Online. Available: www.etg.org.au.

50. Schmitz G, Tibbles C. Genitourinary emergencies in the nonpregnant woman. Emerg Med Clin N Am 2011;296:21–635.

51. Ross J. Pelvic inflammatory disease. Clinical evidence. 2008:1606. Online. Available: http://www.ncbi.nlm.nih.gov/pmc/articles/PMC2907941/; 28 Aug 2011.

52. Therapeutic Guidelines Limited. Post–sexual assault prophylaxis. Revised June 2010. etg34. Online. Available: www.etg.org.au.

53. Therapeutic Guidelines Limited. Postcoital (emergency) contraception. Revised June 2010. etg34. Online. Available: www.etg.org.au.

54. Commonwealth Department of Health and Ageing. National guidelines for post-exposure prophylaxis after non-occupational exposure to HIV. 2007. Online. Available: http://www.ashm.org.au/images/publications/guidelines/2007nationalnpepguidelines2.pdf; 3 Sep 2011.

55. Lukens TW. Abdominal and pelvic pain in the nonpregnant female. In: Tintinalli J, Stapczynski J, Ma O, et al, editors. Tintinalli's emergency medicine: a comprehensive study guide. 7th ed. New York: McGraw Hill Medical; 2011. p. 672–6.

56. David O'Callaghan. Endometriosis. An update. Australian Family Physician 2006;35(11):863–7.

57. Lawrence LL. Unusual presentations in obstetrics and gynecology. Emerg Med Clin N Am 2003;21:649–65.

58. Cadogan M, Yazdani A, Taylor J. Pelvic pain. In: Cameron P, Jelinek G, Kelly A, et al, editors. Textbook of adult emergency medicine. 3rd ed. Edinburgh: Elsevier; 2009. p. 603–8.

59. Morrison LJ, Spence JM. Vaginal bleeding in the nonpregnant patient. In: Tintinalli J, Stapczynski J, Ma O, et al, editors. Tintinalli's emergency medicine: a comprehensive study guide. 7th ed. New York: McGraw Hill Medical; 2011. p. 665–72.

60. Brown AFT, Bryan S. Abnormal vaginal bleeding in the non-pregnant patient. In: Cameron P, Jelinek G, Kelly A, et al, editors. Textbook of adult emergency medicine. 3rd ed. Edinburgh: Elsevier; 2009. p. 598–600.

61. Therapeutic Guidelines Limited. Menorrhagia. Revised June 2009. Amended October 2009. etg34. Online. Available: www.etg.org.au.

62. Kaplan BC, Dart RG, Moskos M, et al. Ectopic pregnancy: prospective study with improved diagnostic accuracy. Ann Emerg Med 1996;28:10–7.

63. Mateer JA, Valley VT, Aiman EJ, et al. Outcome analysis of a protocol including bedside endovaginal sonography in patients at risk for ectopic pregnancy. Ann Emerg Med 1996;27:283–9.

64. Saxon D, Falcone T, Mascha EJ, et al. A study of ruptured tubal ectopic pregnancy. Obstet Gynecol 1997;90:46–9.

65. Barnhart KT, Sammel MD, Rinaudo PF, et al. Symptomatic patients with an early viable intrauterine pregnancy: HCG curves redefined. Obstet Gynecol 2004;104:50–5.

Toxicology

1. Answer: A

Once a drug or toxin has been absorbed and has the potential to exert significant toxicity, a number of methods can be considered to enhance elimination of the drug from the body. These can be non-extracorporeal or extracorporeal methods.

Non-extracorporeal methods of enhanced toxin elimination are:

- MDAC (gastrointestinal dialysis)
- peritoneal dialysis

Extracorporeal methods of enhanced elimination are:

- haemodialysis (HD)
- haemoperfusion (HP)
- exchange transfusion
- CVVH
- continuous arterio-venous haemofiltration (CAVH).

Methods such as CVVH and CAVH may cause less haemodynamic instability than HD and HP, but the toxin clearance rates achieved can be slower.

The most commonly used extracorporeal elimination method is HD. However, the most effective method to remove a toxin from the body is maintenance of optimal renal, liver, lung and cardiovascular functions through good supportive care. **Therefore HD and HP should be considered in specific toxicities where aggressive resuscitation and supportive care alone are less likely to be lifesaving.**[1–3]

2. Answer: D

The specific toxic substances that are likely to be removed by HD and HP are described in the following mnemonic.

COP, I'VE STUMBLED

Carbamazepine

Osmolal gap – increased

Propylene glycol

Isopropanol

Valproic acid

Excess acid (severe metabolic acidosis of toxic origin)

Salicylates

Theophylline

Uraemia (due to nephrotoxic drugs)

Methanol

Barbiturates

Lithium

Ethylene glycol/ethanol

Diethylene and triethylene glycols

Methanol and ethylene glycol, sodium valproate, salicylates and lithium are the most commonly encountered severe toxicities that are amenable to removal by HD.

HP provides a higher rate of clearance for theophylline than HD; however, both can be considered.

In metformin toxicity severe life-threatening lactic acidosis can develop:

- in patients who are on therapeutic doses of metformin but who develop acute renal failure from other causes
- less commonly, in patients who have taken a very large toxic dose.

HD is very useful in severe metformin toxicity because it rapidly clears lactic acidosis and removes metformin thereby reducing the lactate production.

HD is not indicated in systemic iron toxicity. Desferrioxamine chelation therapy is the treatment of choice in that situation.[2,4]

3. Answer: D

MDAC can be considered for enhanced elimination of specific drugs or substances from the body after its absorption. Current available evidence suggests that MDAC can accelerate drug clearance and is able to achieve clearance rates as good as that can be achieved from haemodialysis for specific drugs. There are two proposed mechanisms of action:

- For drugs metabolised in the liver, it interrupts enterohepatic circulation.
- MDAC gets a patient's gastrointestinal mucosa to work as a 'dialyser' (gastrointestinal dialysis).

The most common indication for the use of MDAC is life-threatening carbamazepine overdose.

For carbamazepine toxicity, because of high protein binding, MDAC in combination with HP is favoured for enhanced elimination.

MDAC increases clearance in the following toxicities and therefore may be useful:

- carbamazepine
- dapsone
- phenytoin
- phenobarbitone
- piroxicam
- theophylline
- yellow oleander.

After the initial dose of activated charcoal, further reduced doses are given every 2 hours for a maximum duration of 6 hours. Airway protection is generally indicated prior to commencement of MDAC.

Activated charcoal is not indicated for lithium and iron overdoses, as these metals are poorly bound to activated charcoal.[1,5]

4. Answer: C

Few drugs that are excreted through the kidneys and that are weak acids with small volumes of distribution can be eliminated more rapidly by manipulation of urine pH to alkalinity. In alkaline urine these weak acids are more ionised and therefore prevents their renal absorption, promoting more rapid elimination from the body.

Urine alkalinisation increases urinary elimination of the following agents:

- salicylates (recommended for moderately severe ingestions)
- phenobarbitone (however, MDAC is a superior method of elimination).

Urine alkalinisation should be considered as first-line treatment for patients with moderate to severe salicylate poisoning who do not meet the criteria for haemodialysis.

Administration of bicarbonate to alkalinise the urine results in alkalaemia. Hypokalaemia is the most common complication but can be corrected by giving intravenous potassium supplements. Alkalotic tetany can occur occasionally, but hypocalcaemia is rare.

Volume overload can occur in urinary alkalisation due to bicarbonate therapy. Dehydration is not a typical complication. Hyponatraemia is not a complication of urinary alkalisation. Forced diuresis can cause hyponatraemia. The term urine

alkalinisation emphasises urine pH manipulation rather than a diuresis as the prime objective of treatment.[3,6,7]

5. Answer: A

Sodium bicarbonate is used for immediate correction of life-threatening acidosis in cyanide poisoning, isoniazid overdose and toxic alcohol poisoning. Sodium bicarbonate prevents cardiotoxicity secondary to fast sodium channel blockade in TCA, propranolol, flecainide and quinidine toxicities etc. and it prevents redistribution of drugs to the central nervous system (CNS) in severe salicylate toxicity. It also increases urinary solubility of drugs (in methotrexate toxicity) and enhances urinary drug elimination (in salicylate and phenobarbitone toxicities).

In carbamazepine toxicity, sodium bicarbonate is used to treat the rare event of ventricular dysrhythmias and it is not used for life-threatening acidosis.[8]

6. Answer: B

Causes of high AG metabolic acidosis can be remembered by the following mnemonic.

CAT MUDPILES

Carbon monoxide, cyanide

Alcohol, alcoholic ketoacidosis

Toluene

Metformin, methanol

Uraemia

Diabetic ketoacidosis

Phenformin, paracetamol, propylene glycol, paraldehyde

Iron, Isoniazid

Lactic acidosis

Ethylene glycol

Salicylates

The four major groups of conditions that can cause high AG metabolic acidosis are:

- ketoacidosis
- lactic acidosis
- drugs and toxins
- renal failure.

Frusemide is a diuretic and it causes urinary acid loss leading to metabolic alkalosis.[9]

7. Answer: A

In a patient with suspected poisoning, an increased OG is most likely to be due to the presence of unmeasured osmotically active molecules of a toxic alcohol such as acetone, methanol, ethylene glycol, isopropyl alcohol and propylene glycol. In a poisoned patient, concomitant alcohol ingestion can also cause such an increase. In addition, other non-toxicological medical conditions can cause an increased OG due to increased osmotically active molecules. The presence of a high AG metabolic acidosis and increased OG is highly suggestive of toxic alcohol ingestion in a suspected patient.

The osmolality can be calculated from routine biochemistry results:

calculated osmolality (mOsm/kg) = 2 x Na + urea + glucose + ethanol

(Na, urea, glucose and ethanol concentrations should be in SI units i.e. in mmol/L.) However, the measured osmolality should be specifically requested from the laboratory. This measures additional osmotically active molecules that are present.

osmolar gap = measured osmolality – calculated osmolality

Additionally, a normal OG does not exclude toxic alcohol poisoning.[10]

8. Answer: A

A number of drugs can cause QT prolongation in a poisoned patient. This list includes:
- antiarrhythmics (e.g. flecainide, sotalol)
- tricyclic antidepressants
- citalopram
- antipsychotics (e.g. haloperidol, droperidol)
- antihistamines
- erythromycin.

QT prolongation on the 12-lead ECG is associated with increased risk for development of torsades de pointes in these patients. This polymorphic ventricular tachycardia can degenerate rapidly into a ventricular fibrillation causing cardiac arrest. **Bradycardic patients with QT prolongation are more at risk.** Chan *et al.* described a QT nomogram where the QT interval can be plotted against the heart rate. If this point is located above the 'at risk' line the patient is more likely to develop torsades de pointes.[11,12]

9. Answer: D

The glomerular filtration rate (GFR) decreases by approximately 50% from age 30 to 80 years. Elderly patients may be on a variety of drugs that can potentially be toxic in the presence of poor renal function. Drugs with a narrow therapeutic window include:
- antimicrobials (aminoglycoside, imipenem, vancomycin and pyrazinamide)
- benzodiazepines with active metabolites (diazepam, chlordiazepoxide)
- digoxin
- metformin
- salicylates
- lithium.

These should be prescribed with caution in elderly and in patients with diminished renal function.[13]

10. Answer: A

Toddlers are more likely to accidentally ingest medications and other toxic and nontoxic substances that are easily accessible. Some of these medications and substances can produce significant toxicity in toddlers when ingested in small quantities such as 1–2 tablets or a mouthful, as the dose ingested per kilogram of body weight can be high. Furthermore, the onset of toxicity may be delayed for certain agents. **It is therefore recommended that a toddler who ingested an unidentified tablet should be observed for at least a 12-hour observation period.**

Mercury from a thermometer is unlikely to cause significant toxicity in a toddler. One tablet of a sulphonylurea can produce significant hypoglycaemia in a 10 kg toddler. Few tablets of tricyclic antidepressant can produce seizures, cardiac arrhythmias, hypotension and coma. A sip or mouthful of camphor can cause a reduced level of consciousness, hypotension and seizures.

Other drugs and substances that can potentially cause significant toxicity in small quantities in toddlers include:
- CCBs
- propranolol
- amphetamines
- opioids
- theophylline
- hydrocarbons
- organophosphates
- paraquat.[14,15]

11. Answer: D

Inadvertent intravascular administration is the most common cause of local anaesthetic systemic toxicity. This can occur infrequently during regional nerve blocks. In addition, systemic toxicity may occur in susceptible individuals such as patients with cardiac ischaemia, conduction abnormalities or heart failure, during intravenous or intraarterial administration at therapeutic doses. **CNS symptoms generally precede cardiovascular effects in toxicity. If a patient develops any neurological symptom during or shortly after local anaesthetic administration, the patient should be closely monitored for development of cardiovascular toxicity-bradycardia or other cardiac arrhythmias, hypotension, cardiovascular collapse and asystolic cardiac arrest.** Bupivacaine is highly cardiotoxic therefore close attention is required during its use. Methaemoglobinaemia may occur following administration of lignocaine or prilocaine and is not dose related. Children are more susceptible to develop methaemoglobinaemia than adults after both local and topical administration.[16]

12. Answer: A

ILE is a preparation used in parenteral nutrition and is currently being investigated as an antidote for toxicity secondary to highly lipid soluble drugs. **The current recommendation for the use of ILE is for cardiovascular collapse or cardiac arrest secondary to local anaesthetic toxicity once adequate resuscitative measures have been initiated.** It may also be considered in cardiac arrest refractory to standard resuscitative measures due to toxicity from highly lipid-soluble beta blockers and CCBs (such as propranolol and verapamil) and tricyclic antidepressants. Other beta-blockers and CCBs are not lipid soluble and therefore ILE is not indicated. The described mechanism of action for ILE is the formation of 'a lipid sink' where the intravascular lipid phase created by ILE sequester lipophilic toxins results in a reduction of the toxin concentration at the binding site.[16–19]

13. Answer: C

This patient has signs and symptoms consistent with anticholinergic syndrome. Common signs and symptoms of anticholinergic effects can be remembered with the mnemonic: *Red as a beet, dry as a bone, blind as a bat, mad as a hatter, and hot as a hare*.

The mnemonic refers to the symptoms of flushing, dry skin and mucous membranes, mydriasis with loss of accommodation, altered mental status (AMS) and fever or hyperthermia, respectively. Tachycardia and urinary retention are present.

All drugs mentioned, except digoxin, can lead to anticholinergic effects in overdose. Digoxin causes bradyarrhythmias, hypotension, nausea, vomiting and lethargy.[20]

14. Answer: C

The most common ECG finding in tricyclic antidepressant (TCA) poisoning is *sinus tachycardia*, usually due to peripheral anticholinergic effects. TCAs block fast sodium channels in the myocardium and slow phase 0 depolarisation of the action potential. Subsequently, ventricular depolarisation is delayed, which leads to a *prolonged QRS duration*.

QRS complexes of more than 160 ms (four small squares) have a 50% chance of developing ventricular arrhythmias, whereas a QRS duration >100 ms (2.5 small squares on ECG), is associated with an increased risk of seizures.

Additionally, TCAs affect the right fascicle of the heart leading to *right axis deviation.* A large R wave in lead aVR is a highly sensitive screening tool for tricyclic antidepressant exposure. Furthermore, a high amplitude of this R wave has been associated with an increased risk of toxic effects. **Data suggest that the finding of a large R wave in lead aVR may be even more predictive of seizure and arrhythmia than prolongation of the QRS complex.** Liebelt *et al* found that an R wave of more than 3 mm in lead aVR was 81% sensitive and 73% specific for the development of seizures and arrhythmias.[21,22]

Other ECG changes associated with TCA poisoning include:
- prolongation of the PR and QT intervals
- atrioventricular (AV) blocks
- ventricular ectopy
- nonspecific ST-T changes
- the Brugada pattern, including right bundle branch block (RBBB) and a downsloping ST segment elevation in leads V1–V3.

15. Answer: B

Venlafaxine and desvenlafaxine are selective serotonin and noradrenaline reuptake inhibitors (SNRI). **Seizures occur in 14% of patients with venlafaxine overdose but occur in <4% in SSRI overdose and are mainly associated with citalopram**. Importantly, the onset of seizures may be delayed for up to 16 hours following overdose of venlafaxine. Therefore, all patients must be observed for at least 16 hours after ingestion with intravenous access in place. The risk of seizures is important to recognise in venlafaxine overdose. The patient who is at a high risk for seizures is anxious, sweaty, tremulous, tachycardic with mydriatic pupils and has clonus. Such patients should be prophylactically treated with intravenous benzodiazepines to control their tachycardia and this generally prevents seizures.

Cardiovascular toxicity is not common with either agent. Citalopram and escitalopram may cause dose dependent QT prolongation but torsades de pointes is rare. Minor dose-dependent QRS and QT prolongation may occur with venlafaxine overdose but seldom causes dysrhythmias. However, ingestion of very large doses (>7 g) of venlafaxine, may cause cardiovascular toxicity with hypotension and cardiac arrhythmias.

Mild serotonin syndrome may develop in some patients after a SSRI overdose. **In both SSRI and venlafaxine overdose, severe serotonin syndrome occurs only if coingested with other serotonergic drugs.**

Irrespective of the dose taken, the overdose of SSRI is usually not life threatening, whereas overdose with venlafaxine may be life threatening and is usually dose dependent.[23,24]

16. Answer: B

Serotonin syndrome is a toxic state caused mainly by excess serotonin (5HT) within the CNS, causing excessive stimulation of serotonergic receptors. It results in a variety of mental, autonomic and neuromuscular changes, which can range in severity from mild to life threatening. Most cases are self-limiting. Severe serotonin syndrome is nearly always caused by a drug interaction involving two or more 'serotonergic' drugs, at least one of which is usually a SSRI or monoamine oxidase inhibitor (MAO). Management involves withdrawal of the offending drugs, aggressive supportive care and occasional use of serotonin antagonists such as cyproheptadine. Treatment of the condition for which the serotonergic drugs were prescribed should be reviewed.

Numerous drugs are implicated in the development of serotonin syndrome, of which the most important ones are:
- antidepressants
  - SSRI: citalopram, escitalopram, fluoxetine
  - SNRI: venlafaxine
  - TCA
  - MAO-inhibitors: moclobemide
- analgesics: tramadol, fentanyl, pethidine
- drugs of abuse: amphetamines, MDMA (ecstasy), tryptophan.

Although it is possible for levodopa to cause serotonin syndrome, as it releases 5HT from stored vesicles, it is more commonly associated with neuroleptic malignant syndrome.[25–28]

17. Answer: D

The hallmark feature of acute lithium toxicity is acute gastrointestinal symptoms including vomiting and diarrhoea, leading to significant fluid losses. The hallmark feature of chronic toxicity is neurotoxicity, which may lead to permanent neurological damage. Acute toxicity is typically due to deliberate overdose, whereas chronic toxicity typically occurs in patients who are on chronic lithium therapy when renal excretion of lithium is impaired. Although rare, a delayed onset of neurotoxicity may occur in acute toxicity if renal functions are impaired due to any cause, including significant fluid losses. In chronic toxicity the neurological symptoms can progress from tremor, hyperreflexia, weakness and ataxia to agitation, muscle rigidity and hypertonia. In severe neurotoxicity altered level of consciousness, convulsions and coma may occur.

In chronic toxicity serum lithium levels do not correlate well with the clinical severity. However, when an unwell patient who is on lithium presents to the ED, serum lithium level should be done as this may aid in early diagnosis. In both toxicities serum lithium levels are important to confirm the diagnosis and to monitor the progress of treatment. The neurological symptoms may persist even after the lithium level returns to normal.

The mainstay of treatment in acute toxicity is fluid resuscitation and maintaining hydration to

achieve normal renal function with good urine output and normal electrolyte balance. This enhances lithium excretion from the body. Similarly, in chronic toxicity it is important to maintain good hydration and renal function to enhance renal lithium excretion. However, enhanced elimination with haemodialysis may be necessary in the face of neurotoxicity and established renal failure.

Cardiac monitoring is not indicated in lithium toxicity unless for other reasons including coingestants.[29,30]

18. Answer: C

The threshold single dose of paracetamol ingestion that could produce hepatotoxicity is variable both in adults and children, but is considered as 150 mg/kg in adults and 200 mg/kg in children. The risk of hepatotoxicity from a single acute ingestion when untreated is predictable when a serum paracetamol level obtained 4–15 hours from the time of ingestion is plotted on the Rumack-Matthew nomogram. When this level is >300 mg/L at 4 hours the probability of hepatotoxicity reaches 90% when not treated.

Hepatotoxicity is defined if the peak AST or ALT exceeds 1000 IU/L. With toxic serum paracetamol levels due to single ingestions, the probability of hepatotoxicity depends on the time taken to commence NAC from the time of ingestion. If the time of commencement of NAC is within 8 hours, 100% survival can be expected. The benefits are reduced when NAC is commenced 8–24 hours from the time of single ingestion. Usually there is no demonstrable benefit when NAC is commenced >24 hours later.

In a patient who presents >8 hours from the time of a single ingestion, a toxic paracetamol level together with elevated hepatic transaminase levels indicate early hepatotoxicity. When a patient presents >24 hours from the time of a single ingestion, if the serum paracetamol level is normal and has normal transaminases, the risk of developing hepatotoxicity is minimal.

A child <8 years of age who has accidentally taken <200 mg/kg of paracetamol as a single dose or over a period of 8 hours does not require decontamination or serum paracetamol or liver function tests done.[31,32]

19. Answer: B

NAC is the intravenous sulfhydryl donor used in paracetamol toxicity in Australasia. It protects against paracetamol-induced hepatotoxicity. It is given as three infusions of fixed duration over a 20-hour period and this duration can be extended further in relevant patients. The contraindications for the antidote are almost non-existent. It can be used in a pregnant woman with paracetamol toxicity. It should be started immediately without waiting for serum paracetamol results for any patient who had taken a toxic dose (>150 mg/kg for an adult) and presenting >8 hours later. Beyond the usual 20-hour infusion, NAC should be continued in patients:

- who have evidence of hepatotoxicity as shown by the ALT and/or AST rise
- in late presenters
- in patients who had taken paracetamol at supratherapeutic doses repeatedly.

The incidence of mild anaphylactoid reaction is 10–50% and usually occurs during the initial infusion or shortly after that. The typical symptoms are flushing, rash, mild hypotension and angioedema at times and should be treated accordingly. If the patient gets severe symptoms the NAC infusion can be ceased temporarily until symptoms resolve and it should be restarted early when the patient is stable.[32,33]

20. Answer: D

In large ingestions of aspirin, as well as with enteric-coated tablets, delayed absorption may occur mainly due to bezoar formation in the stomach and the intestine. If the serum salicylate level is rising after the initial dose of activated charcoal a second dose is indicated after a few hours.

These patients typically have a mixed metabolic acidosis and respiratory alkalosis. Alkalaemia should be maintained to prevent salicylate from entering the CNS because it increases ionisation of aspirin. Urinary alkalinisation increases the renal excretion of aspirin.

For the abovementioned reason, even after intubation alkalaemia should be maintained with hyperventilation. Ventilatory settings should not be adjusted to correct this alkalaemia. Lack of meticulous attention to maintain alkalaemia can be catastrophic to the patient.

Aspirin has a low volume of distribution (it is distributed mainly in the intravascular compartment), low protein binding, a low molecular weight and high water solubility, and therefore it can be eliminated with HD. Patients should be considered for HD after intubation if the indication for intubation is severe salicylate toxicity and not coingestants.[34,35]

21. Answer: D

Predictors of potentially lethal acute digoxin toxicity are:

- total dose ingested >10 mg in an adult (in a child >4 mg)
- serum potassium >5.5 mmol/L (predicts >100% mortality without treatment)
- serum digoxin level >15 nmol/L (>12 ng/mL).

Any hyperkalaemia is significant in acute digoxin toxicity and is an indication for the use of digoxin immune Fab as a temporising measure. Temporising options for hyperkalaemia treatment, while awaiting Fab, are sodium bicarbonate intravenously as a bolus and insulin-dextrose treatment. When treating severe hyperkalaemia in acute digoxin toxicity, calcium gluconate should not be used as a membrane stabiliser as it may worsen the cardiotoxicity.

Some patients may have taken digoxin with other cardiotoxic drugs or the initial history of the digoxin overdose may not have been available. In such patients a therapeutic trial of digoxin immune Fab may be helpful.

Serum digoxin levels are not clinically valuable after the patient had digoxin immune Fab as laboratories typically measure both bound and unbound digoxin resulting in very high serum levels.[36]

22. Answer: A

Digoxin immune Fab is a life-saving antidote in both acute and chronic digoxin toxicity. They are fragments of IgG antibody molecules against digoxin produced in sheep. These molecules bind directly to intravascular and interstitial digoxin and 1 ampoule of Fab binds 0.5 mg of digoxin. **The appropriate Fab dose can be calculated using the ingested dose of digoxin in acute toxicity or steady state serum digoxin level in chronic toxicity.** However, in clinical practice empiric doses are often used in suspected patients.

Suggested empiric doses in acute toxicity are:

- 5 ampoules for a haemodynamically stable patient
- 10 ampoules for an unstable patient
- 20 ampoules can be used in cardiac arrest

Then, repeat 5 ampoules every 30 minutes until the reversal of toxicity.

The suggested empiric dose in chronic toxicity is 2 ampoules initially. Then, repeat 2 ampoules every 30 minutes until the reversal of toxicity. Five ampoule can be administered in a cardiac arrest.

Treatment of patients with chronic digoxin toxicity with non-life-threatening features with immune Fab is cost effective. Non-life-threatening cardiac arrhythmias and moderate–severe gastrointestinal symptoms should be treated, especially in patients with renal impairment.

The end points of treatment in any situation are the return of normal cardiac conduction and rhythm and resolution of gastrointestinal symptoms.[37]

23. Answer: D

Severe toxicity secondary to CCB drug ingestion is due to:

- blockade and delays in the cardiac conduction system
- loss of myocardial contractility
- loss of vascular smooth muscle tone.

These result in hypotension and bradydysrhythmias with profound cardiovascular collapse.

The non-dihydropyridine CCBs are verapamil and diltiazem. Verapamil has moderate effects on both cardiac conduction and vascular smooth muscle tone in therapeutic dosage. These effects are exaggerated in toxic dosages of verapamil, especially in toddlers, with resultant hypotension and bradydysrhythmias. Additionally, verapamil is the most potent negative inotropic of all CCB, and causes equal depression of heart contraction and vascular smooth muscle dilation at any concentration with subsequent profound hypotension. In children, initially there may not be any specific clinical features that could indicate severe toxicity. The most common clinical effect is altered mental status.

The dihydropyridine CCBs include nifedipine, amlodipine, felodipine and the most newer agents. They bind more selectively to vascular smooth muscle calcium channels than to cardiac calcium channels. Therefore, in mild to moderate overdoses these CCBs can cause reflex tachycardia secondary to relative hypotension caused by the lax vascular smooth muscle. This is not a feature in severe toxicity and these agents may cause complete heart block, depressed myocardial contractility and vasodilation, which ultimately results in cardiovascular collapse.

Severe CCB toxicity may lead to hyperglycaemia because a reduced release of insulin from pancreatic islet cells.[15,38]

24. Answer: A

Isolated overdose with a beta-blocker, except sotalol and propranolol, causes minimal or no toxicity in most healthy adults. The risk of toxicity is increased in patients with underlying cardiovascular disease, those who take other potential cardiotoxic drugs and in the elderly.

Overdoses with sotalol and propranolol are serious and potentially harmful to adults. Similarly, the risk of toxicity is high if even 1–2 tablets of sotalol or propranolol are taken by a child, whereas this risk seems to be minimal in children ingesting other beta-blockers.

The onset of features of toxicity usually occurs early within a few hours unless due to sustained release formulations. **PR interval prolongation on ECG with or without bradycardia is the earliest sign of toxicity.**[39]

25. Answer: C

Sotalol toxicity can cause QT prolongation leading to polymorphic VT (torsades de pointes). Patients who manifest torsades de pointes can be treated with intravenous magnesium initially and then be started on an isoprenaline infusion. Patients who do not respond to the above will require overdrive pacing.

Bradyarrhythmias, including sinus bradycardia, junctional rhythms and all heart blocks, and hypotension are the other significant cardiovascular issues. An initial fluid load is important in these patients. Atropine can be used as a temporising measure for bradycardia. Isoprenaline or adrenaline intravenous infusion should be considered for persistent bradycardia and hypotension.

Propranolol toxicity and not sotalol toxicity causes QRS widening (similar to tricyclic overdose) therefore will require NaHCO$_3$ to control ventricular arrhythmias. Additionally, Propranolol toxic patients often require early intubation and ventilation, whereas this is a less likely scenario in sotalol overdose.[39]

26. Answer: C

In severe CCB toxicity sudden cardiovascular collapse with cardiac arrest may occur in a patient who becomes shocked with bradycardia and hypotension. A shocked patient can soon be resistant to all treatments such as atropine, intravenous calcium, inotropes, vasopressors and cardiac pacing. **Therefore early consideration for initiation of HIET is now being advocated for severe CCB toxicity.** This is supported by more than 70 case reports of the use of this treatment.

HIET seems to help overcome the metabolic derangement, that is, the metabolic starvation state affecting the heart in severe CCB toxicity. Insulin enhances myocardial contractility, causing positive inotropy. However, insulin does not have any chronotropic activity and may cause vasodilation and therefore it may be best used with inotropes in severe toxicity.

HIET has been described as a safe treatment option with predictable and easily correctible adverse effects that may include hypoglycaemia, hypokalaemia, hypomagnesaemia and hypophosphataemia. The early detection of these potential adverse effects is important. Hypoglycaemia has been reported in only 16% of the published cases. As severe CCB toxicity may cause hyperglycaemia, in some patients hypoglycaemia may not occur despite high doses of insulin.[40]

27. Answer: C

In sulphonylurea toxicity the resultant hypoglycaemia typically occurs within 8 hours from the time of ingestion and it usually remains prolonged and severe. Hypoglycaemia is more severe in non-diabetics than in diabetics.

The specific antidote for hyperinsulinaemia induced by sulphonylurea is octreotide. Octreotide suppresses endogenous insulin release from pancreatic islet cells.

Therefore early commencement of octreotide *at the onset of hypoglycaemia* **is recommended in these patients.** Octreotide can be commenced with an appropriate IV bolus dose followed by a continuous intravenous infusion for at least 24 hours. When a patient is on an octreotide infusion normoglycaemia can usually be maintained without the necessity to have a concurrent glucose infusion.

There is no indication to commence octreotide when there is no hypoglycaemia. Therefore, there is no place for prophylactic octreotide in these patients.

Intermittent boluses of high concentrated glucose (e.g. 50% glucose 50 mL) with a background 5–10% dextrose infusion to maintain euglycaemia is not the best way to manage hypoglycaemia in these patients. **Intermittent glucose boluses stimulate endogenous insulin secretion and therefore potentially cause rebound hypoglycaemia.**[41,42]

28. Answer: C

The majority of patients remain asymptomatic following an acute overdose of thyroxine. Symptoms are not likely to occur following ingestion of <10 mg in adults and <5mg in children. The majority of patients experience mild to moderate symptoms after 2–7 days post-ingestion and therefore immediate cardiac monitoring or drug levels check in the first three days are not indicated. Clinically significant thyrotoxicosis is not reported in children after unintentional ingestion.[43]

29. Answer: A

Eucalyptus oil is a type of commonly available essential oil and is a hydrocarbon. Both ingested and inhaled hydrocarbons can cause CNS depression, coma and seizure in large overdoses. The onset of these symptoms usually occurs within 1–2 hours. Aspiration of hydrocarbons may produce a chemical pneumonitis characterised by initial coughing and subsequent tachypnoea, hypoxia, wheeze and pulmonary oedema. The initial symptoms of this may appear 4–6 hours later and gradually get worse. **Consequently gastrointestinal decontamination is contraindicated and activated charcoal does not bind hydrocarbons.** For chemical pneumonitis oxygen, bronchodilators, non-invasive ventilation (NIV) or intubation may be required. Seizure control should be achieved with intravenous benzodiazepines.

Eucalyptus or other essential oil of 10 mL or more in an adult and 5 mL or more in a child may cause severe CNS toxicity leading to rapid coma and seizures.[44]

30. Answer: B

In most acute carbon monoxide (CO) poisonings (e.g. deliberate inhalation of car exhaust fumes) reaching hospital, although the concentration of CO is high, the duration of exposure is usually limited. Consequently, the risk of development of long-term neuropsychological sequelae is low. The opposite is true for low-concentration long-duration accidental exposures in occupational or domestic situations.

In moderate to severe toxicity the patient presents more with generalised neurological features than focal features. These may include initial transient loss of consciousness, headache, nausea, visual disturbances, ataxia, confusion, seizures and coma. Ischaemic cardiac injury may occur but is uncommon.

The required duration of normobaric oxygen treatment is not well established for symptomatic patients. It is recommended that symptomatic patients receive 100% oxygen until all symptoms have resolved. The use of hyperbaric oxygen is controversial except in some high-risk patients such as pregnant women.[45,46]

31. Answer: D

Cyanide toxicity is not common. However, when it occurs, and if severe, the majority of patients die before reaching hospital. Patients who reach hospital who show signs of toxicity should be treated emergently with an antidote and provision of supportive care.

Several antidotes are commercially available but dicobalt edetate seems to be the antidote most widely available in Australia. Its efficacy has not been established in cyanide poisoning. There should be definitive clinical evidence of cyanide poisoning including worsening metabolic acidosis (due to lactic acidosis) or impaired consciousness present when administering dicobalt edetate. If administered to a patient without cyanide poisoning it can cause serious direct toxic effects including hypotension, convulsions and oedema of the face and larynx.

Intravenous hydroxycobalamin (vitamin B12) has more evidence for efficacy than other antidotes. It causes minimal adverse effects. **Hydroxycobalamin is recommended as the first-line therapy in severely poisoned patients and for a patient in cardiac arrest due to suspected cyanide toxicity.** The recommended dose is 5 mg over 15 minutes with repeat dosing up to 15 mg. Hydroxycobalamin is expensive and may not be available widely in EDs.

Sodium thiosulphate is effective in the treatment of mild to moderately poisoned patients and also as a diagnostic trial in suspected cases. Its efficacy has not been proven and as a second line treatment should be used with other cyanide antidotes in severe cases.[47–52]

32. Answer: B

Widely used household products contain corrosive substances that may result in injury to young children because of poor storage practices. Among those household substances, oven and drain cleaners (potassium hydroxide and sodium hydroxide) have high potential to cause mucosal burns. Household bleaches are relatively safe and generally cause minor injury. Dishwashing powders and tablets are highly alkaline and cause immediate burns. This may be due to the prolonged surface contact expected form powders and tablets.

The absence of oral burns does not exclude oesophageal and gastric burns and therefore does not predict a good outcome. Endoscopy provides the best guide in assessing the early risk of perforation and late sequelae of corrosive burns. About 10–15% of patients with oesophageal burns have no oropharyngeal burns. When there are oral burns one-third of patients have oesophageal burns. Alkalis tend to cause more oesophageal burns than acids do. Acids tend to cause gastric burns.

All symptomatic children should be kept nil by mouth until endoscopic assessment. In children with relatively limited symptoms attempts at neutralisation should be avoided but dilution of corrosive with drinking water is acceptable, especially for acids.[53–54]

33. Answer: B

Serious toxicity after ingestion of concentrated H_2O_2 solutions (>10%) is associated with:
- direct corrosive injury
- systemic gas embolism
- distension of hollow viscera.

The latter two being the consequence of the release of O_2 gas.

The direct corrosive injury to the gastrointestinal tract can cause ulceration of oral mucosa, vomiting, haematemesis and melaena. Also laryngeal oedema and laryngospasm may lead to respiratory distress and airway obstruction. Early airway management is essential in these patients.

Rapid deterioration of neurological function and seizures often occur due to venous and arterial gas embolisation. Features of massive distension of hollow viscera due to liberation of large volumes of gas will be evident.

Direct damage to the eye occurs when it is directly exposed to H_2O_2. Visual disturbances and blindness is not a feature of hydrogen peroxide ingestion.[55]

34. Answer: B

Organophosphates inhibit acetylcholinesterase, leading to increased acetylcholine levels at cholinergic receptors (both muscarinic and nicotinic).

Along with bradycardia, the muscarinic effects of acetylcholine excess can be remembered by the following mnemonic.

DUMBBELS

Diarrhoea

Urination

Miosis

Bronchorrhoea

Bronchospasm

Emesis

Lacrimation

Salivation

The nicotinic effects are:
- muscle fasciculation
- tremor
- muscle weakness
- paralysis
- tachycardia

Atropine is the antidote used as a muscarinic antagonist. It does not act on the nicotinic receptors and therefore there is no improvement of muscle weakness with atropine.

In organophosphate poisoning large doses (up to 100 mg) of atropine may be required. The recommended regime is atropine 1.2 mg IV initially as a bolus, doubling the dose every 5 minutes. **The end points of treatment with atropine are drying of airway and oral secretions, resolution of bradycardia and achieving good air entry with resolution of bronchospasm.** Fully dilated pupils means excessive anticholinergic toxicity due to over administration of atropine and along with this other anticholinergic toxic features may be found. No further atropine should be administered while these toxic features are present.[56–57]

35. Answer: C

The list of drugs that could cause severe cardiotoxicity leading to cardiac arrest is not exhaustive. **Cardiac sodium, potassium and calcium channel blockers and beta-blockers are among the major groups of drugs that cause cardiac arrest in a poisoned patient.** Advanced life support guidelines applied to a poisoned patient who is in a cardiac arrest are similar to that applied to other patients who are in cardiac arrest. Treatment with specific antidotes in adequate doses should be considered very early. However, the clinical effectiveness of antidotes has not been verified with high level evidence. CPR should be continued for a prolonged period, sometimes up to 4 hours, until the cardiac toxicity of the drug dissipates and the patient recovers. Timely and adequate CPR although prolonged does not seem to adversely affect the neurological outcome in these poisoned patients.[58]

36. Answer: A

Button batteries lodged in the oesophagus, nose and the ears should be removed urgently, ideally within 6 hours. A button battery >1.5 cm diameter is likely to become lodged in the oesophagus of a young child when ingested. If lodged for sufficient time it can cause severe local burns to the mucosa and acute perforation and haemorrhage.

Most children are asymptomatic at presentation or they may develop symptoms related to oesophageal burns (e.g. pain and dysphagia) early. In some the symptoms can be delayed for several days. **If suspicious of ingestion of a button battery, all children should be assessed with plain chest and abdominal films to confirm or exclude the diagnosis and to locate the battery**. If it is lodged above the diaphragm, the child should be referred for urgent endoscopic removal and inspection of the oesophagus for injury to be done within 6 hours from the time of ingestion. Carbonated drinks should not be tried. An asymptomatic child with a button battery located below the diaphragm but within the stomach can be managed expectantly. Plain X-ray should be repeated in 24 hours to ensure the battery has passed the pylorus. If it has not passed the pylorus, especially if it is a larger battery, it may require endoscopic removal. Once the battery passes the pylorus it is less likely to cause complications and

close follow up with repeat X-ray is not generally indicated.[59-60]

37. Answer: B

Classically, five overlapping stages of iron toxicity are described. **However, clinically, iron toxicity can be described as gastrointestinal toxicity (mainly due to direct corrosive effects) and systemic toxicity.**

The dose of elemental iron accidentally ingested by young children is often not large enough to cause systemic toxicity. They frequently present asymptomatically. A further small number may present with gastrointestinal symptoms. It is important to calculate the possible amount of elemental iron ingested.

- If this is <20 mg/kg, no intervention is required and child can be discharged.
- 20–60 mg/kg of elemental iron is likely to cause gastrointestinal symptoms but not systemic toxicity.
- Systemic toxicity is caused by >60 mg/kg elemental iron dose.

In addition to calculating the possible ingested elemental iron dose, abdominal X-ray may help to quantify the ingested amount, especially when the child has taken iron tablets, which are usually radio-opaque. Systemic toxicity is unlikely to occur in the absence of gastrointestinal toxicity (e.g. vomiting, diarrhoea, abdominal pain). In the assessment of evidence for systemic toxicity, the following can be considered in the context of child's clinical symptoms:

- Serum iron level 4–6 hours from the time of ingestion (peak level): >90 micromol/L (500 microgram/dL) predicts systemic toxicity. The level should be repeated if a sustained release preparation has been taken.
- Arterial or venous blood gas: a high AG metabolic acidosis due to lactic acidosis.
- Falling venous bicarbonate level: this can be used as a surrogate when serum iron levels are not readily available.

Iron toxicity occurs when serum iron exceeds the total iron binding capacity (TIBC) by saturating transferrin and ferritin. However, TIBC measurements are not valuable in the assessment of systemic toxicity.[61-62]

38. Answer: A

Acquired methaemoglobinaemia is a well-recognised toxicity syndrome secondary to accidental or deliberate exposure to drugs and toxins that act as oxidisers of iron in the haem moiety of haemoglobin from the ferrous (Fe^{2+}) to ferric (Fe^{3+}) form. Generally local anaesthetics, nitrates and nitrites, dapsone, rifampicin and sulfa drugs and some Asian food additives are implicated. Methaemoglobinaemia can be caused by recreational exposure to amyl nitrite and other alkyl nitrites contained in air fresheners and video head cleaners ('poppers'). Methaemoglobin is unable to bind oxygen therefore the oxygen-carrying capacity of the blood is significantly reduced with left shifting of oxygen dissociation curve. This results in tissue hypoxia.

In the ED, methaemoglobinaemia is a clinical diagnosis based on a suggestive clinical history and the examination findings, supported by arterial blood gas (ABG) results. A grey-blue discoloration of the skin is typical while blood drawn for investigations shows a chocolate-brown discoloration. However, this blood does not become red with exposure to oxygen or air.

Methaemoglobin interferes with pulse oximetry readings and these should be interpreted with caution as the pulse oximeter will report a falsely elevated value while patient remains severely hypoxic. Methaemoglobin is able to absorb light at both 660 and 940 nm wavelengths, similar to oxyhaemoglobin. This false absorption of light by methaemoglobin plateaus oxygen saturation on pulse oxymeter around 85%. Therefore, the patient may be severely hypoxic with severe methaemoglobinaemia but pulse oximetry may remain around 85%.

Similarly, the calculated arterial oxygen saturation (SaO_2) obtained by a blood gas analyser will produce a falsely elevated result as the blood gas analyser uses the partial pressure of oxygen for the calculation. The partial pressure of oxygen is a measure of dissolved, not bound oxygen, and remains normal. In summary, the SaO_2 obtained with ABG remains very high and pulse oximetry reading may remain at 85% in severe methaemoglobaemia creating an *increased oxygen saturation gap*.

Definitive identification of methaemoglobin requires co-oximetry, which is capable of differentiating between oxyhemoglobin, deoxyhemoglobin, carboxyhemoglobin and methemoglobin.

Methylene blue is the recommended antidote that acts as a reducing agent. NAC has been investigated for use as a reducing agent in methaemoglobinaemia but has given conflicting results. Exchange transfusion and hyperbaric oxygen as other potentially beneficial treatment options may be considered in life-threatening toxicity.[63–65]

39. Answer: A

Body packers ('swallowers' or 'mules') are people who illegally carry drugs, mostly cocaine, heroin, amphetamines and MDMA, concealed within their bodies. The packets are made of various materials, but most often are from condoms, balloons and plastic. A single person may carry up to 100 small packets containing life-threatening quantities of the drug. The body packer swallows these packets and uses constipating agents to slow the transit time of the packets through the intestine. After entering the country of destination, body packers use laxatives, cathartics or enemas to help pass their cargo rectally. Body packers usually present to EDs with drug-induced toxic effects (due to rupture of packets releasing a potentially lethal quantity of drugs), intestinal obstruction or for medical assessment after detention or arrest. Contrast CT scan of the abdomen is considered the investigation of choice in suspected cases. Urine toxicology, if positive, indicates the need for further investigation. Plain abdominal X-ray may indicate the presence of multiple packets in the intestine and is reported to be sensitive. However, neither negative urine toxicology nor abdominal X-ray can exclude the diagnosis.[66–68]

40. Answer: D

One of the earliest manifestations of envenoming in a patient bitten by a brown snake is early collapse or syncope, often with subsequent recovery until the onset of other features. A positive SVDK test for brown snake venom does not indicate systemic envenoming; however, this helps in choosing the correct monovalent antivenom if the patient develops clinical features of envenoming. Although brown snake venom contains a presynaptic neurotoxin, significant neurological manifestations do not occur when envenomed.[69]

41. Answer: B

Brown snake venom contains potent procoagulants, cardiotoxins and presynaptic neurotoxins. VICC is the hallmark of brown snake envenoming and can cause death due to uncontrolled haemorrhage. The onset is usually early after the bite and presents as bleeding from the gums and venepuncture sites, as well as intracerebral haemorrhage. **The INR and D-dimer are elevated in VICC, whereas fibrinogen is consumed and its levels are almost undetectable.**

In addition to VICC envenomed patients may have thrombocytopenia and microangiopathic haemolytic anaemia. Apart from brown snake envenoming, tiger snake and taipan envenoming are also likely to cause VICC.[69]

42. Answer: D

Important species of black snakes such as the mulga snake cause myotoxin-induced rhabdomyolysis leading to generalised myalgia, weakness, elevated creatine kinase (CK), myoglobinuria and renal failure. Although venom of these snakes contains anticoagulants (not procoagulants), these anticoagulants do not generally cause significant clinical problems or abnormalities of the coagulation profile. Bites from red-bellied and blue-bellied black snakes rarely cause significant systemic envenoming features. Minor myolysis may occur but features of paralysis or coagulopathy do not.

Clinical features due to neurotoxicity and rhabdomyolysis are uncommon with brown snake envenoming, whereas these features are more prominent with taipan and tiger snake envenoming.

Tiger snake envenoming causes VICC similar to brown snake envenoming. In addition to procoagulants, the venom also contains pre- and postsynaptic neurotoxins and myolysins. In contrast to brown snake envenoming, neurotoxicity and rhabdomyolysis are prominent features and usually develop over the ensuing hours.[69-72]

43. Answer: B

In an envenomed patient the choice of antivenom depends on patient's clinical symptoms, the laboratory results, the SVDK test result (which indicates the genus of the snake involved), and knowledge of distribution of snakes in the geographical location.

Monovalent antivenom is the preferred type of antivenom as it significantly reduces the protein load given to a patient. A single ampoule of polyvalent antivenom contains one ampoule from each of the monovalent antivenom available. The indications for use of polyvalent antivenom include the following:

- When there are clinical features of severe life-threatening envenoming and the SVDK result is not immediately available.
- Mixing three or more monovalent antivenom is required to cover all the possible snakes found in the geographical location.
- SVDK cannot be done.

The rate of anaphylaxis and anaphylactoid reactions is 1% for monovalent antivenom and 5% for polyvalent antivenom. As this prevalence is low, prophylactic treatment is not required irrespective of the type of antivenom used.

There is a risk of developing serum sickness from both types of antivenom.[73]

44. Answer: B

Redback spider antivenom is indicated in cases of redback spider bite with refractory local pain or with features of systemic envenoming. These features include:

- initial local pain becoming regional or generalised
- autonomic dysfunction with local or generalised sweating
- tachycardia
- mild hypertension.

The antivenom can also be trialed in patients who had a suspected redback spider bite when that diagnosis is uncertain. Pregnancy is not a contraindication. Children receive the same dose as adults as reversal of venom is the principle of treatment. The antivenom dose does not depend on the age of the patient. However, when using antivenom on children the volume needed to dilute may need to be adjusted. Antivenom can be given intravenously as a diluted preparation with close monitoring. It is equally effective intramuscularly when given undiluted.

Acute allergic reactions are uncommon and occur more frequently with intravenous than intramuscular administration. When such a reaction does occur the antivenom infusion should immediately be stopped, oxygen and fluids given, and if needed, IM adrenaline administered. The antivenom infusion may be recommenced cautiously when the clinical manifestations are controlled. Rarely, it might be necessary to administer an ongoing adrenaline infusion to complete the antivenom administration.[74,75]

45. Answer: A

Patients often give a history of witnessing a painful bite by a big black spider with large fangs. Local erythema and swelling are not features of funnel-web spider bite. Funnel-web spider bite is potentially life threatening. Severe envenoming features rapidly develop within 30 minutes to two hours. Clinical features include:

- general: agitation, vomiting, headache and abdominal pain
- autonomic: sweating, salivation
- cardiovascular: tachy- or bradycardia, hypo- or hypertension, pulmonary oedema
- neurological: paraesthesia, fasciculation, muscle spasm, coma.

Young children may present with inconsolable crying and vomiting.[76]

46. Answer: C

The major box jellyfish, *Chironex fleckeri* (with 40 or more tentacles each of which may be up to 2 m long), is found in tropical waters of Australia, from Gladstone in Queensland to Broome in Western Australia. The major box jellyfish envenoming has caused more than 70 fatalities in Australia and children are at greater risk because the ratio of body surface area that can be in contact with the jellyfish is higher compared with their body mass. Systemic envenoming can occur within 5 minutes, causing cardiac arrest and death. The venom is mainly cardiotoxic and dermatonecrotic.

When tentacles contact bare skin the nematocytes (stinging cells) fire venom into the skin very rapidly, usually to a large area.

The clinical features of stings include:

- immediate severe localised pain
- the patient vigorously attempts to remove the tentacles from the skin (this will release more nematocytes onto the skin, making the situation worse)
- the appearance of welts within minutes in the local area of contact (later: skin blistering and necrosis)

- cardiac arrest within 5 minutes due to direct cardiotoxicity (in severe envenoming).

Treatment includes:

- removing the patient from the water and restrain to prevent removal of tentacles
- liberal use of vinegar, which will neutralise nematocytes (if vinegar is not available remove any remnants of tentacles with the pads of the fingers, which is not harmful to the first aider, and wash the area with salt water, not fresh water)
- ice pack and simple analgesia for an awake patient
- prolonged CPR for a patient with collapse and cardiac arrest
- box jellyfish antivenom
- magnesium sulphate.[77–79]

47. Answer: C

Irukandji syndrome is a clinical syndrome resulting from massive endogenous catecholamine surge secondary to envenoming by a seemingly innocuous contact with a 2 cm diameter box jellyfish called *Carukia barnesi*. This syndrome occurs in the tropical waters of northern Australia extending from Fraser Island in Queensland through northern territory waters to Broom in north-western Western Australia. Irukandji-like syndromes have been reported in tropical waters in other parts of the world. In north Queensland and north-western Australia the number of cases with Irukandji syndrome predominate over the number of cases of envenoming by the box jellyfish *C. fleckeri*. However, in the Northern Territory jellyfish envenoming is mainly by *C. fleckeri*. Only one definitive fatality has been reported in Australia.

Clinical features of Irukandji syndrome include:

- initial minor local sting lesions from relatively innocuous contact with the jellyfish
- onset of severe systemic features within minutes
- 'sense of impending doom'
- restlessness
- nausea, vomiting and diaphoresis
- severe and often cyclical pain affecting the chest, back, limbs, or generalised pain
- hypertension
- ECG abnormalities: atrial and ventricular ectopics, AV conduction abnormalities, ST elevation, T wave changes, ventricular tachycardia
- troponin elevation.

Most symptoms resolve quickly and in the majority this syndrome is not life threatening. The minority of cases develop life-threatening symptoms possibly secondary to uncontrolled hypertension:

- severe pain resistant to opioids
- acute pulmonary oedema
- transient cardiomyopathy
- cardiogenic shock
- intracerebral haemorrhage.

There is no strong evidence basis for current treatments of this syndrome. Vinegar is the recommended first aid. Intravenous opioids for severe pain, antiemetics and urgent/emergent management of severe hypertension are the mainstay of treatment. Although it is unproven, magnesium sulphate is an option in patients with severe pain that is refractory to analgesia.

There is no antivenom available for Irukandji syndrome.[80,81]

48. Answer: D

In Australia tick paralysis in humans is nearly always caused by *Ixodesholocyclus* species, which secretes a pre-synaptic toxin in its saliva. This species of ticks are confined to a narrow coastal strip along the east coast of Australia. Tick paralysis typically occurs in children <3 years of age but may occur in both older children and adults. Paralysis occurring after a tick bite is rare and careful removal of the tick as early as possible after a bite reduces this risk significantly.

The initial symptoms can be non-specific (unsteady gait and drowsiness). This may slowly progress over several days to a symmetrical ascending flaccid paralysis. Ptosis, extraocular muscle paralysis, and facial paralysis may be seen. The ascending paralysis may involve respiratory muscles causing ventilatory failure requiring ventilatory support. **The presentation of tick paralysis is initially similar to Guillain-Barré syndrome; however, in Guillain-Barré syndrome cranial nerve involvement is less common.**

This condition should be suspected in any child who presents with the above symptoms and has visited the endemic area. Another differentiating factor is finding a paralytic tick attached to the child's skin. This should be removed promptly. There is no specific treatment available and supportive care should be continued until child recovers.[82]

49. Answer: C

Acute gastrointestinal toxicity presenting as diarrhoea and vomiting occurs in most patients with mushroom poisoning. In children, a benign outcome can usually be expected following accidental ingestion. Most patients recover from gastrointestinal toxicity with good supportive care including attention to fluid losses. Although cyclopeptide hepatotoxicity is the cause of most mushroom-related deaths, it is rare in Australia and New Zealand. The **cyclopeptide hepatotoxicity should be suspected if the onset of gastrointestinal symptoms occurs more than 6 hours after the time of ingestion.** In such patients, as well as patients with prolonged symptoms, liver function tests are required.

In addition to gastrointestinal toxicity, various types of mushrooms can produce specific clinical syndromes of which cholinergic, hallucinogenic, glutaminergic, hepatotoxic and nephrotoxic syndromes are only a few.

Cardiac monitoring is not usually required in the management of affected children.[83]

50. Answer: D

Scombroid toxicity is the most common fish-related toxicity and may occur as sporadic single or multiple cases. It is caused by consumption of histamine and other biogenic amines in contaminated fish belonging to many families. The suspect mechanism is the production of histamine and other biogenic amines in the dead fish by the action of bacteria. The bacterial histidine decarboxylase is thought to act on endogenous histidine in dead fish, converting it to histamine. Cooking of fish does not prevent scombroid poisoning. The severity of symptoms seems to correlate with the amount of fish consumed and therefore the amount of histamine. Typically the onset of symptoms is within 1 hour from the time of consumption. In the majority of cases, these symptoms can be mild and self-limiting. However, in some patients, symptoms can be quite severe or life threatening, requiring emergent care.

The symptoms are:

- cutaneous: flushing, urticaria
- gastrointestinal: abdominal cramps, diarrhoea, vomiting
- respiratory: bronchospasm, respiratory distress
- vascular: angioedema, hypotension.

The syndrome can be confused with fish allergy or anaphylactic reaction. However, the treatment is similar to treatment of those conditions (i.e. with antihistamines, adrenaline, bronchodilators and intravenous fluids).[84-85]

References

1. Snook C, Handel D. Principles of elimination enhancement. In: Hadad and Winchester's clinical management of poisoning and overdose. 4th ed. Philadelphia: Saunders Elsevier 2007. p. 44–53.

2. Arias J, Borron S. Haemodialysis and haemoperfusion. In: Hadad and Winchester's clinical management of poisoning and overdose. 4th ed. Philadelphia: Saunders Elsevier 2007. p. 53–61.

3. Murray L, Daly F, Little M, et al. Toxicology handbook. 2nd ed. Enhanced elimination. Sydney: Churchill Livingstone Elsevier; 2011. p. 24–9.

4. Murray L, Daly F, Little M, et al. Toxicology handbook. 2nd ed. Metformin. Sydney: Churchill Livingstone Elsevier; 2011. p. 273–5.

5. Murray L, Daly F, Little M, et al. Toxicology handbook. 2nd ed. Gastrointestinal decontamination. Sydney: Churchill Livingstone Elsevier; 2011. p. 17–24.

6. Hack J, Hoffman R. General managemnt of poisoned patients. In: Tintinalli J, Stapczynski J, Ma O, et al, editors. Tintinalli's emergency medicine: a comprehensive study guide. 7th ed. New York: McGraw Hill Medical; 2011. p. 1187–93.

7. Proudfoot AT, Krenzelok EP, Vale JA. Position paper on urinary alkalization. J ClinTox 2004;42:1:1–26.

8. Murray L, Daly F, Little M, et al. Toxicology handbook. 2nd ed. Sodium bicarbonate. Sydney: Churchill Livingstone Elsevier; 2011. p. 224–8.

9. Murray L, Daly F, Little M, et al. Toxicology handbook. 2nd ed. Acid–base disorders. Sydney: Churchill Livingstone Elsevier 2011. p. 109–13.

10. Murray L, Daly F, Little M, et al. Toxicology handbook. 2nd ed. Oswmolality and the osmolar gap. Sydney: Churchill Livingstone Elsevier; 2011. p. 107–9.

11. Chan A, Isbister G, Kirkpatrick C, et al. Drug-induced QT prolongation and torsades de pointes: evaluation of a QT nomogram. Q J Med 2007;100:609–15.

12. Murray L, Daly F, Little M, et al. Toxicology handbook. 2nd ed. The 12 lead ECG in toxicology. Sydney: Churchill Livingstone Elsevier; 2011. p. 113–8.

13. Ahronheim J, Howland M. Geriatric principles. In: Flomenbaum N, Goldfrank L, Hoffman, et al, editors. Goldfrank's toxicological emergencies. 8th ed. New York: McGraw Hill, 2006. p. 501–8.

14. Murray L, Daly F, Little M, et al. Toxicology handbook. 2nd ed. Poisoning in children. Sydney: Churchill Livingstone Elsevier; 2011. p. 120–5.

15. Ranniger C, Roche C. Are one or two dangerous? Calcium channel blocker exposure in toddlers. J Emerg Med 2007;33(2):145–54.

16. Murray L, Daly F, Little M, et al. Toxicology handbook. 2nd ed. Local anaesthetic agents. Sydney: Churchill Livingstone Elsevier; 2011. p. 265–8.

17. Cave G, Harvey M, Graudins A. Review article: intravenous lipid emulsion as antidote: a summary of published human experience. Emerg Med Austral 2011;23:123–41.

18. Weinberg G. Intravenous lipid emulsion: why wait to save a life? Emerg Med Austral 2011;23:113–5.

19. Murray L, Daly F, Little M, et al. Toxicology handbook. 2nd ed. Intravenous lipid emulsion. Sydney: Churchill Livingstone Elsevier; 2011. p. 400–1.

20. Murray L, Daly F, Little M, et al. Toxicology handbook. 2nd ed. Anticholinergic syndrome. Sydney: Churchill Livingstone Elsevier; 2011. p. 72–6.

21. Liebelt EL, Francis PD, Woolf AD. ECG lead aVR versus QRS interval in predicting seizures and arrhythmias in acute tricyclic antidepressant toxicity. Ann Emerg Med 1995;26(2):195–201.

22. Murray L, Daly F, Little M, et al. Toxicology handbook. 2nd ed. The 12-lead ECG. Sydney: Churchill Livingstone Elsevier; 2011. p. 113–8.

23. Murray L, Daly F, Little M, et al. Toxicology handbook. 2nd ed. Selective serotonin reuptake inhibitors. Sydney: Churchill Livingstone Elsevier; 2011. p. 340–3.

24. Murray L, Daly F, Little M, et al. Toxicology handbook. 2nd ed. Venlafaxine and desvenlafaxine. Sydney: Churchill Livingstone Elsevier; 2011. p. 364–8.

25. Chan BS, Graudins A, Whyte IM, et al. Serotonin syndrome resulting from drug interactions. Med J Aust 1998;169:523–5.

26. Murray L, Daly F, Little M, et al. Toxicology handbook. 2nd ed. Serotonin syndrome. Sydney: Churchill Livingstone Elsevier; 2011. p. 66–72.

27. Mills KC, Bora KM. Atypical antidepressants, serotonin reuptake inhibitors, and serotonin syndrome. In: Tintinalli J, Stapczynski J, Ma O, et al, editors. Tintinalli's emergency medicine: a comprehensive study guide. 7th ed. New York: McGraw Hill Medical; 2011. p. 1198–203.

28. Carbone JR. The neuroleptic malignant and serotonin syndromes. Emerg Med Clin North Am 2000;18(2):317–25.

29. Murray L, Daly F, Little M, et al. Toxicology handbook. 2nd ed. Lithium: acute overdose. Sydney: Churchill Livingstone Elsevier; 2011. p. 260–3.

30. Murray L, Daly F, Little M, et al. Toxicology handbook. 2nd ed. Lithium: chronic poisoning. Sydney: Churchill Livingstone Elsevier; 2011. p. 263–5.

31. In: Murray L, Daly F, Little M, et al. Toxicology handbook. 2nd ed. Paracetamol: acute overdose. Sydney: Churchill Livingstone Elsevier; 2011. p. 302–12.

32. Daly F, Fountain J, Murray L, et al. Guidelines for the management of paracetamol poisoning in Australia and New Zealand – explanation and elaboration. Med J Austral 2008;188: 296–301.

33. Murray L, Daly F, Little M, et al. Toxicology handbook. 2nd ed. N-acetylcysteine. Sydney: Churchill Livingstone Elsevier; 2011. p. 403–6.

34. Minns A, Cantrell F, Clark R. Death due to acute salicylate intoxication despite dialysis. J Emerg Med 2011;40(5): 515–7.

35. Murray L, Daly F, Little M, et al. Toxicology handbook. 2nd ed. Salicylates. Sydney: Churchill Livingstone Elsevier; 2011. p. 336–40.

36. Murray L, Daly F, Little M, et al. Toxicology handbook. 2nd ed. Digoxin: acute overdose. Sydney: Churchill Livingstone Elsevier; 2011. p. 222–8.

37. Murray L, Daly F, Little M, et al. Toxicology handbook. 2nd ed. Digoxin immune Fab. Sydney: Churchill Livingstone Elsevier; 2011. p. 381–3.

38. Minns AB, Tomaszewski C. Calcium channel blockers. In: Tintinalli J, Stapczynski J, Ma O, et al, editors. Tintinalli's emergency medicine: a comprehensive study guide. 7th ed. New York: McGraw Hill Medical; 2011. p. 1269–73.

39. Murray L, Daly F, Little M, et al. Toxicology handbook. 2nd ed. Beta-blockers. Sydney: Churchill Livingstone Elsevier; 2011. p. 168–71.

40. Nickson C, Little M. Early use of high-dose insulin euglycaemic therapy for verapamil toxicity. Med J Austral 2009;191(6):350–2.

41. Murray L, Daly F, Little M, et al. Toxicology handbook. 2nd ed. Sulfonylureas. Sydney: Churchill Livingstone Elsevier; 2011. p. 346–8.

42. Murray L, Daly F, Little M, et al. Toxicology handbook. 2nd ed. Octrotide. Sydney: Churchill Livingstone Elsevier; 2011. p. 408–10.

43. Murray L, Daly F, Little M, et al. Toxicology handbook. 2nd ed. Thyroxine. Sydney: Churchill Livingstone Elsevier; 2011. p. 352–3.

44. Murray L, Daly F, Little M, et al. Toxicology handbook. 2nd ed. Hydrocarbons. Sydney: Churchill Livingstone Elsevier; 2011. p. 237–240.

45. Murray L, Daly F, Little M, et al. Toxicology handbook. 2nd ed. Carbon monoxide. Sydney: Churchill Livingstone Elsevier; 2011. p. 196–200.

46. Weaver L. Carbon monoxide poisoning. N Engl J Med 2009;360:1217–25.

47. Australian Resuscitation Council and New Zealand Resuscitation Council. Guideline 9.5.1 emergency management of a victim who has been poisoned. Online. Available: www. resus.org.au.

48. Braitberg G. Cyanide. In: Cameron P, Jelinek G, Kelly A, editors. Textbook of adult emergency medicine. 3rd ed. Churchill Livingston Elsevier; 2009. p. 955–8.

49. Murray L, Daly F, Little M, et al. Toxicology handbook. 2nd ed. Cyanide. Sydney: Churchill Livingstone Elsevier; 2011. p. 219–22.

50. Murray L, Daly F, Little M, et al. Toxicology handbook. 2nd ed. Dicobaltedetate. Sydney: Churchill Livingstone Elsevier; 2011. p. 379–80.

51. Murray L, Daly F, Little M, et al. Toxicology handbook. 2nd ed. Hydroxycobalamin. Sydney: Churchill Livingstone Elsevier; 2011. p. 396–8.

52. Murray L, Daly F, Little M, et al. Toxicology handbook. 2nd ed. Sodium thiosulphate. Sydney: Churchill Livingstone Elsevier; 2011. p. 422–4.

53. Gunja N, Mead H, Cheng N. Specific poisons. In: Cameron P, Jelinek G, Everitt I, et al, editors. Textbook of paediatric emergency medicine. 2nd ed. Edinburgh: Churchill Livingston Elsevier; 2012. p. 426–35.

54. Murray L, Daly F, Little M, et al. Toxicology handbook. 2nd ed. Corrosives. Sydney: Churchill Livingstone Elsevier; 2011. p. 216–9.

55. Murray L, Daly F, Little M, et al. Toxicology handbook. 2nd ed. Hydrogen peroxide. Sydney: Churchill Livingstone Elsevier; 2011. p. 244–6.

56. Murray L, Daly F, Little M, et al. Toxicology handbook. 2nd ed. Organophosphorous agents (organophosphates and carbamates). Sydney: Churchill Livingstone Elsevier; 2011. p. 298–302.

57. Murray L, Daly F, Little M, et al. Toxicology handbook. 2nd ed. Atropine. Sydney: Churchill Livingstone Elsevier; 2011. p. 372–3.

58. Gunja N, Graudins A. Management of cardiac arrest following poisoning. Emerg Med Austral 2011;23:16–22.

59. Murray L, Daly F, Little M, et al. Toxicology handbook. 2nd ed. Button batteries. Sydney: Churchill Livingstone Elsevier; 2011. p. 184–5.

60. Cameron P, Jelinek G, Everitt I, et al, editors. Textbook of paediatric emergency medicine. Ingested foreign bodies. Edinburgh: Churchill Livingston Elsevier; 2006. p. 188–90.

61. Murray L, Daly F, Little M, et al. Toxicology handbook. 2nd ed. Iron. Sydney: Churchill Livingstone Elsevier; 2011. p. 250–4.

62. Cameron P, Jelinek G, Everitt I, et al, editors. Textbook of paediatric emergency medicine. Specific poisons. Edinburgh: Churchill Livingston Elsevier; 2006. p. 500–18.

63. Wilkerson G. Getting the blues at a rock concert: a case of severe methaemoglobinaemia. Emerge Med Austral 2010;22:466–9.

64. Harvey M, Cave G, Chanwai G. Fatal methaemoglobinaemia induced by self-poisoning with sodium nitrite. Emerge Med Austral 2010;22:463–5.

65. Farmer BM, Nelson LS. Dyshemoglobinemias. In: Tintinalli J, Stapczynski J, Ma O, et al, editors. Tintinalli's emergency medicine: a comprehensive study guide. 7th ed. New York: McGraw Hill Medical; 2011. p. 1326–30.

66. Bulstrode N, Banks F, Shrotria S. The outcome of drug smuggling by 'body-packers' - the British experience. Ann R Coll Surg Engl 2002;84:358.

67. Farmer JW, Chan SB. Whole body irrigation for contraband body packers. J Clin Gastroenterol 2003;37:147–50.

68. Murray L, Daly F, Little M, et al. Toxicology handbook. 2nd ed. Body packers and stuffers. Sydney: Churchill Livingstone Elsevier; 2011. p. 104–7.

69. Murray L, Daly F, Little M, et al. Toxicology handbook. 2nd ed. Brown snake. Sydney: Churchill Livingstone Elsevier; 2011. p. 433–4.

70. Murray L, Daly F, Little M, et al. Toxicology handbook. 2nd ed. Black snake. Sydney: Churchill Livingstone Elsevier; 2011. p. 430–2.

71. Murray L, Daly F, Little M, et al. Toxicology handbook. 2nd ed. Tiger snake. Sydney: Churchill Livingstone Elsevier; 2011. p. 439–42.

72. Murray L, Daly F, Little M, et al. Toxicology handbook. 2nd ed. Taipan. Sydney: Churchill Livingstone Elsevier; 2011. p. 442–5.

73. Murray L, Daly F, Little M, et al. Toxicology handbook. 2nd ed. Approach to snakebite. Sydney: Churchill Livingstone Elsevier; 2011. p. 36–43.

74. Murray L, Daly F, Little M, et al. Toxicology handbook. 2nd ed. Redback spider. Sydney: Churchill Livingstone Elsevier; 2011. p. 459–60.

75. Murray L, Daly F, Little M, et al. Toxicology handbook. 2nd ed. CSL redback spider antivenom. Sydney: Churchill Livingstone Elsevier; 2011: 486–8.

76. Murray L, Daly F, Little M, et al. Toxicology handbook. 2nd ed. Funnel-web (big black) spider. Sydney: Churchill Livingstone Elsevier; 2011. p. 461–2.

77. Centre for Disease Control. Chironex fleckeri (box jellyfish). Centre for Disease Control. Department of Health and Families. Northern Territory Government. Online. Available: www.nt.gov.au/health.

78. Murray L, Daly F, Little M, et al. Toxicology handbook. 2nd ed. Box jellyfish (Chironexfleckeri). Sydney: Churchill Livingstone Elsevier; 2011. p. 452–4.

79. CSL. Box jellyfish antivenom. Australian CSL antivenom handbook. 2nd ed. Parkville. CSL Ltd 2001. Online. Available: www.toxinology.com.

80. Nickson C, Waugh E, Jacups S, et al. Irukandji syndrome case series From Australia's tropical Northern Territory. Ann Emerg Med 2009;54:395–403.

81. Murray L, Daly F, Little M, et al. Toxicology handbook. 2nd ed. Irukandji syndrome. Sydney: Churchill Livingstone Elsevier; 2011. p. 454–5.

82. Murray L, Daly F, Little M, et al. Toxicology handbook. 2nd ed. Ticks. Sydney: Churchill Livingstone Elsevier; 2011. p. 465–7.

83. Murray L, Daly F, Little M, et al. Toxicology handbook. 2nd ed. Approach to mushroom poisoning. Sydney: Churchill Livingstone Elsevier; 2011. p. 44–9.

84. Ward D. 'Mass allergy': Acute scombroid poisoning in a deployed Australian Defence Force health facility. Emerg Med Austral 2011;23:98–102.

85. Hall M. Something fishy: Six patients with an unusual cause of food poisoning. Emerg Med Austral 2003;15: 293–5.

1. Answer: B

Cooling is the cornerstone of good outcomes in heat-injured patients and must be done in an appropriate manner. **Studies show that the degree of organ damage correlates with the degree and duration of temperature elevation above 40°C, therefore a reasonable clinical goal is to rapidly reduce the temperature to below 40°C within 30 minutes to an hour after the start of therapy.** Cooling techniques should be stopped when the temperature reaches 38–39°C to avoid overshoot hypothermia. Lowering the body temperature to <38°C with cooling techniques is not recommended as dropping of the central temperature continues even after the technique is discontinued. This is due to a delay in the establishment of an equilibrium between the cold skin and the core. The amount of 'core afterdrop' can exceed >2°C.

Evaporative cooling is an effective and safe external cooling technique. The temperature of the water used to moisten the skin must be tepid (15°C). Warm, forced air is essential for effective evaporation and crucial to maintaining good peripheral perfusion and preventing shivering by warming the skin. If the skin temperature is reduced below 30°C, shivering will result in more heat production, and peripheral vasoconstriction will impair evaporation. In addition to cooling procedures, it is imperative that the clinician institute the judicious use of sedation and/or muscle paralysis to control agitation, suppress shivering, reduce energy expenditures, and make the patient receptive to sometimes unpleasant therapies. In general, intravenous benzodiazepines are the easiest and safest first-line drugs used for sedation.[1,2]

2. Answer: D

The main distinguishing feature between heatstroke and heat exhaustion is *central nervous system* involvement. *Hyperthermia* (>40–41°C) is another cardinal feature of heatstroke. *Anhidrosis*, due to thermoregulatory failure, was traditionally included in the definition of heatstroke; however, sweat is present in >50% of patients with heatstroke and therefore does not exclude the diagnosis of heatstroke. Patients with heat exhaustion do not manifest signs of central nervous system involvement. Additionally, their temperature may be normal or elevated but usually not >40°C. While *multiorgan dysfunction* with disseminated intravascular coagulation, acute renal failure, lactic acidosis, hypokalemia (followed by hyperkalemia later on) and rhabdomyolysis are common with heatstroke, it is unlikely to occur in heat exhaustion.

Currently, only physical methods of cooling are recommended in the management of heatstroke. **There is no role for antipyretics, either salicylates or paracetamol, in the setting of heatstroke because their efficacy depends on a normally functioning hypothalamus.** In addition, overzealous use of paracetamol could potentiate hepatic damage, and salicylates may promote bleeding tendencies.[1,2]

3. Answer: C

Osborn waves consist of an extra positive deflection, with a dome or hump configuration, at the end of the QRS complex at the R-ST junction (J point) on the ECG. They are best seen at the inferior and lateral precordial leads. These waves become more prominent as the body temperature drops and they regress gradually with rewarming. **Osborn waves are characteristic of hypothermia; however, they are not pathognomonic of hypothermia** as they are also seen in 'normothermic' patients. The differential diagnosis includes common electrocardiographic variants such as early repolarisation as well as other pathological conditions such as hypercalcaemia, Brugada syndrome, brain injury, subarachnoid haemorrhage, cardiopulmonary arrest from oversedation, and vasospastic angina. Although Osborn waves may have some arrhythmogenic implications, its arrhythmogenic potential is still unclear and not fully understood. Further studies are needed to determine the true significance of the Osborn waves under various conditions in which they can be observed.[3–8]

4. Answer: B

Onset of any symptoms during or in the hours after diving should be regarded as decompression illness

(AGE and DCS) until proven otherwise. **Distinguishing AGE from decompression sickness is difficult but differentiation between these disorders before recompression is unnecessary since recompression in a hyperbaric chamber is indicated for both.** 'Nitrogen narcosis' is due to the anaesthetic effect of nitrogen dissolved in lipid membranes; symptoms are similar to those of alcohol intoxication and occur at depth. It is immediately reversible on ascent.

The optimal position to manage an injured diver is not known but current consensus is for horizontal orientation in a position that helps care of the patient. Traditionally, the head-down position (Trendelenburg) has been advocated to reduce bubble embolisation to the brain but is not effective and can promote cerebral oedema. The diver should be prevented from sitting or standing up, to avoid bubbles redistributing from the left ventricle to the brain. One hundred percent oxygen should be provided until recompression in a hyperbaric chamber can be performed. Recompression in a hyperbaric chamber is indicated even if the diver becomes asymptomatic with normobaric oxygen therapy, otherwise many will relapse. The relapse may be more severe than the original presentation.[9–11]

5. Answer: D

Decompression illness is a clinical condition associated with barotrauma of ascent and caused by intravascular or extravascular bubbles that are formed as a result of reduction in environmental pressure (decompression). The term covers both AGE, in which alveolar gas or venous gas emboli (via cardiac shunts or via pulmonary vessels) are introduced into the arterial circulation, and DCS, which is caused by in-situ bubble formation from dissolved inert gas, mostly nitrogen. *AGE* usually occurs on ascent or soon after surfacing and is not related to depth, as it can arise after ascent from very shallow depths, nor time spent under water. *DCS* usually occurs after prolonged exposure at depth, when the dive is long enough to saturate tissues, and is uncommon at depths of <10 m.

Boyle's law states that at a constant temperature, the pressure and volume of an ideal gas are inversely related. This pressure-volume relationship is important in the aetiology of injuries due to barotrauma and

produces the volume change of bubbles in the tissues and circulation that are associated with recompression therapy. *Dalton's law* states that the total pressure exerted by a mixture of gases is the sum of the partial pressures of each gas. Therefore, the partial pressure of a given component of a gas mixture will increase as the ambient pressure increases. *Henry's law* states that at equilibrium, the quantity of a gas in a liquid is proportional to the partial pressure of the gas. These last two gas laws best explain the uptake of inert gas into tissues when breathing compressed air at depth.[9–12]

6. Answer: C

The terminology around drowning used to be very confusing. In 2002 the International Liaison Committee on Resuscitation (ILCOR) agreed on recommendations for unified drowning-related definitions and guidelines for reporting data. **The term 'drowning' now refers to a process resulting in primary respiratory impairment from submersion/immersion in a liquid medium and implies a liquid–air interface is present at the entrance of the victim's airway, preventing the victim from breathing air; the victim may die or live after the event.**

Although differences observed between freshwater and saltwater aspirations in electrolyte and fluid imbalances are frequently discussed, they are rarely of any clinical significance for people who have experienced drowning. Most patients have fluid aspiration of <4 mL/kg. Fluid aspiration of at least 11 mL/kg is required for alterations in blood volume to occur, and aspiration of more than 22 mL/kg is required before significant electrolyte changes develop. **Electrolyte abnormalities are usually minimal and transient except in prolonged arrest.** Additionally, life-threatening changes in serum electrolytes are seldom seen, regardless of the type of water.

Multiple studies have been performed to evaluate prognostication rules but a decision tool has not been successfully and consistently validated. Various factors are often associated with a poor prognosis. These include a submersion time >10 minutes, resuscitation time >15–25 minutes, time to effective life support >10 minutes, Glasgow Coma Scale (GCS) <5, and pH on presentation <7.1. **Ultimately, there are no indicators at the rescue site or in the hospital that** are absolutely reliable with respect to death or survival. Furthermore, there are no established rules or consistent algorithms regarding length of resuscitation and therefore the decision to terminate resuscitation is an individual decision made on a case-by-case basis.

The Conn and Modell classification (1980) is a useful classification of the mental status after drowning: category A – awake; category B – conscious but obtunded; and category C – comatose. This classification provides an approximate estimate of the prognosis and can guide management.[12–14]

7. Answer: D

The effects of an electrical current passing through the body are determined by several factors: the type of current, voltage, tissue resistance, current path and contact duration. In addition, the amperage of current affects the severity of injury. In Australia, the vast majority of household current is alternating current (AC) with a frequency of 50 Hz, as this is optimal for the transmission and use of electricity. As such, household current lies within the dangerous frequency range (40–150 Hz). It also spans the vulnerable period of the cardiac electrical potential, and is therefore capable of causing ventricular fibrillation. Voltage is the driving force behind the current. **Most deaths are caused by low-voltage (<1000) exposure and are usually due to ventricular fibrillation occurring at the time of exposure.** Household voltage in Australia is 240 V.

Although delayed arrhythmias are possible and predominantly seen in patients with a past medical history of cardiac disease, they are rare and usually transient in survivors. Death due to delayed arrhythmia is exceptionally rare. **Therefore, cardiac monitoring is not indicated if a patient is asymptomatic and has a normal ECG on presentation and in general can be safely discharged home.**

The most common mode of electrical shock in young children is from chewing or biting on electrical cords. Arcing of the current through the lips causes oral burns, with the oral commissure frequently involved. The burn may be full thickness, involving the mucosa, submucosa, muscle, nerves and blood vessels. Significant oedema and eschar formation follow within hours after the injury. Vascular injury to the labial artery is not immediately apparent because

of vascular spasm, thrombosis and overlying eschar. The eschar usually falls off after 2–3 weeks, being replaced by granulation tissue and scarring that may cause considerable deformity. **Severe bleeding from the labial artery occurs in up to 10% of cases when the eschar separates, usually after 5 days, but can occur up to 2 weeks after the injury.**

Prediction of injuries from a knowledge of the current path is unreliable. Children who sustain hand wounds from electrical outlet injuries with no other injury and no evidence of cardiac or neurological involvement can be discharged after local wound care is provided and their home situation deemed safe.[15–19]

8. Answer: A

Lightning causes a massive countershock to the myocardium and usually takes the form of *asystole*. Interestingly, sinus rhythm may return spontaneously due to the inherent automaticity of the heart. A secondary hypoxic cardiac arrest with deterioration to ventricular fibrillation and asytole may occur with concurrent *respiratory arrest* due to transient paralysis of the medullary respiratory centre and thoracic muscle spasm. **Immediate institution of basic CPR in the field for those in asystole prevents secondary hypoxic cardiac arrest during the interval until cardiac function resumes spontaneously. This principle of first resuscitating those who appear dead is called reverse triage.** There are reports of excellent recovery after lightening-induced cardiac arrest. Additionally, transient autonomic disturbances may cause fixed, dilated pupils with an often unconscious patient after a lightning injury and therefore should not indicate a poor prognosis or brain death after a lightening strike.

Burns due to lightning are common (up to 90%), but despite the massive energy and heat that lightning generates, its short duration and flash-over effect play a protective role. As a result, deep burns occur in only 5% of victims. Lichtenberg figures (feathering, ferns or keraunographic markings) are cutaneous marks that are considered pathognomonic of lightning, but it is unclear whether they are actual burns. They may appear immediately but more often a few hours after injury. Burns are usually superficial and heal remarkably easy.

Transient paralysis (*keraunoparalysis*) and autonomic instability causing hypertension and peripheral vasospasm have been described primarily in the context of electrical injury due to lightning. Keraunoparalysis is characterised by flaccidity and complete loss of sensation of the affected limbs. Peripheral pulses are generally impalpable and the affected limb takes on a mottled, pale, blue appearance. Keraunoparalysis is self-limiting and resolves within 1–6 hours. If it does not resolve in a few hours, other causes should be considered.[15-18]

9. Answer: A

AMS is a clinical syndrome characterised by headache, dizziness or light-headedness, gastrointestinal disturbances, and sleep disturbance. As the illness progresses, headache becomes more severe and vomiting and oliguria develop. **The onset of ataxia and altered level of consciousness heralds high-altitude cerebral oedema (HACE) and requires immediate descent and treatment.** Left untreated, severe AMS may progress to life-threatening HACE or HAPE. Graded ascent with adequate time for acclimatisation is the best prevention. Low-dose acetazolamide, at a dose of 125 mg bd, also provides effective prophylaxis against AMS.

The major predisposing factors are the rate of ascent and high sleeping altitude. It is not related to physical fitness or gender. In addition, age has little influence on susceptibility, with children being as susceptible as adults. Those older than 50 years of age tend to have less AMS.

Mild AMS is usually self-limiting and improves with an extra 12–26 hours of acclimatisation if ascent is halted. Immediate descent is warranted if symptoms worsen and low-flow oxygen should be administered if available. Acetazolamide is very helpful in speeding acclimatisation and aborting illness, especially when used early. The dosage regimen varies: 5 mg/kg/d orally in two or three divided doses is sufficient for prevention or treatment. Dexamethasone, 4 mg po/IM/IV every 6 hours is also effective and can be used as an alternative but is best reserved for cases of moderate to severe AMS.

HAPE is a non-cardiogenic pulmonary oedema associated with markedly elevated pulmonary vascular resistance and pulmonary artery pressure. Rapid and controlled descent, with administration of oxygen, is the mainstay of therapy and is sufficient in most

cases. **Nifedipine reduces pulmonary artery pressures and seems to be an effective adjunctive therapy in the treatment of HAPE, whereas dexamathasone has no proven value.** The recommended dose of nifedipine is 10–20 mg orally 6-hourly or 20–30 mg extended release 12-hourly.[6,20,21]

10. Answer: A

Characteristic and relatively predictable signs and symptoms develop when a significant proportion of the body is exposed to a high level of penetrating radiation over a short period of time; these signs and symptoms are collectively referred to as acute radiation syndrome (ARS). **The patient may initially be asymptomatic and a rapid decline in lymphocytes is one of the best early indicators of the extent of the radiation injury** and plotting it on a nomogram may help to predict the clinical course.

Four distinct phases are seen in the unfolding of ARS. **In general, the higher the dose, the shorter is the duration of each phase and the more severe are the symptoms.**

1. *Prodromal phase*: transient period of self-limiting symptoms. An autonomic nervous system response initiates gastrointestinal symptoms with nausea and vomiting, as well as anorexia and possibly diarrhoea (depending on dose) are the classic symptoms for this stage, which occur from minutes to days following exposure.

2. *Latent phase*: in this stage, the patient looks and feels generally healthy for a few hours or even up to a few weeks.

3. *Manifest illness phase*: symptoms depend on the specific syndrome and last from hours up to several months. Divided into three dose-dependant subsyndromes, in increasing order of severity.

   • Hematopoietic syndrome (dose >2 Gy)
     • prodrome within 2 days
     • latent period of 1–3 weeks, followed by
     • pancytopenia with subsequent infection and bleeding
   • Gastrointestinal syndrome (dose >6 Gy)
     • prodrome within hours
     • short latent period of <1 week, followed by
     • reappearance of gastrointestinal symptoms with severe nausea, vomiting, diarrhoea, and

abominal pain due to damage of the intestinal mucosal barrier with massive fluid losses resulting in profound volume loss, electrolyte disturbances, gastrointestinal bleeding and fulminant enterocolitis

- Cardiovascular/CNS syndrome (dose >20–30 Gy)
  - prodrome within minutes with no latent phase
  - leakage of fluid into tissue causing refractory hypotension and neurological symptoms

4. *Recovery or death.*[22–24]

References

1. Prendergast HM, Erickson TB. Procedures pertaining to hypothermia and hyperthermia. In: Roberts JR, Hedges JR, editors. Clinical procedures in emergency medicine. 5th ed. Philadelphia: Elsevier; 2009. p. 1235–58.

2. Waters TA, Al-Salamah MA. Heat emergencies. In: Tintinalli JE, Kelen GD, Stapczynski JS, editors. Emergency medicine: a comprehensive study guide. 7th ed. New York: McGraw-Hill; 2011. p. 1339–44.

3. Dutto L, Allione A, Ricca M, et al. A spiked arrowhead in severe hypothermia: the Osborn wave. BMJ case reports Published 1 Jan 2009. Online. Available: http://casereports.bmj.com/content/2009/bcr.06.2008.0141.full.

4. Alhaddad IA, Khalil M, Brown EJ. Osborn waves of hypothermia. Circulation 2000;101:e233–44.

5. Maruyama M, Kobayashi Y, Kodani E, et al. Osborn waves: history and significance. Indian Pacing and Electrophysiology Journal 2004;4(1):33–9.

6. Brookes J, Dunn R. Environmental injury. In Dunn R, Dilley S, Brookes J, editors. The emergency medicine manual. 5th ed. 2010. p. 1039–53.

7. Rogers I. Hypothermia. In: Cameron P, Jelinek G, Kelly A, editors. Textbook of adult emergency medicine. 3rd ed. Edinburgh: Elsevier; 2009. p. 852–5.

8. Bessen HA, Ngo B. Hypothermia. In: Tintinalli JE, Kelen GD, Stapczynski JS, editors. Emergency medicine: a comprehensive study guide. 7th ed. New York: McGraw-Hill; 2011. p. 1335–9.

9. Smart DR. Dysbarism. In: Cameron P, Jelinek G, Kelly A, et al, editors. Textbook of adult emergency medicine. 3rd ed. Edinburgh: Elsevier; 2009. p. 856–64

10. Snyder B, Nueman T. Dysbarism and complications of diving. In: Tintinalli JE, Kelen GD, Stapczynski JS, editors. Emergency medicine: a comprehensive study guide. 7th ed. New York: McGraw-Hill; 2011. p. 1367–71.

11. Vann RD, Butler FK, Mitchell SJ, et al. Decompression illness. Lancet 2011;377(9760):153–64.

12. Brookes J, Dunn R. Marine related injury. In: Dunn R, Dilley S, Brookes J, editors. The emergency medicine manual. 5th ed. 2010. p. 1023–38.

13. Mountain D. Drowning. In: Cameron P, Jelinek G, Kelly A, et al, editors. Textbook of adult emergency medicine. 3rd ed. Edinburgh: Elsevier; 2009. p. 872–6.

14. Rose M, Denmark TK. An evidence- based approach to the evaluation and treatment of drowning and submersion injuries. Pediatric Emerg Med Practice 2011;8(6). Online. Available: http://www.ebmedicine.net; 6 Sep 2011.

15. Koumbourlis AC. Electrical injuries. Crit Care Med 2002;30(11)(suppl.):S424–30.

16. Fatovich D. Electrical shock and lightning injury. In: Cameron P, Jelinek G, Kelly A, et al, editors. Textbook of adult emergency medicine. 3rd ed. Edinburgh: Elsevier; 2009. p. 877–81.

17. Brookes J, Dunn R. Electrical injuries. In: Dunn R, Dilley S, Brookes J, editors. The emergency medicine manual. 5th ed. 2010. p. 1055–9.

18. Fish RM. Lightning injuries. In: Tintinalli JE, Kelen GD, Stapczynski JS, editors. Emergency medicine: a comprehensive study guide. 7th ed. New York: McGraw-Hill; 2011. p. 1391–4.

19. Price TG, Cooper MA. Electrical and lightning injuries. In: Marx JA, Hockberger RS, Walls RM, editors. Rosen's emergency medicine: concepts and clinical practice. 7th ed. Philadelphia: Elsevier; 2010. p. 1893–902.

20. Rogers I, O'Brien D. Altitude illness. In: Cameron P, Jelinek G, Kelly A, et al, editors. Textbook of adult emergency medicine. 3rd ed. Edinburgh: Elsevier; 2009. p. 889–92.

21. Hackett PH, Hargrove J. High-altitude medical problems. In: Tintinalli JE, Kelen GD, Stapczynski JS, editors. Emergency medicine: a comprehensive study guide. 7th ed. New York: McGraw-Hill; 2011. p. 1404–10.

22. Catlett CL, Baker Rogers JE. Radiation injuries. In: Tintinalli JE, Kelen GD, Stapczynski JS, editors. Emergency medicine: a comprehensive study guide. 7th ed. New York: McGraw-Hill; 2011. p. 56–61.

23. Centers for Disease Control and Prevention. Radiation emergencies. Online. Available: http://www.bt.cdc.gov/radiation/pdf/arsphysicianfactsheet.pdf; 10 Sept 2011.

24. Mark PD. Radiation incidents. In: Cameron P, Jelinek G, Kelly A, et al, editors. Textbook of adult emergency medicine. 3rd ed. Edinburgh: Elsevier; 2009. p. 865–72.

1. Answer: B

The MSE begins from the moment the clinician first observes a patient and not at the start of the formal interview. The observations of mental state are important and often more revealing than a small sample of behaviour observed during the interview. The main parts of MSE are:

- behaviour
- speech
- mood
- affect
- formal thought content
- perceptual ideation
- cognition
- insight and judgement.

Under the category of speech, suicidal and homicidal ideation and deliberate self-harm thoughts and acts may be included. The symptoms you observe can be confirmed by asking relevant questions. It is best to ask open-ended questions. **Reaching a working diagnosis is an important outcome of the MSE.**

Hallucination is a perception and it occurs in the absence of a sensory stimulus. Command hallucinations are often significant because they order patients to do things. These orders can vary from reminders about simple everyday tasks to dangerous acts of violence. The commands may be directed at the patient to harm themselves or others. A patient may or may not be able to resist these command hallucinations.

Affect is related to mood. Mood is described by the patient but affect is what is observed, for example, the patient might state that his/her mood is good, but you may observe that the patient's face does not show much emotion or facial expression and it looks flat. There may be poor eye contact and diminished body language. This is described as flattened affect. This is more common in schizophrenia and more so if the illness is chronic.[1,2]

2. Answer: B

Evidence shows that one in four females suffers from depression at some time in their lives and most fall into the category of mild depression. This can be successfully treated via an outpatient clinic or the patient's general practitioner. *Diagnostic and statistical manual of mental disorders IV – text revision* (DSM-IV TR) diagnostic criteria for a major depressive episode are given below and the patient must have a total of five symptoms for at least 2 weeks and one of the symptoms must be depressed mood or loss of interest:

- depressed mood
- markedly diminished interest or pleasure in all or almost all activities
- significant (>5% body weight) weight loss or gain, or increase or decrease in appetite
- insomnia or hypersomnia
- psychomotor agitation or retardation
- fatigue or loss of energy
- feelings of worthlessness or inappropriate guilt
- diminished concentration or indecisiveness
- recurrent thoughts of death or suicide.

Most of these presentations are triggered by stressful situations and it helps to enquire about such triggers. If the patient expresses any suicidal ideation, the detailed assessment of the suicidal risk is important. If this risk is appropriately judged to be containable, starting medication is not the first priority in the ED. If antidepressant medication is started in the ED, its effects and any adverse effects cannot be followed up by the clinician. Therefore **the most important part of treatment planning that should be done in the ED is to identify a proper referral pathway.**[3]

3. Answer: C

Late-life depression is an important presentation to the ED. **Approximately 10% of adults 65 years of age or older presenting to primary care settings have clinically significant depression.** It is often masked by other chronic medical conditions and if not proactively sought it could be missed and left untreated. **Depression is often under-diagnosed in men and ethnic minorities. One reason for this is that depressive symptoms are considered as a normal part of ageing.**

Depression is common in women, in patients with chronic medical conditions, patients reporting insomnia, and in patients who have experienced stressful life events such as loss of a spouse, functional decline or social isolation. These patients often present with other problems including worsening of their existing medical illnesses. In a scenario such as that described, it is important to differentiate depression from grief. Depressive symptoms last longer than normal grief. Persistence of major depressive symptoms in a patient who experienced a loss of a loved one more than 2 months previously should increase the suspicion for this diagnosis.

If untreated, late-life depression is associated with a poor quality of life, with poor social and physical functioning, poor adherence to treatment regimes, and worsening of the medical problems. This also increases morbidity and mortality in older people including from completed suicide.

Evidence-based management strategies are:
- pharmacologic management – SSRIs are a popular choice; serotonin and noradrenaline reuptake inhibitors (SNRIs) can be used in some patients, especially those who have neuropathic pain
- psychotherapy
- exercise programs
- electroconvulsive therapy (ECT).

Overall, depression in older people is a diagnosis which should actively be considered in patients who present to the ED with suggestive symptoms. These patients should be appropriately referred to psychiatry services for management and follow-up.[4]

4. Answer: B

Approximately 2% of ED visits are due to patients with suicidal ideation. Suicidal attempts are at least 10 times more prevalent than completed suicide. One of the important factors for an emergency clinician to consider is that suicidal ideation is commonly associated with mental illness, and can successfully be treated with appropriate psychiatric interventions. In addition, many suicide attempts occur during an acute situational crisis, such as a personal loss. These acute crises are usually time-limited and may be resolvable or treatable.

Most people who attempt suicide have one or more risk factors. **Individuals with the highest risk include those with psychiatric disorders, alcohol or substance abuse, adolescents, elderly and people suffering from certain chronic illnesses (e.g. chronic painful conditions, epilepsy, Huntington's disease, cerebrovascular accident (CVA), multiple sclerosis, dementia or AIDS).** There is a high risk for completing suicide among homosexual and bisexual men.

About 70–90% of individuals who completed suicide have DSM-IV TR diagnoses, mainly Axis I diagnoses. These Axis I diagnoses include depression (60–70% of people), schizophrenia (10%), substance abuse disorders and panic disorders. Other mental health diagnoses associated with completed suicide include BPD and antisocial personality disorder. Impulsivity is described as the common reason for increased completed suicide prevalence in these Axis II diagnoses. In schizophrenia, completed suicide is especially associated with the time of their first diagnosis, as well as after recovery from an exacerbation. When a patient first becomes aware of having this severe mental illness they tend to be highly vulnerable to take their life.[5,6]

People with high intelligence have better coping strategies to deal with major stressors and therefore they are less likely to complete suicide than people who are less intelligent.

5. Answer: B

The SAD PERSONS is a quick and useful guide to detect suicidal risk in an acute setting such as the ED. This comprises:

Sex (males have a higher risk of completing suicide)

Age (<19 or >45)

Depression and hopelessness

Previous attempt or psychiatric care

Excessive alcohol or drug use

Rational thinking loss

Separated, divorced or widowed

Organised or serious attempt

No social supports

Stated future intent.

This rough guideline covers many of the high-risk issues and can be easily used in a busy setting.

Patients should be assessed in a sympathetic but direct manner using 'a graduated approach'. Assessing or estimating the suicidal risk of a patient is one of the most challenging clinical judgement situations. All information about risk factors gathered during interview with the patient and other sources should be applied to the patient's clinical presentation and its severity. **The risk factors are generally cumulative and worsen the overall risk; however, they should be evaluated against the presence of any protective factors (factors that mitigate the risk). These potential protective factors include:**

- availability of social supports (family and friends)
- availability of coping skills (ability to tolerate loss, rejection, shame, etc.)
- sense of responsibility to family
- love and care for children
- presence of reasons for living and optimism
- full-time employment
- positive therapeutic relationships.

Two of the most important predictors of suicide are *current suicidal ideation* **and** *severity of previous suicidal attempts*. This information gives valuable insights into the patient's thinking and behaviours towards suicide. Some patients do not admit to suicidal ideation. However, one way the clinician could explore this is by enquiring about the patient's future. Current suicidal ideation with clear and well-conceived plan increases risk. The information that should be gathered in suicidal risk assessment includes:

- intensity of current and recent suicidal ideation and the frequency of such thoughts
- active or passive intent of those thoughts (e.g. a patient with high intent is actively planning to kill themselves)
- the motivation to kill themselves
- any suicidal plan and the lethality of the plan (e.g. a plan with a high lethality and irreversibility makes the patient high risk)
- any preparation or rehearsal of the plan
- the patient's perception or belief about the lethality of the plan
- previous suicidal attempts and self-harm – of the patients who present to hospital after non-fatal self-poisoning or self-injury, 1–6% die by suicide within the following year
- lethality of previous attempts

- previous attempts with a low chance for rescue and discovery.[5,7,8]

6. Answer: B

BPD is a common emergency psychiatric presentation and has a load of about 15–25% in psychiatric inpatients. In primary care situations the prevalence is four times higher than in general population. BPD is the most common personality disorder and many sufferers don't seek treatment. Current evidence doesn't suggest a higher prevalence among either sex. Patients with BPD usually present for treatment after deliberate self-injury or suicidal attempts. These result in at least one ED visit every 2 years on average.

For the diagnosis of BPD, at least five of the nine criteria in the DSM-IV must be met. *Recurrent suicidal threats or acts and self-injury* **with a combination of** *strong preoccupation with expected rejection and abandonment* **are the strongest indicators. These patients feel they need to be connected to someone who they believe really cares.** This preoccupation sets unrealistic expectations and the need for continuous validation by others. The unrealistic expectations and perceived rejections or abandonments by others lead to breakdown of positive relationships.

The patient at one time perceives themselves as a 'good person who has been mistreated by others' (therefore anger predominates during such times) and at other times perceives themselves as a 'bad person with a life not worth living' (therefore self-injurious or suicidal behaviour predominates during such times).

The completed suicide rate in BPD patients is 8–10%. For young women, this rate is considered very high. The self-injurious behaviour (cutting or self-poisoning) is a way of coping through their perceived sense of despair and their inability to gain control of this perceived despair. However, front-line emergency medicine staff see this more as a wilful and manipulative behaviour than signs of an illness. In reality the majority of these patients are low-functioning individuals due to their illness.

BPD is considered to be heritable and the rates are similar to those reported with hypertension. Treatment mainly consists of therapies other than medications. Psychotherapy is a main form of treatment along with dialectical behaviour therapy and mentalisation therapy.[9]

7. Answer: D

BPD is a very common presentation to the ED, with a high level of time and resource requirements in its management. **These patients often have comorbid illnesses and therefore may present to the ED in a variety of presentations.** Although a BPD patient occasionally presents with a psychotic illness (such as paranoid schizophrenia) other presentations are more common. **Most patients with BPD (84.5%) meet criteria for diagnoses such as mood disorders, anxiety disorders and substance misuse. PTSD may be a comorbid illness in these patients.** With respect to comorbid mental disorders, there are differences between female and male patients, with disorders associated with substance misuse being more common in men and eating disorders more common in women.[9]

8. Answer: D

Rapid tranquilisation (neurolepting) is an important aspect of emergency psychiatry. It has to be used appropriately. As this treatment is given without the patient's consent it has to be appropriately supported clinically at that time and needs to be followed up with patient consent later. Rapid tranquilisation must be done in a non-punitive manner with established norms of preserving patient respect and dignity. A written ED guideline should be followed.

Managing agitated patients is complex. Although verbal interventions, with logic and rational explanations, should be attempted first to obtain the patient's cooperation, often such interventions fail in severely agitated patients such as the patient described in this scenario. A confident show of strength with several staff members and security staff may settle patients at times. Some patients may agree to take oral medications. However, once the decision has been made to use rapid tranquilisation, the initiation of such treatment has to be rapid so as to help prevent potential risks to the patient and the staff.

Current options in sedation include both antipsychotics (droperidol, olanzapine) and anxiolytics (benzodiazepines). Both traditional and novel antipsychotics are useful. Rapidly dissolving oral formulations are available for some of the newer antipsychotics (olanzapine). They may be as effective as parenteral formulations if patient cooperation can be obtained.[10]

9. Answer: C

PTSD is a long-lasting anxiety response following a traumatic or catastrophic event. Patients with this condition have poor sleep, hypervigilance and severe anxiety at night, which often leads them to seek help during this time. Patients from certain cultures may present with somatic problems when they are psychologically distressed.

Important symptoms of PTSD include:
- images, dreams or flashbacks of the traumatic event
- avoidance of cues that act as reminders of the traumatic event
- amnesia about important aspects of the traumatic event
- intense arousal and anxiety on exposure to trauma cues
- social withdrawal
- concentration and memory difficulties
- nightmares and disturbed sleep
- being easily startled.

An important management principle when dealing with a patient with PTSD is to ensure the safety of the patient and to validate the symptoms. Detailed questioning should be avoided as it may trigger severe symptoms.[11]

10. Answer: D

Anorexia nervosa is an eating disorder that usually begins in adolescence but can occur in adulthood.
Two types have been described:
- food restricting
- binge eating and purging.

Features of anorexia nervosa include:
- determined dieting
- phobic avoidance of food
- compulsive exercise
- a disturbed body image with a distorted perception of body weight
- an overvaluation of slimness
- a heightened desire to lose more weight
- a fear of fatness
- purging with or without binge eating (in a subgroup of patients)
- resultant sustained low weight
- psychiatric conditions that may coexist – major depression, anxiety disorders, obsessive-compulsive disorder, substance abuse.

Medical complications that should be assessed in the ED include (these can be used as physiological indications for hospital admission):

- dehydration
- bradycardia
- cardiac arrhythmia
- hypotension or postural hypotension
- other cardiovascular abnormalities
- hypothermia (body temperature <36.1°C)
- symptomatic hypoglycaemia
- hypokalaemia or hypophosphataemia
- weight <75% of the expected weight
- any rapid weight loss of several kilograms within a week
- lack of improvement or rapid worsening while in outpatient treatment.

Deaths secondary to medical complications mainly result from cardiac arrhythmias. Early interventions to restore weight can reduce the risk of arrhythmias.

Another very important complication in adolescents is loss of brain white and grey matter during severe weight loss. Although white matter restores with proper weight restoration, grey matter loss persists and results in permanent cognitive impairment.

Death from suicide is higher than the general population in these patients and therefore assessment regarding suicidal risk is important where appropriate.

Treatment in anorexia nervosa is focused on prompt weight restoration while attending to medical complications and psychological issues. Better outcomes have been observed when patients are treated in specialised eating disorder units than in general medical units.[12]

11. Answer: A

Although somatoform disorders are not common psychiatric conditions they are important as these patients occasionally present to the ED. Lack of awareness regarding these disorders may lead to difficulties in detection and appropriate interventions. **Four types of specific disorders are collectively called somatoform disorders. They are:**

- somatisation disorder
- conversion disorder
- pain disorder
- hypochondriasis.

The symptoms of somatoform disorders are not under the voluntary control of the patient. They genuinely believe their symptoms are due to real physical disease. This is not the case in malingering and factitious disorder, where the symptoms are under the conscious control of the patient.

Somatisation means the patient's experience and communication of their psychological distress manifests as physical complaints or symptoms without identifiable pathology to explain the symptoms. Depression and anxiety disorder are often present in these patients. They often present with multiple symptoms rather than a few specific symptoms. Most patients may not strictly fulfil the DSM-IV diagnostic criteria for somatisation disorder. The diagnosis is usually not made but can be suspected in the ED.

The following seven symptoms can be used as a rapid screening test for somatisation in the ED setting:

- dysmenorrhoea
- a sensation of a 'lump' in the throat
- vomiting
- shortness of breath
- burning in the sex organs
- painful extremities
- amnesia lasting hours to days.

In a *conversion disorder* there is a sudden and dramatic onset of a single symptom without associated pathophysiological or anatomical explanation. The typical symptoms are that of a non-painful neurological disorder such as pseudoseizure, syncope, coma, paralysis of a single limb, tremors and sensory loss in a limb. Patients describe these symptoms with apparent lack of concern for their gross symptoms.

The presence of physical symptoms that are disproportionate to demonstrable organic disease is a characteristic of *hypochondriasis*.[13]

12. Answer: D

Neuroleptic malignant syndrome is a rare but potentially fatal condition associated with the use of dopamine antagonists. **It most commonly occurs as an idiosyncratic reaction to antipsychotic medication but can be due to abrupt discontinuation of antiparkinsonian medication** (e.g. by abrupt withdrawal of the dopamine precursor levodopa). The estimated incidence is two per 1000 patients treated with typical antipsychotics. Atypical antipsychotics such as olanzapine, risperidone, clozapine and aripiprazole can also cause this syndrome. **It has a mortality rate of 10–20%.** The onset of symptoms can be rapid or gradual. The development of symptoms is not dose dependent. Other symptoms include:

- muscular rigidity
- elevated temperature (due to muscular contraction causing heat generation and impaired temperature control)
- autonomic dysfunction (tachycardia, increased BP or labile BP)
- altered level of consciousness (mutism, confusion to coma)
- rhabdomyolysis (increased CK and myoglobin) leading to acute renal failure
- leukocytosis
- elevated hepatic transaminases.

Early identification of the condition is paramount. **Patients who are on antipsychotics who have increased risk to develop neuroleptic malignant syndrome include those who are dehydrated, severely ill patients, catatonic patients and those who have had neuroleptic malignant syndrome previously.** When some or all of the above features are present in a patient who is on antipsychotic medication, the diagnosis should be actively considered until proven otherwise and the offending agent should be promptly withdrawn.

These patients often require aggressive supportive therapy including intravenous fluid resuscitation and measures to control temperature. Early consideration should be given for intubation as this will reduce contraction of muscles and production of heat and fever. Use of drugs such as dantrolene (along with supportive care) should be considered, especially in patients with severe muscular rigidity.[14,15]

13. Answer: D

The range of postpartum psychiatric disorders is wide and includes:

- postnatal blues
- postnatal depression
- postpartum psychosis
- PTSD
- anxiety disorders
- disorders of infant–mother relationships
- morbid preoccupations
- obsessions of child harm.

The first three conditions are the most common. 'Postnatal blues' is a very common mild disorder that requires no treatment. The onset is soon after child birth and is short lasting (hours to 2 days). Postnatal depression is most appropriately described as depression that has its onset within 3–6 months following childbirth. This is less frequent than postnatal blues but it may be the most frequent major psychiatric disorder seen after childbirth. In addition to maternal morbidity and mortality, postnatal depression can lead to reduced interaction with children and family.

It is more likely to be present in mothers with previous depression, little family or social supports, unplanned pregnancy, high parity, complications during pregnancy and/or delivery. It can also be triggered by difficult temperament of the baby and presence of colic or reflux. Common presenting features are continuing postnatal blues symptoms, negative feelings about the baby, not wanting to hold baby, lack of eye contact, inability to sleep or excessive sleep, feeding difficulties, and anger and frustration about life circumstances. These symptoms may lead to child neglect. When treated, postnatal depression has a good prognosis.

With obsessions of child harm after child birth, the mother experiences repeated thoughts about harming the child but may take precautions. The mother may avoid staying alone with the child. This is another area that should be explored in the above scenario.

Morbid preoccupations may occur in the postpartum period. Some of these are due to the mother's perception about body image. She may become distressed about the changes in her body due to the pregnancy and childbirth such as weight gain, stretch marks and scars. However, this is the least likely issue in this scenario.[16,17]

14. Answer: B

Amphetamine-induced psychotic disorder or intoxication delirium is usually seen in individuals who have used high amounts of amphetamine over a prolonged period. It can also be seen as a recurrence in individuals who had previous similar episodes. The recurrence can frequently occur as a result of re-exposure to small amounts of amphetamine. In the very acute stage, in addition to mood and delusional symptoms, the psychotic patient may have disturbances to their consciousness with confusion and disorientation (a delirium syndrome). After recovery from both the psychotic and delirium syndromes these patients typically have amnesia to the whole or part of the episode.

In addition to psychosis, amphetamines may induce manic or hypomanic symptoms during intoxication, and depression during withdrawal. Other issues include amphetamine-induced sleep disorder, anxiety disorder, sexual dysfunction and other psychological and physical symptoms. Among the psychological symptoms, mood swings, lack of concentrating ability, paranoia and hallucinations are frequent. Amphetamine-induced aggression and violent episodes are important management issues in the ED.[18]

15. Answer: B

Olanzapine is frequently used in acutely agitated psychiatry patients in the ED. It is a serotonin and dopamine receptor blocker (specifically 5 HT_{2A} and D_2 receptors). It is available in oral, rapid dispersible (wafer) and intramuscular preparations. In the ED, **the rapid dispersible preparation is particularly valuable in settling acutely agitated patients due to its rapid absorption through the oral mucosa and resulting rapid somnolence.** Both oral and rapid dispersible preparations are considered bioequivalent.

Olanzapine is a first-line antipsychotic agent and effective in the treatment of schizophrenia because it is effective for both positive and negative symptoms. This may be less important in an acutely agitated patient but its ability to cause somnolence seems to be important. Olanzapine has a favourable side-effect profile – it causes somnolence and orthostatic hypotension but causes less extrapyramidal side effects than with haloperidol.[19,20]

References

1. Yager J, Gitlin M. Clinical manifestations of psychiatric disorders. In: Sadock B, Sadock V, editors. Kaplan and Sadock's comprehensive textbook of psychiatry. 8th ed. Philadelphia: Lippincott Williams and Wilkins; 2005. p. 964–1002.
2. Hockberger R, Richards J. Thought disorders. In: Marx J, Hockberger R, Walls R, et al, editors. Rosen's emergency medicine: concepts and clinical practice. 7th ed. Mosby Elsevier; 2009. p. 1430–6.
3. American Psychiatric Association. Diagnostic and statistical manual of mental disorders (4th edn) – text revision. Washington DC: American Psychiatric Association.
4. Unutzer J. Late-life depression. N Engl J 2007; 357:2269–76.
5. Sudak H. Suicide. In: Sadock B, Sadock V, editors. Kaplan and Sadock's comprehensive textbook of psychiatry. 8th ed. Philadelphia: Lippincott Williams and Wilkins; 2005. p. 2243–453.
6. Colucciello S. Suicide. In: Marx J, Hockberger R, Walls R, et al, editors. Rosen's emergency medicine: concepts and clinical practice. 7th ed. Mosby Elsevier; 2009. p. 1463–71.
7. Wong F, Wolanin A, Smallwood P. The suicidal patient. In: Riba M, Ravindranath D, editors. Clinical manual of emergency psychiatry. Arlington: American Psychiatric Publishing Inc; 2010. p. 33–53.
8. Hawton K, Heeringen K. Suicide. Lancet 2009;373: 1372–81.
9. Leichsenring F, Leibing E, Kruse J, et al. Borderline personality disorder. Lancet 2011;377:74–84.
10. Slaby A, Dubin W, Baron D. Other psychiatric emergencies. In: Sadock B, Sadock V, editors. Kaplan and
Sadock's comprehensive textbook of psychiatry. 8th ed. Philadelphia: Lippincott Williams and Wilkins; 2005. p. 2453–71.
11. Treatment Protocol Project. Recognition and management of anxiety disorders. In: Management of mental disorders: volume 1. 4th ed. Sydney: World Health Organization. Collaborating Centre for Evidence in Mental Health Policy; 2004. p. 211–64.
12. Yager J, Andersen A. Anorexia nervosa. N Engl J 2005;353:1481–8.
13. Winter A, Purcell T. Somatoform disorders. In: Marx J, Hockberger R, Walls R, et al, editors. Rosen's emergency medicine: concepts and clinical practice. 7th ed. Mosby Elsevier; 2009. p. 1452–7.
14. Marder S, van Kammen D. Dopamine receptor antagonists (typical antipsychotics). In: Sadock B, Sadock V, editors. Kaplan and Sadock's comprehensive textbook of psychiatry. 8th ed. Philadelphia: Lippincott Williams and Wilkins; 2005. p. 2817–38.
15. Levine M, LoVecchio F. Antipsychotics. In: Tintinalli J, Stapczynski J, Ma O, et al, editors. Tintinalli's emergency medicine: a comprehensive study guide. 7th ed. New York: McGraw Hill Medical; 2011. p. 1207–11.
16. Brockington I. Postpartum psychiatric disorders. Lancet 2004;363:303–10.
17. Treatment Protocol Project. Affective disorders. In: Management of mental disorders: Volume 1. 4th ed. Sydney: World Health Organization. Collaborating Centre for Evidence in Mental Health Policy; 2004. p. 145–210.
18. Jaffe J, Ling W, Rawson R. Amphetamine (or amphetamine-like)-related disorders. In: Sadock B, Sadock V, editors. Kaplan and Sadock's comprehensive

textbook of psychiatry. 8th ed. Philadelphia: Lippincott Williams and Wilkins; 2005. p. 1188–200.

19. van Kammen D, Marder S. Serotonin-dopamine antagonists (atypical or second generation antipsychotics). In: Sadock B, Sadock V, editors. Kaplan and Sadock's comprehensive textbook of psychiatry. 8th ed. Philadelphia: Lippincott Williams and Wilkins; 2005. p. 2914–38.

20. Medicines.org.au. Zyprexa (olanzapine) product information v11.0. Online. Available: www.medicines.org.au.

1. Answer: D

A neonate will lose about 10% of birth weight in the first week of life; this is a combination of initial osmotic diuresis post birth, passage of meconium, as well as initial slow introduction of breast or bottle feeding. **Birth weight is usually regained at 10–14 days.** General weight gain is 30 g per day or 1% of birth weight per day. Poor weight gain is an important indicator of a chronic organic process such as congenital heart disease, metabolic disease, malabsorption and chronic infection.

The average intake is 60–90 mL per feed or 10 minutes per breast every 2–3 hours. Breastfed infants need to feed more often (1.5 to every 2 hours) because breast milk is easier to digest and leaves the stomach sooner than formula. Ten wet nappies per day are usual, with 1 stool per day to 1 stool per week for breastfed babies.

The heart rate in a newborn is often elevated to 180–200 bpm in settings of stress but this is usually a variable sinus tachycardia. Normal BP is 60–90 systolic and normal saturation is between 94–100%.[1]

2. Answer: D

When reviewing neonatal morbidity and mortality registries, most infant deaths were due to four causes (classified according to the International Classification of Diseases):

- congenital malformations
- disorders relating to prematurity and unspecified low birth weight
- sudden infant death syndrome (SIDS)
- newborns affected by maternal complications of pregnancy[81]

Birth weight is classified as small for gestational age (SGA), intra-uterine growth restriction (IUGR), low birth weight (<2500 g) and very low birth weight (<1500 g). SGA infants have a birth weight <10th percentile for gestational age, whereas IUGR is defined as a fetus whose estimated weight is below the 10th percentile for its gestational age and whose abdominal circumference is below the 2.5th percentile. At term, the cutoff birth weight for IUGR is 2500 g.

Approximately 70% of fetuses with a birthweight below the 10th percentile for gestational age are constitutionally small; in the remaining 30%, the cause of IUGR is pathologic.

GBS infection occurs in neonates born to women colonised with *Streptococcus agalactiae*. There are two main types of GBS disease; early-onset disease (occurs during the first week of life) and late-onset disease (occurs from the first week through three months of life). For early-onset disease, GBS most commonly causes sepsis, pneumonia and sometimes meningitis. A strong index of suspicion coupled with a rigorous guideline approach is required to decrease the incidence of early onset GBS disease. Most birth suites have protocols designed to identify GBS-positive women who are eligible for parenteral antibiotics if they have prolonged rupture of membranes beyond 12 hours. Neonates born to these mothers are observed carefully. Typically, if a mother who tested positive for GBS received antibiotics during labour, the baby will be observed to assess their need for septic screening because of concerns about early-onset disease. Similar illnesses are associated with late onset GBS disease but meningitis is more common with late-onset GBS disease than with early-onset GBS disease. Late onset disease is more difficult to screen for, although most sepsis/fever algorithms have a low threshold for screening for bacterial illness in a <3-month-old child. Treatment is with parenteral antibiotics, usually ampicillin and gentamicin.

TTN is a benign condition usually occurring in term neonates born after a caesarean section who develop an oxygen requirement with moderate respiratory distress. It usually has its onset at 6–24 hours after birth and may last for up to 72–96 hours. Its aetiology is uncertain, but it is postulated that the usual forces at play during a vertex vaginal delivery are absent from a caesarean birth, with residual fluid retention in the interstitium of the neonatal lung with resultant respiratory distress. It usually resolves after a few days.[2-5]

3. Answer: B

Jaundice occurs in most newborn infants and is usually benign, but because of the potential toxicity of bilirubin, **newborn infants must be risk stratified to identify those who might develop severe hyperbilirubinemia and, in rare cases, acute bilirubin encephalopathy or kernicterus**. The following are risk factors for development of severe hyperbilirubinaemia and acute bilirubin encephalopathy:

- Major risk factors include
  - predischarge TSB or TcB level in the high-risk zone
  - jaundice observed in the first 24 hours
  - blood group incompatibility with positive direct antiglobulin test, other known haemolytic disease (glucose-6-phosphate dehydrogenase deficiency), elevated end-tidal CO_2 concentration
  - gestational age <36 weeks
  - previous sibling received phototherapy
  - cephalohaematoma or significant bruising
  - exclusive breastfeeding, particularly if nursing is not going well and weight loss is excessive
  - East Asian race
- Minor risk factors include
  - predischarge TSB or TcB level in the high intermediate-risk zone
  - gestational age 37–38 weeks
  - jaundice observed before discharge
  - previous sibling with jaundice
  - macrosomic infant of a diabetic mother
  - maternal age ≥25 years
  - male gender

Indications for formal testing of serum bilirubin levels includes those babies with risk factors for progression to severe hyperbilirubinaemia, progressive jaundice, and babies who appear unwell, that is lethargy, poor feeding, dehydration, failure to thrive or evidence of sepsis. The total serum bilirubin should be plotted on the treatment nomogram for jaundiced babies to assess their need for admission for phototherapy.[6–8]

Refer to answer 4 for a further discussion on the causes of jaundice.

4. Answer: C

The following is a useful guide in determining the causes of jaundice classified by time of onset:

- *First 24 hours:* jaundice within 24 hours is probably pathological

It may be due to erythroblastosis fetalis, concealed haemorrhage, sepsis or congenital infections, including syphilis, cytomegalovirus, rubella and toxoplasmosis. Haemolysis (e.g. G6PD-deficiency or ABO incompatability) is suggested by a rapid rise in serum bilirubin concentration (>0.5 mg/dL/hr), anaemia, pallor, indirect (unconjugated) hyperbilirubinaemia, reticulocytosis, hepatosplenomegaly, and a positive family history.

- *First few days*: usually physiologic

Early-onset breastfeeding jaundice and Crigler-Najjar syndrome are seen initially on the second or third day. Crigler-Najjar syndrome is a familial non-haemolytic icterus syndrome with a uniformly poor prognosis and ongoing kernicterus risk throughout life. Jaundice appearing after the third day and within the first week may suggest bacterial sepsis or urinary tract infection; it may also be due to other infections, notably syphilis, toxoplasmosis, cytomegalovirus, and enterovirus.

- *After week 1*

Wide differential including breast milk jaundice, septicaemia, congenital atresia or paucity of the bile ducts, hepatitis, galactosemia, hypothyroidism, cystic fibrosis, and congenital haemolytic anaemia crises-related to red blood cell morphology and enzyme deficiencies.

- *Persistent jaundice* during the first month of life includes hepatitis, cytomegalic inclusion disease, syphilis, toxoplasmosis, familial non-haemolytic icterus, congenital atresia of the bile ducts and galactosemia.

Rarely, physiologic jaundice may be prolonged for several weeks, as in infants with hypothyroidism or pyloric stenosis.[6–8]

5. Answer: D

The most common bacterial causes of neonatal meningitis are GBS, *E. coli* and *L. monocytogenes*. *S. pneumoniae*, other streptococci, non-typable *H. influenzae*, both coagulase-positive and coagulase-negative staphylococci, *Klebsiella*, *Enterobacter*, *Pseudomonas*, *Treponema pallidum* (syphilis) and

Mycobacterium tuberculosis may also produce meningitis.

TORCHES infections (agents that cross the placenta; *Toxoplasmosis gondii*, rubella, CMV, herpes, syphilis) may be asymptomatic at birth or may have mild symptoms to multisystem involvement. Clinical signs that raise suspicion of an intrauterine infection (and help distinguish these infections from acute bacterial infections that occur during labour and delivery) include intrauterine growth restriction, microcephaly/hydrocephalus, intracranial calcifications, chorioretinitis, cataracts, myocarditis, pneumonia, hepatosplenomegaly, direct hyperbilirubinaemia, anaemia, thrombocytopenia, hydrops fetalis, and skin manifestations. Encephalitis is commonly caused by CMV, enteroviruses, herpes simplex virus (HSV), rubella, toxoplasmosis and treponemal organisms. Adverse late outcomes include sensorineural hearing loss, visual disturbances (including blindness), seizures and neurodevelopmental abnormalities.

Neonates with bacterial sepsis may have nonspecific signs and symptoms or focal signs of infection. Integrated Management of Childhood Illness (IMCI) criteria for bacterial sepsis include convulsions, respiratory rate >60 breaths/min, severe chest indrawing, nasal flaring, grunting, bulging fontanel pus draining from the ear, redness around the umbilicus extending to the skin, temperature >37.7°C (or feels hot) or <35.5°C (or feels cold), lethargic or unconscious, reduced movements, not able to feed, not attaching to the breast, no suckling at all, crepitations, cyanosis and a reduced digital capillary refill time. The initial manifestation may involve only one system, such as apnoea alone or tachypnoea with retractions or tachycardia, or it may be an acute catastrophic manifestation with multiorgan dysfunction. Redness of the umbilicus suggests omphalitis – a neonatal infection where the umbilical stump is colonised by bacteria from the maternal genital tract or the environment. Infection may remain localised or may spread to the abdominal wall, the peritoneum, the umbilical or portal vessels, or the liver. Abdominal wall cellulitis or necrotising fasciitis with associated sepsis and a high mortality rate may develop in infants with omphalitis. Prompt diagnosis and treatment are necessary to avoid serious complications.

Normal, uninfected infants 0–4 weeks of age may have the following elevated CSF findings: protein 0.84 ± 0.45 g/L, glucose 2.5 mmol/L ± 0.5 mmol/L, leukocyte count 11 ± 10 per mm³ with the 90th percentile being 22, proportion of polymorphonuclear leukocytes is 2.2 ± 3.8% with the 90th percentile being 6. Newborn CSF is often xanthochromic because of the frequent elevation of bilirubin and protein levels in this age group. Normal opening pressure ranges from 10 to 100 mm H_2O in young children, 60 to 200 mm H_2O after eight years of age, and up to 250 mm H_2O in obese patients. Elevated CSF protein values and leukocyte counts and hypoglycorrhachia may develop in preterm infants after intraventricular haemorrhage. Many noninfectious processes, like certain inflammatory disorders, seizures and malignancy, as well as nonpyogenic congenital infections (toxoplasmosis, CMV, HSV, syphilis producing an aseptic meningitis), can also produce alterations in CSF protein value and leukocyte count. Hypoglycorrhacia (low glucose level in CSF) is also caused by chemical meningitis, inflammatory conditions, subarachnoid haemorrhage and hypoglycemia. Elevated levels of glucose in the blood is the only cause of having an elevated CSF glucose level. There is no pathologic process that causes CSF glucose levels to be elevated.[9–12,82]

6. Answer: C

Substance abuse during pregnancy results in poor maternal nutrition, acute withdrawal shortly after birth, and long-term effects on physical growth and neurodevelopment. Heroin and methadone are the drugs most frequently associated with withdrawal. **Manifestations of withdrawal usually begin within the first 48 hours; rarely, symptoms may appear as late as 4–6 weeks of age. Tremors and hyperirritability are the most prominent symptoms.** Other signs include wakefulness, hyperacuoio, hypertonicity, tachypnoea, diarrhoea, vomiting, high-pitched cry, fist sucking, poor feeding with weight loss (disorganised sucking) and fever. The diagnosis is generally established from the history and clinical findings. Meconium testing is more accurate than neonatal urine drug testing.

The usual cause of neonatal collapse presenting to the ED is sepsis. A careful consideration of potential differentials should be born in mind:

Cardiac

Congenital: hypoplastic left heart syndrome, other structural disease, persistent pulmonary hypertension of the newborn (PPHN)
Acquired: myocarditis, hypovolemic or cardiogenic shock, PPHN

Gastrointestinal

Necrotising enterocolitis
Spontaneous gastrointestinal perforation
Structural abnormalities

Haematologic

Neonatal purpura fulminans
Immune-mediated thrombocytopenia
Immune-mediated neutropenia
Severe anaemia
Malignancies (congenital leukaemia)
Hereditary clotting disorders

Metabolic

Hypoglycaemia
Adrenal disorders: adrenal haemorrhage, adrenal insufficiency, congenital adrenal hyperplasia
Inborn errors of metabolism: organic acidurias, lactic acidoses, urea cycle disorders, galactosemia

Neurologic

Intracranial haemorrhage: spontaneous, due to child abuse
Hypoxic-ischemic encephalopathy
Neonatal seizures
Infant botulism

Respiratory

Respiratory distress syndrome
Aspiration pneumonia: amniotic fluid, meconium or gastric contents
Lung hypoplasia
Tracheoesophageal fistula
Transient tachypnea of the newborn[10,13]

7. Answer: D

In neonates and paediatric patients, SIRS manifests as temperature instability, respiratory dysfunction (altered gas exchange, hypoxaemia, acute respiratory distress syndrome), cardiac dysfunction (tachycardia, delayed capillary refill, hypotension) and perfusion abnormalities

(oliguria, metabolic acidosis). Increased vascular permeability results in capillary leak into peripheral tissues and the lungs, with resultant pulmonary and peripheral oedema. Disseminated intravascular coagulation (DIC) results in the more severely affected cases. The cascade of escalating tissue injury may lead to multisystem organ failure and death.

To make the diagnosis of SIRS, the presence of at least two of the following four criteria, one of which must be abnormal temperature or leukocyte count, must be present:

- **Core temperature of >38.5°C or <36°C**
- **Tachycardia**, defined as a mean heart rate
  - >2 SD above normal for age in the absence of external stimulus, chronic drugs, or painful stimuli; or
  - otherwise unexplained persistent elevation over a 0.5- to 4-hour time period; or
  - for children <1 year old: bradycardia, defined as a mean heart rate <10th percentile for age in the absence of external vagal stimulus, beta-blocker drugs, or congenital heart disease, or
  - otherwise unexplained persistent depression over a 0.5-hour time period
- **Mean respiratory rate >2 SD above normal for age** or mechanical ventilation for an acute process not related to underlying neuromuscular disease or the receipt of general aneesthesia
- **Leukocyte count elevated or depressed for age** (not secondary to chemotherapy-induced leukopenia) or >10% immature neutrophils[14,15]

8. Answer: B

Tepid sponging is not recommended for children with fever according to the 2007 National Institute for Health and Clinical Excellence (NICE) guidelines for managing feverish children.[16]

The risk of serious bacterial illness (SBI) is higher in young infants <3 months of age. Additionally, the clinical clues that are often used to detect serious illness are not reliable in this age group. **Although UTI is the most common SBI identified, 1–3% of febrile infants have bacteremia and/or bacterial meningitis.** While ill-looking children 1–3 months of age require a full septic work-up, empiric antibiotics and admission, there is some debate about the management and disposition of children in the age group of 1–3 months who appear well. Various strategies (Rochester, Philadelphia and Boston criteria) have been tested to identify a set of low-risk criteria based on clinical and laboratory findings. If these criteria are met, it may allow for less aggressive treatment, withhold empirical antibiotic therapy, or allow management as an outpatient. Unlike the other studies, the Rochester criteria did not include spinal fluid analysis as a routine part of their low-risk criteria, based the attainment of urine cultures upon the results of urinalyses, and included infants younger than 1 month. An extensive discussion of each criteria is beyond the scope of this book. **There are, however, no conclusive data to support omission of LP from routine evaluation of fever in this age group.** While awaiting further definitive evidence, it is the author's opinion that the safest approach for most emergency clinicians is to investigate these children fully, including LP and coverage with empiric antibiotics.

PCV7 provides protection against *S. pneumoniae* but is ineffective against GBS. Furthermore, **PCV7 is probably not as effective in this age group, as only the first dose of vaccination would have been given.** PCV7 is usually given at 2, 4 and 6 months.

The omission of LP in the setting of positive urine in infants <3 months is controversial. The difference in management of a UTI versus meningitis in an infant <3 months is usually in the length of treatment with intravenous antibiotics, with meningitis needing a prolonged length of treatment – 14 days in most cases. The traditional theory states that if a UTI is found during septic work-up, it is a reflection of bacteremic seeding to the urine rather than ascending urine infection, and therefore the infant needs to have CSF culture to exclude this bacteremic seeding to the CSF. There is little evidence for this postulation. Small retrospective studies have shown that healthy, nontoxic-appearing infants with evidence of UTI have bacteremia rates of 6–10%. These studies indicate that risk for serious complications, such as meningitis, is low, and repeatedly show that CSF is negative for pathogens in these patients with UTI diagnoses. These studies conclude that it would appear to be safe, less invasive, and more cost-effective to administer intravenous antibiotics and monitor these patients and to perform LPs only in patients with positive findings on BC or in those whose urine cultures yield a pathogen likely to be associated with meningitis (namely GBS). The author's conclusion is that this area needs more study to prospectively prove that this is a safe and valid approach. Anecdotally, it is the practice of many paediatric emergency clinicians to omit LP in the setting of a positive UTI, commence empiric antibiotic cover and admit to the ward under a paediatrician who can observe the clinical course and LP at a later stage if concerns of meningitis are raised. This is the practice of the author, in well-appearing non-septic infants 2–3 months age with confirmed UTI on a valid clean catch, catheter or suprapubic urine specimen.

The safest approach once again depends on the clinical experience of the ED clinician in this area; this entails a full septic screen for all under 3 months including LP.[16–21]

9. Answer: D

Current evidence supports the use of screening for serious bacterial infection with full septic work-up including LP, and if all indices are normal, patients can be discharged with or without antibiotics. Routine follow-up care in the ED in 12 hours is mandatory.

Although most of the emphasis in the management of fever focuses on the detection of underlying SBI, it must not be forgotten that certain viruses, in particular HSV, may cause high morbidity and mortality. Congenital HSV infection should be suspected in full-term infants younger than 4 weeks and in premature infants (<32 weeks' gestation) younger than 8 weeks who have any of the following symptoms: history of HSV lesions in the mother in the third trimester; skin lesions suspicious for HSV on the infant, ill-appearing; seizure associated with the current illness; abnormal liver function test (more than 100 for the AST/ALT); and CSF pleocytosis (bloody, uninterpretable CSF should be considered case by case). **It is important to remember that most (60–80%) of the mothers of HSV-positive babies have no known history of HSV infection and a high index of suspicion should be maintained.** Acyclovir (60 mg/kg per day, given in divided doses via intravenous infusion) should be empirically administered to all children with suspected congenital HSV infection as mentioned above.

GBS disease is unlikely at this age but can occur up to 90 days after birth. There are two clinical types:

early onset (<7 days) and late onset (7–90 days). Vaginal or rectal colonisation occurs in up to approximately 30% of pregnant women and is the usual source for GBS transmission to newborn infants. In the absence of maternal chemoprophylaxis, approximately 50% of infants born to colonised women acquire GBS colonisation, and 1–2% of these infants develop invasive disease.

The IT ratio (immature:total neutrophil) has been in use in neonatal nurseries for two decades as a part of neonatal risk stratification to assess for sepsis. The Philadelphia criteria group was able to improve their sensitivity and negative predictive value (NPV) to 100% for risk stratifying infant 2–3 months into a low-risk group by including the band: total neutrophil count to their screening technique.[17,22,23]

10. Answer: C

The current approach to fever with no focus in a child in the age category of 3–36 months who is well appearing, is to perform appropriate urine screening and careful observation in the ED, with a follow-up visit arranged in 12–24 hours either within the ED or with the child's GP. The approach to these children is dramatically different now after the introduction of PCV7 in the late 1990s. **In this 'post PCV7' era, the rate of invasive pneumococcal bacteremia and subsequently SBI is <1%, making empiric screening for SBI and testing with WCC and BC cost-ineffective.** Furthermore, the incidence of *E. coli*, *Neisseria* and *Salmonella* are all now increased within this <1% occult bacteremia category, and WCC screening is not sensitive for the detection of bacteria other than streptococcus. A WCC that is negative (i.e. <15,000) will therefore have a significant false negative if *Neisseria* or *Salmonella* are the offending organisms causing bacteremia. Clinical observation of the child in the ED may be more sensitive.

There is still a definite correlation between high fever >39°C and bacterial, specifically pneumococcus infection. However, the rate of this infection is so low that it makes it statistically more likely that fever >39°C is going to be due to viral causes.[16–18, 22,24–27]

11. Answer: D

The most accurate method to measure temperature is via a rectal thermometer, particularly in high-risk groups such as infants 0–3 months of age, as axillary,

oral or tympanic thermometers are unreliable in this age group. The rectal route should not be used in patients who are potentially immunocompromised due to the risk of mucosal damage, bacteremia or transmission of infection. However, parental acceptance and ease of use in the ED settings may require that axillary and tympanic methods be used instead of this gold standard. The author's approach to this dilemma is tympanic thermometers for older children, and axillary checks for infants. Electronic or infrared versions are equally accurate.

On average, axillary temperature measurement using an electronic thermometer underestimates body temperature by at least 0.5°C and in some children may underestimate by as much as 2°C. **In neonates the axillary route appears to be more accurate, with a difference from rectal temperature of around 0.5°C and a sensitivity of 98%.** Tympanic measurement differs on average from body temperature by 0.3°C, with a sensitivity to detect fever ranging from 51% to 97%. Some studies reported that tympanic measurements are difficult or inaccurate in infants under the age of 3 months due to the different anatomy – a smaller, shorter canal where the infrared beam may not access the tympanic membrane accurately.[16,22]

12. Answer: D

Ceftriaxone is contraindicated in neonates due to concerns about it displacing bilirubin from protein binding sites and inducing kernicterus, as well as the risk of calcium precipitation in neonates with intravenous infusion. Cefotaxime is recommended instead.

A 3-year-old unimmunised child is assumed to have a susceptibility to pneumococcus and haemophilus b (HIB), which predates the era of HIB and PCV7 vaccination. For this reason it is prudent to perform screening for bacteremia even if the child is well appearing. If the screening WCC is negative, the child can be discharged with defined follow-up arranged in 12 hours in the ED, for clinical review as well as BC results.

In children over 3 months of age, C-reactive protein, interleukin and procalcitonin have repeatedly been shown to be of limited value to an ED clinician attempting to risk stratify children who appear well and have fever without source.[17,18,22,25,27–29]

13. Answer: C

Defervescence after paracetamol administration has not been shown to reliably exclude bacteremia and therefore a response to paracetamol does not predict a benign course in these children. The use of antipyretics such as ibuprofen and paracetamol are useful in lowering the temperature of the child more rapidly (compared with the child's natural sinusoidal temperature variance), allowing for two important management points: symptomatic relief, as the child may be less irritable, and assessment of the child in the afebrile state. Many children are labeled 'toxic' by inexperienced ED clinicians because they are assessed when febrile. Often with time or antipyretics, the fever settles and the child becomes animated and alert. If the child is not septic or toxic, antipyretics should be administered and the child observed in the ED. Urine screening with a clean catch urine or catheter specimen to exclude UTI should be performed. If the child is observed to remain well and alert in the ED, their risk of serious bacterial illness is extremely low (<1%) and WCC and BC are not indicated.

Listeria affects the neonatal population.[17,18,24,25]

14. Answer: A

The most common cause of petechiae in children is due to mechanical causes. **Petechiae from tourniquetting, retching or violent coughing and vomiting is typically confined to the skin above the nipple line in the distribution of the superior vena cava (SVC), whereas petechiae caused by serious bacterial illness can have any distribution.** This is the only group of well-appearing children with an obvious mechanical cause who should not need immediate investigation.

The incidence of meningococcal infection is 7–11% in patients hospitalised with fever and petechiae. The rate of bacteremia of any cause was found to be much lower (1.9%) in an ED population; however, most studies have looked at this scenario during the pre-vaccination era. The differential diagnosis of fever and petechiae also includes disseminated intravascular coagulation, rickettsial disease, pneumococcal bacteremia, *Streptococcus pyogenes* infection, various viral infections, idiopathic thrombocytopenic purpura, Henoch-Schönlein purpura, and leukaemia. Due to the wide differential

and potential for serious infection, most children will need investigation with WCC, BC and coagulation studies.

Empirical antibiotic therapy (ceftriaxone) should be considered in all children presenting with fever and petechiae, even if an outpatient disposition is anticipated.[22]

15. Answer: B

The approach to a child with fever includes the following.

- Identify if there are signs of shock/septic shock. If shock is present, resuscitate first, followed by work-up. Evidence of shock should be aggressively treated with fluid resuscitation. An intravenous or intraosseous line should be placed and the initial resuscitative fluid should be 20 mL/kg of isotonic crystalloid. This should be repeated to a total of 60–100 mL/kg if the signs of hypovolaemia persist, after which the use of a vasopressor should be considered. Every effort should be made to obtain appropriate specimens for culture (blood and urine), even in a critically ill child prior to antibiotic administration. LP may be deferred in a critically ill child until stabilisation occurs. Empirical antibiotic therapy should be directed at the most likely causative organisms based on age.
- If no shock is present, carefully search for the source of the infection and, if found, manage it as per local protocols.
- If no source is found, assess if the child is 'toxic' versus 'nontoxic' using a systematic clinical score (such as the NICE guidelines traffic light scoring system) or discuss with a senior clinician.
- If toxic, perform a septic work-up and consider admission and empiric antibiotics.
- If nontoxic, perform urine screening and observe the child in the ED for signs of deterioration.
- If the child remains well, discharge them with follow-up arranged within 12–24 hours with a GP or within the ED.[16,18,22]

16. Answer: D

Classic KD presents with a fever for >5 days (present from the start of the illness) and 4 out of 5 criteria (polymorphous rash, conjunctival injection, mucous membrane changes, peripheral

TABLE 22.1 SYMPTOM PROFILE OF VARIOUS CONDITIONS

	Fever	Rash	Adenopathy	Conjunctivitis	Oral	Peripheral	Other
KD	– Present in 99% of cases – >5–30 days – Unresponsive to antipyretic treatment – Usually >38.5°C	– Present in 80% of cases – Polymorphous – Diffuse – Present from the start of the illness	– Present in 50% of cases – Cervical – Painful – Singular	– Present in 90% of cases – Nonexudative – Perilimbal sparing	– Present in 90% of cases – Red lips – Red fissured strawberry tongue	– Present in 65% of cases – Red hands, feet – Oedema – Desquamation at days 14–21	– Present in 10% of cases – Pyuria – Arthritis
Me	– >40°C – Falls after 5 days	– Morbilliform – Starts at hairline – Fades by day 7	Generalised	Nonexudative	Koplik	– Brown staining before day 7 – Desquamation only in severe cases – not on the hands	
SF	– >40°C – Lasts 5 days – Responds to penicilin	Starts on day 2 in groin/axillae then spreads	– Severe – Extensive	Not seen	– Strawberry tongue – Pharyngitis	Desquamation at days 7–10	
Ru	<37.5°C	Pink macules on face and trunk spreading to the arms and legs in 5 days	– Cervical – Suboccipital – Post auricular	Not seen	N/A	No desquamation	
RI	– 40°C – 3–5 days	– As defervescence occurs by day 4, a fine maculopapular rash on the trunk/neck spreads to the arms and legs lasting – 1–2 days	– Cervical – Suboccipital – Postauricular	Not seen	N/A	N/A	
SJIA	>40°C for 2 weeks	Fleeting pink macular	Generalised and painless	Not seen			Arthritis – mono or polyarticular – Hepatomegaly – Serositis

KD: Kawasaki disease; Me: measles; SF: scarlet fever; Ru: rubella; RI: roseola infantum; SJIA: systemic juvenile idiopathic arthritis.

extremity changes, cervical lymphadenopathy), whereas in atypical or incomplete KD the full criteria are not met. Other findings (not included in the criteria) include sterile pyuria, arthritis (10%), reactive thrombocytosis, normocytic normochromic anemia, transaminitis, hydrops of gallbladder, hyponatremia, aseptic meningitis (which may explain severe irritability) and erythema of the Bacillus Calmette-Guérin (BCG) vaccination site (50%).

This patient has signs satisfying the criteria for incomplete KD (fever as well as oral, conjunctival and rash features). Adenopathy and peripheral changes are absent. The child also has one supplemental criteria – sterile pyuria. The next step will be inflammatory markers. If raised, the rule is a low threshold to commence on intravenous immunoglobulin as well as high-dose aspirin to avoid the coronary complications of KD. The risk of coronary artery aneurysm formation is 15–25% if untreated.

Measles is unlikely in this case because the fever and rash usually settles by day 5. Other characteristics include a morbiliform rash that normally appears in the hairline and face first, generalised adenopathy, non-exudative conjunctivitis and Koplik spots in the mouth. Peripheral features are rare and usually appear after day 7. Desquamation only occurs in severe cases and not in the hands.

Scarlet fever is unlikely. Although pharyngitis and a strawberry tongue are characteristic, conjunctivitis is not a feature, and a good response is the rule with penicillin administration. For the same reason, titres to streptococcal antigen are unlikely to be elevated. The fever usually settles within 5 days and the rash starts from day 2 onwards, initially in the groin and axilla. Adenopathy is usually extensive and severe and desquamation may occur at day 7–10.

Rubella, roseola infantum and systemic juvenile idiopathic arthritis may also mimic KD and should be included in the differential diagnosis.[30–31]

Table 22.1 outlines the clinical profiles of the various conditions.

17. Answer: D

This child has the typical IM-like syndrome associated with adenovirus infection. **Adenoviruses cause prolonged fever and IM-like syndromes and should be included, along with cytomegalovirus,** toxoplasmosis and HIV, as a cause of heterophile-negative IM, especially if peripheral blood counts reveal neutrophilia rather than atypical lymphocytosis. In addition, many of the features associated with KD, including high fever, pharyngitis, lymphadenitis, conjunctivitis and rash, as well as laboratory findings of acute inflammation, such as elevated sedimentation rate and C-reactive protein levels, have been described in children with virologically proven adenovirus disease.

Concurrent infections are common in patients with KD, found in up to 40% of patients. Concomitant viral infection is associated with a higher frequency of coronary artery dilatation. A diagnosis of an infectious condition does not preclude a concurrent diagnosis of KD.[32–33]

18. Answer: B

Infants <1 year or children >5 years of age are more likely to have incomplete KD than those between one and 4 years of age. **Children with incomplete KD are also at risk for cardiovascular sequelae.** Cervical lymphadenopathy is the cardinal manifestation most often absent in children with either complete or incomplete KD. Adenopathy is missing in up to 90% of children with incomplete disease versus 40–50% of those who met criteria for KD. Rash is not present in 50% of children with incomplete disease compared with 7–10% of children with typical KD. Peripheral extremity changes are absent in approximately 40% of incomplete KD cases. In comparison, only 15% of those with typical KD fail to develop palmar erythema, dorsal oedema or periungual desquamation. Mucous membrane changes are most characteristic of KD and present in more than 90% of children with either typical or incomplete disease.

The current approach to treatment is outlined in guidelines published by the American Heart Association and American Academy of Pediatrics, which strongly favour treatment with intravenous immunoglobulin and aspirin, even in doubtful cases. The reason for this is that the treatment is safe, and the complications of coronary artery aneurysms in untreated 'doubtful' or incomplete cases are truly disastrous. Children with a variety of other febrile conditions may receive IVIG treatment using these abovementioned guidelines. All children with incomplete KD, or fever >5 days who are young, should have a full lab work-up, including CRP and ESR, and one should have a low threshold to progress to urgent echocardiography to further evaluate the risk of coronary artery complications. The following steps summarise the approach to fever >5 days and suspected incomplete KD:

- Establish fever >5 days with 2–3 clinical criteria for KD.
- If consistent with potential KD, assess lab tests.
- If CRP and ESR elevated, assess supplementary lab criteria.
- If more than three of the following present: albumin >3.0 g/dL, anaemia for age, elevation of ALT, platelets after 7 days >450 000/mm³, WCC 15 000/mm³, and urine 10 white blood cells (WBC) or high-power field, proceed to treat with IVIG and aspirin, then arrange echo. If <three supplemental citeria, arrange echo. If positive echo criteria, treat with IVIG and aspirin. If echo is negative, admit and discuss with KD expert.

The message is clear: take care in assessing the patient but have a low threshold to treat if you think the diagnosis could be KD.[30–31]

19. Answer: D

A *suprapubic aspirate (SPA)* is the recommended gold standard test for diagnosing a UTI in children, particularly those who are young (<6 months) or unwell. It has high sensitivity and specificity and reliably rules out UTI in the setting of an unwell child with a fever without a source. The current recommended practice is to perform SPA with ultrasound guidance. The presence of five or more WBC/high-power field suggests an infection. The presence of 10 or more WBC/µL is also consistent with infection. Any growth of organisms is deemed to confirm a UTI as the bladder is meant to be sterile. An exception to this is culture positive *Staphylococcus epidermidis*, which usually represents a false positive from skin contamination. A catheter specimen of urine is the next best alternative (and favoured in the US), but is not as accurate and requires a pure growth of >1000 CFU to confirm a UTI. Midstream clean-catch urine specimens are adequate for older children who can provide them. More than 100,000 CFU/mL in a midstream clean-catch urine specimen is defined as a UTI.

A *bag specimen* is not reliable for the exclusion or diagnosis of UTI. It has a high false positive (60%) and a high false negative (15%) and should not be used to exclude UTI if the pretest likelihood of UTI is high, or when no obvious focus of infection has been found.

A urine specimen that is found to be positive on *dipstick* for nitrite, leukocyte esterase or blood may indicate a UTI. Dipstick tests have sensitivities approaching 85–90%. Dipstick tests should not be used as a rule-out test due to their high false negative rate of up to 20%. This may be due to a number of reasons, including infections with nitrite negative organisms, or very early infections where a sufficient inflammatory reaction has not yet resulted in a leukocytosis. Dipstick tests also produce false positive results in many other disorders including renal diseases, URTI and sterile pyuria (for example with abdominal pathology or KD.)

A *renal ultrasound* is usually performed in young children after a first UTI, especially those under 4 years of age. The main purpose of ultrasound is to exclude urinary tract obstruction or anatomical abnormality, in addition to assessment of previous renal scarring from possible vesicoureteric reflux. Unwell children or those under the age of 6 months require an inpatient ultrasound to exclude renal abscess or anatomical abnormality such as posterior urethral valves. Most other children <4 years should have their imaging as outpatients.

MCUG is utilised to visualise vesicoureteric reflux disease. The requirement to diagnose vesicoureteral reflux (VUR) is controversial and individual paediatricians have their preference for ordering or omitting this test. It may be done in children under 6 months of age (especially boys), and may be necessary for older children according to circumstances. MCUG should not be arranged from the ED, and discussion of the pros and cons of this with the parents can be undertaken at outpatient review.[34–35]

20. Answer: B

Bonsu et al studied the use of peripheral WBC counts as a screen for need for LP in infants 3–89 days old. Of the 22 cases of bacterial meningitis, 41% had peripheral WBC counts between 5000 and 15,000 (low risk according to Philadelphia and Rochester criteria), and 64% had peripheral WBC counts between 5000 and 20,000 (low risk according to Boston criteria). **They concluded that LPs of febrile infants should not be omitted based on the results of peripheral WBC counts.**[25]

The common causes of bacterial meningitis in children 1 month to 12 years of age are *N. meningitidis*, *S. pneumoniae* and *H. influenzae* type b. Specific *host defense defects* due to altered immunoglobulin production in response to encapsulated pathogens result in increased risk of bacterial meningitis (e.g. IgG subclass deficiency). Defects of the complement system (C5–C8) have been associated with recurrent meningococcal infection. Splenic dysfunction (sickle cell anaemia) or asplenia (due to trauma, or congenital defect) is associated with an increased risk of pneumococcal, *H. influenzae* type b (to some extent) and, rarely, meningococcal sepsis and meningitis. *Congenital or acquired CSF leak* across a mucocutaneous barrier, such as cranial or midline facial defects (cribriform plate), or CSF leakage through a rupture of the meninges due to a basal skull fracture into the cribriform plate or paranasal sinus, is associated with an increased risk of pneumococcal meningitis. **The risk of bacterial meningitis caused by *S. pneumoniae* in children with cochlear implants is more than 30 times the risk in the general population.**

Meningococcal routine vaccination in Australia only involves protection against meningococcal C. Infections by strains A, C, W135 and Y are vaccine preventable in older children and adults. They are polysaccharide vaccines that give short-term protection against serogroups A, C, W135 and Y and are mainly used for travellers to regions where serogroup A and W135 infections are prevalent, but they can also be used in outbreak control. **The B strain currently causes most cases of *Neisseria*-related meningitis and there is no vaccine against this serotype.**[9,17,25,36]

21. Answer: D

Meningitis presents in two patterns:
- several days of fever accompanied by upper respiratory tract symptoms, followed by nonspecific signs of CNS infection such as increasing lethargy and irritability or, less commonly
- fulminant rapidly progressive manifestations of shock, purpura, DIC and reduced levels of consciousness often resulting in progression to coma or death within 24 hours.

Meningeal irritation is manifested as nuchal rigidity, back pain, Kernig's sign (flexion of the hip 90 degrees with subsequent pain with extension of the leg) and Brudzinski's sign (involuntary flexion of the knees and hips after passive flexion of the neck while supine). However, Kernig's and Brudzinski's signs are not reliable in those younger than 12–18 months. *Increased ICP* is suggested by headache, emesis, bulging fontanel or diastasis (widening) of the sutures, oculomotor (anisocoria, ptosis) or abducens nerve paralysis, hypertension with bradycardia, apnoea or hyperventilation, decorticate or decerebrate posturing, stupor, coma or signs of herniation. **Papilloedema is uncommon in uncomplicated meningitis and suggests a more chronic process such as intracranial abscess, subdural empyema or occlusion of a dural venous sinus.** Cranial neuropathies of the ocular, oculomotor, abducens, facial and auditory nerves may also be due to focal inflammation. **Around 10–20% of children with bacterial meningitis have focal neurologic signs.** *Seizures* (focal or generalised) occur in 20–30% of patients with meningitis.[9]

22. Answer: C

Many organisms other than the typical bacterial agents cause meningitis syndromes: *Mycobacterium tuberculosis*, *Nocardia* spp, *Treponema pallidum* (syphilis) and *Borrelia burgdorferi* (Lyme disease); fungi, such as those endemic to specific geographic areas (*Coccidioides*, *Histoplasma* and *Blastomyces*) and those responsible for infections in compromised hosts (*Candida*, *Cryptococcus* and *Aspergillus*); parasites, such as *Toxoplasma gondii* and those that cause cysticercosis; and, most frequently, viruses (enteroviruses – coxsackie, echo, entero, herpes viruses, varicella, Epstein-Barr virus (EBV), CMV, influenza, measles, mumps and rubella).

Focal infections of the CNS including brain abscess and parameningeal abscess (subdural empyema, cranial and spinal epidural abscess) may also be confused with meningitis. In addition, noninfectious illnesses can cause generalised inflammation of the CNS. Relative to infections, these disorders are uncommon and include malignancy, collagen vascular syndromes and exposure to toxins.

Careful examination of the CSF may indicate the specific cause with specific stains (Kinyoun carbol fuchsin for mycobacteria, India ink for fungi), cytology, antigen detection (*Cryptococcus*), serology (syphilis, West Nile virus, arboviruses), viral culture (enterovirus) and polymerase chain reaction (HSV, enterovirus and others). **PCR of the CSF has a sensitivity of 95 to 100% for HSV type 1, EBV and enterovirus. There is a wide range of variability in the sensitivity (54 to 100%) for PCR testing for tuberculous meningitis, with a specificity of 94–100%**, and it could replace acid-fast bacillus smear and culture as the test of choice. PCR is also sensitive for acute neurosyphilis but not for more chronic forms.[9,12,37]

23. Answer: C

This child's clinical findings suggest a viral URTI with a high temperature, and her likelihood of recurrent febrile seizure is 30%. Febrile convulsions are the most common seizure disorder in childhood and usually have an excellent prognosis. They are rare before 9 months and after 6 years of age. Febrile seizures have a genetic origin; the febrile seizure gene has been mapped to chromosomes 19p and 8q13–21. **The most important task is to determine the cause of the fever and to rule out meningitis or encephalitis**; these two serious conditions can usually be excluded on clinical grounds when children emerge from their short postictal state and return to a normal physiological well state. If any doubt exists about the possibility of meningitis, an LP with examination of the CSF is indicated, especially in children <12 months, if seizures are complex or sensorium remains clouded after a short postictal period. Viral infections are most frequently the cause of febrile convulsions.

A simple febrile convulsion is diagnosed in the presence of a:
- generalised tonic–clonic (GTC) seizure, that is
- brief in duration <15 minutes, and
- occurs once in 24-hour period
- without any signs of serious infection, and
- no clinical findings suggesting CNS infection, metabolic or traumatic cause, and
- normal developmental milestones

About 30% of children have recurrent febrile seizures with a subsequent febrile illness. Factors associated with increased recurrence risk include: age <12 months; lower temperature before seizure onset; a positive family history of febrile seizures; and complex features. Most children with febrile seizures have a similar risk of epilepsy as the general population (1%). The risk of subsequent epilepsy increases if atypical features are present, or if independent risk factors for epilepsy exist.

The height of fever is no longer strongly statistically correlated with a bacterial illness, due to the current low prevalence of streptococcal bacteremia after the introduction of PCV7 immunisation. Furthermore, antipyretics have not been shown to prevent seizure recurrences. Their role is restricted to improve comfort for the child. Seizures lasting >5 min should be terminated with a benzodiazepine as a first-line therapy. Anticonvulsant prophylaxis for preventing recurrent febrile convulsions is controversial and no longer recommended for most children. In selected cases where parental anxiety is very high and recurrent febrile seizures have occurred, some paediatricians and neurologists still advocate the use of oral diazepam as prophylaxis during a febrile illness. The side effects of this approach are usually minor, but this is certainly a controversial prophylactic measure and not a practice that is widespread.[16,38]

24. Answer: D

This boy presents with a simple febrile seizure in the setting of clinical findings suggestive of otitis media. The treatment for his viral otitis media is a nonsteroidal anti-inflammatory drug (NSAID) of which ibuprofen is well studied in this setting.

Children satisfying the criteria for simple febrile convulsions do not routinely require further investigations, aside from a blood sugar, and can usually be discharged home with appropriate follow-up. The yield from 'baseline blood tests' is extremely low, and electrolyte analysis is only indicated if a history of vomiting, diarrhoea or poor oral intake is present. Laboratory testing such as serum electrolytes should be individualised and are generally unwarranted. An underlying metabolic disorder would usually not present for the first time at age 3, and the patient would normally have some other features in the history to suggest such a disorder including failure to thrive, vomiting, abnormal development, features of malaise and previous seizures.

It is rare for bacterial meningitis to be diagnosed on a routine LP after a simple febrile seizure. If the only indication for performing an LP is the seizure, meningitis will be found in <1% of patients and less than one-half of these will have bacterial meningitis. A more appropriate option would be to arrange careful observation of the child within the ED or a short stay admission ward to detect other clinical features of invasive bacterial disease. The American Academy of Pediatrics recommends an LP in the setting of febrile seizures and:

- meningeal signs or symptoms or other clinical features that suggest a possible meningitis or intracranial infection
- in infants between 6 and 12 months if the immunisation status for *H. influenzae* type B or *S. pneumoniae* is deficient or undetermined
- when the patient is on antibiotics as this can mask the signs and symptoms of meningitis

It is the author's opinion that an LP should be considered if the febrile seizure is atypical or febrile status epilepticus (seizure >30 minutes) is the presenting seizure type.

Similarly, an electroencephalogram (EEG) and neuroimaging is not warranted after a simple febrile seizure. Patients with symptoms falling outside of the definition of simple febrile seizure have an atypical or complex febrile seizure and should be admitted for further investigation.[39,40]

25. Answer: B

Standard protocols suggest the following sequence of therapies is effective:

- Maintain airway and provide oxygen, assess ventilation.
- Consider IV glucose if hypoglycemic or unable to rapid test glucose.
- Consider IV pyridoxine in neonates or if isoniazid toxicity suspected.
- Repeat benzodiazepines once or twice in succession and if there is no response in 5 minutes
  - midazolam IV, intranasal, buccal or IM, or
  - diazepam PR or IV.

- Try phenytoin loading 15–20 mg/kg IV if there's no response after 15 minutes.
- Administer phenobarbitone 15–20 mg/kg IV or IM if there's no response after 20 minutes.

Consider anaesthetic agents (thiopentone, propofol, isoflurane) or other anticonvulsants. Once anaesthetic agents are considered for termination, definitive airway management with intubation and mechanical ventilation is mandated.

Phenytoin loading is reduced in the setting of patients who are known to be on phenytoin where there is some risk of toxicity. Normal doses should be used if phenytoin level is known to be low.

Intravenous sodium valproate has been shown to be efficacious in the management of refractory status epilepticus (SE). Intravenous Keppra is a drug that also shows promise in the management of refractory SE. Other novel approaches to the management of SE include:

- midazolam infusion with or without intubation and ventilation
- clonazepam IV
- paraldehyde IV: loading dose followed by infusion. A 5% solution of paraldehyde is prepared by adding 1.75 mL of paraldehyde (1 g/mL) to D_5W to a total volume of 35 mL. The drug is incompatible with plastic and therefore a glass bottle should be used.

At this stage in management, patients should usually be cared for in an ICU setting, preferably with EEG monitoring available to detect non-convulsive status.[41–45]

26. Answer: D

Neonatal seizures often present in a subtle way and often carry a poor prognosis. Unlike seizures in older children, neonatal seizures are less likely to be idiopathic and need a more extensive evaluation. The differential diagnosis includes:

- trauma (always suspect non-accidental injury)
- sepsis (regardless of a fever history)
- metabolic disorders
  - electrolyte abnormalities
  - glucose abnormalities
  - inborn error of metabolism
- drug withdrawal or overdose

The clinical findings in this case are suggestive of raised intracranial pressure; a non-accidental injury should always be excluded. In this particular case, a work-up to cover the above differentials would include an urgent brain CT scan to exclude acute or acute on chronic subdural haemorrhage.

This neonate needs resuscitative care with oxygen and fluid. Neonatal status epilepticus is best terminated with phenobarbitone loading as first choice, followed by benzodiazepines as second-line therapy if this fails. BP assessment in neonates is notoriously inaccurate, as is the fundoscopic exam, therefore cushings triad (bradycardia, hypotension, papilloedema) may be hard to define and the drowsiness and bradycardia may be enough evidence for mannitol administration to prevent or ameliorate raised intracranial pressure and possible uncal or tonsillar herniation.

A trial of pyridoxine is an excellent option once obvious traumatic, infective or metabolic causes have been excluded, and particularly if the seizures have been ongoing and have not responded to the standard status epilepticus regimes. It is commonly commenced in an ICU or paediatric ward scenario.[1,44,46]

27. Answer: D

In general, anticonvulsants are commenced after a patient has had two or more seizures. This decision is usually taken in conjunction with the child's follow-up team such as neurologist, paediatrician or GP. Factors that are included in this decision are:
- exclusion of organic causes of seizure
- the age of the patient
- the type of seizure and risk of recurrence
- comorbid medical and psychosocial factors
- the benefit from the drug outweighing its side effect profile

Table 22.2 summarises the most common anti-convulsants used in paediatric epilepsy syndromes.

Topiramate is an anticonvulsant that is specific as adjunctive therapy for partial seizures or Lennox-Gastaut syndrome. Levetiracetam (Keppra) is indicated for adjunctive therapy in partial seizures, GTC and juvenile myoclonic seizures.[47]

28. Answer: B

This child presents with combination of subtle seizures and myoclonic seizures. Five seizure types are common in neonates: subtle, tonic, clonic, spasms and myoclonic. Often there is no EEG seizure correlation with the clinical picture. It is rare for neonates to have GTC seizures, as the immature neonatal central nervous system (CNS) is unable to sustain such neurological activity. 'Subtle' seizures are much more common and include chewing, lip smacking, bicycling, eye deviation or blinking – these are usually not correlated on an EEG. Myoclonic seizures are rapid jerking, single or repetitive, and suggest severe underlying pathology. Tonic seizures – focal or generalised with sustained tonic activity – are often due to HIE in neonates. Clonic seizures – focal or multifocal – with rhythmic jerking of limb or limbs often relate to metabolic abnormality such as hypoglycemia. Spasms are sudden generalised jerks lasting 1–2 seconds that are distinguished from generalised tonic spells by their shorter duration.

The above clinical picture suggests a hypoxic perinatal event in an at-risk population (premature, low birth weight with initial low Apgar score). *HIE* is a common complication of premature births. HIE is the cause of 50–60% of all neonatal seizures, with perinatal asphyxia the most common mechanism causing HIE in neonates. At birth, these infants may

TABLE 22.2 COMMON ANTI-CONVULSANTS USED IN PAEDIATRIC EPILEPSY SYNDROMES

| | Generalised | | | | Partial | |
	GTC	Absence	Myoclonus	Atonic	SPS	CPS
Carbamazepine	√				√	√
Phenytoin	√				√	√
Valproate	√	√	√		√	√
Clonazepam			√	√		
Ethosuximide		√				

be depressed and may fail to breathe spontaneously. In the ensuing hours, they remain hypotonic or change from a hypotonic to a hypertonic state, or their tone may appear normal. Hypotonia, lethargy and decreased spontaneous movements are classic signs. Upper motor neuron (UMN) brisk tendon reflexes and hypotonia are hallmarks of this condition.

Intracranial haemorrrhage is the second most common cause of neonatal seizures. Intracerebral haemorrhage is often related to prematurity, while subdural haematoma and subarachnoid haemorrhage are associated with term babies and birth trauma or non-accidental injury (NAI). The obvious complication to rule out in this setting is birth trauma with intracranial haemorrhage – a head ultrasound followed by definitive brain CT is indicated. NAI with subdural or extradural haemorrhage is another important differential to consider.

Meningitis is a possible diagnosis in this scenario, but the absence of fever is against this as the likeliest diagnosis. After a head CT has excluded focal pathology, an LP is indicated. Additionally, any of the antenatal or peripartum infectious agents included in the TORCHES infections (toxoplasmosis, rubella, CMV, herpes and syphillis) may cause seizures in the neonate and a full septic work-up is always indicated.

While *hypoglycaemia* can cause seizures, the BSL of 3.1 is not classified as hypoglycaemia requiring correction. A sugar <2.7mmol/L would require 5 mL/kg 10% dextrose as an immediate IV bolus. Other causes of seizures include hypocalcaemia, hypomagnesemia, hypo- or hypernatraemia, kernicterus, inborn errors of metabolism, mitochondrial defects and pyridoxine dependency, which may respond to a trial of pyridoxine and drug withdrawal syndromes related to narcotic or amphetamine abusing mothers.[47]

29. Answer: C

There is some disagreement in the literature, and also within paediatric neurology circles, about which is the anticonvulsant of choice in status epilepticus in neonates. A suggested regime is as follows.

- Initial seizure termination
  - Lorazepam 0.05 mg/kg IV can be used either as the initial drug or as second-line treatment in a newborn who did not respond to treatment

with phenobarbital and phenytoin. The anticonvulsant effect is seen within 5 minutes and the effect can last 6–24 hours. It does not usually cause hypotension or respiratory depression.

- Second dose of benzodiazepine
  - Midazolam 0.1 mg/kg IV or 0.2 mg/kg IM, IN or buccal. More experience with midazolam infusions is slowly making its way into the literature with promise.
  - Diazepam 0.1–0.2 mg/kg IV may be considered. However, diazepam is highly lipophilic, distributes very rapidly into the brain and then is cleared very quickly out; therefore, there is a risk of recurrence of seizures. Additionally, there is a risk of apnoea and hypotension, particularly if the patient has received a barbiturate and these features make it a less suitable agent.
- Phenobarbitone 10–20 mg /kg IV – traditionally considered by many to be the drug of first choice in neonatal seizures.
- Phenytoin 15–20 mg/kg, although kinetics very difficult to predict in neonates. If a total loading dose of 40 mg/kg of phenobarbital is not effective, then a loading dose of 15–20 mg/kg of phenytoin can be administered intravenously. The rate must not exceed 0.5–1 mg/kg/min in order to prevent cardiac problems. Phenytoin should not be mixed with dextrose solutions. Owing to its reduced solubility, potentially severe local cutaneous reactions, interaction with other drugs and possible cardiac toxicity, intravenous phenytoin is not widely used.

Consideration of novel drugs in discussion with paediatric neurology. Topiramate and levetiracetam have been reported to be the drugs of second and third choice for many paediatric neurologists. Further studies are needed to confirm efficacy and safety profiles in neonates.

- Trial of IV pyridoxine. Pyridoxine dependency, a rare, inherited autosomal recessive disorder, must be considered when generalised clonic seizures begin shortly after birth with signs of fetal distress in utero. These seizures are particularly resistant to conventional anticonvulsants such as phenobarbital or phenytoin. When pyridoxine-dependent seizures are suspected, pyridoxine or pyridoxal phosphate should be administered intravenously, ideally during the performance of an EEG. The seizures abruptly cease, and the EEG normalises in the next few hours. Some cases of pyridoxine dependency do not respond dramatically to the initial bolus of IV pyridoxine. Therefore, a 6-week trial of oral pyridoxine or preferably pyridoxal phosphate is recommended for infants in whom a high index of suspicion is present.[47]

30. Answer: B

This child has features suggesting a diagnosis of DKA in the setting of an intercurrent upper respiratory tract infection. Her vital signs are not suggestive for shock, but rather support the likelihood of acidosis; increased respiratory rate due to compensatory respiratory alkalosis, and a delayed capillary refill, which accompanies acidosis. She has some features of dehydration, likely due to her osmotic diuresis. The biochemical criteria for the diagnosis of DKA include:

- hyperglycaemia – blood glucose >11 mmol/L
- venous pH <7.3 and/or bicarbonate <15 mmol/L
- associated glycosuria, ketonuria and ketonaemia

There is no universal agreement as to the exact definition of DKA, nor is there exact agreement as to how to grade the severity of DKA. The Australian Society of Paediatrtic Endocrinology (ASPEG) uses the following classification based on the severity of acidosis:

- mild: venous pH <7.25–7.3, bicarbonate 10–15 mmol/L
- moderate: venous pH 7.1–7.24, bicarbonate 5–10 mmol/L
- severe: venous pH <7.1, bicarbonate <5 mmol/L

Fluid management in DKA in children is always balanced against their increased risk of cerebral oedema. Cerebral oedema may develop as a complication of the disease process as well as the theoretical pathogenesis due to the rapid administration or excessive volume of fluid. For this reason, fluid deficit and maintenance is replaced over 48 hours. **There is currently a strong trend away from bolus fluid management in children with DKA**, unless shock is evident, in which case caution is advised when administering a fluid bolus, and the current recommendation is not to exceed a bolus of 20 mL/kg (without prior consultation with an intensivist or paediatric endocrinologist).

Urine output is a poor marker of good renal perfusion due to the profound osmotic diuresis present anyway, which once more makes estimation of fluid requirements in DKA challenging.[48]

31. Answer: A

Although poorly understood, the risk factors for cerebral oedema in DKA include presentation with new onset type 1 diabetes, younger age, elevated serum urea nitrogen and/or severity of dehydration at presentation, severity of acidosis, greater hypocapnia at presentation (after adjusting for degree of acidosis) and an attenuated rise in serum sodium during treatment for DKA. Bicarbonate treatment to correct acidosis has also been associated with cerebral oedema, but whether this is due to a de novo effect, or simply a reflection of the severity of DKA, is unclear.

The use of hypotonic fluids, however, is associated with greater rises in intracranial pressure compared with isotonic fluids. **Therefore, the use of solutions with salt content <0.45% NaCl, which contain a large amount of electrolyte-free water, is likely to lead to a rapid osmolar change, movement of fluid into the intracellular fluid (ICF) compartment and may increase the risk of cerebral oedema.** The failure of the serum sodium to rise or development of hyponatraemia during intravenous fluid administration has been shown to precede cerebral oedema.[48–52]

32. Answer: C

Factors associated with DKA in children with newly diagnosed type 1 diabetes include younger age (those aged <5 years are at greatest risk), children with a first degree relative with type 1 diabetes, and those from families of lower socioeconomic status. High-dose glucocorticoids, antipsychotics, diazoxide and immunosuppressive drugs have been reported to precipitate DKA in individuals not previously diagnosed with type 1 diabetes. The risk of DKA in established type 1 diabetes is increased in children and young people with poor metabolic control or previous episodes of DKA.

The most common precipitating factors in the development of DKA include infection, often as a result of inadequate insulin therapy during intercurrent illness and insulin omission. Adolescent girls, children with psychiatric disorders (e.g. eating disorders) and those from families of lower socioeconomic status are also at increased risk. DKA is rare in children whose insulin is administered by a responsible adult.

Insulin should be commenced after fluid rehydration has commenced. Administration of intravenous fluid prior to insulin results in substantial falls in blood glucose, because the resultant increase in glomerular filtration rate (GFR) leads to increased urinary glucose excretion. The aims of fluid and sodium replacement therapy in DKA are:

- restoration of circulating volume
- replacement of sodium and water deficits over at least 36–48 hours
- restoration of GFR with enhanced clearance of glucose and ketones from the blood
- avoidance of cerebral oedema, which may be caused by fluid shifts from the extracellular fluid (ECF) to the ICF compartment

Following initial resuscitation (if required), subsequent fluid management should be with 0.9% saline. If hypernatraemia is present, consider the use of 0.45% saline.

Abdominal pain may be a prominent complaint in children experiencing DKA. The abdominal pain may be severe enough to mimic an acute 'surgical abdomen'. The exact cause of the abdominal pain associated with DKA is not known. One theory involves prostaglandins. Prostaglandins I2 and E2, which are generated in adipose tissue, are increased during DKA.[48,52,53]

33. Answer: A

Young or partially treated children and pregnant adolescents may present in DKA with near-normal glucose values ('euglycaemic ketoacidosis'), where ketosis and abnormal acid–base measurement satisfy part of the diagnostic criteria. Relative normoglycaemia may be seen in patients who were given or took insulin before being seen in the ED, those who were starving or had reduced food intake, and those who have impaired gluconeogenesis from liver failure.

In a study of children with DKA where their WCC was reviewed, it was found that neither the absolute WBC count, nor the differential or the presence of leukocytosis were associated with bacterial infections. Leukocytosis was common regardless of the absence of infection, the presence of a presumed viral infection, or the presence of a bacterial infection. The mechanism for this postulated to be due to the general adrenergic drive present in DKA.

A serum measurement of beta-hydroxybutyrate is the preferred method of measuring ketones in children with suspected or confirmed DKA. The nitroprusside method for measuring ketones in the urine only measures acetoacetic acid and acetone, not beta-hydroxybutyrate, the dominant acid in DKA. Because beta-hydroxybutyrate is converted to acetoacetic acid during successful treatment of DKA, acetoacetic acid levels rise, which may lead to confusion as to whether the acidosis is improving or worsening. Recent studies indicate that advances in point of care 'fingerprick' ketone measurement are more accurate than traditional urine ketone assessment.

Hypocalcaemia is usually not a feature of DKA. The differentiation of DKA from ethylene glycol (EG) is largely based on the clinical progression of EG poisoning through various stages, as well the specific finding of an osmolality gap in the first stage of EG poisoning. Measurement of EG in serum or urine will confirm the diagnosis.

Urinalysis may be diagnostic with calcium oxalate crystalluria, highly suggestive of EG poisoning. Fluorescein is added to many commercial antifreeze preparations hence fluorescence of urine or gastric contents with a Wood lamp supports EG poisoning early after ingestion.[53–57]

34. Answer: D

This 4-month-old boy (by corrected age) presents with typical features suggestive of bronchiolitis. However, he also has chronic failure to thrive (FTT) (babies gain on average 20–30g per day for the first 2–3 months of life) and this, coupled with recurrent respiratory tract illnesses, suggests that he has an underlying disorder. His tachycardia, sweaty appearance and FTT is suggestive of heart failure and possible cardiac pathology, hence his need for CXR.

Bacterial pneumonia is a clinical diagnosis; this child appears well, interactive and is apyrexial (i.e. he appears non-toxic). Furthermore, no asymmetrical findings are present – the hallmark of bacterial lobar consolidation in children. The presence of wheeze makes bacterial lobar pneumonia very unlikely.

Bronchiolitis is a clinical diagnosis based on typical features including cough, tachypnoea, feeding difficulties and inspiratory crackles – wheezing may be associated but is not an essential feature. The upper age for bronchiolitis is limited to 12 months of age in the Australasian and English literature, whereas European and North American publications include cases up to age of 3 years – this may explain 'bronchodilator response' in some studies. The differential diagnosis should always be considered and include:

- asthma in young children with atopy
- cystic fibrosis or congenital lung disease
- recurrent aspiration or inhaled foreign body
- exacerbation or unmasking of cardiac disease and heart failure
- atypical bacterial infections (i.e. pertussis, mycoplasma, chlamydia)
- sepsis with tachypnoea

A risk assessment should always be performed on children with bronchiolitis to identify those in which a severe course of illness is anticipated. These risk factors include:

- prematurity (gestational age <37 weeks)
- low birth weight
- age <6–12 weeks
- chronic pulmonary disease (bronchopulmonary dysplasia, cystic fibrosis, congenital anomaly)
- haemodynamically significant congenital heart disease
- immunodeficiency
- neurologic disease

Routine NPA (nasopharyngeal aspirate) testing is of little clinical value in the well bronchiolitic. There is some value in doing this test where patients are being admitted to an inpatient ward; cohorting patients with the same viruses may decrease the rate of nosocomial spread. Routine suctioning and toilet of the nasal passage with saline is common practice, but it has not been studied in any prospective or randomised trials to assess if it is beneficial.

A CXR is not routinely indicated in children with bronchiolitis. Radiography may be useful when the hospitalised child does not improve at the expected rate, if the severity of disease requires further evaluation, or if another diagnosis is suspected. Although many infants with bronchiolitis have abnormalities that show on chest radiographs, data are insufficient to demonstrate that chest radiograph abnormalities correlate well with disease severity. Further, obtaining a CXR could affect the emergency clinician's decision to start antibiotics. This child needs a CXR to ascertain why he has had recurrent respiratory illnesses, FTT and to evaluate specifically for heart failure.[58–60]

35. Answer: B

This child requires an ordered approach to aid diagnosis and management. The 'hyperoxia test' essentially trials whether high-dose oxygen makes a differences to the saturations recorded on pulse oxymetry. If it does, this likely reflects a pulmonary cause, rather than a pure cardiac lesion. Classic congenital heart disease does not respond to the hyperoxia test.

The initial evaluation involves a systematic approach with three major components. First, consider two major groups based on the presence or absence of cyanosis, which can be determined by examination aided by pulse oximetry. Second, these two groups can be further subdivided according to whether the chest radiograph shows evidence of increased, normal, or decreased pulmonary vascular markings. Finally, the ECG can be used to determine whether right, left or biventricular hypertrophy exists. The character of the heart sounds and the presence and character of any murmurs further narrow the differential diagnosis. The final diagnosis is then confirmed by echocardiography, CT or MRI, or cardiac catheterisation.[61]

36. Answer: D

Children often present to the ED with innocent murmurs when auscultation is carried out under nonbasal circumstances (high cardiac output because of fever, infection, anxiety).

Features suggestive of pathologic murmurs include diastolic murmurs, pansystolic, grade III or higher, harsh, located at the left upper sternal border, and associated with an early or midsystolic click or an abnormal second heart sound.

The most common innocent murmur is a medium-pitched, vibratory or 'musical,' short systolic ejection murmur along the left lower and midsternal border with no significant radiation to the apex, base or back. The intensity of the murmur often changes with respiration and position and may be attenuated in the sitting or prone position.

Innocent pulmonic murmurs are also common and occur due to turbulence during ejection into the pulmonary artery. They are higher pitched, blowing, brief early systolic murmurs of grade I–II in intensity and are best detected in the second left parasternal space with the patient in the supine position.

A venous hum is another common innocent murmur heard during childhood due to turbulence of blood in the jugular venous system; they have no pathologic significance and may be heard in the neck or anterior portion of the upper part of the chest. It usually has a soft humming sound heard in both systole and diastole; it can be exaggerated or made to disappear by varying the position of the head, or it can be decreased by lightly compressing the jugular venous system in the neck. These manoeuvres are sufficient to differentiate a venous hum from the murmurs produced by a patent ductus arteriosus.[62]

37. Answer: B

This child presents with classic features of heart failure. The child is acyanotic and appears to have increased blood flow to the lungs (on CXR and clinically evidenced by pulmonary oedema). **The most common lesions in this group are those that cause left-to-right shunting: atrial septal defect, ventricular septal defect (VSD), AV septal defects (AV canal), and patent ductus arteriosus.** There is communication between the systemic and pulmonary sides of the circulation, which results in shunting of fully oxygenated blood back into the lungs. The direction and magnitude of the shunt across such a communication depend on the size of the defect, the relative pulmonary and systemic pressure and vascular resistances, and the compliances of the two chambers connected by the defect.

A large VSD will have little shunting and few symptoms during the initial weeks of life but as pulmonary vascular resistance declines in the next several weeks, the volume of the left-to-right shunt increases, and symptoms begin to appear, usually at 2–4 months of age. Fluid leaks into the interstitial space and alveoli and causes pulmonary oedema. If left untreated, pulmonary vascular resistance eventually begins to rise and, by several years of age, the shunt volume will decrease and eventually reverse to right to left (Eisenmenger physiology, where pulmonary hypertension supercedes with resultant cyanosis and fixed split second heart sound).

Additional lesions that impose a volume load on the heart include regurgitant lesions and the cardiomyopathies. Regurgitation through the AV valves is most commonly encountered in patients with partial or complete AV septal defects (AV canal, endocardial cushion defects). In these lesions, the combination of a left-to-right shunt with AV valve regurgitation increases the volume load on the heart and often leads to more severe symptoms. Isolated regurgitation through the tricuspid valve is seen in mild to moderate forms of Ebstein's anomaly.

In contrast to left-to-right shunts, heart muscle function is decreased in the cardiomyopathies. Cardiomyopathies may affect systolic contractility or diastolic relaxation, or both. Decreased cardiac function results in increased atrial and ventricular filling pressure, and pulmonary oedema occurs secondary to increased capillary pressure. The major causes of cardiomyopathy in infants and children include viral myocarditis, metabolic disorders and genetic defects.

TOF is a cyanotic lesion that results from pulmonary outflow tract obstruction and results in cyanotic spells with decreased pulmonary blood flow. **Patients with TOF do not present with pulmonary oedema.** The other components of TOF include an over-riding aorta, VSD and right ventricular (RV) hypertrophy.[61]

38. Answer: B

Salbutamol has been shown in a Cochrane review to be ineffective in the management of bronchiolitis. It found bronchodilators other than adrenaline had no effect on the rate of hospitalisation or other longer term outcomes although it may produce small short-term improvements.[83] The American Academy of Pediatrics still advocates the use of salbutamol as a trial in infants with a history of response to bronchodilator or a strong family history of asthma or atopy, in the age group over 6 months, despite a paucity of evidence in its favour. The small potential benefit of routine short-acting bronchodilator treatment must be weighed against the potential negative effects associated with these agents.

A transient decrease in saturation is common after the administration of a bronchodilator, as its first effect is on the pulmonary vasculature, which causes vessel dilation, while the airway remains bronchconstricted with poor airflow. This results in a worsening of the ventilation-perfusion mismatch, albeit transiently, until the airway also dilates to improve airflow to the now already dilated capillary bed, ultimately improving gaseous exchange.

Steroids are of no benefit in bronchiolitis. Another Cochrane review determined that systemic corticosteroids have no impact on clinical scores, admission rates, length of stay or readmission rates and should not be used routinely in the management of bronchiolitis.[84]

Three percent hypertonic saline may be useful. Four small trials assessed in a 2008 Cochrane review, have shown to improve clinical scores and reduce the length of stay. This supports a beneficial adjunctive role for hypertonic saline in the treatment of bronchiolitis. However, there is not enough data to make an evidence-based recommendation.[58–60,63–65]

39. Answer: B

The treatment for bronchiolitis remains controversial and is mainly supportive. **Infants with respiratory distress are at increased risk of aspiration.** It may be necessary to suspend oral feeding because of concerns about pulmonary aspiration. However, whether nasogastric or intravenous fluids are most efficacious is still uncertain. Two large prospective randomised controlled trials are currently comparing the two therapies to assess which is most efficacious.

Nebulised adrenaline, which has both β2-agonist and α-agonist activity, has also been proposed as a useful therapy in bronchiolitis as it might reduce airway oedema. **However, an Australian randomised controlled trial and a Cochrane review failed to demonstrate any clinically significant benefit for the use of nebulised adrenaline for infants admitted to hospital with bronchiolitis.**[85] Additionally, adrenaline cannot be instituted as outpatient therapy. The American Academy of Pediatrics still suggests a carefully monitored trial of α-adrenergic or β2-adrenergic medication as an option but emphasises that therapy should be continued only if there is a documented positive clinical response to the trial using an objective means of evaluation.[58]

A Cochrane review found no evidence to support the use of *physiotherapy* in the care of infants with bronchiolitis[69] (see Table 22.3).

Nasal continuous positive airway pressure has been shown to be efficacious in the setting of rising oxygen

TABLE 22.3 SUMMARY OF COCHRANE REVIEWS OF TREATMENT OPTIONS IN BRONCHIOLITIS

Intervention	Year of Cochrane review	Conclusion
Physiotherapy	2005	No benefit
Systemic corticosteroids	2007	No benefit
Inhaled corticosteroids	2007	No benefit
Bronchodilators	2006	No significant benefit: not recommended
Nebulised adrenaline	2004	No benefit
Nebulised 3% hypertonic saline	2008	Useful: improved clinical scores
Antibiotics	2007	No benefit
Ribavirin	2004	No benefit

requirements in an infant who is tiring, where it is useful for reducing the need for endotracheal intubation. More data with larger trial numbers is needed to further confirm these findings.[59,60,66–70]

40. Answer: B

Assessing the severity of presenting signs and symptoms during an acute asthma episode is crucial in determining the initial management strategy (see Table 22.4). This child satisfies the criteria for severe/life-threatening asthma and requires immediate management with oxygen and continuous nebulised salbutamol and three doses of nebulised ipratropium. Current trends in life-threatening asthma management support the use of intravenous salbutamol as well as concurrent or subsequent use of intravenous magnesium sulfate. Aminophylline has fallen out of favour in recent years due to its poor side effect profile (specifically nausea and vomiting), despite the fact that studies have shown good efficacy in the management of acute severe and life-threatening asthma. For this reason it is usually recommended only in the intensive care setting. There is no role for empiric antibiotics when sepsis is not suspected. Most exacerbations of asthma will be viral induced.[71]

TABLE 22.4 INITIAL ASSESSMENT OF ACUTE ASTHMA IN CHILDREN

Symptoms	Mild	Moderate	Severe and life threatening*
Altered consciousness	No	No	Agitated Confused/drowsy
Oximetry on presentation (SaO$_2$)	94%	90–94%	<90%
Talks in	Sentences	Phrases	Words Unable to speak
Pulse rate	<100 beats/min	100–200 beats/min	>200 beats/min
Central cyanosis	Absent	Absent	Likely to be present
Wheeze intensity	Variable	Moderate to loud	Often quiet
PEF**	>60% predicted or personal best	40–60% predicted or personal best	<40% predicted or personal best Unable to perform
FEV1	More than 60% predicted	40–60% predicted	<40% predicted Unable to perform

Source: National Asthma Council Australia. Managing acute asthma in children. In: Asthma management handbook 2006; Table 5, p. 44. Online. Available: http://www.nationalasthma.org.au/cms/images/stories/amh2006_web 5.pdf; May 2011.
*Any of these features indicates that the episode is severe. The absence of any feature does not exclude a severe episode. These tests are usually not used in the assessment of acute asthma in children.
**Children under 7 years old are unlikely to perform PEF or spirometry reliably during an acute episode.

41. Answer: D

Wheezing is common in children with the highest incidence in preschool children. Epidemiological studies have demonstrated three different phenotypes; the majority of children will stop wheezing before the age of 3 (transient wheezers), some will wheeze beyond this age (persistent wheezers) and a small group will only start wheezing at 3 years of age (late onset wheezers). Few children continue to wheeze beyond 6 years.

In infants, wheezing is often not due to asthma but rather due to acute viral bronchiolitis or transient early wheeze. Therefore, the response to inhaled bronchodilators is not generally as beneficial as in older children. Young children aged 2–5 years usually do not have classical asthma but rather a viral-induced wheeze associated with a respiratory tract infection. These children are well in-between episodes, are non-atopic and have a good prospect of outgrowing the tendency to wheeze in later childhood. The standard approach for these patients is to use bronchodilators as needed. Neither inhaled nor oral steroids appear to be helpful. Leukotriene receptor antagonists (LTRA) may be useful both as a long-term preventive agent and as an 'episode modifier'.

From the author's perspective, the simplest approach to wheeze in children is to categorise by age:

- 0–12 months: bronchiolitis is the common cause of wheeze. Poor response to salbutamol is the rule and there is no role for steroid therapy.
- 12–24 months: viral-induced wheeze or transient wheezing in infancy is common. Salbutamol response is variable and the risks of regular steroid use far outweigh the unlikely gain (as the pathogenesis does not involve chronic inflammation). Some role for LRTA in this age group.
- >24 months: Unclear if recurrent episodes represent the previous diagnoses or progression to asthma. Salbutamol response is the rule and steroids as a short course is indicated. Differentiation into persistent or intermittent asthma is important, as well as formal lung testing to confirm the diagnosis in the >6-year age group. Persistent asthma and frequent intermittent asthma require consideration for preventer medication.

All of these groups still require the exclusion of other pathologies such as heart failure, foreign body aspiration, gastroesophageal reflux disease (GERD), suppurative lung disease, atypical pneumonia, cystic fibrosis and structural abnormalities to ensure the wheeze is not due to an organic cause. This exclusion of other causes can be done with careful history taking and good clinical examination.[71,72]

42. Answer: C

This girl has symptoms suggestive of asthma. She would be classified as persistent asthma due to her interval symptoms and would benefit from preventer medication. Exclusion of other causes of wheeze is an important consideration. This girl is unlikely to have a chronic lung disease such as cystic fibrosis or bronchiectasis as there is no evidence of FTT and no productive sputum. Nevertheless, a CXR is indicated due to the chronic nature of her symptoms, as well as formal lung function testing to confirm an obstructive lung disease pattern.

In the majority of children, the diagnosis of asthma is based on a history of recurrent or persistent wheeze in the absence of any other apparent pathology. Cough, shortness of breath, or both often accompany wheeze due to asthma. A history of associated eczema, urticaria or a history of asthma in a first-degree relative supports the diagnosis. In young children, asthma can be confirmed by a clinical response to an inhaled bronchodilator. In children aged ≥7 years, spirometry can be used reliably to confirm the diagnosis.

Classification of childhood asthma is based mainly on the clinical pattern (see Table 22.5). The pattern of asthma determines the need for preventive therapy in children. Children with intermittent, infrequent asthma can be managed with bronchodilators as needed. They do not require any long-term preventive medications. However, children of any age with frequent intermittent or persistent asthma will require preventative medication that is effective in reducing asthma attacks. In children with frequent intermittent and mild persistent asthma, inhaled cromones, oral leukotriene receptor antagonists (LTRAs) or low-dose inhaled corticosteroids (ICS) are recommended. For children with moderate-to-severe persistent asthma, an ICS is the preferred option. Long-acting beta$_2$-agonists (LABAs) can be prescribed in children in combination with ICS (salmeterol in children >5 years or eformoterol in children >12 years). However, there is limited evidence for their efficacy and safety in children. The National Asthma Council Australia suggests a stepwise approach to drug therapy in children – starting treatment at the step most appropriate to the level of asthma severity and step up or down as necessary. The goal is to decrease treatment to the least medication necessary to maintain control.[71]

TABLE 22.5 CLASSIFICATION OF ASTHMA IN CHILDREN OVER 5 YEARS OLD

	Daytime symptoms between exacerbations	Night-time symptoms between exacerbations	Exacerbations	PEF or FEV1*	PEF variability**
Infrequent intermittent	Nil	Nil	Brief, mild, occur less than every 4–6 weeks	>80% predicted	<20%
Frequent intermittent	Nil	Nil	>2 per month	At least 80% predicted	<20%
Mild persistent	>1 per week but not every day	>2 per month but not every week	May affect activity and sleep	At least 80% predicted	20–30%
Moderate persistent	Daily	>1 per week	At least twice per week; restricts activity or affects sleep	60–80% predicted	>30%
Severe persistent	Continual	Frequent	Frequent; restricts activity	≥60% predicted	>30%

Source: National Asthma Council Australia. Managing acute asthma in children. In: Asthma management handbook 2006; Table 2, p. 14. Online. Available: http://www.nationalasthma.org.au/cms/images/stories/amh2006_web_5.pdf; May 2011.
*Predicted values are based on age, sex and height.
**Difference between morning and evening values.

43. Answer: D

This child most likely has post viral cough syndrome with irritation of her upper airways, activation of cough receptors and therefore worse coughing at night (due to cold air, and lying flat with upper airway secretions causing irritation). Symptomatic management with upper airway soothing agents such as honey or warm drinks may be of benefit, although the course is usually 4–8 weeks with spontaneous resolution in time. Pneumonia is unlikely, as this child appears completely well. Cough can be the predominant symptom of asthma, but it is extremely rare for cough to be the only symptom. When cough is due to asthma, it is usually accompanied by some wheeze and episodes of shortness of breath.

Most children with chronic cough require some diagnostic work-up including a CXR, sputum examination and a nasopharyngeal aspirate polymerase chain reaction (NPA-PCR) for pertussis or other specific viral testing. Exclusion of pertussis by NPA-PCR, empiric treatment with azithromycin and a screening CXR are usual initial steps in the ED. The most important management point is reassurance to parents after thorough clinical assessment, with an end point at 2 months of ongoing symptoms requiring referral to a respiratory clinician for more complicated work-up, including tests for cystifibrosis, aspiration syndromes and gastroesophageal reflux.[71,73–75]

44. Answer: B

Bacterial pneumonia beyond the neonatal period generally has a sudden onset with associated high fever (often temperature >39°C). Cough may or may not be present, but children often appear relatively toxic with tachypnoea disproportionate to the fever. Confined rales or wheezes and localised decreased breath sounds commonly occur in older children, although the physical examination in a younger child may be completely unrevealing.

S. pneumoniae is the most common bacterial agent causing pneumonia in children. Risk factors for developing infection from *S. pneumoniae* include immune deficiency, chronic renal disease, functional or anatomic asplenia, and Aboriginal or Torres Strait Islander decent.

S. aureus pneumonia is less common and tends to cause a more severe pneumonia, with more than 70% of all cases occurring in the first year of life. Children with foreign body aspiration, immunosuppression, or skin infections may be at increased risk for *S. aureus* pneumonia. Progression of the disease is rapid, and empyema (90%), pneumatocele (50%), pneumothorax (25%) and bacteremia are common complications.

H. influenzae incidence has decreased by 90% since the introduction of immunisation but it still causes clinically important respiratory disease (mostly non-type B strains). Most cases now occur in older children. *H. influenzae* pneumonia has a higher incidence of associated pleural effusions (25–75%) and bacteremia (75–95%). Other foci of infection are more common and include meningitis, epiglottitis, septic arthritis, pericarditis, soft tissue infection, and otitis media.

Group A streptococcal pneumonia may occur sporadically and may occur as a complication of varicella. It is typically a severe illness with rapid progression to toxicity and a high fatality rate.

M. pneumonia accounts for 10 to 20% of all pneumonias and traditional teaching was that it affected 5–18 year olds. However, it clearly plays a significant role in younger children but is still rare in infants <1 year old. Classically, the onset is gradual and insidious, but some patients also may present with abrupt onset of symptoms similar to its bacterial counterpart. Prodromal symptoms include fever, headache and malaise followed several days later by a nonproductive, hacking cough. Patients also may present with pertussis-like illness. Other symptoms of infection may include hoarseness, sore throat and chest pain; coryza is unusual. Children with mycoplasmal pneumonia generally appear nontoxic. Patients may have rales, with wheezing occurring less often. Pharyngitis, cervical lymphadenopathy, conjunctivitis and otitis media may occur occasionally. Rash is present in 10% of patients and may be urticarial, erythema multiforme, maculopapular or vesicular. Myooplasma is generally a benign and self-limited infection but does play a significant role in exacerbating asthma, and can be the inciting infection leading to bronchiectasis. The radiographic findings typically are more impressive than the physical exam; involvement is usually unilateral and in the lower lobes. The radiographic findings may include lobar consolidation, scattered segmental infiltrates or interstitial disease. Pleural effusions may occur but are uncommon. The WBC count is usually normal; the erythrocyte sedimentation rate tends to be elevated. Mycoplasma infection is often diagnosed clinically and treated empirically. Diagnosis may be confirmed with acute and convalescent antibody titers; however, patients may take 4–6 weeks to seroconvert, and some patients may fail to mount an immune response. Culture is not routinely available; PCR diagnosis from throat swabs is available at selected labs. Complications are varied but unusual and include haemolytic anaemia, myopericarditis, neurologic disease (meningoencephalitis, Guillain–Barré syndrome, transverse myelitis, cranial neuropathy), arthritis and rash.[76]

45. Answer: D

GBS and gram-negative bacilli predominate in neonates. Ureaplasma urealyticum and Listeria monocytogenes may cause illness in infants younger than 3 months. This is the rationale for empiric neonatal antibiotic cover (for fever without source) with ampicillin and gentamicin with penicillins preferred over cephalosporins in covering listeria.

S. pneumoniae is the leading bacterial cause of pneumonia in all age groups beyond the newborn period, although the spectrum of invasive pneumococcal disease is changing after the introduction of Prevenar (PCV7), which is a heptavalent protein conjugate vaccine against the seven leading invasive strains of *S. pneumoniae*. A drastic reduction in all invasive pneumococcal disease has been seen between 2001–2005, with staphylococcus increasing in frequency as an invasive respiratory organism.

Respiratory syncytial virus (RSV) and parainfluenza are the most common viral agents in infants younger than 1 year. Viruses that may be responsible for neonatal pneumonia include rubella, CMV and HSV. Other viral agents include influenza, adenovirus, rhinovirus, enterovirus, measles, varicella and EBV.

Chlamydia trachomatis is a unique cause of pneumonia in infants 3–19 weeks old. *Bordetella pertussis* classically occurs in children younger than 1 year but also occurs in older children and adolescents. *M. pneumoniae* is one of the most common causes of pneumonia among children older than 5 years and may play a role in younger children but the incidence is much less. *Chlamydia*

pneumoniae is more common in children older than 5 years but also may cause infection in younger children.

An immunocompromised host is susceptible to all the aforementioned causes of pneumonia, as well as mixed and opportunistic infections including bacterial, viral (CMV, varicella), protozoan (*Pneumocystis carinii*), and fungal disease. *Pseudomonas aeruginosa*, *Legionella pneumophila*, *P. carinii*, and rickettsial infections need mention as well. The incidence of *M. tuberculosis* has in recent years increased with the co-infection of hosts with HIV disease, as well as resurgence in developed countries among the poor and dispossessed.[76]

46. Answer: D

A well-appearing child with cough and rales may be diagnosed clinically and treated as an outpatient. A child who appears ill or in whom the diagnosis is unclear requires further evaluation.

An arterial blood gas (ABG) should be considered in a child with severe respiratory distress. Serum electrolytes, blood urea nitrogen, and creatinine are useful in assessing the degree of dehydration and guiding fluid management when clinically relevant. The leukocyte count may be helpful in differentiating aetiology – peripheral WBC counts >15,000/mm³, with predominance of mature and immature granulocytes, suggest bacterial infection, with pneumococcal pneumonia typically producing the highest WBC counts. Normal to elevated WBC counts with lymphocytosis may be seen in viral infections, and eosinophilia suggests chlamydial disease. Increased WBC counts with extreme lymphocytosis typically are associated with pertussis. BC is not very useful because they are positive in only 1 to 10% of cases of bacterial pneumonia.

Sputum cultures may be useful in adolescents but are not useful in younger children because contamination by organisms of the upper respiratory tract is common. Bacterial cultures of upper respiratory secretions are of no value as they reflect only colonisation.

Patients with pleural effusions should have lateral decubitus radiographs to assess effusion size and loculation. Ultrasound is a useful ED modality to confirm fluid in the chest cavity. CT scan is useful to provide greater detail of effusions and lung abnormalities in critically ill children with complicated pneumonia. Thoracentesis for diagnostic and therapeutic purposes is important. Although most suggestive of bacterial infection, parapneumonic effusions also occur with mycoplasmal and occasionally with viral infections. Bronchoscopy with bronchoalveolar lavage may be useful in a severely ill child. Nasopharyngeal viral cultures, antigen detection for specific viral or bacterial agents, and serum antibodies for specific agents may be helpful in determining certain aetiologic agents. Skin testing for tuberculosis should be considered for patients with lobar pneumonia, pulmonary effusions or hilar adenopathy, especially in immunocompromised children or children who have recently immigrated from less developed countries.

Occasonally dehydration can result in a normal CXR, with rehydration revealing an obvious consolidation. Bacterial pathogens usually have alveolar infiltrates in a lobar distribution but may produce diffuse interstitial infiltrates. Viral and chlamydial infections tend to appear as diffuse interstitial infiltrates with associated hyperinflation and atelectasis. Chest radiographs also identify multilobar disease, pleural effusions, pneumatoceles and pneumothorax. Hilar adenopathy may indicate tuberculosis or malignancy. Children without comorbid conditions, who are without fever, unilateral wheezing or tachypnea, are unlikely to have pneumonia and a chest radiograph is unnecessary. Further, a Cochrane review demonstrated that for non-ill-appearing children with <14 days of symptoms and clinical signs of pneumonia, chest radiography does not reduce subsequent hospitalisation rate, nor duration of symptoms. Routine chest radiography is not beneficial in ambulatory children over 2 months with acute lower respiratory infections.[76,77]

47. Answer: C

In severe croup, there is stridor at rest but the loudness of the stridor is a poor guide to severity. Severe upper airway obstruction is characterised by signs of severe respiratory distress, cyanosis and reduced air entry. However, the stridor is usually soft and may be expiratory as well as inspiratory.

Principles of management include the following:

- Avoid agitating the patient. The child is best nursed on mother's lap and should be disturbed as little as possible.
- Caution is needed in administering oxygen in these settings as this may mask the signs of impending complete obstruction.
- Do not give steam or mist therapy; they are proven to be of no benefit in this setting.
- **Any form of steroid, regardless whether it is given orally, intravenously or intramuscularly, is effective in croup, but in severe settings, dexamethasone IM or IV is recommended. An alternative is prednisolone IV, oral or NG.** Steroids have been shown to lessen the duration of illness, amount of time in hospital and the amount of adrenaline nebuliser therapy required.
- **Administer adrenaline 1:1000, 0.5 mL/kg/dose (max 5–6 mL) by inhalation as required.** Outside intensive care settings, a doctor must be in attendance whenever adrenaline is given for croup, because the need for adrenaline indicates potential imminent airway obstruction.
- In intensive care, adrenaline can be given repeatedly every hour or two if required to give the dexamethasone time to take effect.
- The child should be intubated if he or she has severe obstruction, or has a poor response to inhaled adrenaline. Do not wait until the child is exhausted or very severely obstructed. **If intubation must be performed in the ED, an endotracheal tub (ETT) 1 mm smaller than that the calculated for age should be used to accommodate the subglottic oedema and airway narrowing.**[78,79]

48. Answer: A

A rudimentary understanding of developmental milestones is important, particularly when trying to assess if a child is toxic and unwell (assess if smiling), or if assessing traumatised children and establishing their risk of non-accidental injury when reviewing mechanism of injury and if injuries are developmentally appropriate (see Table 22.6). Other important scenarios for reviewing milestones include the assessment of failure to thrive or neurological disease.[80]

TABLE 22.6 DEVELOPMENTAL MILESTONES

Age (months)	Gross motor	Visual motor	Language, social and adaptive
1	Raises head slightly from prone position	Birth: visually fixes 1 month: has tight grasp, follows to midline	Alerts to sound Regards face
2	Holds head in midline, lifts chest off table	Follows object past midline	Smiles socially (after being stroked or talked to) Recognises parent
3	Supports on forearms in prone position, holds head up steadily	Holds hands open at rest, follows in circular fashion	Coos (produces long vowel sounds in musical fashion) Reaches for familiar people or objects, anticipates feeding
4	Rolls front to back	Reaches with arms in unison, brings hands to midline	Laughs, orients to voice Enjoys looking around
5	Rolls back to front, sits supported	Transfers objects	Says 'ah-goo,' orients to bell (localises laterally)
6	Sits unsupported, puts feet in mouth in supine position	Unilateral reach, uses raking grasp	Babbles Recognises strangers
7	Creeps		Orients to bell (localises indirectly)
8	Sits, crawls		'Dada' indiscriminately
9	Pivots when sitting, pulls to stand, cruises	Uses pincer grasp, waves bye-bye, holds bottle,	'Mama' indiscriminately, understands 'no'. Starts to explore environment, plays gesture games (e.g, patty cake) 10 months: 'Dada' and 'Mama' discriminately
12	Walks alone	Uses mature pincer grasp, releases voluntarily	Uses 2 words comes when called, cooperates with dressing
15	Creeps up stairs	Scribbles in imitation, builds tower of 2 blocks	Uses 4–6 words Uses spoon, uses cup independently, points to 5 body parts,
18	Runs	Scribbles spontaneously, builds tower of 3 blocks	2-word combinations, 7–20 words
21	Squats in play	Builds tower of 5 blocks	Uses 50 words, 2-word sentences. Asks to have food and to go to toilet
24	Walks up and down steps without help	Imitates stroke with pencil, builds tower of 7 blocks	Uses pronouns (I, you, me appropriately), follows 2-step commands

49. Answer: B

A knowledge of the normal variation with age of physiological parameters is important in assessing if a child is toxic or unwell (see Table 22.7). Normal heart rate varies with age. Tachycardia can be a product of fever, anxiety, pain or fear but is also the first and most sensitive sign of cardiovascular compromise in the paediatric patient. When measuring the heart rate, the quality of the pulse can be extremely helpful. The quality of the brachial and radial pulses or the femoral and dorsalis pedis pulses palpated concurrently provides important information to differentiate cardiovascular compromise from benign causes of tachycardia. Bradycardia can be an ominous sign in an ill patient heralding cardiopulmonary failure and impending cardiac arrest. In this patient, a mild tachycardia is probably due to a raised temperature, especially since other parameters of sepsis – CRT, appearance, RR – are normal. Repeated examination and vital sign review is important to complete a full

TABLE 22.7 NORMAL PAEDIATRIC VITAL SIGNS FOR AGE

Age (years)	Respiratory rate (breaths/minute)	Heart rate (beats per minute)
<1	30–60	100–160
1–2	24–40	90–150
2–5	22–34	80–140
6–12	18–30	70–120
>12	12–16	60–100

Adapted from Dieckmann R, Brownstein D, Gausche-Hill M, editors. Pediatric education for prehospital professionals. Sudbury: Mass, Jones & Bartlett, American Academy of Pediatrics, 2000:43–45.

assessment, that is, normalisation of HR when apyrexial would confirm the initial hypothesis.

Blood pressure measurement should be obtained in ill patients of all ages. Infants and young children have excellent compensatory measures for maintaining blood pressure in the presence of significant loss of circulatory volume. Compensatory mechanisms include an increase in heart rate and systemic vascular resistance. When these compensatory mechanisms fail and blood pressure drops below normal, the patient moves from a state of compensated to decompensated shock. Obtaining an accurate blood pressure in infants and small children requires the appropriate selection of the blood pressure cuff. A properly-sized cuff should cover approximately two-thirds of the circumference of the upper arm and extend at least 50% of the length of the upper arm. The lower limit for acceptable BP in children older than 1 year can be quickly estimated by using the following formula: systolic BP (mmHg) = 70 + (2 x age in years). The pulse oximetry waveform can also be used to determine systolic BP. Observing for the return of a plethysmographic waveform of the pulse oximeter as the BP cuff is deflated has been shown to correlate closely with conventional methods of BP measurement.[80]

Lower limits of systolic BP as suggested by the American Heart Association in the ECC guidelines 2000:

- 0–28 days: 60 mmHg
- 1–12 months: 70 mmHg
- 1–10 years: 70 mmHg + (2 x age in years).[86]

50. Answer: C

It is not unusual for infants to have periodic breathing with episodes of apnoea lasting up to 20 seconds. Their central control of ventilation matures with age and 'periodic breathing' is much less common by 6 months of age. These episodes may be benign but these babies usually require a careful history, examination and focused investigation to exclude signs of CNS disease (intracranial haemorrhage, seizures, meningitis, signs of NAI – clinical exam), early sepsis (clinical exam, temperature observation with septic screen if febrile, urine MCS), metabolic or electrolyte abnormality (BSL, U/E, venous gas and ammonia if appears encephalopathic) or dehydration due to poor feeding or GI losses. Obvious respiratory causes can be ruled out by careful respiratory exam, and cardiac/congenital heart disease likewise. Drug ingestion or medications taken by a breastfeeding mother should also be considered. A period of observation is usually required to ascertain if the baby is well, to support the diagnosis of benign physiological apnoea of the newborn. To be considered abnormal, periodic breathing must be associated with a drop in heart rate or oxygen saturation, or symptoms of peri-oral cyanosis or unresponsiveness.

The large surface area-to-weight ratio in young infants can result in heat loss and temperature instability. However, the need to maintain thermoregulation and normothermia needs to be balanced with the potential benefits in maintaining a hypothermic state in the 34–35°C range, in a child with an out-of-hospital arrest. More data is needed to establish whether hypothermia will deliver the same improvements in mortality and morbidity for children as the evidence suggests for adult out-of-hospital cardiac arrest.

Newborns are obligate nose breathers. Older infants are often preferential nose breathers, and nasal obstruction from secretions can result in significant airway compromise. An irritable and crying infant may just be learning to mouth-breathe when the nose is obstructed.

Because of the elasticity of the cervical spine in young children, spinal cord injuries without radiographic abnormalities (SCIWORA) can occur. These injuries result in ligamentous instability, which if ignored may result in significant morbidity or mortality.[80]

References

1. Mody AP, Silverman BK. Problems in the early neonatal period. In: Fleisher GR, Ludwig S, editors. Textbook of pediatric emergency medicine. 6th ed. Philadelphia: Lippincott Williams & Wilkins; 2011. p. 902–1010.

2. Carlo WA. Prematurity and intrauterine growth restriction. In: Kliegman RM, Behrman RE, Jenson HB, et al, editors. Nelson textbook of pediatrics. 19th edn. Philadelphia: Saunders Elsevier; 2011. p. 552–63.

3. Carlo WA. Overview of mortality and morbidity. In: Kliegman RM, Behrman RE, Jenson HB, et al, editors. Nelson textbook of pediatrics. 19th ed. Philadelphia: Saunders Elsevier; 2011. p. 531–40.

4. Peleg D, Kennedy CM, Hunter SK. Intrauterine growth restriction: identification and management. American Family Physician. Online. Available: http://www.aafp.org/afp/980800ap/peleg.html.

5. Centers for Disease Control and Prevention. Prevention of perinatal group B streptococcal disease. Revised guidelines from CDC, 2010. MMWR 2010; 59(RR-10):1–36. Online. Available: http://www.cdc.gov/groupbstrep/about/newborns-pregnant.html.

6. Ambalavanan N, Carlo WA. Jaundice and hyperbilirubinemia in the newborn. In: Kliegman RM, Behrman RE, Jenson HB, et al, editors. Nelson textbook of pediatrics. 19th ed. Philadelphia: Saunders Elsevier; 2011. p. 600–12.

7. Bhutani VK, Johnson LH, Sivieri EM. Predictive ability of a predischarge hour-specific serum bilirubin for subsequent significant hyperbilirubinemia in healthy term and near-term newborns. Pediatrics 1999;103:6–14.

8. Bhutani VK, Johnson LH, Keren R. Diagnosis and management of hyperbilirubinemia in the term neonate: for a safer first week. Pediatr Clin North Am 2004;51:843–61.

9. Prober CG, Dyner L. Central nervous system infections. In: Kliegman RM, Behrman RE, Jenson HB, et al, editors. Nelson textbook of pediatrics. 19th edn. Philadelphia: Saunders Elsevier; 2011. p. 2086–98.

10. Stoll BJ. Infections of the neonatal infant. In: Kliegman RM, Behrman RE, Jenson HB, et al, editors. Nelson textbook of pediatrics. 19th edn. Philadelphia: Saunders Elsevier; 2011. p. 629–48.

11. Vergnano S, Sharland M, Kazembe P, et al. Neonatal sepsis: an international perspective. Arch Dis Child Fetal Neonatal Ed 2005;90:F220–4.

12. Seehusen DA, Reeves MM. Cerebrospinal fluid analysis. Am Fam Physician 2003;68(6):1103–9.

13. Stoll BJ, Klegman RM. Substance abuse and neonatal abstinence (withdrawal). In: Kliegman RM, Behrman RE, Jenson HB, et al, editors. Nelson textbook of pediatrics. 19th ed. Philadelphia: Saunders Elsevier; 2011. p. 579–99.

14. Adams-Chapman I, Stoll BJ. Systemic inflammatory response syndrome. Semin Pediatr Infect Dis 2001;12:5–16.

15. Goldstein B, Giroir B, Randolph A, et al. International pediatric sepsis consensus conference: definitions for sepsis and organ dysfunction in paediatrics. Pediatric Critical Care Medicine 2005;6(1):2–8.

16. National Institute for Health and Clinical Excellence. NICE clinical guideline 47: Feverish illness in children. Assessment and initial management in children younger than 5 years. Issue date: May 2007. Developed by the National Collaborating Centre for Women's and Children's Health. Online. Available: http://www.nice.org.uk/CG047; 13 Jun 2011.

17. Baker MD, Avner JR The febrile infant: what's new? Clin Ped Emerg Med 2008;9:213–20.

18. The Royal Children's Hospital Melbourne. Clinical practice guidelines. Febrile child under 3 years. Online. Available: http://www.rch.org.au/clinicalguide/cpg.cfm?doc_id=5181.

19. Ashouri N, Butler J, Ofelia M, et al. Urinary tract infection in neonates: how aggressive a workup and Therapy? Posted: 03/25/2003: Cliggott Publishing, Division of CMP Healthcare Media. Online. Available: www.medscape.com/viewarticle/450299.

20. Crain E, Gerschel JC. Urinary tract infections in febrile infants younger than 8 weeks of age. Pediatrics 1990;86:363–7.

21. Nield LS, Kamat D. Fever without a focus. In: Kliegman RM, Behrman RE, Jenson HB, et al, editors. Nelson textbook of pediatrics. 19th ed. Philadelphia: Saunders Elsevier; 2011. p. 896–902.

22. Mick NW. Pediatric Fever. In: Marx JA, Hockberger RS, Walls RM, editors. Rosen's emergency medicine: concepts and clinical practice. 7th ed. Philadelphia: Elsevier; 2009. p. 2094–103.

23. Lachenauer CS, Wessels MR. Group B streptococcus. In: Kliegman RM, Behrman RE, Jenson HB, et al, editors. Nelson textbook of pediatrics. 19th ed. Philadelphia: Saunders Elsevier; 2011. p. 925–8.

24. Baker RC, Tiller T, Bausher JC, et al. Severity of disease correlated with fever reduction in febrile infants. Pediatrics 1989;83(6):1016–9.

25. Bonsu BK, Harper MB. Identifying febrile young infants with bacteremia: Is the peripheral white blood cell count an accurate screen? Ann Emerg Med 2003;42(2):216–25.

26. Baraff LJ. Management of fever without source in infants and children. Ann Emerg Med 2000;36:602–14.

27. Mahajan P, Stanley R. Fever in the toddler-aged child: old concerns replaced with new ones. Clin Ped Emerg Med 2008;9(4):221–7.

28. Baker MD, Bell LM, Avner JR. The efficacy of routine outpatient management without antibiotics of fever in selected infants. Pediatrics 1999;103:627–31.

29. Hsiao AL, Baker MD. Fever in the new millennium: a review of recent studies of markers of serious bacterial infection in febrile children. Curr Opin Pediatr 2005;17:56–61.

30. Maconochie IK. Kawasaki disease. Arch Dis Child Educ Pract Ed 2004;89:ep3–ep8.

31. Newburger JW, Takahashi M, Gerber MA, et al. Diagnosis, treatment, and long-term management of Kawasaki disease: a statement for health professionals from the Committee on Rheumatic Fever, Endocarditis and Kawasaki Disease, Council on Cardiovascular Disease in

the Young, American Heart Association. Circulation 2004;110:2747–71.

32. Demmler GJ. Adenoviruses. In: Long S, Pickering LK, Prober CG, editors. Long: principles and practice of pediatric infectious diseases. 3rd ed. Philadelphia: Churchill Livingstone; 2008. p. 1052–5.

33. Jordan-Villegas A, Chang ML, Ramilo O, et al. Concomitant respiratory viral infections in children with Kawasaki disease. Pediatr Infect Dis J 2010;29:770.

34. Quigley R. Diagnosis of urinary tract infections in children. Curr Opin Pediatr 2009;21(2):194–8.

35. The Royal Children's Hospital Melbourne. Clinical practice guidelines: urinary tract infection. Online. Available: http://www.rch.org.au/clinicalguide/cpg. cfm?doc_id=5241.

36. Burgess M. Meningococcal vaccines. Australian Prescriber 2003;26:56–8.

37. The Royal Children's Melbourne Clinical practice guidelines. CSF interpretation. Online. Available: http://www.rch.org.au/clinicalguide/cpg.cfm?doc_id=5185.

38. Mikati MA. Seizures in childhood. In: Kliegman RM, Behrman RE, Jenson HB, et al, editors. Nelson textbook of paediatrics. 19th ed. Philadelphia: Saunders Elsevier; 2011. p. 2013–39.

39. Carrol W, Brookfield D. Lumbar puncture following febrile convulsion. Arch Dis Child 2002;87:238–40.

40. Duffner PK, Berman PH, Baumann RJ, et al. Subcommittee on febrile seizures. Neurodiagnostic evaluation of the child with a simple febrile seizure. Pediatrics 2011;127:389–94.

41. Gorelick MH, Blackwell CD. Neurologic emergencies. In: Fleisher GR, Ludwig S, editors. Textbook of pediatric emergency medicine. 6th ed. Philadelphia: Lippincott Williams & Wilkins; 2010. p. 1011–32.

42. Yu K, Mills S. Safety and efficacy of intravenous valproate in pediatric status epilepticus and acute repetitive seizures. Epilepsia 2003;44(5):724–6.

43. Wolfe TR, Macfarlane TC. Intranasal midazolam therapy for pediatric status epilepticus. Am J Emerg Med 2006;24:343.

44. Rubin DH, Halpern Kornblau D, Conway EE Jr. Neurologic disorders. In: Marx JA, Hockberger RS, Walls RM, editors. Rosen's emergency medicine: concepts and clinical practice. 7th ed. Philadelphia: Elsevier; 2010. p. 2218–44.

45. Kemp CA, McDowell JM, Bogovic A, et al. Paediatric pharmacopoeia. 13th ed. Melbourne: The Royal Children's Hospital; 2002.

46. Holsti M. Seizures and status epilepticus in children. In: Tintinalli JE, Stapczynski JS, Ma OJ, et al, editors. Emergency medicine: a comprehensive study guide. 7th ed. New York: McGraw-Hill; 2011. p. 872–80.

47. Mikati M A, Obeid M. Conditions that mimic seizures. In: Kliegman RM, Behrman RE, Jenson HB, et al, editors. Nelson textbook of paediatrics. 19th ed. Philadelphia: Saunders Elsevier; 2011. p. 2039.

48. Australasian Paediatric Endocrine Group. Clinical practice guidelines: Type 1 diabetes in children and adolescents. Department of Health and Ageing, NHMRC. Online.

Available: http://www.nhmrc.gov.au/_files_nhmrc/ publications/attachments/cp102.pdf.

49. Glaser N, Barnett P, McCaslin I, et al. The Pediatric Emergency Medicine Collaborative Research Committee of the American Academy of Pediatrics. Risk factors for cerebral edema in children with diabetic ketoacidosis. NEJM 2001;344:264–9.

50. Edge JA, Hawkins MM, Winter DL, et al. The risk and outcome of cerebral oedema developing during diabetic ketoacidosis. Arch Dis Childhood 2001;85:16–22.

51. Hale PM, Rezvani I, Braunstein AW, et al. Factors predicting cerebral edema in young children with diabetic ketoacidosis and new onset type 1 diabetes. Acta Paediatrica 1997;86:626–31.

52. Agus M. Endocrine emergencies. In: Fleisher GR, Ludwig S, editors. Textbook of pediatric emergency medicine. 6th ed. Philadelphia: Lippincott Williams & Wilkins; 2011. p. 758–82.

53. Stewart C. Guidelines for the ED management of pediatric diabetic ketoacidosis (DKA). Emergency Medicine Practice 2006;3(3). Online. Available: http://www.ebmedicine.net.

54. Flood RG, Chiang VW. Rate and prediction of infection in children with diabetic ketoacidosis. Am J Emerg Med 2001;19:270–3.

55. Wiggam MI, O'Kane MJ, Harper R, et al. Treatment of diabetic ketoacidosis using normalization of blood 3-hydroxybutyrate concentration as the endpoint of emergency management. A randomized controlled study. Diabetes Care 1997;20(9):1347–52.

56. Noyes KJ, Crofton P, Bath LE, et al. Hydroxybutyrate near-patient testing to evaluate a new end-point for intravenous insulin therapy in the treatment of diabetic ketoacidosis in children. Pediatr Diabetes 2007;8(3): 150–6.

57. Burn MJ. Alcohol-related agents and conditions – ethylene glycol. In: Wolfson AB. Harwood-Nuss' Clinical practice of emergency medicine. 4th ed. Philadelphia: Lippincott Williams & Wilkins; 2009. p. 1454–8.

58. American Academy of Pediatrics, Subcommittee on Diagnosis and Management of Bronchiolitis. Diagnosis and management of bronchiolitis. Pediatrics 2006;118(4):1774–93.

59. Fitzgerald DA. Viral bronchiolitis for the clinician. Journal of Paediatrics and Child Health 2011;47(4):160–6.

60. Seiden JA, Scarfone RJ. Bronchiolitis: an evidence-based approach to management. Clin Ped Emerg Med 2009;10:75–81.

61. Bernstein D. Evaluation of the infant or child with congenital heart disease. In: Kliegman RM, Behrman RE, Jenson HB, et al, editors. Nelson textbook of pediatrics. 19th ed. Philadelphia: Saunders Elsevier; 2011. p. 1549–51.

62. Bernstein D. History and physical examination. In: Kliegman RM, Behrman RE, Jenson HB, et al, editors. Nelson textbook of pediatrics. 19th ed. Philadelphia: Saunders Elsevier; 2011. p. 1529–36.

63. Gadomski AM, Bhasale AL. Bronchodilators for bronchiolitis. Cochrane Database Syst. Rev 2006; CD001266.

64. Kuzik BA, Al-Qadhi SA, Kent S, et al. Nebulized hypertonic saline in the treatment of viral bronchiolitis in infants. J Pediatr 2007;151(3):266–70, 270 e1.

65. Sarrell EM, Tal G, Witzling M, et al. Nebulized 3% hypertonic saline solution treatment in ambulatory children with viral bronchiolitis decreases symptoms. Chest 2002;122:2015–20.

66. Kugelman A. Intravenous fluids versus naso/orogastric-tube feeding in hospitalized infants with bronchiolitis. Israel: Trial. Bnai Zion Medical Center, Ministry of Health; 2010.

67. Oakley, E. The CRIB Study: A prospective randomised trial comparing nasogastric with intravenous hydration in children with bronchiolitis. Melbourne: The Royal Children's Hospital.

68. Wainwright C, Altamirano L, Cheney M, et al. A multicenter, randomized, double-blind, controlled trial of nebulized epinephrine in infants with acute bronchiolitis. N Engl J Med 2003;349:27–35.

69. Hartling L, Wiebe N, Russell K, et al. Epinephrine for bronchiolitis. Cochrane Database Syst Rev 2004;(1): CD003123.

70. McKiernan C, Chua LC, Visintainer PF, et al. High flow nasal cannulae therapy in infants with bronchiolitis. J Pediatr 2010;156(4):634–8.

71. National Asthma Council Australia. Managing acute asthma in children. In: Asthma management handbook 2006;43–6. Online. Available: http://www.nationalasthma. org.au/cms/images/stories/amh2006_web_5.pdf; May 2011.

72. Martinez FD, Wright AL, Taussig LM, et al. Asthma and wheezing in the first 6 years of life. NEJM 1995;332(3): 133–8.

73. Stevenson MD, Ruddy RM. Asthma and allergic emergencies. In: Fleisher GR, Ludwig S, editors. Textbook of pediatric emergency medicine. 6th ed. Philadelphia: Lippincott Williams & Wilkins; 2011. p. 649–70.

74. Bolte RG. Emergency department management of pediatric asthma. Clin Ped Emerg Med 2004;5(4):256–69.

75. Boat TF, Green TP. Chronic or recurrent respiratory symptoms. In: Kliegman RM, Behrman RE, Jenson HB, et al, editors. Nelson textbook of pediatrics. 19th ed. Philadelphia: Saunders Elsevier; 2011. p. 1445.

76. Stocker DM, Kirelik S. Pediatric respiratory emergencies: disease of the lungs. In: Marx JA, Hockberger RS, Walls RM, editors. Rosen's emergency medicine: concepts and clinical practice. 7th ed. Philadelphia: Elsevier; 2009. p. 2127–37.

77. Swingler GH, Zwarenstein M. Chest radiograph in acute respiratory infections. Cochrane Database Syst Rev 2008;(23):CD001268.

78. Shann F. Croup. Paediatric intensive care guidelines. The Royal Children's Hospital Melbourne. Intensive Care Unit. 3rd ed. Collective Pty Ltd; 2008.

79. Cantor RM, Wittick L. Upper airway emergencies. In: Strange GR, Ahrens WR, Schafermeyer RW, editors. Pediatric emergency medicine. 3rd ed. New York: McGraw Hill; 2009. p. 353–60.

80. Wiebe RA, Scott SM. General approach to the pediatric patient. In: Marx JA, Hockberger RS, Walls RM, editors. Rosen's emergency medicine: concepts and clinical practice. 7th ed. Philadelphia: Elsevier; 2010. p. 2083–93.

81. World Health Organization. Perinatal mortality: guidelines for certification and rules for coding. In: International statistical classification of diseases and related health problems. 10th revision. 2010. p. 115-20. Online. Available: http://www.who.int/classifications/icd/en/.

82. World Health Organization. Handbook : IMCI integrated management of childhood illness. Online. Available: http://whqlibdoc.who.int/publications/2005/9241546441. pdf

83. Patel H, Platt R, Lozano JM, et al. Glucocorticoids for acute viral bronchiolitis in infants and young children. Cochrane Database Syst. Rev 2007; CD004878.

84. Zhang L, Mendoza-Sassi RA, Wainwright C, et al. Nebulized hypertonic saline solution for acute bronchiolitis in infants. Cochrane Database Syst Rev 2008; CD006458.

85. Perrotta C, Ortiz Z, Roque MG. Chest physiotherapy for acute bronchiolitis in paediatric patients between 0 and 24 months old. Cochrane Database Syst. Rev 2005; CD004873.

86. ECC Guidelines. Part 10: Pediatric Advanced Life Support. Circulation 2000;102:I-291–I-342, doi:10.1161/01.CIR.102. suppl_1.I-291. Online. Available: http://circ.ahajournals. org/content/102/suppl_1/I-291

1. Answer: B

Disaster planning is organised on an integrated approach to deal with any circumstance (all-hazard, all-agency). However, standard codes are nationally applied to a number of specific circumstances – red, (fire), blue (cardiac arrest), black (personal injury threat), yellow (internal emergency), brown (external emergency), purple (bomb threat) and orange (evacuation).

Australian disaster planning is coordinated under aegis of Emergency Management Australia (EMA), a branch of the Attorney-General's Department of the Australian Government. EMA supports a comprehensive approach to emergency management, pursuing a cooperative and collaborative relationship with government agencies, and encouraging this all-hazard, all-agency approach to disaster planning. A tiered response is organised, with integrated plans existing at local, state and federal levels. Disaster planning is structured around five management activities: strategic, planning, logistics, operational and financial management.

A major incident is defined as an incident causing so many *live* casualties that special arrangements are necessary to deal with them. The level meeting this standard will depend on the location and type of injuries, as well as the availability of local healthcare resources.

The process of disaster planning addresses four phases of an incident: prevention, preparation, response and recovery.[1]

See also <http://www.ema.gov.au/www/emaweb/emaweb.nsf/Page/Emergency_Management>.

2. Answer: A

The following mnemonic can be used to announce and report an incident.

METHANE

Major incident standby/declared

Exact location

Type of incident

Hazards present

Access for rescue vehicles

Numbers of cases (and severity/type) such as multiple paediatric or burn cases

Emergency services present or required.

In past disasters, communication failures have been a recurring feature. However, the first priority in managing the scene of a disaster is to establish chains of command between and within services in order to organise the other aspects of care. There is another mnemonic to recall the key elements of a disaster response.

CSCATTT

Command and Control

Safety

Communications

Assessment

Triage

Treatment

Transport

Decontamination processes should be carried out on site prior to transport. This is to avoid contaminating healthcare facilities, which puts the safety of staff and all patients at risk. Nevertheless, contaminated patients may make their own way directly to hospitals, and this hazard must be recognised at an early stage.

Triage processes apply a rapid sieve and sort process, to identify how the most benefit can be brought to the greatest number of patients. The triage *sieve* identifies the order of transfer to treatment areas. A subsequent *sort* using more detailed physiological criteria determines the order of transport to hospital.[1]

3. Answer: D

Key initial steps in managing an incipient surge of patients are the establishment of control over and around the department in order to ensure arriving patients are directed to appropriate clinical areas, and to limit access by non-patient groups such as relatives and the media. This is in keeping with the CSCATTT concept described previously (answer 2).

Surge capacity includes four elements (4 Ss):
- **s**taff
- **s**tuff (equipment)
- **s**tructure (physical and management)
- **s**pace.

Available bed spaces are only one element of a hospital's ability to deal with a surge. All patients arriving during the management of an incident should be tracked using the same (dedicated) documentation system, since they involve deploying the same ED and hospital resources. ED staff are best utilised within the ED – it is possible that potentially contaminated or untreated patients will make their own way to the hospital, arriving prior to anticipated ambulance transfers. Inpatient staff should be engaged to retrieve patients who are already in the ED to their own areas prior to arrival of new patients. **Surge management requires a whole-of-hospital response, not one confined to the ED.**[1]

4. Answer: D

The first two ambulance officers become the transport collection officer and the casualty collection officer. Between them they are responsible for organising the casualty clearing system for removing all patients from the scene. The casualty collection officer carries out initial triage using a triage sieve, delivering minimal first aid.

The senior medical officer on site is the scene medical officer, who has responsibility for management of medical resources at the site and liaises with central coordination. The scene medical officer does not triage or treat patients themselves. Disaster teams – small groups of medical and nursing staff – operate under the direction of the scene medical officer; their activities are confined to life-saving procedures such as airway management, haemorrhage control and support, and analgesia. They do not provide more complex interventions such as intubation or CPR.[1]

5. Answer: D

There is an ongoing legal requirement for controlled drugs to be used under monitored and documented circumstances, whether in hospital or in the field. A chain of accountability must follow the transport and use of these medications.

Key personnel at a disaster scene should be wearing labelled vests or tabards that are easily identifiable. This allows key personnel in each service to recognise each other at a distance, and to liaise more effectively. Rescuers must have sturdy protective clothing and boots to avoid adding to the casualty load; individuals who are inappropriately dressed should be denied access to the site, regardless of their expertise. Radio communications should be controlled via a communications officer in the command post, with all site rescuers operating on the same frequency.[1]

6. Answer: A

The 1-2-3 of safety refers to the order of priority in considering safety on site:
- self
- scene (bystanders and rescuers)
- casualties.

This prevents rescuers from becoming injured, and therefore adding to casualty load while reducing caring staff.

In a suspected chemical, biological or radionuclear exposure, the area immediately around the contamination is referred to as the 'hot zone'. Security is set up to control access to this area via a specific point allowing only staff equipped with PPE. Surrounding this is the warm zone in which decontamination of casualties and staff is performed under the supervision of a decontamination officer. The cold zone in turn surrounds this. The size of these zones will depend on the scale and nature of the potential threat, and may alter by subsequent circumstances (e.g. change in wind or rain). These zones are controlled by the police.

Noxious agents have four routes of access into the body: inhalation, skin, eye and ingestion. PPE and decontamination processes must take this into consideration. Decontamination should involve cutting off patients' clothing rather than lifting it over their face and airway, then applying a rinse-wipe-rinse technique using dilute detergent solution.

Patients requiring decontamination should not be transferred into the cold zone because of the risk they then pose to healthcare staff and the public. PPE places significant restrictions on the senses, and cannot be worn while driving or caring for a patient in an ambulance.[1]

7. Answer: C

Smallpox virus spreads by person-to-person droplet transmission. Infection via pharynx results in widespread centripetal vesicular skin rash, high fever and severe abdominal pain. Diagnosis is made by electron microscopy findings in association with clinical features. The discovery of a single suspected case should be treated as an international health emergency.

Anthrax is a naturally occurring aerobic, gram-positive bacillus which can cause respiratory, cutaneous or gastrointestinal infections. Mortality is high, due to bacterial toxins provoking a secondary lymphadenitis, causing haemorrhagic necrosis of exposed tissue. Person-to-person transmission has not been reported. While most strains are penicillin sensitive, the possibility of deliberately engineered attack has led to a recommendation of prolonged combination chemotherapy, primarily including ciprofloxacin.

Pneumonic plague is a rapidly progressive, frequently fatal febrile illness, considered to be the most likely form of a deliberate exposure. It carries a high risk of respiratory droplet transmission, and is rapidly fatal if not treated within 24 hours with double-agent chemotherapy, including streptomycin or gentamicin.

Botulinus toxin blocks peripheral cholinergic synapses, resulting in a flaccid paralysis that characteristically first presents in the bulbar muscles. Treatment is largely supportive, including ventilation and parenteral nutrition.[2]

8. Answer: A

Most modern chemical warfare agents (e.g. sarin) are organophosphates. Toxicity can be acute, intermediate, or delayed, depending on the agent used. They cause actions at the autonomic ganglia. The toxidrome can be prompted by the following mnemonic.

MUDDLES

Muscular paralysis/fasciculation

Urination

Defecation

Diaphoresis

Lacrimation

Excitation

Salivation (and meiosis)

Respiratory paralysis may require supportive ventilation for days.

Atropine is first-line treatment for organophosphate toxicity, reversing non-neuromuscular and central nervous system (CNS) manifestations including bradycardia. However, the toxidrome of sarin, while an organophosphate, is not responsive to atropine. Pralidoxime is most effective early in post-sarin exposure.

In treating cyanide exposure, which causes toxicity by inhibiting cellular respiration, the drug of choice is intravenous hydroxycobalamin, which forms a stable compound that is then renally excreted. Mustard gas is a vesicant agent, liquid at room temperature, which attacks the skin and mucosal surfaces and poses an ongoing threat to treating staff. Death is most commonly due to pulmonary destruction. However, the toxic agent is not present in blister fluid.[3,4]

9. Answer: D

In the event of a nuclear accident, radioactive iodine might be released into the environment. **Potassium iodate tablets block the uptake of radioactive iodine by the thyroid gland, therefore reducing the risk of developing thyroid cancer.**

Irradiated patients are not radioactive, and so do not pose a threat to staff. Patients exposed to particulate radioactive material – such as following an explosion – may still have radioactive material on their person, and so should be considered as requiring decontamination until declared clear by a radiation safety officer. Haemopoetic syndrome – due to bone marrow suppression – displays developing symptoms of bleeding, depressed white cell count (WCC) resulting in impaired immune response and fatigue by 3 weeks post exposure. Treatment is supportive. Gastrointestinal symptoms of vomiting, bloody diarrhoea and ileus denote an exposure of >2–10 Gy, and result in 50% mortality due to renal, hepatic and pulmonary injuries.[5]

10. Answer: C

In the initial triage sieve of mass casualties, the priority of healthcare is shifted from 'the best care for every patient' to 'do the greatest good for the greatest number'. The process is to determine which patients should be taken to different treatment areas, and in which order.

- All ambulant patients are prioritised P3, regardless of injury.
- Patients with non-patent airways must be considered dead, in order to optimise resources where they can be of benefit.
- Patients with respiratory rate <10 or >29 are P1 (top priority), as are those with a cap refill >2s or pulse >120.
- Everyone else is assigned a P2.

All patients will then be reassessed at the casualty clearing station using the triage sort, a more detailed physiology-based assessment.

Triage exercises may be used to practise the triage sieve or sort processes used in a disaster situation. This can be done as a paper exercise for individuals, or with a group allowing discussion of decisions and processes.

Table-top exercises are run for small groups, and may be useful for assessing or rehearsing particular aspects of a plan such as identifying areas of a hospital or site for strategic planning. This works best when the group comprises individuals who represent different groups or specialties, and are useful in demonstrating command, control and communication processes.

A large multiagency exercise with live casualties provides a realistic way of testing out-of-hospital responses, and the casualties used can be progressed through to be used in an in-hospital exercise. However, it is difficult to perform this without disrupting hospital function, and conducting the process can be expensive, complex, and requires much forward planning and coordination.[1]

References

1. Brookes J, Dunn R. Disaster medicine. In: Dunn R, et al, editors. The emergency medicine manual. 5th ed. Tennyson: Venom Publishing; 2010. p. 378–85.
2. Dilley S, Dunn R. Biological warfare agents. In: Dunn R, et al, editors. The emergency medicine manual. 5th ed. Tennyson: Venom Publishing; 2010. p. 783–90.
3. Dunn R. Chemical agents. In: Dunn R, et al, editors. The emergency medicine manual. 5th ed. Tennyson: Venom Publishing; 2010. p. 1391–406.
4. Dunn R. Biological warfare agents. In: Dunn R, et al, editors. The emergency medicine manual. 5th ed. Tennyson: Venom Publishing; 2010. p. 1407–12.
5. Dunn R. Other mechanisms of injury. In: Dunn R, et al, editors. The emergency medicine manual. 5th ed. Tennyson: Venom Publishing; 2010. p. 1220–1.

1. Answer: C

ACEM provides recommendations on the minimum size and number of treatment areas in the configuration of an ED in Australia and New Zealand. These must be considered in relation to the projected activity, casemix and population served by an individual department.

Ambulatory and ambulance entrances should be separate, for reasons of security, control of patient flow and traffic safety. Paediatric areas require adequate space to accommodate not only the patient, but also adult carers, family and storage for toys, books and other distractants.[1]

2. Answer: C

ACEM also provides recommendations for minimum equipment in each type of clinical area. A single central staff area enables better communication between, and coordination of, staff members.

Isolation rooms require negative ventilation to minimise the risk of spread of infection. Decontamination rooms should be accessible directly from outside the ED at the ambulance bay, with self-contained decontamination facilities rather than having hazardous patients in the waiting rooms with other patients. Consultation rooms should ideally be adapted to be multipurpose because specialisation of rooms imposes limits on patient flow. However, if a room is adapted for ophthalmology problems (with blacked-out or absent windows), equipment should include both a vision screen for testing vision, as well as a slit lamp for examining the different structures of the globe.[1]

3. Answer: A

A clinical practice guideline is a systematically developed statement to support clinicians and patients when making decisions about appropriate healthcare in specific circumstances. **It is the result of summarising the current body of evidence on a particular issue, and translating it into a tool to improve the care of individual patients, or appropriate use of resources.** Collating the evidence on a particular issue may be hampered by a lack of available literature on a topic. Available evidence should be graded on its quality, and all available evidence considered – not every topic has been researched via a randomised controlled trial. The ultimate quality of the produced guideline is dependent on the rigor of the development process, rather than the distinction of the authors.

A guideline should be considered in the specific setting and patient to which it is being applied, rather than as a blanket protocol of action. Much research may be carried out on otherwise healthy subjects with single conditions, or study populations very different from those attending our EDs. This must be taken into consideration when applying any guideline. New research and new medical practices constantly evolve. For this reason, It has been estimated that the effective half-life of a clinical guideline is around 6 years; the intention to review it by a certain date should be declared at publication.[2]

4. Answer: C

Primary uses of ED information systems are as tools to manage the ED by tracking the progress of patients, plus storage and retrieval of clinical data as required. They may also be used to provide data for wider purposes such as:

- management of complaints/compensation claims
- process development
- planning financial strategy
- research.

Manual (paper) systems have some advantages in terms of low cost, ease of use and reliability in the face of power supply issues. However, most Australasian EDs are so large that computerised systems offset these benefits, as well as displaying other advantages:

- Data is accessible simultaneously over multiple sites within and external to the ED.
- Data can be updated 'live'.
- Clinical notes cannot be lost or mislaid.
- Systems can be designed specifically to
  - collect particular information of interest (e.g. injury surveillance)
  - interact with other hospital systems (e.g. medical imaging or pathology)

- implement local clinical guidelines and protocols.

However, additional costs to consider include not only introduction but maintenance of both software and hardware, training of staff to maintain consistent practice, and ongoing development to ensure it supports expansion and changing practice within the department. Procedures to support data security, data integrity and back-up during power loss are required.[2]

5. Answer: D

Effective appraisal of staff is a powerful tool for developing behaviours and performance desirable to the ED activity. However, in order to do so, it is important to understand what incentives – financial, time-based, recognition – are important to the individual being appraised.

Logbooks are useful for recording caseload and the frequency of procedures; however, they indicate activity rather than provide any information on quality of care. Individuals involved in appraisals are prone to a number of potential errors, including personal tendencies to mark higher or lower than average, or submit similar appraisals regardless of performance. They may also be biased by:
- otherwise positive behaviours (halo error)
- perceiving the subject in a false light based on
  - preconceived assumptions (prejudice)
  - assumed similarities to the appraiser (similarity error).

For these reasons, appraisals are most effectively conducted involving multiple appraisers, drawing on multiple sources of information about performance.[3]

6. Answer: C

In planning a shift-based roster, the following features have been found to have beneficial effects on health and work/life balance:
- rapid rotation through the shift pattern (maximum of four shifts each block)
- forward (clockwise) rotation – subsequent shifts start progressively later in the day
- self-scheduling of shifts – providing staff with a sense of control over working patterns.

The adaptation of circadian rhythm to night shift takes around two weeks – a biological argument may be made for staff working permanent night shift (this may, however, create difficulties in obtaining balance in staff rosters, and involving night staff in communication and business management).

The Australian Medical Association has a voluntary code of practice relating to risk assessment of roster patterns in which backward rotation, speed of rotation and longer shift lengths are regarded as higher risk patterns.[3]

7. Answer: C

Stress is dependent on an individual's perception of lack of control over a situation. A study of Australian emergency clinicians found that perception of control over hours worked and varied clinical activities was positively associated with work and life satisfaction but negatively associated with work stress and measures of wellbeing. Effective strategies are person- and context-specific, for example, being around family may be a positive or negative experience, depending on circumstances. **Effective time management – such as organising one's tasks in a Do, Defer, Drop or Delegate system – may promote a sense of personal control and reduce stress. This can be positive in both personal and professional arenas.**

Burnout is a form of low-grade stress that may be recognised by features including depersonalisation, compassion fatigue, and negative perceptions of one's own work and accomplishments. It has a very high incidence in medical staff in Australian EDs. Risk factors include:
- male gender
- trainee level
- work stressors – long shifts, lack of control over work conditions, excessive workload
- personal stressors – fatigue and an unhealthy lifestyle.[3]

8. Answer: A

Complaints may be useful in highlighting areas of ED performance in which patient satisfaction has not been met. Rather than an indicator of poor treatment, it may simply be that there is a disparity between a patient's expectations and their management process, which has not been adequately addressed or explained. A senior staff member addressing this in person at the time of the event is often able to resolve the issue without the complaint progressing further. Issues relating to responsibility of other departments should be redirected to the appropriate manager.

While many staff may be distressed when informed of a complaint, these consistently occur in relation to a few areas – most commonly, in communication with or attitude of staff, access to services, and inadequate/incorrect treatment. The majority of treatment complaints relate to issues that are simple to address by implementing CQI systems, such as missed fractures or inadequate analgesia.

Complaints should be adequately and carefully investigated, then responded to within a set time frame. Most complaints can be resolved by:

- acknowledging the patient's distress
- an expression of regret regarding the distress experienced – this does not imply an acceptance of fault
- an explanation of what occurred and why, addressing specific concerns raised
- an explanation of what will be done to prevent future recurrence of such an episode.

These steps will resolve most complaints to everyone's satisfaction. Complaints can be a powerful tool to identify issues needing attention within the ED – such as interaction with inpatient specialties, delivery of services or access block – and drive necessary changes.[2,4]

9. Answer: C

Clinical handover is the transfer of professional responsibility and accountability for some or all aspects of care for a patient, or group of patients, to another person or professional group. Poor communication between healthcare professionals has been found to be a key contributory factor in over 70% of sentinel events. In emergency medicine, its functions include:

- ensuring the safe transfer of both department and patients
- providing information about departmental issues
- communication
- debriefing, team-building and socialisation
- teaching.

Factors shown to improve the transfer of clinical information include:

- a minimum dataset
- having a standard operating protocol that includes

- consistent scheduled times
- consistent handover process
- consistent pattern of information delivery – e.g. SBAR, ISOBAR – the speaker is able to organise their thoughts better, while the listener is better attuned to receiving information and recognises when information is missing
- protected time/environment, including sound hygiene
- senior supervision
- education of staff regarding risk management and importance of establishing processes.

Some authorities advocate bedside handover, involving the patient in processes. Advantages include improved patient satisfaction (as they are aware of changeovers and are seen by a senior doctor), pick-up of errors/misinformation, and earlier decision making. However, some functions of handover – discussion of errors, discipline and teaching – are less well performed at the bedside, and the process may act as a focus for some problematic or aggressive patients.[5–8]

10. Answer: D

Violence is rarely entirely unpredictable. Paying attention to verbal and non-verbal behaviours will help staff anticipate potential problems, and modulate their own responses to affect the situation.

Several red flags for violent escalation are identifiable here: change in the group's perception of staff role from helpful to being an obstacle, provocative and demanding behaviour, and physical restlessness. Further concerns might be behavioural, such as a shortened attention span, increased verbal aggression (taunting, sarcastic), and changes in speech – raised volume, higher pitch and more rapid intonation. They may also try to enlist the rest of the waiting room as an audience ('Oh, we're *sorry* you're too busy'), which may cause further escalation as the aggressive individuals may feel a need to 'win' the confrontation, or lose face.

Attempting to communicate with a number of agitated people in a public place may provide a focus for aggressive action. Separating the concerned individual (the brother) from the audience and communicating with him in a quiet, controlled environment achieves a number of positive actions.

People who are aggressive may provoke automatically negative and forceful responses. However, a number of stresses may be acting on such an individual: unfamiliarity with the environment and with the behaviour expected; lack of information; and anxiety over his sibling's condition (there is also the question of mechanism of injury yet to be established). Providing him with clear, current information may relieve these anxieties and reduce his aggression risk. This in turn can assist in defusing the hostility of his companions. Information must be calmly expressed in simple, clear terms, stated repeatedly to overcome his situational short attention span.

This conversation should take place in a private but not isolated area. Surrounding ED staff should be aware of the location of both staff and the relative. Security staff should be advised at an early stage of the potential hazard.[9,10]

11. Answer: C

Successful negotiation has much in common with complaint management, and aggression management. Effective practices are based on seeking positive relationships with counterparts, rather than arguing, intimidating or losing your temper. These practices include:[11]

- wanting to hear what the other person has to say
- working to resolve conflict (separate the person from the problem)
- seeking a neutral negotiating environment
- respecting adversaries as speakers for their cause, with valid values and viewpoints – even if different from yours
- remembering you could be wrong, or partly wrong.

Negotiation may be considered in four stages:
- Preparation
  - Identify clear objectives.
  - Identify a range of settlement options – ideal/acceptable/bottom line.
  - Consider tradable issues rather than a list of demands.
  - Establish initial common ground.
  - Establish that both negotiators have appropriate authority to address what is being bargained – are you dealing with the correct person?
- Debate
  - Listen as much as you speak – try to hear what the other person is saying.

- Check your understanding of their wants by regular recapping.
- Bargain
  - Move from proposing hypothetical situations – 'What if I..?' to exploring hypothetical tradable wants such as 'If you … then I …', and listen to the responses.
  - Avoid one-sided concessions.
  - Summarise constantly to avoid misunderstandings (*But you said…*).
- Agreement
  - Establish what has been agreed – be prepared to counter-bargain or walk away if the offer is unacceptable.
  - Once final agreement has been reached, this should be documented in writing ASAP to avoid backtracking or further issues being raised.

12. Answer: C

A business plan is a yearly framework agreed between the ED management team and the hospital management, setting out expected performance for the coming year, and the facilities available to support that performance. The four main components are *finance, activity, quality and efficiency*. It should be based on as much accurate information as possible about the past year's activity, in order to set future projections. Once the plan is implemented, regular monitoring should continue to identify and remedy any variance.

The financial aspect, the budget plan, is used to project financial outcomes for the coming year. It is usually developed on the basis of the previous year's financial activity, with every variance from that plan accounted for. Up to 85% of ED costs are fixed, with the largest single field related to staff wages. Purchases of new equipment over $5000 requires a business case including tenders to be prepared and submitted to hospital management. Capital expenditure refers to items with recurrent use over many years (e.g. infrastructure, buildings or monitoring equipment).

Activity may be expressed in terms of total attendances and triage mix, admissions by triage category, top diagnosis-related groups (DRGs) in any observation ward, and other relevant activity such as interhospital transfers. Quality and efficiency may be assessed by defined clinical indicators – such as waiting times per ATS triage category, access block, ambulance bypass – established internally or by external authorities such as ACEM or the Australian Council on Healthcare Standards (ACHS). Morbidity and mortality rates, written complaint rates and patient 'Did Not Wait' rates also constitute measures of quality.[12]

13. Answer: B

CQI begins with the concept that things can be done better than they are being done now.
Improving quality within an ED requires several elements, including defining clinically meaningful outcomes. Accepted elements of a CQI program for an ED may include ongoing improvements in clinical quality, cost efficiency and service quality. These three elements are not necessarily entirely compatible.

Improving quality in a specific setting requires setting standards, establishing weak points in processes, designing and implementing changes to address these weaknesses, and reviewing the process to ensure processes have improved. This should then be repeated to continue the process of advancing towards an ideal situation. The PDSA cycle is a cyclical tool to support ongoing developmental changes in a process in a stepwise fashion.

Clinical indicators from bodies such as ACHS are intended as clinically meaningful measures of healthcare. They address major areas of care, focusing on various aspects of that area such as the percentage of acute myocardial infarction patients receiving thrombolysis within 1 hour, or time to analgesia or antibiotics. However, their utility may be limited by being factors that are relatively easy to measure, rather than being actual indicators of quality. In addition, investigating an improvement in one aspect of care may miss consequent deterioration in other areas due to the same intervention.[2]

14. Answer: A

Overcrowding occurs when the ED function is impaired by the number of patients waiting or undergoing assessment, treatment or disposition exceeds either the physical or staffing capacity of the department.[13] If this occurs, emergency clinicians have a responsibility to advise hospital management that patient care could be compromised. Hospital management then has a responsibility to restore a safe working environment.[4]

If ambulances cannot safely offload patients and return to external activity, community emergency response capacity is reduced. Bed availability is a feature not only of physical bed numbers, but of how those beds are used. Improving GP services is advocated in the hope of diverting primary care-related problems away from the ED. However, there is little evidence that this is an effective strategy. Likewise health advice lines, while popular with the public, have not been shown to reduce ED attendance, and may in some circumstances make patients more likely to attend hospital.[15]

15. Answer: B

Access block is defined as a total ED time from arrival to transfer, admission or death of over 8 hours.[16] Studies have shown correlation with a number of adverse impacts on healthcare, including inpatient stay, mortality and time to clinical treatments such as analgesia or antibiotics.

Access block is mainly due to systemic lack of capacity throughout a health system (i.e. a symptom of whole-system hospital overload). While strategies aimed purely at improving ED function may show short-term benefits, these are unlikely to be maintained without addressing in-hospital bed management. Some strategies such as over census beds (transferring patients awaiting beds to inpatient wards) may be effective in spreading the clinical load but may encounter resistance difficult to reach acceptance. Hospital-wide measures are dependent on leadership from senior hospital management. Facility planning should aim for an access block of 10% or less.[2,15]

16. Answer: B

SSUs, observation wards, or clinical decision units are a recent development within emergency medicine, in which selected populations of patients are admitted to an area adjacent to the ED and under the control of ED senior staff for a specified period of time (usually <24 hours). While having dedicated staff promotes consistency of practice, rotating ED nursing staff through the unit promotes skill maintenance and establishes the unit as a part of the broader ED.

Decisions regarding admission should be coordinated by a single senior emergency clinician. Using the SSU as a strategy for managing access block runs the risk of spreading the block to this area and impairing the ability of the unit to function. **Patients being transferred to the unit should have a defined condition or management protocol, including a specific end point at which the patient is to be admitted or discharged.** Primary responsibility for patients within the ED remains with the emergency clinician responsible for the department until they are physically transferred to another clinical area and handed over.[14,17]

17. Answer: C

Observation medicine is a model of care within the discipline of emergency medicine for patients requiring an extension of traditional ED services. Key principles specific to the model include:

- early access to diagnostics, specialist advice, observation and reassessment to inform rapid decision-making and treatment
- evidence-based pathways and protocols to guide delivery of care and reduce variation
- collaboration between multidisciplinary clinicians and specialists with external stakeholders such as GPs or community service providers
- efficiency in streamlining the care of selected patients, reducing service duplication and avoidable use of inpatient resources.

Units depend on frequent patient review promoting rapid decision making. As such, they require the regular or ongoing presence of experienced emergency clinicians. Coordination of support services can be cohorted in this setting. Complex patients with multiple problems are not appropriate for this setting due to the workload involved.[17]

18. Answer: A

A post-sedation patient has a stable condition with anticipated complete resolution within a defined time period.

Patients with diabetes will require ongoing monitoring and regular blood investigations. The COPD patient, if requiring admission, is unlikely to recover to discharge status within an appropriate time period. Recurrent pneumothorax will require insertion of a chest drain and subsequent medical admission for over 24 hours.[17]

19. Answer: D

Australian privacy legislation is controlled by a federal Act which defines 10 national privacy principles:[18]

- Collection – only data required to assist healthcare is collected.
- Use and disclosure – patients should receive an explanation of how data may be used or disclosed to a third party.
- Data quality – steps must be taken to ensure data collected is accurate and secure.
- Data security – data must be safe from loss, corruption, or unauthorised access.
- Openness – an explanation should be provided as to how data is handled.
- Access and correction – patients have a right to access and correct their records. This does not mean that they have the right to read their notes or results on demand or without medical explanation, as misinterpretation or poor comprehension may be detrimental to their physical or mental wellbeing. However, patients do not have to provide a reason for their request, and have a right of access even if the report specifies otherwise.
- Identifiers – hospitals must have unique identifiers for each patient.
- Anonymity – where practicable, patients should have to option of accessing healthcare services without identifying themselves.
- Transborder data flows – obligations exist when transferring health information to other countries.
- Sensitive information – health data should not be collected or shared without the patient's consent, except in some situations where required by law such as where there is a potential risk to the patient or others, or in the investigation of a criminal act.

Similar legislation exists in New Zealand and the United Kingdom.

20. Answer: B

Medical errors are a 'failure of a planned action to be executed as intended (error of execution)' or 'use of a wrong plan to achieve an aim (error of planning)'. In international studies, approximately one in 10 patients admitted to hospital experienced an adverse event, of which half were due to medical errors. The majority of these occurred within 24 hours of arrival to hospital.

Factors specific to the ED increase the possibility of medical error – relating to staff, clinical situation, physical environment (including overcrowding), and complex interactions with multiple other systems.

Areas of error, rather than being unpredictable, occur at points found repeatedly across EDs:

- patient identification errors
- triage-related errors
- hospital-acquired infections
- delays and misinterpretation of radiology and pathology tests
- medication errors
- communication errors (at handover, admission or discharge).

The majority of errors result in minor or no harm to the patient. However, since these 'near misses' are valuable in identifying weak points in a system, an effective incident reporting system should be part of a ED clinical risk management (CRM) system, which contributes to CQI programs.[19,20]

More than 30 cognitive (thinking) and affective (emotional) dispositions have been recognised as contributing to imperfect decision making in emergency clinicians.[21] A number of strategies have been identified to counteract these, including cognitive forcing – reducing potential to make wrong decisions, and reducing alternatives to correct decisions. **It is recognised that incidents are often due less to individual poor performance of staff, but rather to an accumulation of multiple gaps in the healthcare system as in Reason's Swiss-cheese model.**[22]

RCA is a component of CRM systems. It is a systematic process of examining an adverse event, following the care of a patient at each phase of their journey through and beyond the ED, and examining why failures of care occurred rather than apportioning blame.

21. Answer: A

For negligence to be proven, a number of points must be established:

- that there existed a duty of care
- that there has been a breach of that duty of care
- that this resulted in harmful consequences – physical or psychological
- that the harm was due directly to the breach.

Duty of care is a legal obligation to conform to a particular standard of conduct for the protection of unreasonable risks. Reasonable care is the standard of care that might be expected of the average practitioner of the class to which the healthcare practitioner belongs. It includes a duty to possess and exercise proper skill, to maintain competence and current knowledge in their field.

In allegations of breach of duty of care, the subsequent event must involve both foreseeability and probability of harm. This is not clear in this situation from the information given. Damage to a plaintiff is considered in terms of physical harm or psychological injury, rather than emotional distress. While this patient had a life-threatening illness, and a breach of care has not been excluded, the precipitating cause of death was not a direct consequence of such a breach.[23]

22. Answer: B

Consent may be implied (e.g. arriving at hospital seeking assistance), verbal or written. The level of consent must be commensurate with the seriousness of a proposed procedure, or the consequence of declining treatment. For example, consent for a surgical procedure must be obtained in writing, with evidence that the procedure, possible side effects, complications and purpose have all been explained, and the patient has had a chance to ask questions. This is then signed by both patient and doctor.

In order for consent to be valid, five elements must be established. It must be:

- informed
- specific
- freely given (without any coercion)
- covering what is actually done
- associated with established competence to consent or decline.

Assessment of competence is based on a number of factors:

- communication – Can the patient receive information the doctor wishes to present?
- comprehension – Can they understand the information?
- credibility – Do they believe the information (and the staff)?
- retention – Can they remember the information long enough to consider it?
- conclusion – Can they synthesise the information to reach a logical conclusion, whether this fits with the healthcare staff's values or not?

The patient's judgement as to what is in her own best interest may differ from that of the treating team but constitute a valid viewpoint. When in doubt, enlist another staff member or senior, and document the decision-making process clearly. Where there is disagreement, discuss with the hospital legal advisors at an early stage.[24]

23. Answer: A

While hospital staff have a duty to provide each patient with the best clinical care and support, there is no legal obligation to report a victim of domestic abuse without the patient's consent, unless concern exists that a vulnerable adult or child may also be at risk in the domestic environment. Where concern exists that the public may be endangered, this outweighs the duty of non-disclosure protecting patients' confidentiality.[23]

A medical practitioner who believes that a patient is unsafe to possess a firearm by reason of illness, disability or deficiency, is legally obliged to inform the officer in charge of their jurisdiction's firearms section at the earliest point after this belief is formed.[23]

The Communicable Disease Network Australia & New Zealand coordinates the surveillance of more than 50 communicable diseases, including AIDS, diphtheria, leptospirosis, measles, mumps and most sexually transmissible diseases.[25]

24. Answer: D

Victims of sexual assault have the right to access an appropriately trained forensic practitioner. Clinical care takes precedent over forensic considerations. Forensic examination is carried out at the request of the police service for collection of evidence, rather than for any therapeutic benefit, and therefore requires specific consent to be obtained. Specimen handling should follow the legal concept of 'chain of evidence'. The forensic examination is to collect evidence regarding three areas:
- proof of sexual contact
- consent or the use of force
- identification of the assailant.

Proof of sexual contact is established by detecting semen or spermatozoa on or within the victim or their clothing. It is not necessary to prove sexual contact to prove sexual assault. Evidence of force might be detection of physical injuries.[26]

25. Answer: D

Provision of healthcare information requires signed consent from the patient, unless required by the coroner. In providing a report, it is important to confine statements to actual fact rather than speculation, and to confine reporting to one's own area of expertise. Where opinion has been requested, this should be clearly differentiated from reporting of facts. Reports should be written in the understanding that the author may be called upon in future to speak to their report in court.[23]

Components should include:
- the solicitor's references
- the author's name, designation, qualifications, experience
- the patient details
- the purpose of report
- information the report is based on – limitations of information
- assumptions made
- medical factors
- the patient's history and examination findings
- diagnostic reports
- provisional diagnosis
- management
- prognosis (with regard to ongoing complications or impairment)
- signature and date.

26. Answer: B

An expert witness is someone identified by the court as having qualifications and experience relevant to the legal issue before the court. They are an independent member, engaged with the purpose of assisting the court, rather than as an advocate for a particular party. They are permitted to advance opinion in their field of expertise, which is legally admissible.[23]

27. Answer: B

Brain death is said to be present in a patient with irreversible cessation of function of brainstem function, and is diagnosed via repeated clinical examinations. Testing for brain death must be carried out with the patient at normal body temperature and BP, no indication of endocrine or metabolic dysfunction, and in the absence of sedatives or muscle relaxants.

Confirmation is reached via absence of reflexes including corneal, pupillary, spinociliary, vestibulocochlear, oculocephalic and cough. There should also be absent responses to pain, atropine injection, and absent respiratory effort at PCO_2 over 60 mmHg with adequate oxygenation. In consideration for organ transplant, examinations should be carried out by at least two experienced doctors, neither of whom are on the transplant team, one of whom has not been directly involved with the patient's current care.[27]

28. Answer: C

Requirements for coronial notification vary between jurisdictions; however, relevant situations usually include those in which:

- the body is found, or died, in the jurisdiction
- the death occurred in unexplained or unknown circumstances
- the patient was in specific circumstances such as police custody, a detention centre, or in an approved treatment centre for treatment of drug addiction
- deaths occurring unexpectedly as the result of a surgical, invasive or diagnostic procedure (including the administration of an anaesthetic), are also reportable.

A coronial inquiry may only be instituted if the death has been reported. The responsibility of the coroner is to confirm the identity of the deceased, the details and cause of a death, and any individuals contributing to the death. The coroner may comment on any matter relating to the death, in terms of public health or safety, or administration of justice. They may not include a finding that any person is guilty of an offence – such reports should be passed to the Director of Public Prosecutions for consideration of action.[28]

29. Answer: A

An advance health directive allows a patient to determine medical treatments in advance. It may prevent interventions likely to have been unwanted by the patient. It should include specific elements:

- It must have been completed while the patient was sound of mind.
- It must specify particular circumstances under which it should be activated.
- It must specify which treatments the patient does and does not wish to receive if they are unable to provide consent.

Another person is usually named as guarantor of the document.

Any decisions made on the ongoing care of the patient should be made following inspection of her advanced directive. This allows confirmation that it is applicable to current situation, and provides information as to what treatment is acceptable to the patient. It is therefore reasonable to continue supportive care as indicated until the document is available. **An advanced health directive is legally invalidated in cases of self-harm and attempted suicide, although the patient may still be assessed as capable of consenting to or refusing treatment** (see answer 22).[23]

30. Answer: B

AHPRA was formed by an Act of Parliament in 2009. All registered doctors in Australia must provide an annual statement, including declarations on the existence of any impairment, and whether there have been any issues in meeting the standards of the Medical Board of Australia.

An impairment includes any physical or mental impairment, disability, condition or disorder (including substance abuse or dependence) that currently affects, or is likely to detrimentally affect, a registered health practitioner's capacity to safely practise.

Practitioners and employers are mandated by law to report certain notifiable conduct relating to registered health practitioners or students. Registered practitioners who fail to report appropriately may face disciplinary action by their national board. Notifiable conduct includes:

- intoxication by alcohol or drugs while practising or training in the profession
- engagement in sexual misconduct in connection with the practice or training of the profession
- impairment that places the public at risk of substantial harm
- a significant departure from accepted professional standards, placing the public at risk of harm.

In the current situation, the doctor has not been intoxicated while working, and indeed, has absented herself from the workplace rather than do so. However, the reported pattern of recurrent absences and inappropriate attitude to certain patients raises concerns about the doctor's wellbeing, as well as being a possible issue with discipline or unacceptable values. Chronic low-grade stress – burnout – may be difficult to recognise initially, but changes in behaviour, loss of empathy, and dependence on drugs and alcohol are features of concern. Suspension may remove the doctor from a situation of risk while further assessment is made; however, it may also be seen as 'proof' of wrong-doing.

When a health-related notification is received by AHPRA, the health practitioner or student may be subject to a health assessment by a relevant national board to ensure appropriate action is taken, if required, to protect the public. AHPRA is a regulatory body; assistance for the practitioner can be found via the Medical Association for each state.[29]

References

1. Australasian College for Emergency Medicine. G15: Guidelines on emergency department design. Online. Available at: http://www.acem.org.au/media/policies_and_guidelines/G15_ED_Design.pdf; 5 Jun 2011.

2. Dunn R, Brookes J. Clinical systems management. In: Dunn R, et al, editors. The emergency medicine manual. 5th ed. Tennyson: Venom Publishing; 2010. p. 339–66.

3. Dunn R, Brookes J. Staff management. In: Dunn R, et al, editors. The emergency medicine manual. 5th ed. Tennyson: Venom Publishing, 2010. 23 p. 367–72.

4. Yuen A. Complaints. In: Cameron P, Jelinek G, Kelly A, et al, editors. Textbook of adult emergency medicine. 3rd ed. Sydney: Churchill Livingstone Elsevier; 2009. 27 p. 835–40.

5. Australasian College for Emergency Medicine. G21: Guideline on clinical handover in the emergency department. Online. Available at: http://www.acem.org. au/media/policies_and_guidelines/Clinical_Handover_in_ the_EM.pdf; 5 Jun 2011.

6. Australian Commission on Safety and Quality in Health Care. Clinical handover: critical communications. MJA 2009:190.

7. Australian Medical Association. Safe handover: safe patients. Guidance in clinical handover for clinicians and managers. Online. Available at: http://www.ama.com.au/ node/4064; 5 Jun 2011.

8. Paterson, ES et al. Handoff strategies in settings with high consequences for failure: lessons for health care operations. International Journal for Quality in Health Care 2004;16:125–32.

9. Dunn R, Brookes J. Patient safety. In: Dunn R, et al, editors. The emergency medicine manual. 5th ed. Tennyson: Venom Publishing; 2010. 10 p. 161–77.

10. Neate S, Phillips G. The challenging patient. In: Cameron P, Jelinek G, Kelly A, et al, editors. Textbook of adult emergency medicine. 3rd ed. Sydney: Churchill Livingstone Elsevier; 2009. p. 680–91.

11. Dunn R, Brookes J. Professional skills. In: Dunn R, et al, editors. The emergency medicine manual. 5th ed. Tennyson: Venom Publishing; 2010. 11 p. 178–96.

12. Ashby RH. Business planning. In: Cameron P, Jelinek G, Kelly A, et al, editors. Textbook of adult emergency medicine. 3rd ed. Sydney: Churchill Livingstone Elsevier; 2010. p. 823–6.

13. Australasian College for Emergency Medicine. S57; ACEM statement on emergency department overcrowding. Online. Available at: http://www.acem.org.au/media/ policies_and_guidelines/S57_-_Statement_on_ED_Overcr. pdf; 5 Jun 2009.

14. Australasian College for Emergency Medicine. S18: Statement on responsibility for care in emergency departments. Online. Available at: http://www.acem.org. au/media/policies_and_guidelines/responsibility_care.pdf; 5 Jun 2009.

15. Richardson D. Emergency department overcrowding and access block. In: Cameron P, Jelinek G, Kelly A, et al, editors. Textbook of adult emergency medicine. 3rd ed. Sydney: Churchill Livingstone Elsevier; 2009. p. 803–6.

16. Australasian College for Emergency Medicine. P02: ACEM policy on standard terminology. Online. Available at: http://www.acem.org.au/media/policies_and_guidelines/ P02_-_Standard_Terminology_16.04.09.pdf; 5 Jun 2011.

17. Williams A. Emergency department observation wards. In: Cameron P, Jelinek G, Kelly A, et al, editors. Textbook of adult emergency medicine. 3rd ed. Sydney: Churchill Livingstone Elsevier; 2009. 26(6) p. 800–2.

18. Yuen A. Privacy and confidentiality. In: Cameron P, Jelinek G, Kelly A, et al, editors. Textbook of adult emergency medicine. 3rd ed. Sydney: Churchill Livingstone Elsevier; 2009. 25(4) p. 771–5.

19. Sprivulis P. Patient safety. In: Cameron P, Jelinek G, Kelly A, et al, editors. Textbook of adult emergency medicine. 3rd ed. Sydney: Churchill Livingstone Elsevier; 2009. p. 806–9.

20. Vinen John. Clinical risk management in the emergency department. In: Cameron P, Jelinek G, Kelly A, et al, editors. Textbook of adult emergency medicine. 3rd ed. Sydney: Churchill Livingstone Elsevier; 2009. p. 840–7.

21. Croskerry P, Sinclair D. Emergency medicine: A practice prone to error? CEMJ 2001;3:271–6.

22. Reason J. Human error: models and management. BMJ 2000;320:768–70.

23. Dunn R, Brookes J. Medicolegal medicine. In: Dunn R, et al, editors. The emergency medicine manual. 5th ed. Tennyson: Venom Publishing; 2010. p. 373–7.

24. Brentnall E, Parker HL. Consent and competence – the Australian and UK perspectives. In: Cameron P, Jelinek G, Kelly A, et al, editors. Textbook of adult emergency medicine. 3rd ed. Sydney: Churchill Livingstone Elsevier; 2009. p. 767–71.

25. Dilley S, Dunn R. Infection control. In: Dunn R, et al, editors. The emergency medicine manual. 5th ed. Tennyson: Venom Publishing; 2010. p. 730–40.

26. Knox I, Crampton R. Sexual assault. In: Cameron P, Jelinek G, Kelly A, et al, editors. Textbook of adult emergency medicine. 3rd ed. Sydney: Churchill Livingstone Elsevier; 2009. p. 658–64.

27. Dilley S, Dunn R. Neurological assessment. In: Dunn R, et al, editors. The emergency medicine manual. 5th ed. Tennyson: Venom Publishing; 2010. p. 605–29.

28. Dunn R, Brookes J. Dealing with special situations. In: Dunn R, et al, editors. The emergency medicine manual. 5th ed. Tennyson: Venom Publishing; 2010. p. 208–27.

29. AHPRA. AHPRA – notifications and outcomes. Online. Available at: http://www.ahpra.gov.au/Notifications-and-Outcomes.aspx; 8 Jun 2011.

INDEX

....

Page numbers followed by 't' indicate tables, and 'b' indicate boxes.

A

A-a gradient, 53, 238
AAA *see* abdominal aortic aneurysm
AACG *see* acute angle closure glaucoma
abdominal aortic aneurysm (AAA)
  rupture risk and, 71, 284
  ultrasound and, 71, 283
abdominal pain
  acute, 70, 282
  in children, 74, 294–295
  in female of reproductive age, 85, 326
abdominal wound dehiscence, 74, 293
ABG *see* arterial blood gas
abruptio placentae, 83, 322–323
abusive head trauma (AHT), 57, 250
acalculous cholecystitis, 71, 286
access block, 109, 399
ACE *see* angiotensin-converting-enzyme inhibitor
ACEM *see* Australasian College for Emergency Medicine guidelines
acetylcholine excess, 339
Achilles tendon rupture, 67, 276
acidaemia, 238
acid–base disorders
  answers, 233–240
  questions, 51–53
acidosis *see* lactic acidosis; metabolic acidosis
ACL *see* anterior cruciate ligament
ACS *see* acute coronary syndrome
acute angle closure glaucoma (AACG), 76, 302
acute coronary syndrome (ACS), 11–12
  emergency reperfusion and, 11, 134
  pharmacological management of, 12, 136
  STEMI and, 134–135
  see also non-ST segment elevated ACS
acute mountain sickness (AMS), 93, 351
acute post-streptococcal glomerulonephritis (APSGN), 38–39, 202
  streptococcal infection and, 202
acute pulmonary oedema, 12, 136
acute radiation syndrome (ARS), 93, 351–352
  phases of, 351–352
acute renal failure (ARF)
  causes regarding, 37, 198
  clinical features and, 37, 198
  medication precipitating, 37, 198–199
  mortality associated with, 37, 198
  transplantation and, 38, 200
    fever and, 200
acyclovir
  herpes gingivostomatitis, primary, and, 46, 222–223
  varicella and, 44, 219

adenosine, 15, 140
adenovirus infection, 99, 369
adrenal crisis
  diagnosis, 29–30, 176
  hydrocortisone and, 176
  management, 30, 176
adrenal hyperplasia, congenital, 74
adrenal insufficiency, 29, 175–176
adrenaline, high-dose, 4, 118
adult epiglottitis, 78, 306
adult respiratory distress syndrome (ARDS), 3, 116
advanced healthcare directive, 111, 403
AED *see* automated external defibrillator
AF *see* atrial fibrillation
AG *see* anion gap
AGE *see* arterial gas embolism
aggression management, in ED, 108, 397–398
AHT *see* abusive head trauma
alcohol, 26, 168
alcoholic ketoacidosis
  diagnosis, 29, 175
  management, 29, 175
alkalaemia, 238
altitude-related problems, 93, 351
American Society of Anesthesiology (ASA), 55–56, 245–246
amphetamine-induced psychiatric disorders, 96, 358–359
AMS *see* acute mountain sickness
anaemia, 41–42, 208–209
anaesthesia, emergency
  answers, 241–247
  questions, 54–56
anaesthetics toxicity, 87, 333
AnGel®, 247
angiotensin-converting-enzyme (ACE) inhibitor, 37, 198–199
anion gap (AG)
  explained, 51, 234
  metabolic acidosis and, 52–53, 86, 237, 331
ankle
  fracture, 67–68, 276
  sprain, 67, 275
    radiographic assessment of, 67, 275–276
    talar dome fracture and, 67, 276
anorexia nervosa, 95, 356–357
antepartum haemorrhage, 83–84, 323
anterior cruciate ligament (ACL), 67, 274–275
anterior uveitis, 76, 302
anthrax, 393
antibiotics
  clearance, 218
  empiric antibiotic therapy, 47, 224–225

HUS and, 202

  pneumonia regime of, 44, 219

  pyelonephritis regime of, 311

anticholinergic syndrome, 87, 333

anticoagulation therapy, 41, 209

anti-convulsive therapy, 100, 374, 374t

anti-D prophylaxis, 82–83, 319–320

antidepressant toxicity, major tricyclic, 87, 333

anti-hepatitis A virus (anti-HAV), 35, 193

aorta, traumatic rupture of, 61, 259

aortic dissection, 73, 290–291

apnea, neonates and, 104, 387

appendicitis

  MANTRELS score and, 281t

  pregnancy and, 71, 284–285

  signs of, 70, 281

APSGN *see* acute post-streptococcal glomerulonephritis

ARDS *see* adult respiratory distress syndrome

ARF *see* acute renal failure

ARS *see* acute radiation syndrome

arterial blood gas (ABG), 90, 341

arterial gas embolism (AGE), 92, 348–349

arterial occlusion, acute embolic, 72–73, 289

arthritis

  children and, 65, 269–270

  reactive, 46, 222

  septic, 65, 270

ASA *see* American Society of Anesthesiology

ascites, 34, 190

  salt and, 34–35, 190–191

ascitic tap, 35, 192–193

aspiration pneumonitis, 19, 150

aspirin

  ACS and, 12, 136

  overdose, 87–88, 335

asthma

  adult ventilation and, 21, 154–155

  blood gas and, 53, 237–238

  bronchodilator therapy, 20–21, 153

  children and

    assessment, 102, 380, 381t

    salbutamol, 21, 155

  classification of, 382, 382t

  DOPE mnemonic, 155

  intubation and, 3, 21, 116, 154

  life threatening, 20, 153

    invasive ventilation and, 21, 154

  mechanical ventilation and, 3, 116, 116t

  $MgSO_4$ and, 21, 154

  salbutamol and, 21, 155

  wheezing and, 103, 382

asymptomatic bacteriuria, 39, 204

atrial fibrillation (AF), 15–16, 141

  sinus rhythm reversion and, 16, 141

  WPW and, 16, 141–142

atrial flutter, 16, 142

atropine, 89, 339

Australasian College for Emergency Medicine (ACEM) guidelines

  on ED equipment, 107, 395

  on ED layout design, 107, 395

automated external defibrillator (AED), 8, 128

avulsed tooth, 78, 308

  milk and, 308

B

Bacillus cereus, 33, 185

bacterial vaginosis, 314

Barmah Forest virus, 46, 223

benign paroxysmal positional vertigo (BPPV), 24, 167–168

benzodiazepines, 338

beta-blocker

  ACS and, 12, 136

  overdose, 88, 337

bilateral interfacetal dislocation, 252

bilevel positive airway pressure (BiPAP), 3, 115–116

bimanual laryngoscopy, 54, 241

biological emergencies, 105–106, 393

BiPAP *see* bilevel positive airway pressure

black snake bite, 90, 342

bladder outlet obstruction, 310

bleeding disorders, 42

blistering skin disorders, 49, 231

blood gas

  ABG, 90, 341

  asthma and, 53, 237–238

  pneumonia and, 53, 238

  seizure and, 53, 239–240

  VBG analysis, 18, 146

blood transfusion

  anaemia patient, 41, 208–209

  blood type and, 41, 207

  fever and, 41, 208–209

  massive, 41, 207–208

  multi-trauma patient, 41, 207–208

  TXA and, 208

blunt trauma, flail chest and, 59, 256

BNP *see* B-type natriuretic peptide

body packers, 90, 341

body temperature measurement, in children, 98, 366

Boerhaave's syndrome, 72, 289

bomb explosion

  injury categories and, 62, 262–263

  primary blast injury and, 62, 262

borderline personality disorder (BPD), 94–95, 355

  comorbid conditions, 95, 356

  suicide rate and, 94–95, 355

botulinus toxin, 393

botulism, 27, 47, 170, 225

bowel obstruction, 35–36, 194

  bent inner tube and, 70–71, 283

  see also large bowel/colonic obstruction; small bowel obstruction

box jellyfish, 91, 343
   Irukandji syndrome and, 91, 343–344
   sting features, 343
   treatment, 343
Boyle's law, 92, 349
BPD *see* borderline personality disorder
BPPV *see* benign paroxysmal positional vertigo
brain death, 110, 402–403
breast
   carcinoma, 42
   infection, 73, 291–292
bronchiectasis, 19, 150–151
bronchiolitis, in children, 102, 377–378
   in neonate, 102, 380
   treatment options in, 102, 379–380, 380t
bronchodilator therapy, 20–21, 153
bronchoscopy, 147
brown snake bite
   earliest indication of, 90, 341
   VICC and, 90, 342
Brugada syndrome, 15, 140
   isoprenaline and, 140
B-type natriuretic peptide (BNP), 22, 156
bupivacaine, 55, 243–244
burnout, ED staff, 396
burns
   answers, 250–264
   intravenous fluid rate and, 63, 263
   from lightning, 350
   Parkland formula and, 63, 263
   questions, 57–63
   rule of nines and, 62, 263
business planning, ED, 108, 398–399
button battery
   ingestion, 74–75, 296–297
   toxicity, 89–90, 340

C

caesarean section, 62, 262
calcium, 38, 200
calcium channel blocker (CCB)
   HIET and, 88, 337
   overdose, 88, 336–337
Canadian cervical spine rule, 58, 252
Candida albicans, 47
CAP *see* community-acquired pneumonia
carbamazepine toxicity, 86, 331
carbon monoxide (CO) poisoning, 89,
   338
cardiac arrest
   care following, 5, 119
   hypothermia and, 5, 118–119
   pregnancy and, 4–5, 118
   prognostication after, 5, 119–120
cardiogenic shock, 12–13, 136–137
   management, 13, 137
   myocardial infarction and, 13, 137

cardiopulmonary resuscitation (CPR), 3–4, 116–117
   non-shockable rhythm and, 4, 118
   ventilation and, 4, 117
cardiorespiratory arrest, 7, 126
   in children
      compression cycle and, 7, 127
      paediatric arrhythmia and, 7, 126–127
      pulse check and, 7, 127
cardiorespiratory collapse, in neonate, 97, 363–364
cardiotoxic drugs, 89, 340
cardiovascular emergencies
   answers, 133–144
   questions, 11–17
   see also specific disorder
Carukia barnesi, 343–344
CATMUDPILES mnemonic, 238, 331
CCB *see* calcium channel blocker
CD *see* Crohn's disease
ceftriaxone, 98, 366
cellulitis, 76, 301–302
   causes of, 46, 223
   organisms involved in, 302
central retinal artery occlusion (CRAO), 76, 303
   causes and treatment of, 76, 303
central retinal vein occlusion (CRVO), 76, 303
cerebral oedema, 29, 101, 174, 376
cerebrospinal fluid (CSF), 100, 371–372
cervical artery dissection, 25–26, 166–167, 166t
cervical lymphadenitis, 75, 297
cervical spinal cord injury (SCI), 58, 253
cervical spine injuries
   assessment, 58, 252
   in children, 58, 252
      radiographs, 65
   isolated ligament, 68, 277
   unilateral facet joint dislocation, 68, 277
cervicitis, 47, 226
CFS *see* chronic fatigue syndrome
charcoal, multiple dose activated, 86, 330–331
chemical exposures, 106, 393
chest pain, positive LR for, 11, 133
chest trauma, 59–60, 256–257
   EDT and, 60, 258
   myocardial contusion, 60, 257–258
   pneumomediastinum and, 60, 257
   stab wounds, 59–60, 256–257
   sternum, undisplaced fracture of, 60, 257
chickenpox, 44, 219
children
   abdominal pain in, 74, 294–295
   adenovirus infection and, 99, 369
   AHT in, 57, 250
   anti-convulsive therapy and, 100, 374, 374t
   arthritis and, 65, 269–270
   asthma and
      assessment, 102, 380, 381t
      salbutamol, 21, 155

body temperature measurement in, 98, 366

bronchiolitis in, 102, 377–378

   treatment options in, 102, 379–380, 380t

button battery

   ingestion, 74–75, 296–297

   toxicity, 89–90, 340

cardiorespiratory arrest in

   compression cycle and, 7, 127

   paediatric arrhythmia and, 7, 126–127

cellulitis in, 76, 301–302

cervical spine

   injuries in, 58, 252

   radiographs and, 65, 270

congenital heart disease in, 102, 378

conjunctivitis in, 76, 301

corrosive ingestion by, 89, 339

croup, viral, in, 103, 385

defibrillation dose and, 8–9, 129

development milestones in, 103–104, 385, 386t

DKA and, 101, 376

   insulin and fluid rehydration, 101, 376–377

   serum blood sugar levels, 101, 377

ED management and, 245–246

ETCO₂ and, 10, 131

febrile seizures and, 100, 372–373

femur, fracture of, 64–65, 269

fever, approach to, in, 367

heart failure in, 102, 379

heart murmur in, 102, 378–379

humerus

   distal fracture of, 64, 268–269

   supracondylar fracture of, 64, 267–268

with hypertension, 17, 144

iron toxicity and, 90, 340

KD and, 99, 367–370, 368t

LP and, 98, 364–365

meningitis in, 99, 370–371

   clinical manifestation of, 99–100, 371

   CSF and, 100, 371–372

mercury, thermometer, and, 86, 332

mushroom poisoning and, 91, 344

NAI in, 57, 250

nasal foreign body removal in, 78, 306

nasal fractures in, 78, 306–307

nerve screening test for, 267

non-pharmacological pain techniques and, 56, 246–247

osteomyelitis and, 65, 269–270

pain scales and, 56

PCV7 and, 98, 366

petechiae and, 42, 98–99, 367

physeal growth plate injuries in, 64, 267

pneumonia and, 103, 383–384

   acute, 103, 384

   diagnosis, 103, 384–385

post viral cough syndrome in, 103, 383

procedure-related pain and, 56, 247

PSA and, 55–56, 245–246

radius, distal fracture of, 64, 269

SBI in, 98, 364–366

septic shock and, 3–4, 99, 129, 367

SIRS and, 97, 364

skin puncture pain management and, 56, 247

splenic injuries in, 61, 259–260

SVT and, 16, 143

symptom profile, of various conditions in, 368t

toddler's fracture, 65, 269

transient synovitis and, 65, 270

trauma management, 57, 250

   compared with adult, 57, 250

UTIs and, 98–99, 367, 370

   diagnosis in, 40, 205

   epidemiology in, 39–40, 204–205

vital signs, normal, 104, 386–387, 387t

vomiting and, 74, 294

weight estimation in, 8, 128–129

wheezing and, 103, 376–377

Chironex fleckeri, 91, 343

   sting features, 343

   treatment, 343

Chlamydia trachomatis, 203, 226

cholecystitis, 71, 286

cholelithiasis, 71, 285

   gallstone complication and, 71, 285–286

cholera, 46, 223

chronic fatigue syndrome (CFS), 100, 371–372

chronic obstructive pulmonary disease (COPD)

   BNP and, 22, 156

   hypercapnic and normocapnic, 22, 156

   management of acute, 21, 156

   NIV and, 22, 157

   pneumothorax and, 20, 151

   systemic steroids and, 22, 157

CIN *see* contrast-induced nephropathy

clavicle, 65, 271

clinical handover, in ED, 108, 397

clinical practice guidelines, 107, 395

Clostridium difficile, 32–33, 184–185

Clostridium perfringens, 33, 185

CO *see* carbon monoxide poisoning

community-acquired pneumonia (CAP)

   aetiological diagnosis of, 19, 149

   blood cultures and, 19, 149

      volume of blood taken and, 44, 218–219

   severity assessment, 18–19, 148–149, 148t–149t

compartment syndrome

   diagnosis of, 66, 273

   of forearm, 66, 273

complaints, ED management of, 108, 396–397

compression ventilation ratio, 8, 128, 128t

condylar fractures, 268–269

confidentiality, ED and, 109, 400

congenital adrenal hyperplasia, 74, 294–295

congenital heart disease, children and, 102, 378

conjunctivitis, 76, 301

consent, 110, 401–402

continuous quality improvement (CQI), 108, 399

contraception, postcoital (emergency), 85, 326
    progestin-only method, 326
    Yuzpe method, 326

contrast-induced nephropathy (CIN), 37, 199
    parenteral volume repletion and, 199

conversion disorder, 95, 357

COP, I'VE STUMBLED mnemonic, 330

COPD see chronic obstructive pulmonary disease

coronial investigations, 110–111, 403

corrosive ingestion, 89, 339

CPR see cardiopulmonary resuscitation

CQI see continuous quality improvement

CRAO see central retinal artery occlusion

Crohn's disease (CD), 33, 185
    Crohn's Disease Activity Index and, 186
    extraintestinal manifestations of, 185

croup, viral, 103, 385

CRVO see central retinal vein occlusion

CSCATTT mnemonic, 391

CSF see cerebrospinal fluid

cuffed tracheal tube size, 8, 127–128

cyanide
    exposure, 393
    poisoning, 89, 338

cyclopeptide hepatotoxicity, 344

D

Dalton's law, 349

damage control resuscitation (DCR), 63, 264
    aim of, 263–264
    components of, 63, 263–264

decompression sickness (DCS), 92, 348–349
    Boyle's law and, 92, 349

deep venous thrombosis (DVT), 23, 159

defibrillation, 4, 117
    AED, 8, 128
    dose for children, 8–9, 129
    monophasic and biphasic, 4, 117
    VF and, 4, 117–118

dehydration, 32, 182
    hypotonic oral rehydration and, 182–183
    severity classification, 182

delayed primary closure, 73, 292–293

delta gap, 51, 234–235, 235t

delta pressure, 273

dengue, 45, 220

dental emergencies
    answers, 301–308
    questions, 76–79

depression
    diagnostic criteria for, 353
    late life, 94, 353–354
    suicide risk and, 94, 353

dermatological emergencies
    answers, 229–232
    questions, 49–50

development milestones, in children, 103–104, 385, 386t

DGI see disseminated gonococcal infection

diabetes
    foot ulcers and, 28, 172
    hyperglycaemia and, 31, 180, 180t
    hypoglycaemia and, 28, 172–173
    insipidus, 51, 233
    lower limb ulcer and, 29, 175
    ophthalmic complications and, 28, 172
    osteomyelitis and, 29, 175
    unstable blood glucose and, 28, 172

diabetic ketoacidosis (DKA), 101, 174, 376
    cerebral oedema and, 29, 101, 174, 376
    insulin and fluid rehydration and, 101, 376–377
    serum blood sugar levels and, 101, 377
    standard urine ward test and, 28, 173
    water deficit and, 28, 173–174

diaphragmatic injuries, 61, 259

diarrhoea
    bloody, 32, 183–184
        causative agents, 183
    Clostridium difficile related, 32–33, 184–185
    metabolic acidosis and, 52, 237
    travellers', 32, 184

diazepam, 375

dicobalt edetate, 89, 338

diffuse axonal injury, 57, 251

digit replantation, 66, 272–273

Digoxin Immune Fab, 88, 336

digoxin toxicity, 88, 336

dihidropiridine, 336

diphtheria, 48, 226

disaster
    biological emergencies, 105–106, 393
    chemical exposures, 106, 393
    equipment and supplies, 105, 392
    mass casualty incident
        response, 105, 391
        triage, 106, 393–394
    planning, 105, 391
    radiation exposure, 106, 393
    site
        health and safety issues, 105, 392
        roles and responsibilities, 105, 392
    surge capacity planning, 105, 391–392

disaster management
    answers, 391–394
    questions, 105–106

dislocation
    bilateral interfacetal, 252
    hip, 66–67, 274
    Monteggia's fracture, 269
    perilunate, 66, 272
    scapholunate, 66, 272
    shoulder joint, 65, 271
    unilateral facet joint, 68, 277

disseminated gonococcal infection (DGI), 46, 221–222
    sexually active patient and, 49, 230–231
diverticulitis, 70, 281
DKA *see* diabetic ketoacidosis
dobutamine, 122, 122t
dopamine, 121–122, 122t
DOPE mnemonic, 155
drowning, 92, 349–350
drug skin eruptions, 49, 231
duct-dependent congenital heart lesion, 16–17, 143
DUMBBELS mnemonic, 339
duty of care, 109–110, 401
DVT *see* deep venous thrombosis
dyspnoea, 18, 146
dysrhythmias, 15, 140
dysuria-frequency syndrome, 39, 203–204

E

E. coli, 203
ear
    nose, and throat (ENT) emergencies
        answers, 301–308
        questions, 76–79
    pinna of, 78, 307
EBV *see* Epstein-Barr virus
ECG *see* electrocardiogram
eclampsia, 83, 321
ectopic pregnancy, 82, 318
eczema herpeticum, 232
ED *see* emergency department management
EDD *see* oesophageal detector device
EDT *see* emergency department thoracotomy
Elapidae snake bite, 90, 342
electrical injuries
    household current, 92, 350
    lightning, 93, 350–351
electrocardiogram (ECG)
    emergency reperfusion and, 11, 134
    hyperkalaemia and, 52, 236, 236t
    Osborne or J waves on, 92, 348
    pericarditis and, 13, 137–138
electrolyte disorders
    answers, 233–240
    questions, 51–53
EM *see* erythema multiforme
emergency department (ED) management
    of access block, 109, 399
    ACEM guidelines
        on equipment, 107, 395
        on layout, 107, 395
    aggression management and, 108, 397–398
    answers, 395–404
    of burnout, 396
    business planning and, 108, 398–399
    children and, 245–246
    clinical handover and, 108, 397
    clinical practice guidelines, 107, 395

complaints and, 108, 396–397
consent and, 110, 401–402
CQI and, 108, 399
discharge suitability and, 72, 288
information systems and, 107, 395–396
mandatory reporting and, 110, 402
medical errors and, 109, 400–401
negligence and, 109–110, 401
negotiation and, 108, 398
    stages of, 398
OM and, 109, 400
overcrowding and, 108–109, 399
performance appraisals, 107, 396
privacy and confidentiality and, 109, 400
questions, 107–111
reports and, 110, 402
rostering of staff and, 107, 396
SSUs and, 109, 399–400
of staff burnout, 396
stress, work related, and, 107–108, 396
emergency department thoracotomy (EDT), 60, 258
EMLA®, 247
empiric antibiotic therapy, 47, 224–225
endocarditis, 13–14, 138
    blood cultures and, 14, 139
    criteria for, 138b
        major, 138
        minor, 138
    mortality, 139
    right-sided, 139
endocrine emergencies
    answers, 172–180
    questions, 28–31
endotracheal tube placement, 3
end-stage renal disease (ESRD), pericarditis and, 37, 199
    uraemic, 199
end-tidal carbon dioxide (ETCO$_2$), 115
    resuscitation of children and, 10, 131
enoxaparin, ACS and, 12, 136
ENT *see* ear, nose, and throat emergencies
environmental emergencies
    answers, 348–352
    questions, 92–93
epiglottitis, adult, 78, 306
epilepsy syndrome, 100, 374, 374t
epistaxis
    bleeding, 77, 305
    treatment of, 77, 305–306
Epstein-Barr virus (EBV), 47, 225
    oral hairy leukoplakia and, 47, 225–226
errors, medical, 109, 400–401
erythema multiforme (EM), 49, 229
erythema toxicum neonatorum, 230
erythroderma, 49, 230
ESRD *see* end-stage renal disease

ETCO$_2$ *see* end-tidal carbon dioxide
eucalyptus oil, 89, 338
evaporative cooling, 92, 348
expert witness, 110, 402
extracorporeal elimination, of toxins, 86, 330
eye emergencies
    acid and alkali injuries, 77, 304
    answers, 301–308
    dilated pupil and, 77, 303–304
    questions, 76–79
    retrobulbar haematoma, 77, 305

F

Faces Pain Scale, 246
facial trauma
    injury management in, 59, 255
    midfacial fractures and, 58–59, 254–255
    tongue and, 59, 255
    zygomatic fractures and, 58, 254
Fanconi's syndrome, 53, 238
fasting, 55, 245
febrile neutropenia, 42–43, 213
febrile seizures, 100, 372–373
femoral artery pseudoaneurysm, 72, 288
femoral nerve blocks, 55, 244
femur
    fracture, in children, 64–65, 269
    fractured neck of
        in elderly, 66, 273
        imaging of, 66, 274
fentanyl, 244
finger, 68–69, 279
fish-related toxicity, 91, 344–345
Fitz-Hugh–Curtis syndrome, 85, 326
FLACC scale, 246
flail chest, 59, 256
fluid resuscitation, 7, 123
food poisoning, 33, 185
    botulism, 47, 225
foot
    Lisfranc's injury of, 68, 276–277
    ulcers, 28–29, 172, 175
foreign bodies
    in child's nose, 78, 306
    in oesophagus, 74–75, 296–297
forensic examination, sexual assault and, 110, 402
Fournier's gangrene, 81, 314
fracture, 58, 253
    ankle, 67–68, 276
    distal radial
        abnormalities regarding, 65–66, 271–272
        reduction and, 65–66, 271–272
    femur, 64–65, 269
        in children, 64–65, 269
        fractured neck of, 66, 273–274
    Galeazzi's, 269
    hangman, 253

humerus
    distal fracture of, 64, 268–269
    Gartland type fracture of, 64, 268
    supracondylar fracture of, 64, 267–268
    Jefferson, 253
    Monteggia's fracture dislocation, 269
    orbital blowout fracture, 77, 304
        treatment of, 77, 304
    pelvic
        haemodynamically unstable patient and, 61, 260–261
        Young-Burgess classification and, 61, 260, 260t
    radius, 64, 269
    supracondylar
        Gartland type, 64, 268
        of humerus, 64, 267–268
        vascular compromise and, 64, 268
    of talar dome, 67, 276
    teardrop, 58, 253
    toddler's, 65, 269
    undisplaced sternum, 60, 257
funnel-web spider, 91, 343

G

Galeazzi's fracture, 269
gall bladder, 33, 186
    cholelithiasis and, 71, 285–286
gallstones, 71, 285–286
Gartland type fracture, 64, 268
gastroenterological emergencies
    adult, 32
    answers, 182–195
    cow's milk and, 32, 183
    paediatric, 32
    questions, 32–36
gastrointestinal tract (GIT)
    bleeding
        aetiology, 33, 187
        clinical manifestations, 34, 187–188
        investigations, 34, 188
        octreotide and, 34, 189
        variceal, 34, 189–190
    endoscopy and, 34, 188–189
    foreign bodies in, 74–75, 296–297
    rebleeding of, 188–189
GBS *see* group B streptococcus
generalised convulsive status epilepticus, 26, 168
genital infections, 81, 314–315
genitourinary injuries, 61–62, 261
gentamicin, 224–225
GFR *see* glomerular filtration rate
GIT *see* gastrointestinal tract
Glasgow criteria, 287
glaucoma, 76, 302
    see also primary open angle glaucoma
glomerular filtration rate (GFR), 332
goal-directed therapy, 6, 121
gonococcal urethritis, 314

Graves' disease, 30, 177
group B streptococcus (GBS), 97, 361
growth plate injuries
    physeal, in children, 64, 267
    Salter-Harris type I, 64, 267
Guillain-Barré syndrome, 27, 169
gynaecological emergencies
    answers, 317–327
    questions, 82–85

H
H$_2$O$_2$ see hydrogen peroxide
HACE see heralds high-altitude cerebral oedema
haematemesis, octreotide and, 34, 189
haematochezia, 188
haematological malignancies, 43, 214–215
haematuria, 39, 203
    causes, 203, 314
    urine and, 81, 314
haemodialysis (HD)
    of toxins, 86, 330
    vascular access and, 38, 199–200
haemodynamically stable patients
    mortality regarding, 22, 157
    with PE, 23, 159
haemodynamically unstable patients, with pelvic fracture, 61,
        260–261
haemolytic uremic syndrome (HUS), 38, 202
    antibiotics and, 202
    central nervous system irritability and, 202
    forms of, 202
haemoptysis, 18, 147
    bronchoscopy and, 147
haemorrhagic hypovolaemia, 63, 263
haemorrhoids, 73, 291
haemothorax, 59, 256
hallucinations, 353
hand, foot and mouth disease, 49, 231–232
hanging injuries, 59, 256
hangman fracture, 253
hard signs, 59, 255
βHCG testing, 82, 318–319
HD see haemodialysis
head injury
    AHT, 57, 250
    diffuse axonal injury, 57, 251
    hypotension and, 57, 251
    intracranial haemorrhage, 57–58, 252
    intracranial injury and, 57, 251
    motor function and, 57, 250–251
    secondary insult and, 57, 251
headache
    pregnancy and, 83, 320–321
    primary causes of, 24, 162
    SAH and, 25, 164
    secondary causes of, 24, 162
    see also migraine; subarachnoid haemorrhage; temporal arteritis

heart
    block, 14, 139
        atrioventricular, 14, 139
    children
        congenital heart disease in, 102, 378
        failure in, 102, 379
        murmur in, 102, 378–379
        neonate, duct-dependent congenital heart lesion in, 16–17, 143
        stab wound to, 60, 258
        see also specific disorder
heat exhaustion, 92, 348
heat stroke, 92, 348
heat-related illnesses, 92, 348
haematological emergencies
    answers, 207–216
    INR levels and, 41, 209–210
    questions, 41–43
Henry's law, 349
heparin, 41, 210
hepatic encephalopathy, 35, 193
hepatitis B, 45, 221
hepatitis C, 45, 221
heralds high-altitude cerebral oedema (HACE), 351
hernias
    repair indicators, 72, 288
    types of, 72, 287–288
herpes
    gingivostomatitis, primary, 46, 222–223
    simplex infections, 232
        skin and, 50
HG see hyperemesis gravidarum
HHS see hyperglycaemic hyperosmolar state
HIE see hypoxic ischemic encephalopathy
high-dose insulin euglycaemic therapy (HIET), 88, 337
hip
    dislocation, 66–67, 274
    septic arthritis of, 65, 270
HIV see human immunodeficiency virus
Horner's syndrome, 77, 303–304
human immunodeficiency virus (HIV)
    acute infection of, 46, 222
    with gastrointestinal symptoms, 47, 225–226
    ring-enhancing lesions and, 45, 220
    seizure and, 27, 169
    toxoplasmosis and, 45, 220
    transmission risk, from percutaneous exposure, 45, 220–221
humerus
    distal fracture, in child, 64, 268–269
    Gartland type fracture of, 64, 268
    supracondylar fracture, in child, 64, 267–268
HUS see haemolytic uremic syndrome
hydralazine, 13, 137
hydrocarbons, inhaled, 89, 338
hydrocortisone, 176, 179
hydrogen peroxide (H$_2$O$_2$), 89, 339
hydroxycobalamin, 89, 338
hyperaldosteronism, 31, 178–179

hypercalcaemia
  acute life-threatening, 179
  causes of, 179
  hydrocortisone and, 179
  intravenous bisphosphonate and, 179
  management, 31, 43, 179
  rehydration and, 179
  signs and symptoms, 234
  treatment goals, 51, 234
hyperemesis gravidarum (HG), 82, 317
hyperglycaemia, 31, 180, 180t
hyperglycaemic hyperosmolar state (HHS), 29, 174–175
hyperkalaemia
  calcium and, 38, 200
  ECG and, 52, 236, 236t
  intravenous insulin and, 38, 201
hyperleucocytosis, 43, 215
hyperlipidaemia, 51, 233
hypernatraemia, 51, 233
hyperoxia test, 17, 143
hypertension, children with, 17, 144
hypertensive crises, 13, 137
  pharmacological treatment of, 13, 137
hypertonic saline, 6, 122
hypocalcaemia, 53, 239
hypoglycaemia, 28, 172–173
hypokalaemia, 52, 236
hyponatraemia, 53, 238–239
hypopituitarism, 31, 178
hypotension, 30, 57, 176, 251
hypotensive resuscitation, 6, 122–123
hypothermia, 92, 348
  cardiac arrest and, 5, 118–119
  induced, 5, 119
hypothyroidism, 31, 178
hypotonic oral rehydration, 182–183
hypovolaemia, haemorrhagic, 63, 263
hypoxic ischemic encephalopathy (HIE), 101, 374–375

I
IBD see inflammatory bowel disease
idiopathic thrombocytopaenic purpura (ITP), 42
ILE see intravenous lipid emulsion
impaired health practitioner, 111, 403–404
inadvertent intraarterial drug injection
  appropriate next step, 73, 289–290
  diagnosis, 73, 289–290
infection control, 46–47, 224
infectious diseases
  answers, 218–226
  questions, 44–48
infectious flexor tenosynovitis, 68–69, 279
inflammatory bowel disease (IBD), 33, 185
  complications of, 33, 185–186
information systems, ED, 107, 395–396
inotropes, 13, 137
INR see international normalised ratio

inspiratory positive airway pressure (IPAP), 115
international normalised ratio (INR), 41, 209–210
  vitamin K and, 41, 210
intraabdominal injuries, 61, 259
intracerebral haemorrhage, 26, 167
intracranial haemorrhage, 57–58, 252
intracranial injury, 57, 251
intradecidual sign, 317
intraosseous (IO) access, 7–8, 127
  complications of, 9, 129
intravenous lipid emulsion (ILE), 87, 333
intravenous regional anaesthesia, 55, 244
intubation, 115
  asthma and, 3, 21, 116, 154
  of morbidly obese patient, 54, 241–242
  see also rapid sequence intubation
intussusception, 74, 295
IO see intraosseous access
IPAP see inspiratory positive airway pressure
iron toxicity, 90, 340
irritable bowel syndrome, 281
Irukandji syndrome, 91, 343–344
isolated ligamentous injuries, 68, 277
isoprenaline, 122, 122t
  Brugada syndrome and, 140
  torsades de pointes and, 140
ITP see idiopathic thrombocytopaenic purpura

J
jaundice, 72, 287
  lactation and, 97, 362
  newborn period and, 97, 362
Jefferson fracture, 253
jellyfish, 91, 343
  Irukandji syndrome and, 91, 343–344
  sting features, 343
  treatment, 343
jugular venous pressure (JVP), 12, 136

K
Kawasaki disease (KD), in children, 99, 367–369, 368t
  typical and atypical, 99, 369–370
ketamine, 245
ketoacidosis see alcoholic ketoacidosis; diabetic ketoacidosis
knee
  ACL injury, 67, 274–275
  ligamentous injuries of, 67, 274
  meniscal injury, 67, 275

L
Laceraine®, 56, 247
lactation
  drug use in, 83, 322
  jaundiced baby and, 97, 362
  mastitis and, 73, 291–292
lactic acidosis, 5, 120
lactulose, 193

large bowel/colonic obstruction, 70, 283
laryngeal mask airway (LMA), 54, 241
laryngospasm, 54, 241
late-life depression, 94, 353–354
Le Fort fractures, 254
leg pain, 72–73, 289
leukaemia, 43, 215
lid retraction, 30, 176–177
lightning, 93, 350–351
  burns from, 350
lignocaine, 55, 243–244
likelihood ratios (LR), 11, 133
Lisfranc's injury, 68, 276–277
lithium
  diabetes insipidus and, 51, 233
  toxicity, 87, 334–335
liver disease, 34, 190
  ascitic tap and, 35, 192–193
  18-gauge needle and, 35, 191–192
  paracentesis and, 35, 191
  salt and, 34–35, 190–191
liver function tests, 35, 193–194
liver transplant, 36, 194–195
  timing of infection following, 194–195
  transfusion regarding, 36, 195
LMA see laryngeal mask airway
LMWH see low-molecular-weight heparin
LMX4®, 247
lorazepam, 101, 375–376
low-molecular-weight heparin (LMWH), 159
LP see lumbar puncture
LR see likelihood ratios
Ludwig's angina, 78, 307–308
lumbar puncture (LP), 98, 364–365
lumbosacral pain
  lumbar spinal canal stenosis and, 68, 278–279
  without sciatica, 68, 277–278
lyme disease, 46, 222

M

magnesium sulphate (MgSO₄), 21, 83, 154, 321–322
major tricyclic antidepressant toxicity, 87, 333
malaria
  cause of, 45, 220
  diagnosis of, 45, 219
malignant otitis externa, 78, 307
malignant spinal cord compression (MSCC), 43
malrotation, 294
mandatory reporting, 110, 402
MAS see meconium aspiration syndrome
mass casualty incident, 105, 391
  response, 105, 391
  triage, 106, 393–394
mastitis, 73, 291–292
MDAC see multiple dose activated charcoal
measles, 45, 221
mechanical ventilation, 3, 116, 116t

Meckel's diverticulum, 74, 295–296
meconium aspiration syndrome (MAS), 9, 130
medical errors, 109, 400–401
medicolegal issues
  advanced healthcare directive, 111, 403
  coronial investigations, 110–111, 403
  expert witness and, 110, 402
  impaired health practitioner, 111, 403–404
  questions, 107–111
  reports and, 110, 402
melioidosis, 46, 223
meningitis
  in children, 99, 370–371
    clinical manifestation of, 99–100, 371
    CSF and, 100, 371–372
  meningococcaemia and, 44, 218
  neonate and, 97, 362–363
meningococcaemia, 44
  clearance antibiotics and, 218
  meningitis and, 44, 218
meniscal injury, 67, 275
mental state examination (MSE), 94, 353
mercury thermometer, 86, 332
meropenem, 44, 219
mesenteric ischaemia, 70, 281–282
metabolic acidosis, 51–52, 235
  AG
    high, 53, 238
    normal, 52, 237
    wide, 86, 331
  diarrhoea and, 52, 237
  saline therapy and, 52, 237
  sodium bicarbonate and, 86, 331
    complications and, 52, 236
    treatment regarding, 52, 237
metabolic alkalosis
  causes of, 51, 235
  hypokalaemia and, 52, 236
  saline unresponsive, 52, 235–236
metaraminol, 4, 122
methaemoglobinaemia, 90, 341
  ABG and, 90, 341
METHANE mnemonic, 391
methicillin resistant *S. aureus* (MRSA), 19, 150
MgSO₄ see magnesium sulphate
midazolam, 375
midfacial fractures, 58–59, 254–255
migraine, 24, 162
milk, 32, 183, 308
miscarriage, 82, 318
monovalent antivenom, 342
Monteggia's fracture dislocation, 269
MRSA see methicillin resistant *S. aureus*
MSCC see malignant spinal cord compression
MSE see mental state examination
MUDDLES mnemonic, 393

multiple dose activated charcoal (MDAC), 86, 330–331
mushroom poisoning, 91, 344
mycoplasma pneumonia, 47, 225
myocardial contusion, 60, 257–258
myocardial infarction, 12, 135, 135t
  cardiogenic shock and, 13, 137
  troponin assays and, 133, 134t
  see also ST elevation myocardial infarction; thrombolysis in myocardial infarction
myocarditis, 102, 379
myoglobin, 201
myxoedema crisis
  management, 30, 177–178
  underlying infection and, 30, 177

N

NAC *see* N-acetylcysteine
N-acetylcysteine (NAC), 87, 335
NAI *see* non-accidental injury
nasal foreign body removal, 78, 306
nasal fractures, in children, 78, 306–307
nasogastric tube (NGT), 35–36
nasopharyngeal airway, 8, 127
National Institute of Health Stroke Scale (NIHSS), 25, 164
neck
  stab wound to, 59, 255
  zones, 59, 255
necrotising fasciitis, 46, 222
negligence, 109–110, 401
negotiation, in ED, 108, 398
  stages of, 398
neonate
  apnea and, 104, 387
  bronchiolitis in, 102, 380
  ceftriaxone and, 98, 366
  collapse, 97, 363–364
    cardiac, 364
    gastrointestinal, 364
    haematologic, 364
    metabolic, 364
    neurologic, 364
    respiratory, 364
  duct-dependent congenital heart lesion in, 16–17, 143
  HIE in, 101, 374–375
  jaundiced, 97, 362
  lorazepam and, 101, 375–376
  MAS and, 9, 130
  mortality and morbidity causes in, 97, 361
  normal physiological changes in, 97, 361
  pustules in, 49, 230
  resuscitation, 9, 129–130
  seizures and, 100, 373–374
    anticonvulsives and, 375–376
    types of, 374
  sepsis and meningitis and, 97, 362–363

  SIRS and, 97, 364
  ventilation strategies in, 9, 131
nephrotic syndrome, 39, 202–203
neuroleptic malignant syndrome, 95, 357–358
neurolepting, 95, 356
neurological and neurosurgical emergencies
  answers, 162–170
  questions, 24–27
NEXUS, 58, 252
NGT *see* nasogastric tube
NIHSS *see* National Institute of Health Stroke Scale
NIV *see* non-invasive ventilation
non-accidental injury (NAI), 57, 250
non-invasive ventilation (NIV), 3, 22, 115–116, 157
non-pharmacological pain techniques, 56, 246–247
non-ST segment elevated ACS (NSTEAC), 11, 133, 134t
nonsteroidal anti-inflammatory drugs (NSAIDs), 37, 198–199
noradrenaline, 5, 120–122, 122t
NSAIDs *see* nonsteroidal anti-inflammatory drugs
NSTEAC *see* non-ST segment elevated ACS

O

observation medicine (OM), 109, 400
obstetric emergencies
  answers, 317–327
  questions, 82–85
octreotide, 34, 88, 189, 337–338
oesophageal detector device (EDD), 115
oesophagus, foreign bodies in, 74–75, 296–297
OG *see* osmolar gap
olanzapine, 96, 359
OM *see* observation medicine
oncological emergencies
  answers, 207–216
  questions, 41–43
opioids, 55, 244–245
optic neuritis, 76, 302–303
oral hairy leukoplakia, 47, 225–226
orbital blowout fracture, 77, 304
  treatment of, 77, 304
orchitis, 313
organophosphate toxicity, 89, 339, 393
orthopaedic emergencies
  answers, 267–279
  questions, 64–69
orthopnoea, 12, 136
Osborne or J waves, 92, 348
osmolar gap (OG), 86, 332
osteomyelitis, 69, 279
  children and, 65, 269–270
  foot ulcer and, 29, 175
otitis externa, malignant, 78, 307
otitis media, 26, 167
ovarian torsion, 85, 326
overcrowding, ED, 108–109, 399
ovulatory bleeding, 85, 327

P

pacemaker
  code, 16, 142
  electrical and mechanical capture and, 16, 142
  oversensing and, 16, 142–143
paediatrics
  arrhythmia, 7, 126–127
  emergency
    answers, 361–387
    questions, 97–104
  resuscitation
    answers, 126–131
    guidelines, 7, 126
    questions, 7–10
  see also children; neonate
pain management, emergency
  answers, 241–247
  questions, 54–56
pain scales, 56, 246
pancreatitis
  complications of, 71, 286
  Glasgow criteria, 287
  Ranson criteria for, 286
    at 48 hours, 286t
    gallstone-related, 287t
    predicting severity, 287t
    at presentation, 286t
papillary necrosis, 37, 198
paracentesis, liver disease and, 35, 191
paracetamol overdose, 87, 335
  NAC and, 87, 335
parenteral volume repletion, 199
Parkland formula, 63, 263
paroxysmal nocturnal dyspnoea, 12, 136
passive leg raising (PLR), 121
PCI *see* percutaneous coronary intervention
PCV7 *see* pneumococcal conjugate vaccine
PE *see* pulmonary embolism
pelvic fracture
  haemodynamically unstable patient and, 61,
    260–261
  Young-Burgess classification and, 61, 260, 260t
pelvic inflammatory disease (PID), 84, 325
  sexually acquired, 84, 325
peptic ulcer, 70, 282
peptic ulcer disease (PUD)
  aetiology of, 33, 186
  PPI and, 33, 186–187
PERC *see* pulmonary embolism rule-out criteria
percutaneous coronary intervention (PCI), 12, 135–136
percutaneous suprapubic catheterisation (SPC), 80, 310
  complications of, 310
performance appraisals, 107, 396
pericardial tamponade, 13, 138
pericardiocentesis, 7, 123–124
pericarditis, 13, 137
  ECG and, 13, 137–138

ESRD and, 37, 199
  uraemic, 199
perilunate dislocation, 66, 272
peritonsillar abscess, 77, 306
pertussis, 18, 147–148
petechiae, 42, 98–99, 367
pethidine, 244–245
phaeochromocytoma, 31, 179–180
phenobarbitone, 375
phenytoin, 168, 375
physeal growth plate injuries, 64, 267
PID *see* pelvic inflammatory disease
Pieces of Hurt tool, 246
pilonidal sinus, 73, 291
pinna, of ear, 78, 307
plague, 393
pleural effusion, 18, 146–147
PLR *see* passive leg raising
pneumococcal conjugate vaccine (PCV7), 98, 366
pneumomediastinum, 60, 257
pneumonia
  antibiotic regime, 44, 219
  blood gas and, 53, 238
  children and, 103, 383–384
    acute, 103, 384
    diagnosis, 103, 384–385
  mycoplasma, 47, 225
  sepsis and hypotension and, 30, 176
  Staphylococcus aureus caused, 19, 149–150
  see also community-acquired pneumonia
pneumonic plague, 393
pneumothorax, 19, 151
  COPD and, 20, 151
  identification, 20, 151
  intercostal catheter and, 20, 152–153
  reexpansion pulmonary oedema and, 20, 153
  supplemental oxygen and, 20, 152
  trauma, 59–60, 256–257
  ultrasound and, 20, 152
POAG *see* primary open angle glaucoma
poison
  CO, 89, 338
  cyanide, 89, 338
  food poisoning, 33, 185
    botulism, 47, 225
  mushroom, 91, 344
  OG and, 86, 332
  scombroid poisoning, 91, 344–345
  TCA poisoning, 87, 333
  torsades de pointes and, 86, 332
  see also toxicology
post viral cough syndrome, 103, 383
postnatal blues, 358
postpartum haemorrhage (PPH), 84, 324
postpartum psychiatric disorders, 96, 358
posttraumatic stress disorder (PTSD), 95, 356
potassium iodate tablets, 393

PPH *see* postpartum haemorrhage
PPI *see* proton pump inhibitor
PPV *see* pulse pressure variation
preeclampsia, 83, 320–321
preexcitation syndromes, 15, 141
pregnancy
    abruptio placentae in, 83, 322–323
    antepartum haemorrhage and, 83–84, 323
    anti-D prophylaxis after first trimester, 82–83, 319–320
    anti-D prophylaxis in first trimester, 82, 319
    appendicitis and, 71, 284–285
    blurred vision and headache and, 83, 320–321
    cardiac arrest and, 4–5, 118
    drug use in, 83, 322
    eclampsia and, 83, 321
    ectopic, 82, 318
    βHCG testing in early, 82, 318–319
    membrane rupture and, 84, 324
    $MgSO_4$ infusion and, 83, 321–322
    PE diagnosis and, 22, 158
    physiological changes in, 62, 261
    preeclampsia in, 83, 320–321
    shoulder dystocia and, 84, 323–324
    trauma management
        caesarean section and, 62, 262
        motor vehicle crash and, 62, 261–262
    ultrasound findings in early, 82, 317–318
    varicella and, 44, 219
    venous thromboembolism and, 22, 158
    see also obstetric emergencies
priapism
    causes, 80, 311
    management, 80, 311
prilocaine, 55, 244
primary blast injury, 62, 262
primary open angle glaucoma (POAG), 302
privacy, ED and, 109, 400
procedural sedation and analgesia (PSA), 55, 245
    children and, 55–56, 245–246
    fasting and, 55, 245
procedure-related pain, 56, 247
propofol, 54, 242
propranolol, 337
prostatitis, 39, 203, 314–315
    Chlamydia trachomatis and, 203
    E. coli and, 203
    Pseudomonas and, 203
    reinfection and, 203
proton pump inhibitor (PPI), 33, 186–187
proximal left system disease, 11, 134
PSA *see* procedural sedation and analgesia
pseudohyponatraemia, 51, 233
Pseudomonas, 203
Psudomonas aeruginosa, 307
psychiatric emergencies
    answers, 353–359
    questions, 94–96

PTSD *see* posttraumatic stress disorder
PUD *see* peptic ulcer disease
pulmonary aspiration, 19, 150
pulmonary embolism (PE), 22, 157
    fluid resuscitation and, 7, 123
    haemodynamically stable patients with, 23, 159
    pregnancy and, 22, 158
pulmonary embolism rule-out criteria (PERC), 22–23, 158–159
pulse pressure variation (PPV), 121
pupil, dilated, 77, 303–304
pustules, in neonate, 49, 230
pyelonephritis, 281, 310–311
    antibiotic regime for, 311
pyloric stenosis, 74, 294
pyoderma gangrenosum, 49, 229
pyridoxine, 375–376

Q
QTc, prolonged, 52, 236

R
rabies, 45, 221
radiation
    ARS, 93, 351–352
        phases of, 351–352
    exposure, 106, 393
    proctocolitis, 71, 284
radius, distal fracture of, 64, 269
Ranson criteria, for pancreatitis, 286
    at 48 hours, 286t
    gallstone-related, 287t
    predicting severity, 287t
    at presentation, 286t
RAPD *see* relative afferent pupillary defect
rapid sequence intubation (RSI)
    bimanual laryngoscopy and, 54, 241
    pretreatment agents and, 54, 242
    propofol and, 54, 242
    Sellick's manoeuvre and, 54, 241
    suxamethonium and, 54, 242–243
reactive arthritis, 46, 222
redback spider antivenom, 90, 342–343
reexpansion pulmonary oedema, 20, 153
relative afferent pupillary defect (RAPD), 76, 301
renal colic, 80, 310
    admission criteria, 310
renal emergencies
    answers, 198–205
    hyperkalemia and, 38, 200
    questions, 37–40
renal failure, investigations and, 37, 199
renal function, toxic ratio and, 86, 332
renal transplant, 38, 200
reperfusion, 11, 134
respiratory emergencies
    answers, 146–159
    questions, 18–23

resuscitation
  adult
    answers, 115–124
    questions, 3–7
  paediatric
    answers, 126–131
    questions, 7–10
resuscitative thoracotomy, 6, 60, 123, 258
retrobulbar haematoma, 77, 305
Rh D immunoglobulin (RhIG), 82–83, 319–320
rhabdomyolysis, 53, 239
  aetiology of, 38, 201
  diagnosis of, 38, 201–202
  myoglobin and, 201
RhIG see Rh D immunoglobulin
ring-enhancing lesions, 45, 220
rostering, of ED staff, 107, 396
rotator cuff tear, 65, 271
RSI see rapid sequence intubation
rule of nines, 62, 263

S
sacral injuries, 252–253
SAD PERSONS mnemonic, 354
SAH see subarachnoid haemorrhage
salbutamol, 21, 155
salicylate overdose, 30, 177
saline, normal, 53, 238
saline unresponsive metabolic alkalosis, 52, 235–236
salt
  ascites and, 34–35, 190–191
  liver disease and, 34–35, 190–191
Salter-Harris type I growth plate injuries, 64, 267
San Francisco syncope rule, 139
SBI see serious bacterial illness
SBO see small bowel obstruction
scapholunate dislocation, 66, 272
SCD see sickle cell disease
SCI see cervical spinal cord injury
sciatica, 68, 278
  causes of pain in, 278
  medications and, 278
scombroid poisoning, 91, 344–345
scrotal pain, 80–81, 313
seizures
  absence, 27, 168–169
  alcohol and, 26, 168
  blood gas and, 53, 239–240
  febrile, 100, 372–373
  HIV and, 27, 169
  lorazepam and, 101, 375–376
  neonate, 100, 373–374
    anticonvulsives and, 375–376
    types of, 374
  pseudoseizures compared with, 27, 169
  sodium valproate and, 100, 373
  tonic–clonic, 83, 321

selective serotonin reuptake inhibitor (SSRI), 87, 334
Sellick's manoeuvre, 54, 241
sepsis
  goal-directed therapy in, 6, 121
  neonate and, 97, 362–363
septic shock
  children and, 3–4, 99, 129, 367
  noradrenaline or dopamine and, 5, 120–121
serious bacterial illness (SBI), 98, 364–366
serotonin syndrome, 87, 334
sex
  DGI and, 49, 230–231
  PID and, 84, 325
sexual assault
  forensic examination and, 110, 402
  treatment options following, 85, 326
short stay units (SSUs), 109, 399–400
  admission to, 109, 400
shoulder dystocia, 84, 323–324
shoulder joint dislocation, 65, 271
SIADH see syndrome of inappropriate antidiuretic
    hormone
sickle cell disease (SCD), 42
sigmoid volvulus, 70–71, 281, 283
sinus rhythm reversion, 16, 141
SIRS see systemic inflammatory response syndrome
SJS see Stevens-Johnson syndrome
skin puncture pain management, 56, 247
small bowel injury, 61, 260
small bowel obstruction (SBO), 70, 282–283
smallpox virus, 393
snake bite
  antivenom choice for, 90, 342
  black, 90, 342
  brown, 90, 341
    VICC and, 90, 342
  Elapidae, 90, 342
  tiger, 90, 342
sodium bicarbonate, 86, 331
  metabolic acidosis and, 86, 331
    complications and, 52, 236
    treatment regarding, 52, 237
sodium ions, 53
sodium thiosulphate, 89, 338
sodium valproate, 100, 373
somatisation disorder, 95, 357
somatoform disorders, 95, 357
sotalol, 337
  overdose, 88, 337
SPA see suprapubic aspirate
SPC see percutaneous suprapubic catheterisation
spider
  funnel-web, 91, 343
  redback, 90, 342–343
spinal injuries
  spinal shock, 58, 253–254
  teardrop fractures and, 58, 253

young adult and, 58, 254

   see also cervical spine injuries

spinal shock, 58, 253–254

splenic injuries, 61, 259–260

sprain, ankle, 67, 275

   radiographic assessment of, 67, 275–276

   talar dome fracture and, 67, 276

SSRI *see* selective serotonin reuptake inhibitor

SSSS *see* Staphylococcal scalded skin syndrome

SSUs *see* short stay units

ST elevation myocardial infarction (STEMI), 11, 134

   ACS and, 134–135

   mimics of, 134

stab wound

   chest trauma, 59–60, 256–257

   to heart, 60, 258

   to neck, 59, 255

   neck zones and, 59, 255

staphylococcal scalded skin syndrome (SSSS), 49,
   229–230

Staphylococcus, 33, 185

Staphylococcus aureus, 19, 149–150

   MRSA and, 19, 150

STEMI *see* ST elevation myocardial infarction

sternoclavicular joint, 65, 271

sternum, undisplaced fracture of, 60, 257

Stevens-Johnson syndrome (SJS), 49, 229

   TEN and, 49, 229

Streptococcus species, 138

stress, ED work related, 107–108, 396

stroke

   embolic, 25, 164

   ischemic, 25, 164–165

   NIHSS and, 25, 164

   posterior circulation, 25, 165

   thrombolytic therapy and, 41–42, 210

   TIA and, 25, 165

subarachnoid haemorrhage (SAH), 74, 293

   cerebrospinal fluid and, 24, 164

   complications associated with, 24, 164

   diagnosis regarding, 24, 163

   investigation and management, 74, 293–294

   non-contrast CT and, 24, 163

   suspicious headache and, 25, 164

submandibular swelling, 75, 297

submersion events, 92, 349–050

suicide

   BPD and, 94–95, 355

   risk, 94, 353

     assessment, 94, 354–355

     for completed suicide, 94, 354

sulphonylurea overdose, 88, 337–338

supracondylar fracture

   Gartland type, 64, 268

   of humerus, 64, 267–268

   vascular compromise and, 64, 268

suprapubic aspirate (SPA), 370

supraventricular tachycardia (SVT), 14, 140

   adenosine and, 15, 140

   children and, 16, 143

   reentrant, 15, 141

surge capacity planning, 105, 391–392

surgical emergencies

   answers, 281–297

   questions, 70–75

suxamethonium, 54, 242–243

SVT *see* supraventricular tachycardia

syncope, 14, 139

   clinical examination and, 139

   prolonged QTc and, 52, 236

   San Francisco syncope rule and, 139

   unexplained, 139

syndrome of inappropriate antidiuretic hormone (SIADH), 51, 233

systemic inflammatory response syndrome (SIRS), 97, 364

T

tachycardia *see* ventricular tachycardia

talar dome, fracture of, 67, 276

tall-tented T waves, 13, 137

TB *see* tuberculosis

TBI *see* traumatic brain injury

TCA *see* tricyclic antidepressant poisoning

TCP *see* transcutaneous pacing

teardrop fractures, 58, 253

temperature measurement, body, 98, 366

temporal arteritis, 24, 163

TEN *see* toxic epidermal necrolysis

testicular torsion, 80, 311–313

tetralogy of Fallot, 16, 143

thoracic trauma, 59, 256

thoracotomy

   EDT and, 60, 258

   resuscitative, 60, 258

thrombocytopaenia, 42

thrombolysis in myocardial infarction (TIMI), 133, 134t

   contraindications to, 135

thrombolytic therapy, 41–42, 210

thyroid disease, ocular examination in, 30, 176–177

thyroid storm, 30, 177

thyrotoxic crisis, 30, 177

thyroxine overdose, 89, 338

TIA *see* transient ischemic attack

tick paralysis, 91, 344

tiger snake bite, 90, 342

TIMI *see* thrombolysis in myocardial infarction

toddler's fracture, 65, 269

tongue, 59, 255

   laceration, 79, 308

tonic–clonic seizure, 83, 321

tooth

   avulsed, 78, 308

   milk and, 308

   extraction bleeding, 78, 308

TORCHES infections, 363

torsades de pointes, 15, 140
  isoprenaline and, 140
  poison and, 86, 332
tourniquet inflation time, 55, 244
toxic epidermal necrolysis (TEN), 49, 229
  SJS and, 49, 229
toxic ratio, 86, 332
toxicology
  answers, 330–345
  questions, 86–91
toxoplasmosis, 45, 220
TRA see traumatic rupture of the aorta
TRALI see transfusion-related acute lung injury
tranexamic acid (TXA), 208
tranquilisation, 95, 356
transaminases, 193–194
transcutaneous pacing (TCP), 5, 120
transfusion, 63
  liver transplant and, 36, 195
  massive, 264
    monitoring, 264
  see also blood transfusion; damage control
    resuscitation
transfusion-related acute lung injury (TRALI), 6, 123
transient ischemic attack (TIA), 25, 165
transient synovitis, 65, 270
transient tachypnoea of the newborn (TTN), 97, 361
transplant
  liver, 36, 194–195
    timing of infection following, 194–195
    transfusion regarding, 36, 195
  renal, 38, 200
trauma
  answers, 250–264
  hypotensive resuscitation and, 6, 122–123
  questions, 57–63
  resuscitative thoracotomy and, 6, 123
  systems for timely management, 63, 264
traumatic brain injury (TBI)
  diffuse axonal injury and, 57, 251
  hypertonic saline and, 6, 122
  hypotension and, 57, 251
  intracranial haemorrhage and, 57–58, 252
  secondary insult and, 57, 251
traumatic rupture of the aorta (TRA), 61, 259
travellers' diarrhoea, 32, 184
Trendelenburg position, 121
triage, mass casualty incident, 106, 393–394
Trichomonas, 314
tricyclic antidepressant (TCA) poisoning, 87, 333
troponin assays, 133, 134t
Truelove and Witts' classification, 185–186, 186t
TTN see transient tachypnoea of the newborn
tuberculosis (TB), 46, 223–224
tumour, solid, 43
tumour lysis syndrome, 43
TXA see tranexamic acid

tympanic membrane rupture, 62, 262
typhoid, 45, 220

U
UC see ulcerative colitis
ulcerative colitis (UC), 33, 185
  Truelove and Witts' classification of, 185–186, 186t
ultrasound
  AAA and, 71, 283
  early pregnancy findings, 82, 317–318
  pneumothorax and, 20, 152
unilateral facet joint dislocation, 68, 277
unimmunised patients, 48, 226
ureteric stent, 81, 315
ureteric stones, 80, 310
urinary alkalinisation, 86, 331
urinary retention, 81, 313
  causes of, 313
urinary tract infections (UTIs)
  aetiolgoy, 39, 203
  children and, 98–99, 367, 370
    diagnosis in, 40, 205
    epidemiology in, 39–40, 204–205
  diagnosis, 39, 204
urine dipstick testing, 81, 313–314
urogenital trauma, 80, 311–312
  classes of, 312
  grading of, 312t
urological emergencies
  answers, 310–315
  questions, 80–81
uterine bleeding, 85, 327
UTIs see urinary tract infections
uveitis, 76, 302

V
vaginal bleeding, 82, 85, 318, 326–327
vaginitis, 84, 324–325
vapocoolant, 56, 247
varicella, 44, 219
vasoactive agents, 6, 121–122
vasopressors, 4, 118
VBG see venous blood gas analysis
venepuncture, 247
venlafaxine, 87, 334
venom-induced consumptive coagulopathy (VICC), 90,
  342
venous blood gas (VBG) analysis, 18, 146
venous thromboembolism, 22, 158
ventilation
  for asthma
    adult ventilation, 21, 154–155
    invasive ventilation, 21, 154
    mechanical ventilation, 3, 116, 116t
  compression ventilation ratio, 8, 128, 128t
  CPR and, 4, 117
  neonate and, 9, 131

NIV and, 3, 22, 115–116, 157
    obesity and, 54, 241–242
ventricular fibrillation (VF), 4, 117–118
ventricular tachycardia (VT), 14, 139–140
    broad-complex, 14, 140
    SVT and, 14, 140
ventriculoperitoneal shunt, 27, 169–170
vertigo, 26, 167–168
VF *see* ventricular fibrillation
Vibrio, 33, 185
VICC *see* venom-induced consumptive coagulopathy
visual analogue scales, 246
visual loss, 76, 302–303
vital signs, in children, 104, 386–387, 387t
vitamin K, 41, 210
vitiligo, 29, 175–176
vomiting, 74, 294
VT *see* ventricular tachycardia
vulvovaginitis, 84, 324–325

W
warfarin
    adverse effects of, 209
    anticoagulation therapy and, 41, 159, 209
        brands of, 209
        function of, 209
waveform capnography, 115
weight estimation, in children, 8, 128–129
wheezing, 103, 376–377
    asthma and, 103, 382
Wolff-Parkinson-White syndrome (WPW), 15, 141
    AF and, 16, 141–142
wounds, 73, 292–293
    see also abdominal wound dehiscence
WPW *see* Wolff-Parkinson-White syndrome

Y
yellow fever, 45, 220
Young-Burgess classification, 61, 260, 260t
Yuzpe method, 326

Z
zygomatic fractures, 58, 254

Lightning Source UK Ltd.
Milton Keynes UK
UKHW032032061219
354907UK00009B/682/P